Cancer in Children and Young People
Acute Nursing Care

Edited by

Faith Gibson *RSCN, RGN, Onc Cert, Cert Ed, MSc, PhD, FRCN, Senior Lecturer in Children's Cancer Nursing Research, UCL Institute of Child Health and Great Ormond Street Hospital for Children NHS Trust, London*

Louise Soanes *RSCN, RGN, MSc, BSc (Hons), Senior Sister for Children's Services, the Royal Marsden Hospital NHS Trust, Sutton*

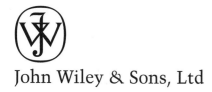

John Wiley & Sons, Ltd

Other Wiley Editorial Offices

John Wiley & Sons Inc., 111 River Street, Hoboken, NJ 07030, USA

Jossey-Bass, 989 Market Street, San Francisco, CA 94103-1741, USA

Wiley-VCH Verlag GmbH, Boschstr. 12, D-69469 Weinheim, Germany

John Wiley & Sons Australia Ltd, 42 McDougall Street, Milton, Queensland 4064, Australia

John Wiley & Sons (Asia) Pte Ltd, 2 Clementi Loop #02-01, Jin Xing Distripark, Singapore 129809

John Wiley & Sons Canada Ltd, 6045 Freemont Blvd, Mississauga, ONT, L5R 4J3, Canada

Wiley also publishes its books in a variety of electronic formats. Some content that appears in print may not be
available in electronic books.

Library of Congress Cataloging in Publication Data

Gibson, Faith.
    Cancer in children and young people / Faith Gibson and Louise Soanes.
        p. ; cm. — (Wiley series in nursing)
    Includes bibliographical references and index.
    ISBN 978-0-470-05867-1 (cloth : alk. paper)
    1. Cancer in children—Nursing. 2. Cancer in adolescence—Nursing. I. Soanes, Louise. II. Title. III. Series.
    [DNLM: 1. Neoplasms—nursing. 2. Neoplasms—therapy. 3. Adolescent. 4. Child.
    5. Oncologic Nursing—methods. 6. Pediatric Nursing—methods. WY 156 G4485c 2007]
    RC281.C4G52 2007
    618.92'994—dc22

                                                                                        2007024695

British Library Cataloguing in Publication Data

A catalogue record for this book is available from the British Library

ISBN 978-0-470-05867-1

Typeset in 9.5/11.5pt Palatino by Integra Software Services Pvt. Ltd, Pondicherry, India
Printed in Singapore by Markono Print Media Pte Ltd
This book is printed on acid-free paper responsibly manufactured from sustainable forestry
in which at least two trees are planted for each one used for paper production.

Contents

Preface

The first edition of this text, entitled *Paediatric Oncology: Acute Nursing Care*, was published in 1999. 'A practical approach focusing on the detailed nursing management of care, underpinned by theory and research' was the main aim of the textbook (Gibson & Evans, 1999, p. 503). We would suggest that this has been achieved. The many 'tattered covers' and well-thumbed copies of the book we see on clinical units show the book has become a familiar companion to many children's cancer nurses in the United Kingdom and beyond. So much so that it is fondly known as simply 'the Red Book'.

In this much awaited second edition we have built on the success of 'the Red Book', taking into consideration comments made to us by nurses in practice and recognising the changes in care over the years. First, you will notice that the title has changed to *Cancer in Children and Young People*. We feel this more appropriately reflects the emphasis of practice where the care of children and young people is perceived as two separate and distinctly different fields of practice within cancer care. In recognition of the many transitions in the cancer journey between acute to chronic care, we have chosen to let go the second part of the original title. Second, you will notice that there is a new part to the book related to long-term follow-up care, late effects and issues about survivorship. By the year 2010, 1 in 715 young people will be survivors of cancer. Despite such positive increases in survival, we know that approximately

60% of this population will have one or more treatment- or disease-related late effects. There are also long-term psychosocial late effects associated with a childhood cancer diagnosis that may impinge on a young person's quality of life, and we felt it important that the new edition should reflect this.

What remains the same is the emphasis on the nurse's role as a key member of the multiprofessional team, embracing the philosophy of family-focused care, respect for the young person's growing autonomy and negotiation of care. There are common threads that run through the text, for example, psychosocial issues, family teaching, health education and involving children and young people in decisions about their care. Like the first edition, the text is presented in sections (though now called parts), that stand alone, with references for each placed at the end of the chapter, so the reader can focus on a particular area of interest without needing to scan the whole text. Some parts include a commentary from practitioners in the field, and these are useful reflections on the contribution of the part to developing practice.

We have welcomed some new authors who have worked tirelessly on the task, and have sought to update each section in terms of new areas of clinical practice as well as research. We acknowledge the work of previous authors, namely Gaynor Young, Louise Hooker, Sarah Palmer, Phillipa Chesterfield, Hilary Brocklehurst, Jane Watson,

Jane Pownall and Linda Scott. We also recognise the contribution of Margaret Evans, one of the pioneer editors, without whom there would not have been a first edition. It is the dedication of all these authors that has resulted in this second edition: balancing work responsibilities and writing is a demanding task, but without these efforts many examples of 'know-how' of expert clinicians would be lost (Benner, 1984, p. 11).

References

Benner P (1984) *From Novice to Expert: Excellence and Power in Clinical Nursing Practice*. Menlo Park, CA: Addison-Wesley

Gibson F & Evans M (1999) *Paediatric Oncology Nursing: Acute Nursing Care*. London: Whurr Publishers

Faith Gibson and Louise Soanes

Foreword

Paediatric oncology is a rapidly developing speciality and has paralleled a time of major improvement in the prognosis for children and adolescents with cancer. The speciality has evolved as a multi-professional area with collaboration between a range of medical specialities together with nursing and paramedical skills. It aims to promote family-centred treatment and involve the child patient wherever possible.

The improved prognosis has been largely due to better diagnostic radiology and histology, new chemotherapeutic drugs together with increased knowledge of how best to use them, and advanced surgical and radiotherapy skills associated with specialisation.

For the last 30–40 years an ever-increasing proportion of children with cancer have been entered into clinical trials, both national, e.g. Medical Research Council and UK Children's Cancer Study Group, and international. These trials have played a major role in developing new and more effective treatment schedules.

This book is written primarily for nurses working in paediatric oncology. It is comprehensive, up to date and well referenced. There is a useful commentary at the beginning of most parts. It covers a wide range of available treatments and emphasises the importance of involving the child and their family. Psychological, social and educational aspects are covered.

With the improved prognosis for childhood cancer, the number of survivors grows. This is recognised by a new Part 5, devoted to long-term follow-up, late effects of disease and its treatment and practical problems that are important in future life.

This, the second edition, albeit with a change of title, follows a successful initial edition published in 1999. It maintains the standard and deserves to be consulted, not only by nursing staff, but by a wide range of those working in the field of cancer in children and young people.

John Martin FRCP, FRCPCH
Formerly Paediatric Oncologist, Royal Liverpool
Children's Hospital Alder Hey
Founding Chairman UK Children's
Cancer Study Group

I am delighted to see the enormous progress that has been made in the management of children with cancer since I first became a paediatric ward sister in 1970. At that time paediatric sub-specialties were largely a thing of the future and generally children's wards catered for a broad mix of sick children. Most consultants were general paediatricians and nursing staff likewise were generic. In those early days we had a few children with renal and other solid tumours who were managed by the surgeons with the help of the radiotherapists, but most of the nursing involvement was with children who unfortunately would die. There were no specialist social workers, although the Malcolm Sargent Cancer Fund for Children would provide some material support.

During the early 1970s the recognition that more could be done for children with cancer and leukaemia led to a centralisation of care, and eventually all children from the region were referred to our centre. As chemotherapy became more specific and sophisticated and later bone marrow transplantation became a reality, nurses, out of necessity, had to become more specialised and knowledgeable about cancer.

Nurses were, however, not only involved in the hands-on care of the sick children but were instrumental, along with social work colleagues, who were now included in the developing paediatric oncology team, in helping develop psycho-social support for children, their parents and siblings. Now childhood cancer was moving from being an acute terminal illness to a long-term condition. This required a change in how we communicated with the children, and the need for openness regarding the disease and treatment was recognised. Consequently nurses with others were at the forefront in developing literature specifically for children and their families.

Very soon it became apparent that a separate ward was needed where expertise could be concentrated and skills developed. This led to the concept of specialist paediatric oncology nurses, and with the need to share experiences with others, the Royal College of Nursing in 1984 facilitated the formation of the Paediatric Oncology Nurses Forum. There was also recognition that in order to facilitate children dying at home there needed to be support for them to do so and Paediatric Oncology Outreach Nursing posts were developed.

How things have changed in such a relatively short period of time. We now have the second edition of this nursing text book devoted to the acute care of children with cancer. We have gone from a situation 35 years ago when the majority of children with cancer died to one where now over 75% can be cured. Developments and improvements in nursing care have played an enormous part in this success story and I look forward to following their contribution over the coming years.

Anne Craft MSc RSCN RGN HV RNT
Former Director of Nursing, Royal Victoria
Infirmary, Newcastle upon Tyne
Founding Chairman Paediatric Oncology
Nurses Forum

Contributors

Nikki Bennett-Rees Clinical Nurse Specialist, Fox BMT Unit, Great Ormond Street Hospital, London

Jamie Cargill Senior Staff Nurse, Haematology, Bristol Royal Hospital for Children, Bristol

Gill Chapman Clinical Nurse Specialist, Children's Pain Management, Leeds Teaching Hospital Trust, Leeds

Sharon Denton Sister, Paediatric Surgery, Leeds Teaching Hospital Trust, Leeds

Ruth Elson Clinical Nurse Specialist for Late Effects, Department of Paediatric Oncology/BMT, Bristol Children's Hospital, Bristol

Faith Gibson Senior Lecturer in Children's Cancer Nursing Research, UCL Institute of Child Health and Great Ormond Street Hospital, London

Lesley Henderson Haemophilia Nurse Specialist, Haemophilia Centre, Great Ormond Street Hospital, London

Chris Henry Clinical Nurse Specialist, Stanmore Hospital, London

Rachel Hollis Senior Sister, Paediatric Oncology, St James's University Hospital, Leeds

Monica Hopkins Advanced Nurse Practitioner, Oncology Unit, Alder Hey Children's Hospital, Liverpool

Sian Hopkins Practice Nurse Educator, Fox BMT Unit, Great Ormond Street Hospital, London

Beverly Horne Senior Sister, Day Care Unit, St James's University Hospital, Leeds

Angela Houlston Senior Sister, Paediatric Oncology Unit, John Radcliffe Hospital, Headington, Oxford

Lindy May Consultant Nurse, Parrott Ward, Great Ormond Street Hospital, London

Susan Mehta Clinical Nurse Specialist for Late Effects, Great Ormond Street Hospital, London

Anthony Penn Paediatric Oncology Research Fellow, Bristol Children's Hospital and Frenchay Hospital, Bristol

Charlie Rogers Senior Staff Nurse, John Radcliffe Hospital, Headington, Oxford

Lin Russell Royal Orthopaedic Hospital, Northfield, Birmingham

Jennie Sacree Barbara Russell Children's Ward, Frenchay Hospital, Bristol

Cornelia Scott Specialist Nurse Paediatrics, Cookridge Hospital, Leeds

Karen Selwood Advanced Nurse Practitioner, Paediatric Oncology Unit, Alder Hey Children's Hospital, Liverpool

Louise Soanes Senior Sister for Children's Services, the Royal Marsden Hospital, Sutton

Joanna Stone Staff Nurse, Children's Unit, the Royal Marsden Hospital, Sutton

Beth Ward Neuro-oncology Outreach Nurse Specialist, Parrott Ward, Great Ormond Street Hospital, London

Helen Webster BMT Nurse Specialist, Alder Hey Children's Hospital, Liverpool

Jinhua Xu-Bayford Clinical Nurse Specialist Gene Therapy, Acute Medical Services Unit, Great Ormond Street Hospital, London

Acknowledgements

We would like to thank the following professionals for their diligence and for generously giving up their time to review and comment upon this revised textbook: Steve Andrews, Jamie Cargill, Mark Gaze, Rob Grimer, Gill Levitt, Anthony Michalski, Julie Mycroft, Kanchan Rao, Charlie Rogers, Lyn Russell, Jennie Sacree, Frank Sarran, Roly Squire and Helen Webster.

Many thanks also to our various friends, colleagues and family members, who once again have lived through the voyage of another book!

Part 1

Chemotherapy

Commentary

Chemotherapy

Jamie Cargill

As the care that children with cancer and their families require becomes ever more complex and demanding, the need of the paediatric oncology nurse to understand therapy and management of the resulting symptoms grows every year. Nurses must therefore draw on the most appropriate body of knowledge in specific instances of care.

The following chapters (Chapters 1–6) provide the paediatric oncology nurse with a platform of knowledge in the pursuit of better practice. It presents the reader with an overview of chemotherapy; from its biological principles and protocol development, to the administration and potential side effects and oncological emergencies that may arise, to advances and future development. It importantly places the child and the family at the centre of its commentary and champions how nurses have been, and will continue to be, at the forefront in the understanding and management of their patients

Chapter 1 introduces the concept of chemotherapy from its infancy at the beginning of the last century, to the understanding of the principles of pharmacokinetics and pharmacodynamics. For all oncology nurses an integral part of their work is the ability to understand protocol development and the use of clinical trials, as parents will rely on this understanding when asked to participate in trials and randomisation. Parents find this randomisation a concept difficult to grasp and are often reluctant to consent in case of failure in the future. The more the nurse can understand what the child and family are experiencing around the time of diagnosis, when often the prognosis is also addressed, the more he or she can support them through this stage.

This chapter is very helpful in that it informs the nurse of the rationale for therapy choice and how protocol development is guided by factors such as toxicity and drug resistance. The authors discuss the recent advancement in protocols which identify where dose reduction could be introduced without reducing the efficacy of treatment. This is an exciting time, but delicate and supportive discussions must be undertaken as parents are very vulnerable at this juncture in the treatment of their child, and will need the understanding and time that an experienced oncology nurse can offer.

Chapters 2 and 3 discuss the classification of chemotherapy and the process of administration. Linking the theory of classification back to practice is often an abstract concept for many oncology nurses, which this chapter goes some way to solving. But paediatric oncology nurses provide far more than the technical administration of chemotherapy. The nurse can empower and educate the child and family by explaining exactly what is going to happen and why. Such specific

Cancer in Children and Young People   Edited by Faith Gibson and Louise Soanes
© 2008 John Wiley & Sons, Ltd

information can help the nurse answer questions, thus helping to reduce fear of the unknown. It is also useful as a reference for others involved in this process, such as the play specialist.

The practical aspects to administration are considered, utilising a step-by-step process, which will be very helpful in standardising competencies and practices. The central venous line, peripheral access, the intrathecal route and administration of chemotherapy are depicted, leading the reader through what can often be a confusing number of legislative requirements. As nurses, we are morally bound by a duty to care to safeguard not just ourselves, but also the patients and parents in the delivery of chemotherapy. Legislation is there to ensure that training and continuing professional development are key factors in maintaining and improving standards of care (NICE, 2005), something that is clear in the text of these chapters. The choice of setting for chemotherapy administration is discussed, with the nurse being at the forefront of changes in both administration methods (altering the route for post-fluid hydration) and the setting (home versus hospital), with the requirement of excellent information (both written and verbal) to ensure effective outcomes.

At the heart of oncology nursing is the ability to control the side effects of therapy. Knowledge of the actual and the potential side effects of treatment ensures that nurses are able to professionally assess, manage and evaluate care given. The education of side effects should always preclude the actual presence of signs and symptoms, as knowledge about treatment and side effects is necessary to ensure active participation of family members in the decision-making process. It is therefore no surprise that throughout Chapters 4 and 5, the constant theme is that of education and information-giving. The authors are able to provide excellent descriptions of practice, which is supported by research and other published literature.

Reviewing existing practice in the management of side effects is pertinent to the care of the paediatric patient. It is, however, clear from current research, that many questions remain to be asked and answered for the management of many of the side effects for children undergoing cancer therapy. Part 1 discusses the lack of validated and reliable assessment tools for children in many areas of care but analyses those that do exist. Internationally accepted assessment scales for measuring the severity and impact of symptoms such as mucositis, nutrition and nausea and vomiting in children are therefore of paramount importance (van der Rijt & van Zuijlen, 2001).

Aside from all the mechanistic and pharmacological interventions, paediatric oncology nurses must not ignore the positive effect of good nursing care, a constant theme in Part 1. Nurses play a pivotal role in the provision and education of care for children and their families during cancer. Nevertheless a gulf still exists between the knowledge base and clinical practice, resulting in confusion, conflicting advice, and uncertainty (Ezzone et al., 1993; Mueller et al., 1995; Collard & Hunter, 2001; Gibson, 2004). Nurses must, however, be accountable for the care they give and whenever possible scientific-based evidence should inform decision-making and underpin the rationale for the care given (Williams et al., 2003).

It is now recognised that nurses are in a prime position to lead in the area of symptom management (Gibson & Nelson, 2000; Soanes et al., 2000). However, there is often a feeling that the nurse's ability to further the scientific credibility of the profession is hampered by the lack of robust and well-designed research studies. There is a requirement from within and outside the nursing profession that clinical nursing practice be based on best available evidence.

For the care of children to benefit from research, it must embrace a range of methodologies to generate new knowledge. Multi-centred, placebo-controlled studies need to be designed and implemented to study the effectiveness of the interventions to reduce the incidence and severity of side effects such as mucositis, pain and nausea and vomiting (Barker, 1999; Scully et al., 2004). As supported by the authors, the role of the paediatric oncology nurse must be included in this changing and challenging time, with such a vast and diverse specialty ultimately aiming to provide the child and family with the highest standards of care. By challenging the innovations that treatment offers and sustaining the accomplishments achieved so far, only then can we be confident that consensus on best practice has been achieved.

Knowing the patient and family is now considered to be a key component of excellent nursing care (Jenny & Logan, 1992) and is considered a 'central theme in nurses' everyday disclosure about their practice' (Tanner *et al.*, 1993, p. 273). The Calman–Hine Report (1995) highlights the importance of working with families and patients with cancer, ensuring a holistic approach to care. The authors always placed the child and the family at the centre of its commentary with nursing knowledge required in providing an understanding of their treatment.

Part 1 provides an excellent reference guide to enhance the knowledge of both nurses and other health professionals in the provision of treatment for childhood cancer. It shows us the challenge for the future: to continue to improve and collaborate within the paediatric oncology multi-disciplinary team in the treatment and management of cancer. It will not come as any surprise to find that this second edition of the 'Little Red Book' will be an essential theoretical textbook to any aspiring oncology nurse working with children.

References

Barker GJ (1999) 'Current practices in the oral management of the patient undergoing chemotherapy or bone marrow transplantation' *Supportive Care Cancer* 7(1): 17–20

Calman K & Hine D (1995) *A Policy Framework for Commissioning Cancer Services: A Report by the Expert Advisory Group on Cancer to the Chief Medical Officers of England and Wales.* London: Department of Health

Collard MM & Hunter ML (2001) 'Oral and dental care in acute lymphoblastic leukaemia: a survey of United Kingdom children's cancer study group centres' *International Journal of Paediatric Dentistry* 11(5): 347–351

Ezzone S, Jolly D, Replogle, K, Kapoor, N & Tutschka PJ (1993) 'Survey of oral hygiene regimens among bone marrow transplant centers' *Oncology Nursing Forum* 20(9): 1375–1381

Foot AB. & Hayes C (1994) 'Audit of guidelines for effective control of chemotherapy and radiotherapy induced emesis' *Archive of Diseases of Childhood* 71(5): 475–480

Gibson F (2004) 'Best practice in oral care for children and young people being treated for cancer: can we achieve consensus?' *European Journal of Cancer* 40(8): 1217–1224

Gibson F & Nelson W (2000) 'Mouth care for children with cancer' *Paediatric Nurse* 12(1): 18–22

Jenny J & Logan J (1992) 'Knowing the patient: one aspect of clinical knowledge' *Journal of Nursing Scholarship* 24(4): 254–258

Mueller BA, Millheim ET, Farrington EA, Brusko C & Wiser TH (1995) 'Mucositis management practices for hospitalized patients: national survey results' *Journal of Pain Symptom and Management* 10(7): 510–520

National Institute for Health and Clinical Excellence (2005) *Improving Outcomes in Children and Young People with Cancer.* London: NICE Cancer Service Guidance

Scully C, Epstein J & Sonis S (2004) 'Oral mucositis: a challenging complication of radiotherapy, chemotherapy, and radiochemotherapy. Part 2: diagnosis and management of mucositis' *Head and Neck* 26(1): 77–84

Soanes L, Gibson F, Bayliss J & Hannan J (2000) 'Establishing nursing research priorities on a paediatric haematology, oncology, immunology and infectious diseases unit: a Delphi survey' *European Journal of Oncology Nursing* 4(2): 108–117

Tanner CA, Benner P, Chesla C. & Gordon DR (1993) 'The phenomenology of knowing the patient' *Journal of Nursing Knowledge* 25(4): 273–280

van der Rijt CC & van Zuijlen L (2001) 'Studies on supportive care in oral mucositis: random or randomised?' *European Journal of Cancer* 37(16): 1971–1975

Williams K, Scheinberg A, Moyer V & Mellis C (2003) 'Using an evidence-based approach to a paediatric problem' *Journal of Paediatric Child Health* 39(2): 139–144

1 Principles of Chemotherapy

Angela Houlston

The history of the development of chemotherapy

Chemotherapy is the term given to refer to any drug or chemical treatment used to treat any disease. Cytotoxic (or anti-neoplastic) chemotherapeutic agents are used to treat malignancy.

The development of cytotoxic chemotherapy at the beginning of the twentieth century revolutionised the treatment of cancer, especially the treatment of disseminated disease such as leukaemia. Crucial to the development of cytotoxic chemotherapy was the discovery that certain chemicals acted chiefly on any rapidly dividing cells, and this includes cancer cells. During the First World War it was noted that soldiers who were exposed to nitrogen gas developed an abnormally low white cell count. A derivative of nitrogen gas, nitrogen mustard was first used as an anti-cancer treatment in the 1940s. Many of the cytotoxic drugs used today were discovered incidentally when developing drugs for other purposes, while others have been developed specifically to interfere with metabolic pathways.

Cell cycle

To understand the principles of chemotherapy and how it works, it is important to have a basic understanding of the normal cell cycle. The cell cycle is an ordered series of events that involves several sequential phases. The purpose of the cell cycle is for cells to reproduce themselves, to replace dead or injured cells and add new ones during tissue growth.

There are two types of cell division, somatic and reproductive, and these have different goals. Somatic cell division involves all cells except for germ cells involved in reproduction. In somatic cell division, each cell duplicates its contents and divides into two identical cells through a nuclear division process called mitosis. The cell cycle consists of two main periods: interphase, when the cell is not dividing, and the mitotic (M) phase when the cell is dividing.

Interphase

The cell replicates its DNA during this period of rapid growth. Interphase has three phases: G^1, S

Cancer in Children and Young People   Edited by Faith Gibson and Louise Soanes
© 2008 John Wiley & Sons, Ltd

and G^2. S phase is concerned with the synthesis of DNA and the G phases are gaps or interruptions in DNA replication.

1. *G^1 phase.* This is the interval or gap between the mitotic stage and the S phase. The cell is preparing for DNA synthesis and is metabolically active through the synthesis of RNA and protein. This stage may last from 8 to 10 hours; however, some cells remain in this phase for a longer time and are considered to be in the G^0 or resting phase.
2. *S phase.* Once a cell enters this phase, it is committed to go through cell division. The S phase is between G^1 and G^2 and lasts approximately 8 hours. This is the phase of DNA synthesis when the DNA replicates, ensuring that the two cells being formed are made of the same genetic material.
3. *G^2 phase.* This is the gap between S phase and mitosis, which will give rise to two daughter cells. This phase may last for 4 to 6 hours. Cell growth continues and enzymes and other proteins are synthesised in preparation for cell division.

M phase (Mitosis)

This phase results in the nucleic and cytoplasmic division that produces two identical, or daughter, cells. This may be broken down into four distinct phases: prophase, metaphase, anaphase and telophase, culminating in cytokinesis or the division of cytoplasm that creates two new cells.

The sequence of events in the cell cycle is shown in Figure 1.1:

G^1 Phase → S phase → G^2 phase → M phase

(Mitosis) → Cytokinesis → two new cells

Most cancer cells are characterised by their ability to divide uncontrollably. Cytotoxic chemotherapy interferes with cell division at various points in the cell cycle, affecting both cancer cells and other rapidly reproducing cells. This knowledge has enabled the development of drugs which either act specifically during one point of the cell cycle (cell cycle phase-specific) or which have some effect during all phases of the cell cycle (cell cycle non-phase-specific). Cell cycle non-specific

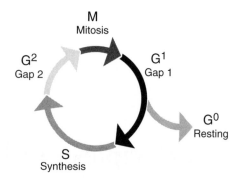

Figure 1.1 The cell cycle.
Source: Tortora & Derrickson; 2005; Fischer *et al.*, 2003; Rang *et al.*, 2003

chemotherapeutic agents (specifically the alkylating agents and platinum compounds) are also effective against cells in the G^0 phase which are not actively dividing. This group of drugs has been particularly effective against slow-growing tumours (Fischer *et al.*, 2003).

Cell cycle time

The overall objective in any cancer treatment plan is patient survival and the eradication of tumour cells, with minimal disruption to normal cell activity. It is known that tumours have a steady, progressive growth pattern which is affected by cell cycle time, growth fraction and cell loss. Chemotherapy has a greater effect on rapidly dividing cells. Cancer cells appear to have an initial rapid, proliferative phase during which time cells will be cycling quite quickly from mitosis to mitosis. The time it takes for each cycle to complete varies between 24 and 120 hours, depending on cell type.

Age and developmental status are known to influence cellular proliferation. Children and young people are growing, so have more body tissues with a dividing cell population; this helps to explain why paediatric malignancies appear to be more receptive to chemotherapy and more susceptible to the adverse side effects that may follow (Ettinger *et al.*, 2002).

Growth fraction

The growth fraction represents the percentage of cells undergoing division at any one time.

During early tumour development (when tumour bulk is small) there is a high fraction of dividing cells and tumours are able to double their size rapidly. As tumours grow in size, the blood, oxygen and nutrient supply become compromised and space for growth is restricted. During this time the cell growth fraction is low and the cycle time is slowed, therefore the doubling time is decreased (Ettinger *et al.*, 2002). Chemotherapy is more effective against rapidly dividing cells, so may be less effective when tumours reach this stage. It is thought, however, that it may be possible to increase both cell growth fraction and cell cycle time by achieving an initial tumour reduction, either through chemotherapy, radiotherapy or surgery. This would stimulate trigger mechanisms on the cell surfaces to recruit cells back into the cycle in an attempt to replace the lost bulk. Once this has been achieved, chemotherapy can once again become effective against reduced tumour bulk (Ettinger *et al.*, 2002). It can be concluded therefore that doubling times can vary greatly between different tumours and that chemotherapy-sensitive tumours tend to grow faster than slow-growing ones that are less sensitive to chemotherapy (Tortorice, 2000).

Pharmacokinetics and pharmacodynamics

Pharmacokinetics is the study of drug absorption, distribution, metabolism and excretion, or the movement of drugs within the body (Ettinger *et al.*, 2002). Pharmacokinetics therefore plays an important role in the successful application of cancer chemotherapy. Although some tumours may be known to be sensitive to a given cytotoxic agent, that agent may still fail to achieve a response. An understanding of how a patient's body is able to deal with a particular drug is essential in determining dose, timing and route of administration. Individual patients may demonstrate variable responses to therapies due to a variety of factors such as altered organ function. The pharmacokinetic behaviour of cytotoxic drugs has not been extensively evaluated in children; however, improved techniques have led to an increased emphasis on measuring the concentration of various drugs through pharmacokinetic studies (Balis *et al.*, 2002).

Pharmacodynamics is the study of the relationship between drug concentration and drug effect. It may therefore be possible to give a particular drug either as a bolus or as an infusion and achieve a completely different therapeutic or toxic effect (Ettinger *et al.*, 2002).

There is a very close link between the antitumour and toxic effects of chemotherapy; this means that the difference between an effective and a toxic dose can be very small. The aim of any chemotherapeutic schedule is therefore to gain the greatest anti-tumour effect with an acceptable level of toxicity (Ettinger *et al.*, 2002; Boddy, 2004).

An understanding of these two principles highlights the importance of careful and regular monitoring of the patient before each course of treatment so that doses can be modified accordingly.

Protocol development and clinical trials

Childhood cancer is very rare; hence the best way to search for better treatments is to conduct multi-institutional trials within a co-operative group, this may be either national or international. In the United Kingdom trials are co-ordinated by the Children's Cancer and Leukaemia Group (CCLG). It is the work of this organisation that has resulted in a 70 % cure rate for all childhood cancers (Sposto, 2004). The advantage of multi-institutional collaboration is that patient accrual is quicker, allowing for faster, reliable conclusions to be made (Ablett, 2004a). Co-ordination of trials reduces duplication and allows prompt evaluation of new agents and ways of giving treatments.

Clinical trials

There are few conditions for which treatment is known to be 100 % effective; this gives great potential for making improvements. Improvements to prescribed treatments can be determined via a clinical trial. A clinical trial is a planned experiment that is designed to discover the most appropriate treatment for patients with a given condition (Ablett, 2004a).

All clinical trials are described in a protocol document. This protocol will outline information relating to the purpose, design and conduct of the trial, including which patients are eligible, which treatments are to be evaluated and how each patient's response will be evaluated. Trial data will be analysed to evaluate the patient outcome with a given treatment regime. The patient outcome may be measured in terms of length of time to death or relapse. As outcomes improve, many childhood cancer trials aim to reduce the morbidity of treatment while maintaining its efficacy (Sposto, 2004).

Any research involving human subjects is subject to strict regulations. The European Union Directive on Good Clinical Practice (GCP) was implemented in May 2004. This is an international ethical and scientific quality standard for designing, conducting, recording and reporting trials that involve the participation of human subjects. GCP affects everyone working in clinical trials, whether in the pharmaceutical industry or academia. Failure to comply with certain elements of the legislation constitutes a criminal offence. These regulations have therefore affected all staff working with clinical trials involving the treatment of childhood cancer and resulted in additional training and working within agreed standard operating procedures (Ablett, 2004b).

Clinical trials fall into four phases:

1. Phase I to determine an acceptable drug dosage
2. Phase II to provide evidence of efficacy of treatment
3. Phase III to compare efficacy/side effects with those of other drugs/treatments
4. Phase IV large-scale epidemiological study (mainly industry).

Phase I studies

Phase I studies are the first trials in humans. They may be viewed as toxicity screening studies, where following testing in laboratories, a new drug is administered to human subjects to determine the maximum tolerated dose and any dose-limiting toxicities. The first human studies are undertaken in adults, but as children often have different tolerance patterns for chemotherapy drugs, the paediatric dose cannot be accurately extrapolated from the results of adult trials. Phase I trials are undertaken in paediatrics, but only children who have failed to respond to conventional treatments

are eligible for entry. Pharmacokinetic data are frequently collected, via serial blood and urine sampling, to determine the absorption, bioavailability and excretion patterns for the new drug.

Phase II studies

These aim to determine the potential efficacy of the new drug in different types of cancer. The maximum tolerated dose is given to a statistically defined number of children with a variety of relapsed or refractory cancers, and response is monitored. The goal of a phase II study is to identify which drugs warrant further study in a given tumour type.

Phase III studies

In childhood cancer, these phase III studies are the large-scale multicentre or international randomised trials into which the majority of children in the United Kingdom will be entered at the time of diagnosis. Large numbers of children will either be given a new drug or previously used drugs in a new combination or at a new dose. These new elements are usually in combination with standard therapy, to determine whether significant survival benefit is achieved by its addition to the previous 'best known' treatment or whether the new treatment is better than the standard one (Ablett, 2004a).

Considerations when planning chemotherapy treatments

Drug resistance

There is a wide variety of therapeutic responses and unacceptable toxicities in patients receiving chemotherapy (Tortorice, 2000). Some cancer cells demonstrate either an intrinsic or an acquired resistance to chemotherapy. Several mechanisms of drug resistance in cancer cells have been identified:

- decreased drug uptake by the cell;
- increased efflux (flow outwards) of drug out of the cell;

- detoxification of drugs in the cell secondary to metabolic changes;
- increased DNA repair;
- alterations in the structure of drug receptor sites or targets;
- decreased sensitivity to apoptosis (programmed cell death);
- multidrug resistance gene from genetic mutation following exposure to particular chemotherapeutic agents.

(Ettinger *et al.*, 2002)

It has been identified that resistant malignant cells contain the gene known as the multidrug resistance (MDR) gene. In intrinsic resistance the MDR gene is present from the onset, whereas the gene is the result of genetic mutation following exposure to chemotherapy in acquired cases. These resistant cells have a protein called P-glycoprotein present on the cell surface. This protein acts as an efflux pump, rapidly pushing through and eliminating the chemotherapeutic agents from within the cell, preventing their therapeutic effect.

In order that the risk of resistance is kept to a minimum, it is recommended that chemotherapy is administered at maximum dose intensity. This means that chemotherapy schedules should be constructed to offer the maximum tolerated dose with the smallest possible interval between doses. Advances in supportive care, such as colony stimulating factors and powerful antibiotics, have helped to make these dose-intensive protocols possible (Balis *et al.*, 2002; Ettinger *et al.*, 2002).

Toxicities

Chemotherapeutic agents have the same cytotoxic effect on both normal and malignant cells. This cell toxicity is often dose-limiting and restrictive. Normal cells need to have the opportunity for recovery between treatments to avoid life-threatening toxicities or those threatening quality of life which may be unacceptable to patients, both in the short and long term. Even in the presence of drug resistance, unacceptable toxicities may still occur because of the toxic effects of chemotherapy on normal cells.

Several toxicities are common to the majority of cytotoxic drugs, for example, myelosuppression,

nausea and vomiting, and alopecia. These acute toxicities are usually reversible. Some drugs also have unique toxicities affecting specific organs or tissues, such as cardiotoxicity which is associated with anthracyclines. Many of these unique toxicities are cumulative and in some cases irreversible (Balis *et al.*, 2002).

The severity of any toxicity is an important factor when planning a treatment protocol. It is usual therefore to combine drugs that have differing side effects, for example, a non-myelosuppressive drug such as vincristine may be combined with myelosuppressive ones without compromising the dose of either drug (Balis *et al.*, 2002).

In the palliative stages of disease, when cure is no longer the aim of treatment, careful consideration needs to be given to ensuring that the balance between an achievable quality of life is weighed up against the toxic side effects of any treatments given. It is possible that toxicity deemed acceptable during active therapy may prove unacceptable for the dying child (Hain and Hardy, 2004).

Treatment approaches

The ultimate aims of treatment for all patients are cure and quality of life. There are many approaches to treatment that will be used to achieve this aim.

Single agent versus combination

It has long been acknowledged that combination drugs regimes significantly increase the chance of complete remission (Balis *et al.*, 2002). This is because combination regimes offer a way to overcome drug resistance to individual agents. When different drugs are used to treat a particular tumour, it is usual to select those that have different toxic effects, as this helps to reduce the treatment-related morbidity.

Adjuvant chemotherapy

Adjuvant chemotherapy is a term sometimes used to describe therapy that is used in addition to other modalities of treatment, such as surgery or radiotherapy. This is particularly effective in patients who have a high risk of relapse at metastatic sites, for example, those with solid tumours (Ettinger *et al.*, 2002).

Neo-adjuvant chemotherapy

This is the term used to describe chemotherapy that is given prior to definitive localised therapy such as surgery or radiotherapy in an attempt to reduce the tumour bulk, thus facilitating less radical surgical or radiotherapeutic interventions. Chemotherapy used in this way will also provide earlier treatment of micrometastatic disease (Balis *et al.*, 2002; Ettinger *et al.*, 2002). It is also possible to identify which chemotherapeutic agents are effective against a particular tumour in a particular patient. Further courses of chemotherapy are frequently prescribed once recovery from definitive localised treatment has been attained.

Dose-intensive regimes

One way of overcoming drug resistance is to ensure that drugs are administered at the maximum drug intensity. Dose intensification can be achieved in two ways. By alternating myelotoxic drugs with non-myelotoxic ones, given at the neutropenic nadir, it is possible to continue cytotoxic onslaught on malignant cells while permitting bone marrow recovery. Another approach is to reduce the duration of marrow aplasia by combining intensive chemotherapy with the administration of colony-stimulating factors (Scurr *et al.*, 2005).

Combination chemotherapy

Drugs used in combination may have an enhanced effect against malignant cells; however, it is not completely understood why this is (Ettinger *et al.*, 2002). Tumour cells do not progress through the cell cycle at the same time, so it is important to select agents that exert their antineoplastic effects at different stages of the cell cycle. The objective of any regime is to achieve maximum tumour cell kill without excessive toxicity. Drugs with

different toxicities will be chosen wherever possible, however, if overlapping toxicities are unavoidable, for example, bone marrow depression, it may be necessary to reduce doses or extend the period of time between cycles (Tortorice, 2000).

Reducing doses

High-dose therapies have been responsible for many of the improvements seen in the treatment of childhood cancers. Randomised studies are now being conducted which set out to identify whether some children can be treated at lower doses without reducing efficacy, for example, the current treatment trial for treating acute lymphoblastic leukaemia (Medical Research Council, 2003) sets out to identify low-risk children by looking at minimal residual disease at various points in the induction period of treatment. The main focus is to attempt to reduce the cumulative, dose-related cardiotoxic effects of the anthracyclines and the risk of infertility and secondary malignancies associated with alkylating agents. It is hoped that the optimum balance between effective treatment and low toxicity can be achieved by reducing the total doses given, by substituting less toxic analogues of effective drugs and, where possible, by avoiding anthracyclines or alkylating agents completely. Children who are participating in these studies will require particularly close monitoring for response, in order that treatment may be modified back to the standard therapy if necessary.

Chemoprotective agents

Cytotoxic chemotherapy is extremely toxic and has many unwanted side effects. Some side effects, such as nausea and vomiting and alopecia, are unpleasant but are reversible and not life-threatening. Bone marrow depression can be life-threatening but is usually reversible, especially if doses are modified. There is a group of toxicities that are potentially life-threatening and can cause irreversible damage to normal cells, for example, the cardiotoxic effects of anthracyclines. Much interest has therefore been generated in the development of drugs that may block the toxic effects of chemotherapeutic agents while maintaining their antineoplastic properties. These developments include both chemoprotective and rescue agents for drugs such as doxorubicin (liposomal preparations and cardio-protective agents), ifosfamide (mesna) and methotrexate (folinic acid) (Boddy, 2004).

Administration schedules

Prolonged drug administration has been explored as an additional way of reducing toxicity. The toxicity associated with peak serum levels in some drugs, such as the anthracyclines, is thought to be reduced by slow administration; this may be over several days. However, the relative benefits of these regimes over shorter infusions have yet to be substantiated, mainly because other short- to medium-term side effects, such as mucositis, are enhanced with prolonged infusion time (Boddy, 2004; Scurr et al., 2005).

References

Ablett S (2004a) An Introduction to Clinical Trials (5th edn). Leicester: United Kingdom Children's Cancer Study Group

Ablett S (2004b) UKCCSG Guide to GCP and the EU Directive on Clinical Trials. Leicester: United Kingdom Children's Cancer Study Group

Balis FM, Holcenberg JS & Blaney SM (2002) 'Chapter 10 – General principles of chemotherapy' in: Pizzo PA & Poplack DG (eds) Principles and Practice of Pediatric Oncology (4th edn). Philadelphia: Lippincott, Williams and Wilkins, pp. 237–308

Boddy AV (2004) 'Chapter 8 – Cancer chemotherapy and mechanisms of resistance' in: Pinkerton R, Plowman PN & Pieters R (eds) Paediatric Oncology (3rd edn). London: Arnold, pp. 142–168

Ettinger AG, Bond DM & Sievers TD (2002) 'Chapter 6 – Chemotherapy' in: Baggott CR, Kelly KP, Fochtman D & Foley GV (eds) Nursing Care of Children and Adolescents with Cancer (3rd edn). Philadelphia: WB Saunders Company, pp. 133–176

Fischer DS, Knobf MT, Durivage HJ & Beaulieu NJ (2003) The Cancer Chemotherapy Handbook (6th edn). Philadelphia: Mosby

Hain R & Hardy J (2004) 'Chapter 33 – Palliative care in paediatric oncology' in: Pinkerton R, Plowman PN & Pieters R (eds) Paediatric Oncology (3rd edn). London: Arnold, pp. 685–703

Medical Research Council Working Party on Leukaemia in Children (2003) UK Acute Lymphoblastic Leukaemia (ALL) Trial, UKALL 2003 (updated 2004, 2005). London: Medical Research Council

Rang HP, Dale MM, Ritter JM & Moore PK (2003) Pharmacology (5th edn). Edinburgh: Churchill Livingstone

Scurr M, Judson I & Root T (2005) 'Chapter 2 – Combination chemotherapy and chemotherapy principles' in: Brighton D & Wood M (eds) Cancer Chemotherapy. London: Elsevier, pp. 17–30

Sposto R (2004) 'Chapter 10 – Design and role of clinical trials' in: Pinkerton R, Plowman PN & Pieters R (eds) Paediatric Oncology (3rd edn). London: Arnold, pp. 189–200

Tortora GJ & Derrickson B (2005) Principles of Anatomy and Physiology (11th edn). New Jersey: Wiley and Sons

Tortorice PV (2000) 'Chapter 18 – Chemotherapy: principles of therapy' in: Yarbo CH, Frogge MH, Goodman M & Groenwald SL (eds) Cancer Nursing: Principles and Practice (5th edn). Massachusetts: Jones and Bartlett, pp. 352–384

2 Chemotherapy Agents

Angela Houlston

Classification of drugs

In general, chemotherapeutic agents are classified according to their chemical structure, biological source or effect on the cell cycle. The most useful classification is by mechanism of action (Pinkerton et al., 2004). There are six major classes of drugs (Table 2.1):

- alkylating agents
- platinum compounds
- antimetabolites
- tubulin-binding drugs
- topoisomerase inhibitors
- miscellaneous agents.

Alkylating agents

These are a group of reactive chemicals which act through the co-valent bonding of an alkyl group, by substituting the hydrogen atoms in the cellular molecules. This causes cross-linking and DNA strand breaks. Through this process damage is caused to the DNA template, RNA, DNA, and protein synthesis is inhibited and replication is unable to take place. The most affected of the nucleic acid bases is guanine, but cytosine and adenine are also known to be affected.

Alkylating agents are classed as cell cycle non-phase-specific and are effective against cells in all phases of the cycle, including the G^0 phase. This means that they have the capacity to affect tumour shrinkage, causing more cells to be recruited back into the active proliferative cycle where they become susceptible to the cell cycle phase-specific agents. This also means that the alkylating agents are effective against both slow-growing and rapidly proliferating tumours.

Platinum compounds

This group of agents contain platinum atoms, which were found to form complexes that arrest cell division. Platinum compounds have a similar mechanism to alkylating agents but in addition to forming interstrand cross-links also attach to bases on the same DNA chain (intrastrand linkages).

Antimetabolites

These are a group of agents which act by mimicking the essential metabolites necessary for DNA

Cancer in Children and Young People   Edited by Faith Gibson and Louise Soanes
© 2008 John Wiley & Sons, Ltd

Table 2.1   Classification of cytotoxic drugs

Drug	Action	Common use
Alkylating Agents		
Busulphan	Causes DNA cross-links; cell cycle non-phase-specific	Leukaemias; Neuroblastoma
Carmustine (CCNU)	Causes DNA cross-links and strand breaks	CNS; Lymphomas
Cyclophosphamide	Causes DNA cross-links	Leukaemias; Lymphomas; Neuroblastoma; Rhabdomyosarcoma; Ewing's Sarcoma and Germ Cell Tumours
Dacarbazine (DTIC)	Causes DNA cross-links and strand breaks; inhibits DNA and RNA synthesis	Sarcomas and Hodgkin's Lymphomas
Ifosfamide	Causes DNA cross-links with DNA and binds to proteins	Sarcomas
Lomustine (CCNU)	Causes DNA cross-links and strand breaks; inhibits DNA and RNA synthesis	CNS and Lymphomas
Melphalan	Causes DNA cross-links, strand breaks and miscoding RNA synthesis	Neuroblastoma; Sarcomas; Leukaemias and Hodgkin's Lymphomas
Procarbazine	Affects pre-formed DNA, RNA and protein	Hodgkin's Lymphomas
Temozolamide	Similar to Dacarbazine, a prodrug-active metabolite is formed by chemical degradation	CNS
Thiotepa	Chromosome cross-links with inhibition of nucleo-protein synthesis	CNS
Treosulphan	A bifunctional alkylating agent similar to Busulphan	Sarcomas
Platinum Compounds		
Carboplatin	Causes interstrand and intrastrand cross-links by reacting with nucleophilic sites on DNA	Germ Cell Tumours; Neuroblastoma; Sarcomas; CNS and Liver Tumours
Cisplatin	Causes interstrand and intrastrand cross-links and prevents cell replication by denaturing the double helix	Germ Cell Tumours; Neuroblastoma; Sarcomas; CNS and Liver Tumours
Antimetabolites		
Clofarabine	Purine nucleoside analogue	Leukaemias
Cytarabine	Pyrimidine analogue incorporated into DNA; slows synthesis and causes defective links and erroneous duplication of early DNA strands; S phase-specific	Leukaemias; Lymphomas and CNS
Fludarabine	Purine antimetabolite	Leukaemias
Gemcitabine	Inhibits DNA synthesis	Neuroblastoma
Methotrexate	Dihydrofolate reductase enzyme inhibitor; results in the inhibition of the precursors of DNA, RNA and cellular proteins. S phase-specific	Leukaemias; Lymphomas; CNS and Osteosarcoma
6-Mercaptopurine	Thiopurine antimetabolite which inhibits *de novo* purine synthesis by converting to monophosphate nucleotides; S phase-specific	Leukaemias and Lymphomas
6-Thioguanine	Thiopurine antimetabolite which inhibits *de novo* purine synthesis by converting to monophosphate nucleotides; S phase specific	Leukaemias and Lymphomas

5-Flurouracil	Inhibits thymidine synthesis; incorporated into DNA and RNA	Colorectal Tumours and Liver Tumours
Tubulin-Binding Drugs		
Vinblastine	Binds to microtubular proteins causing mitotic arrest during metaphase. May also inhibit DNA, RNA and protein synthesis; active in S and M phases	Lymphomas
Vincristine	Bids to microtubular proteins causing mitotic arrest during metaphase; active in S and M phases	Leukaemias; Lymphomas; Wilms' Tumours; Neuroblastoma and Rhabdomyosarcoma
Vinorelbine	Mitotic inhibitor; blocks microtubule polymerisation	Sarcomas
Vindesine	Similar to Vinblastine, binds to microtubular proteins of the mitotic spindle leading to mitotic arrest	Lymphomas
Topoisomerase I Inhibitors		
Iridotecan	Causes DNA strand breaks	Investigational
Topotecan	Causes DNA strand breaks	Investigational
Topoisomerase II Inhibitors		
a) Epipodophyllins		
Etoposide	Inhibits DNA synthesis in S and G^2 phases causing single strand breaks in DNA	Leukaemias; Lymphomas; Neuroblastoma; Rhabdomyosarcoma; Ewing's sarcoma and Wilms' Tumour
Teniposide	Inhibits DNA uptake of thymidine thereby impairing DNA synthesis; works in late S and early G^2 phases	Leukaemias; Lymphomas; Neuroblastoma and Germ Cell Tumours
b) Anthracyclines		
Daunorubicin	Intercalates DNA blocking DNA, RNA and protein synthesis	Leukaemias
Doxorubicin	Binds to DNA base pairs; inhibits DNA, RNA and protein synthesis; S phase-specific	Leukaemias; Lymphomas; Neuroblastoma; Rhabdomyosarcoma; Ewing's Sarcoma and Wilms' Tumour
Epirubicin	Causes DNA strand breaks	Lymphomas and Sarcomas
Idarubicin	Inhibits RNA synthesis; S phase specific	Leukaemias
Mitozantrone	Inhibits DNA and RNA synthesis through intercalation of base pairs; cell cycle non-phase-specific	Leukaemias
c) Miscellaneous		
Amscarine	Intercalates and binds DNA and inhibits topoisomerase II and RNA synthesis; S phase-specific	Leukaemias
L-Asparaginase	Hydrolysis of serum asparagine G^1 phase-specific	Leukaemias
Dactinomycin	Inhibits DNA and RNA synthesis by binding to the guanine portion of DNA; DNA is then unable to act as a template for DNA and RNA; G^1 and S phase-specific	Wilms' Tumour; Ewing's Sarcoma and Rhabdomyosarcoma
Bleomycin	Induces double and single strand breaks in DNA synthesis	Germ Cell Tumour and Lymphomas

Table 2.1   (Continued)

Drug	Action	Common use
Hydroxyurea	Ribonucleotide reductase inhibitor	Leukaemias
13-Cis Retinoeic Acid	A derivative of vitamin A, increases DNA, RNA and protein synthesis, affects cellular mitosis	Neuroblastoma
Cortico steroids	Receptor-mediated lympholysis	Leukaemias and Lymphomas

Sources: Pinkerton, *et al.* (2004) and Pizzo & Poplack (2002).

and RNA synthesis. They are so structurally similar to the metabolites of which they are analogues that they are able to deceive the cells into incorporating them into the metabolic pathways. They are effective either through inhibition of cellular macromolecular synthesis and their building blocks, or through their incorporation into the metabolic pathways which results in a defective end-product.

The antimetabolites are classed as cell cycle phase-specific and are effective in the S phase. They are most cytotoxic against cells which are synthesising DNA and are therefore most effective against rapidly proliferating rather than slow-growing tumours.

Tubulin-binding drugs

This group of drugs is often called the vinca alkaloids and includes a number of agents originally derived from the periwinkle plant. These drugs are all cell cycle-specific, attacking cells at certain phases of division. These drugs interfere with normal microtubule formation and function, causing arrest during mitosis. This results in a lack of mitotic spindle that causes chromosomes to be dispersed throughout the cytoplasm. Tubulin-binding drugs may have some effect on cells in the G^1 and S phase but mainly affect the M phase.

Topoisomerase inhibitors

Topoisomerase enzymes control the manipulation of the structure of DNA, necessary for cell replication. The cytotoxic agents that interfere with the action of the topoisomerase enzymes (Topoisomerase I and II) are classified together. Topoisomerase II inhibitors are placed into three sub-groups: epipodophyllotoxins, anthracyclines and miscellaneous.

1. Topoisomerase I inhibitors – these bind with the DNA enzyme complex causing DNA strand breaks and cell death.
2. Epipodophyllotoxins – this group is derived from plants and is thought to inhibit topoisomerase II and produce DNA strand breaks. They affect cells in late S and early G phases of the cycle.
3. Anthracyclines – the mechanism of action includes covalent binding of DNA and subsequent formation of free radicals. They also cause inhibition of topoisomerase II enzyme which blocks the rejoining of the cleaved DNA strands.
4. Miscellaneous.

Miscellaneous agents

In normal tissues the non-essential amino acid, asparagine, is produced through synthesis of aspartic acid and glutamine by the enzyme, asparagine synthase. This results in a continual production and release of asparagine into the circulation. Normal cells are therefore able to synthesise their own asparagine, which is needed to maintain normal growth and development. Tumour cells are unable to synthesise their own asparagine to facilitate protein synthesis because they lack an enzyme necessary for this synthesis to take place. Instead they rely on this continual circulating pool of asparagine produced by normal cells. By introducing a catalyst, the enzyme L-asparaginase, into this circulating pool of amino acids, asparagine is converted into aspartic acid and ammonia. This effectively starves the tumour cells through rapid depletion of circulating asparagine and inhibits tumour cell protein synthesis. L-asparaginase is cell cycle non-specific.

Corticosteroids have anti-tumour effects and are used in many drug regimes. Steroids bind with macromolecules in the cell cytoplasm and then enter the cell nucleus. The complex then binds with DNA and modifies the transcription process.

References

Pinkerton R, Plowman PN & Pieters R (2004) *Paediatric Oncology* (3rd edn). London: Arnold

Pizzo PA & Poplack DG (eds) *Principles and Practice of Pediatric Oncology* (5th edn) Philadelphia: Lippincott, Williams & Wilkins

3

Administration of Chemotherapy

Angela Houlston

Safe practice with cytotoxic drugs: legislation

The Cancer Plan (DoH, 2000) and the *Manual of Cancer Services* (DoH, 2004) both highlight the need for highly trained professionals to be involved in the administration of chemotherapy. The latter is focused on adult services but makes clear the need for a minimum standard for the training of doctors and nurses who administer chemotherapy. Each hospital Trust must have its own policy and guidelines on the safe handling and administration of cytotoxic drugs. With the advent of Cancer Networks, these policies are becoming network-wide and may also include children's services.

Cytotoxic chemotherapy is a very powerful cancer treatment and errors can be highly significant. There is a very small margin between a therapeutic and a toxic effect, and this has led to the development of national standards (Lomath, 2005). These national guidelines aim to improve patient safety and give measurable standards to ensure consistency of practice and good documentation across the country.

Elimination of errors involving intrathecal chemotherapy is a major target in the NHS programme to improve patient safety. This has resulted in the publication of National Guidelines for the safe administration of intrathecal chemotherapy (HSC 2003/010) (DoH, 2003). This will be discussed in more detail later in this chapter.

Consent

Before commencing a course of chemotherapy treatment or participating in any clinical trial, written consent must be obtained from the child's parent or carer in accordance with the Department of Health Guidance (2001d). The consent form should allow the parent to acknowledge that they have received written information and discussed the risks and intended benefits of the treatment plan.

Safe handling

The same mechanisms that kill cancer cells are toxic to healthy cells (Power, 2004). This has led to concerns regarding the risks to health-care workers involved in the preparation, administration and care of patients receiving cytotoxic chemotherapy.

Cancer in Children and Young People Edited by Faith Gibson and Louise Soanes
© 2008 John Wiley & Sons, Ltd

There is some anecdotal evidence that suggests that nurses who handle chemotherapy may be subject to hair loss and skin or nail problems. There are also reports of tissue damage following eye injuries or skin exposure to chemotherapeutic agents (Power, 2004). Common routes of exposure include contact with the skin or mucous membranes following splash or spill accidents and inhalation from powders and aerosols. The Health and Safety Executive (HSE, 2003) suggests that acute effects such as irritation of the skin and mucous membranes are possible following accidental exposure to cytotoxic drugs. Chronic effects are less well documented because the majority of studies have been conducted on animals. However, it is clear that some cytotoxic drugs are mutagenic and carcinogenic and individuals whose working life includes contact with chemotherapeutic agents are taking unnecessary risks if they do not follow guidelines for safe practice.

The Health and Safety at Work Act (1994) and the Management of Health and Safety at Work Regulations (1999) clearly state the legal duty to protect both employees and the public. The Health and Safety at Work guidelines outline procedures for the safe handling of cytotoxic drugs (HSE, 2003).

However, safe practice involves not only the protection of those directly involved in administration and patient care, but also consideration of other people in the chemotherapeutic environment who may not be aware of the risks and are therefore unable to take appropriate steps to protect themselves. By virtue of their professional knowledge and role, nurses have a duty of care to others. Subsequently, they have a responsibility to support the creation and maintenance of a safety culture, where protection of themselves and their colleagues, patients and their families and other visitors is accorded due respect.

Reconstitution and preparation of chemotherapeutic agents

The principle behind all the recommended safety precautions is to provide physical barriers between the cytotoxic drugs and the possible routes of contamination: inhalation, absorption, ingestion and inoculation. General issues of safe practice will be outlined here, with specific details being discussed with respect to each of the different routes of drug administration.

- *Inhalation* of aerosols can easily occur without the knowledge of the handler; aerosols may be inhaled in liquid or powder form, causing local inflammation of mucous membranes or systemic effects following entry into the blood via the pulmonary circulation.
- *Absorption* can occur through contact with the skin, cornea or mucous membranes through splashes and spills. Some agents can cause rashes, blistering or local necrosis.
- *Ingestion* can take place if traces of drug enter the mouth via the hands, or by food or drinks placed in the area of preparation becoming contaminated.
- *Inoculation* via accidental puncturing of the skin, or if an unhealed, exposed skin injury comes into contact with the drug.

Ideally, all cytotoxic drugs should be prepared centrally in a pharmacy department, using an aseptic technique in a suitable safety cabinet or pharmaceutical isolator, by designated staff who have received training in this area. In the rare event that cytotoxic drugs have to be prepared in the ward environment, recommendations for drug preparation include use of a segregated area, ideally with an isolator, by appropriately trained and experienced staff.

Manipulation of oral and topical medicines, such as the crushing of tablets, should be avoided wherever possible.

Personal Protective Equipment (PPE)

The Personal Protective Equipment at Work Regulations (1992) state that PPE should be provided wherever there are risks to health and safety that cannot be controlled. The Control of Substances Hazardous to Health (COSHH) Regulations (2002) define cytotoxic chemotherapy as hazardous substances that should be subject to a risk assessment to help identify the most appropriate PPE necessary. The following precautions are recommended:

- *Gloves* – it is recommended that protective gloves should be worn if accidental contact with a cytotoxic drug is possible. No material has been found to give unlimited protection (HSE, 2003), however. Singleton and Connor (1999) suggest that any gloves used should be impermeable or minimally permeable to cytotoxic drugs on testing. Traditionally, latex gloves have been recommended but concerns over latex sensitivity have led to nitrile gloves gaining in popularity (Oncology Nursing Society, 2004).

- *Eye and face protection* – it is recommended that visors or goggles are worn if there is any risk of splashing when handling cytotoxic drugs.
- *Respiratory protection* – it is recommended that special respiratory protective equipment is worn if there is any risk of exposure to cytotoxic drugs through aerosol or powder inhalation. Ideally any procedures where this is a risk should be carried out in an enclosed environment such as an isolator.
- *Protective clothing* – gowns and aprons can help to prevent contamination of clothes and the skin. The selection of an appropriate garment is dependent on its lack of absorptive qualities.

When giving drugs to a child, a balance should be maintained between ensuring reasonable protective measures are taken, and the potential for alarming the recipient. By considering logically the possible routes of contamination for the method of administration and related procedures, an approach that is both sensible and safe can usually be achieved; individual hospital Trust policies should be adhered to. Correct and thoughtful administration practices can minimise the risk of accidental contamination. Whatever protection is worn during drug administration, the child and parents require an explanation of the reasons for its use.

Work practices

Certain practices can increase the risk of contamination, for example, priming the intravenous tubing with the hazardous drug instead of saline. The Oncology Nursing Society guidelines (2004) recommend the following work practices to reduce the risk of contamination:

- use of locking connections and intravenous (IV) delivery devices;
- careful use and disposal of any 'sharps';
- avoid spiking IV bags, ideally the tubing should be primed and the bags attached in pharmacy conditions;
- if necessary, prime IV tubing with a non-hazardous solution, for example, saline;
- avoid 'unspiking' IV bags, discard the infusion bags with the tubing still attached;
- perform work below eye level.

Storage

If cytotoxic drugs are not intended for immediate administration, they should be clearly labelled with the name, dose and volume of the drug supplied, method of storage (locked refrigerator or cupboard at room temperature), expiry date and time, and a statement that the drug is cytotoxic. Drugs should then be stored in accordance with local policy.

Disposal of waste

The management and disposal of used or contaminated equipment, body fluids, spillages and unused drugs should be addressed, as these are a potential source of drug exposure:

- *Equipment* – 'Sharps' (needles, ampoules and vials) should be disposed of in an approved container which is clearly labelled and reserved solely for the use of cytotoxic waste. Empty syringes are either disposed of in the sharps container or with other dry clinical waste to be incinerated, including administration sets, bags and disposable protective clothing. Non-disposable equipment should be washed in warm soapy water and dried after use.
- *Unused drugs and solutions* – Whenever possible, cytotoxic drug waste of any kind should be disposed of by high temperature incineration (1000°C). Unused doses of drugs should be returned to the dispensing pharmacy at the earliest opportunity for possible re-use or disposal. Part-used doses of drugs should be

disposed of as hazardous clinical waste, but only if their container can be securely resealed for storage and transportation. Staff should wear protective clothing when disconnecting cytotoxic infusions, disposing of equipment and waste and washing non-disposable equipment. These procedures should not be delegated to others (e.g. trainee nurses) without first providing adequate education.

- *Body fluids* – Body fluids may contain potentially hazardous amounts of cytotoxic drugs or their active metabolites and most drugs are eliminated by renal or faecal excretion. Body fluids should therefore be handled promptly and with caution, wearing gloves and an apron at all times. Care should also be taken when handling vomit, wound drainage fluid and blood (HSE, 2003). As a general rule, body fluids should be assumed to be contaminated during chemotherapy and for a minimum of two days and up to seven days afterwards, although each drug has a different excretion rate. The excretion pattern varies as well, for example, some drugs are excreted unchanged in the urine; for others only a trace appears in the urine. It is important that parents are made aware of this fact so that they can be supplied with gloves for changing nappies and/or soiled bed linen and for dealing with their child's body fluids, both in and out of hospital.

Spillage and contamination

All staff should be familiar with the procedures required to deal with spills and accidental contamination (HSE, 2003):

- *Spillage* – Any spillage of a cytotoxic drug must be cleared up immediately. Access to the spillage area should be restricted and protective clothing must be worn. A specially prepared spill kit will give prompt access to the appropriate equipment to safely clear up any spills. All the waste should be disposed of in an identified cytotoxic disposal bag for incineration. If airborne powder or aerosol is involved, it is recommended that a face mask or particulate respirator is also worn to prevent inhalation and

that damp paper towels are used for wiping surfaces. Parents giving chemotherapy in the home need information about management of accidental spillage.

- *Contamination* – If contamination of the skin or eyes occurs, then immediate action must be taken. Skin should be washed thoroughly with copious amounts of soap and water and then dried. Eyes should be irrigated with 0.9% sodium chloride and eye wash using freeflowing irrigation to the eye. An eye bath should NOT be used as the contained fluid may spread the cytotoxic agent around the enclosed area within the eye bath. Further medical attention should be sought immediately if any visible trauma to the skin or eyes develops and reference to any individual drug recommendations should be followed. Any incidents should be reported to the Occupational Health Department, supported by written documentation according to local hospital incident reporting policy. If contamination to clothing or bed linen occurs, these should be changed immediately and treated according to the local policy for soiled linen.

Safe practice during pregnancy

Older studies, carried out in the 1980s, have shown links between occupational exposure to chemotherapy and miscarriages, menstrual dysfunction and infertility. However, it is important to point out that more recent studies have shown no statistically supported association; this may be due to an increased awareness and better use of PPE (NHS, 2002).

Safe practice with cytotoxic drugs, using recommended protection and excellent technique, should theoretically prevent exposure and therefore rule out the risk to the foetus. However, for ethical reasons, it is unlikely that research will ever be conducted to provide conclusive proof that absolutely no risk to the foetus exists if precautions are taken. Evidence seems to indicate that by taking the recommended precautions, pregnant staff can continue to work safely in a paediatric oncology environment, provided a risk assessment takes place and individuals are made aware of their right to choose to opt out of any procedures that involve contact with cytotoxic drugs (NHS, 2002; HSE, 2003).

Patient support

Decision-making

Advances in health care have led to more treatment options and therefore more decision-making points in every child's cancer journey. With increased options comes an associated uncertainty regarding outcomes. Children are more vulnerable to harm than adults due to their cognitive and emotional development, legal capacity, level of autonomy and dependence on family influences. In most cases parents become surrogate decision-makers for their children. Within paediatric oncology most decisions will be emotionally charged at times of uncertainty and anxiety and good support mechanisms need to be available.

The United Nations Convention on the Rights of the Child (1989) saw a shift from a paternalistic and medically dominated view of decision-making to one that considers the views and best interests of the child. The Children Act (Department of Health, 1989) states that the ascertainable wishes and feelings of children should be sought about matters that affect them. It may be argued that expecting a child to contribute to a health-care decision causes unnecessary pressure; however, they both have a need and a right to be involved in matters that affect their lives. Health-care professionals working with children have a duty to act as the child's advocate in decision-making, ensuring that the child's interests are paramount and that they are always consulted so that any decisions are truly in their best interest.

Setting for chemotherapy administration

Chemotherapy may be administered in many different settings; selection of the most appropriate setting will depend on many factors. Shared Care is growing in popularity as a way of organising care in the United Kingdom. The Principal Treatment Centre is responsible for confirming the diagnosis and prescribing, administering and guiding the family through complex treatment regimes. Treatment for children with acute lymphoblastic leukaemia and some solid tumours is less intense and much of the treatment can be received at the Paediatric Oncology Shared Care Unit (POSCU) or at home, supervised by appropriately trained children's nurses (Edwards et al., 2005).

Inpatient chemotherapy

The majority of chemotherapy regimes have traditionally been administered in the inpatient setting; this allowed for adequate management of toxic side effects as well as time for parental education and support. Protocols that require high doses of chemotherapy and associated support such as hydration and rescue regimes can only be safely managed as an inpatient.

Non-inpatient chemotherapy

Many chemotherapy regimes no longer require an inpatient hospital stay and it is standard to have haematology/oncology day care facilities associated with every inpatient unit. Non-inpatient chemotherapy regimes support the philosophies of home care and parental involvement and are potentially less disruptive to family life (Edwards et al., 2005). It should, however, be acknowledged that some families may feel more isolated at home, especially during the period immediately following diagnosis. Measures should therefore be put in place to ensure that adequate support is provided in the form of both written information and community nursing provision. This is particularly important if parents are to manage their child's chemotherapy side effects confidently without the degree of support and supervision available in hospital.

When proposing to give chemotherapy in the day care or home setting, many issues must be considered. In fact, most of the important factors are those routinely assessed when preparing for the discharge of a child from hospital after inpatient chemotherapy. Details of the specific treatment regime, the circumstances of each child and family, and the services available to them must be considered when planning any package of care. Most children receiving chemotherapy are cared for by their parents at home following each treatment block, and parents are routinely expected to be capable of monitoring their child for the side effects of highly toxic therapy, with the necessary information and support. Through exploring the available options with the multidisciplinary team and the family, the nurse can optimise patient safety and family coping, by ensuring that appropriate input is provided in the best location for each child.

Although care is planned in negotiation with the child and family, the decisions of the professionals about the location of treatment should be based on an assessment of the risks and benefits of the available options. The possibility always exists for coercion by one or other party: professionals may believe that home treatment is always best, and subtly exert pressure on parents; or they may be under pressure themselves from the demand for inpatient beds. Families who are desperate to avoid inpatient care may endeavour to persuade staff to permit home treatment before education and assessment programmes have been completed or in the absence of sufficient professional home support services. Pressure may also be exerted by professionals from other disciplines, and nurses require both knowledge and confidence in order to negotiate effectively and honestly with their colleagues and with families.

Day care chemotherapy

Day care services have gained greater importance in recent years, as the potential for giving more complex chemotherapy in this setting has been recognised. The subsequent effect upon families and service providers has meant that the role of nurses working in this environment has developed a higher profile. Children attending for day care chemotherapy are generally well and they may be considered to be a low priority by a stretched medical team. This has led to the development of nursing roles, such as nurse-led assessment prior to the administration of chemotherapy (Boyer & Whiles, 2004).

In order to facilitate treatment as a day care procedure, some adjustments to standard schedules may be possible, such as oral rather than intravenous post-hydration. Any adjustments must be clearly documented and sanctioned by a doctor.

For day care chemotherapy to be a safe option, it is clear that the child must be well enough to be cared for at home following the treatment and that rapid deterioration is not expected. In some cases the introduction of day care chemotherapy is best delayed until treatment is established and the family have the necessary knowledge and confidence to care for their child at home.

The effective management of nausea and vomiting is a nursing priority for successful day care administration; poor control can prove to be the limiting factor as to whether day care treatment is an acceptable alternative. The child will be travelling between hospital and home after treatment and any nausea or vomiting will be distressing for the child and cause significant problems for parents, particularly on public transport.

Home chemotherapy

It is widely accepted that for many children, home care is the best option. Home chemotherapy for children is often parent-administered, and is almost exclusively limited to oral drugs or low-dose bolus intravenous injection. Home intravenous chemotherapy usually requires a central venous access device and requires scrupulous monitoring by parents or nursing staff. The initiation of parentally led home chemotherapy therefore assumes that the parents are confident carers with regard to the management of their child's central venous access device. The routine administration of vesicant drugs should not be undertaken outside the hospital setting. Other drugs given at home are also limited by safety considerations; a risk assessment for possible reactions, side effects, other adverse events and available emergency support should be carefully made before specific home treatments are offered. While it is possible to administer a variety of treatments at home, it is important that the child receives regular monitoring by the specialist hospital team so a certain number of hospital visits are unavoidable.

Ambulatory chemotherapy

Many cytotoxic drugs are cell cycle phase-specific, attacking the cell during a short period of the replication process. 5-Fluorouracil (5-FU) is commonly administered as a prolonged infusion over several days; this ensures that the maximum numbers of cells are exposed to chemotherapy during their active phase. In such cases it may not be practical to keep the child in hospital throughout the infusion and a small ambulatory pump may be used to administer the chemotherapy safely at home (Legge, 2005). Ambulatory chemotherapy is used more commonly in the adult population than in children.

Administration of chemotherapy

Training

The *Manual of Cancer Services Standards* (DoH, 2004) states that all staff who administer chemotherapy should receive appropriate training and be assessed as competent. A framework that offers guidance for those who provide the training has been developed by the Paediatric Oncology Nurses Forum (PONF) (RCN, 2005). This guidance offers a consistent and equitable approach to the training and assessment of competence of staff involved in the administration of chemotherapy.

Assessment

A thorough nursing assessment must be undertaken before cytotoxic drugs are given. Chordas (2005) summarises the key nursing responsibilities prior to administering chemotherapy:

- Ensure that local policies and procedures are followed.
- Check any pre-treatment investigations are within acceptable limits.
- Review any previous courses to ensure that no problems occurred.
- Ensure that any pre-medication or hydration is administered.

- Read the appropriate section of the relevant treatment protocol.
- Check the surface area and doses are correct, noting any prescribed modifications.
- Administer prescribed, appropriate antiemetics.
- Ensure the family and child are adequately prepared and informed.

Potential and actual problems and planned strategies to overcome them should be documented. The involvement of the child and the family in this process can help them understand the treatment and assist in the process of negotiating the family's desired level of involvement in care. If the agreed roles of the parents, the child and professionals are clearly recorded, and these records are made available to the family, the likelihood of confusion, uncertainty and error should be reduced.

Before starting chemotherapy all children must be assessed to ensure that they are fit enough to commence treatment. This will usually include full blood count, temperature, weight and general well-being. If the child is clinically unwell on nursing assessment, he should be referred to a doctor for a full medical assessment before proceeding with chemotherapy. Monitoring the child's full blood count is a routine test to determine both the degree of bone marrow suppression resulting from the effect of the cytotoxic drugs and to initiate supportive measures as required. The delay between courses of chemotherapy is determined by the specific treatment regime, but usually requires the neutrophil count to have reached $> 1 \times 10^9/l$ and the platelet count to be $> 100 \times 10^9/l$. However, not all drug administration is dependent on the blood count and therefore each treatment protocol should be considered individually. The majority of chemotherapy is prescribed on the body surface area (BSA). Measurement of BSA in children can be particularly difficult so the CCLG has evaluated a way of estimating BSA using weight only. The only exceptions are children who are obese (over the 98th percentile) or severely cachexic (under the 2nd percentile). An alternative formula is available for calculating the doses of chemotherapy in these children (Sharkey *et al.*, 2001; MRC, 2006). Careful monitoring of the child's body surface area must take place throughout the course of treatment as significant changes in height and particularly weight can occur and will alter the dose.

Preparation

Investigations and tests are carried out before the administration of specific drugs to establish a results baseline. The investigations are then repeated after administration of the cytotoxic drugs. Any short-term side effects as a result of the drugs can be monitored and, if necessary, modifications to the drug dosage or even the drugs being given can be made to the next block of treatment. Examples of these tests are: blood biochemistry (to detect electrolyte imbalance and abnormal liver function); audiology tests (to check for ototoxicity); glomerular filtration rate (GFR) and tubular re-absorption of phosphate (TRP) (to detect renal toxicity); and echocardiogram (to detect cardiotoxicity). It is vital that the results of recent tests are found to be satisfactory before any further chemotherapy is given (Table 3.1).

Table 3.1 Investigation results that should be checked before administration of specific drugs (non-haematological toxicities)

Drug	Side effects	Investigation
Busulphan	pulmonary fibrosis	pulmonary function test chest X-ray
Carboplatin	ototoxicity audiology nephrotoxicity	GFR
Cisplatin	ototoxicity audiology nephrotoxicity	GFR
Daunorubicin	cardiotoxicity	echocardiogram
Doxorubicin	cardiotoxicity	echocardiogram
Epirubicin	cardiotoxicity	echocardiogram
Ifosfamide	nephrotoxicity	GFR, TRP
Methotrexate	nephrotoxicity	GFR

It is important to give appropriate antiemetics before chemotherapy and to plan patient care accordingly. Adequate hydration of the patient is necessary to reduce the toxic side effects of some drugs. Pre- and post-hydration fluids are often an important requirement of the treatment regime and during administration, it is therefore important that an accurate fluid balance is recorded.

Routes of administration

Chemotherapy can be given by nearly all accepted drug routes. The most common routes used in the treatment of children are:

- oral
- intravenous
- intrathecal
- intramuscular and subcutaneous.

All drugs should be given in accordance with local operational policies and procedures. The basis of good practice in the administration of chemotherapy is safety and patient comfort. Nurses giving chemotherapy must therefore ensure that they are familiar with the treatment protocol and the needs of the child and family.

The oral route

If at all possible, oral cytotoxic drugs should not be handled, due to their possible absorption through the skin. A non-touch technique is advised and, immediately after dealing with them, the hands should be washed with soap and water. Unfortunately for younger children there are rarely any liquid oral preparations of cytotoxic drugs available due to very small national demand for them and their poor chemical stability. Crushing or breaking tablets disrupts the coating and extra safety measures should be taken. If it is necessary to crush tablets, this should ideally be carried out in a pharmacy department under controlled conditions. Drug preparation at ward level and at home is strongly discouraged, but if unavoidable should only be carried out with an enclosed tablet crusher (Edwards *et al.*, 2005). Alternatively, dispersible tablets can be dissolved in a syringe once the liquid is added. Capsules should be opened with extreme caution as the fine powder is easily lost into the atmosphere, posing risks of both inhalation and inaccurate dosing. For small doses, the original capsules should be divided in a pharmacy department to ensure correct dosing by drug weight. Wherever possible, doctors should prescribe a pattern of doses that avoids having to split capsules. It is essential that families are given appropriate information regarding the correct handling of oral chemotherapy at home.

With the help and advice of nurses and play therapists, even quite young children can be encouraged and taught to swallow small tablets or capsules whole. Children should be discouraged from 'crunching' tablets as particles remaining between the teeth can cause local stomatitis. It is important for the child to have a drink following an oral dose of cytotoxic drugs to remove any residual drug from the mouth and oesophagus.

In childhood acute lymphoblastic leukaemia complete remission is usually followed by relapse unless patients receive prolonged outpatient maintenance treatment based on oral chemotherapy. It is not enough to assume that just because a child has a life-threatening illness they will reliably take their medicines daily (Lilleyman & Lennard, 1996). Nurses need to be aware of this possibility and take action to support compliance with treatment. Good information and education will assist in helping to gain understanding of the importance of compliance with treatment regimes.

The intravenous route

It is common to use a central venous access device (CVAD) to reduce exposure to repeated cannulation and allow chemotherapy to be given safely in all settings. There are three commonly used CVADs:

- *Peripherally inserted central catheter (PICC)* – this is a semi-permanent catheter that is inserted via the ante-cubital veins in the arm, advanced to the central veins with the tip located in the lower third of the superior vena cava.
- *Skin tunnelled catheter (Hickman®)* – the catheter lies in a subcutaneous tunnel exiting midway from the anterior chest wall, the tip lies at the junction of the superior vena cava and the right atrium. This is the most frequently used long-term device.
- *Implantable port (Portacath®)* – this is a totally implanted vascular device which consists of a portal body attached to a silicone catheter, placed subcutaneously in the chest wall. It

requires accessing by a needle and may be left in situ for long periods of time.

(Dougherty, 2005)

It is now widely recognised that there is an increased risk of thrombotic events in children receiving treatment for acute lymphoblastic leukaemia. There have been reports of 5–36.5% of children receiving a thrombotic event during induction chemotherapy (Medical Research Council, 2006). Asparaginase and the presence of a CVAD are accepted as the main predisposing factors so the insertion of a CVAD is not recommended until the completion of induction therapy in this group of children.

When central venous access is not possible or a short course of treatment is prescribed, e.g. for Hodgkin's disease, peripheral access is used. Efforts should be made to reduce the trauma of repeated peripheral venepuncture. Children and teenagers may benefit from being coached in coping techniques, such as relaxation and guided imagery, counting games, story- or joke-telling or bubble blowing, which serves both as a distraction and slow breathing exercise. Computer games can prove very absorbing and children or teenagers can learn to distract themselves while playing with one hand. Remedial work with children who have established needle phobia may prove more challenging and may require the input of a psychologist trained in systematic desensitisation or hypnosis.

When peripheral administration of chemotherapy is necessary, it is important that an appropriate site is chosen. Sites to be avoided are: areas of poor venous circulation; sites previously exposed to radiation; the wrist; antecubital fossa; or bruised, sore areas. The cannula should be well taped in place and the limb splinted to prevent it being dislodged, but not so as to obscure the injection site in order to observe for signs of extravasation. The patency of the vein should be checked before, during and after administration of a cytotoxic drug by testing for backflow of blood. If, at any time, there is no blood return or resistance is felt when trying to give a drug, administration should cease immediately. If the child is to receive several cytotoxic drugs through the same peripheral site, the vesicant drugs and bolus injections must be given first. Care should be taken to dilute the drug adequately according to the manufacturer's recommendations in order to avoid high tissue concentrations and the method of administration should be carefully checked, i.e. infusion, bolus. Peripheral infusion of vesicant drugs should be undertaken with extreme caution and continuous supervision is recommended; for this reason overnight administration is not advisable if it can be avoided.

The vein should always be flushed well after the administration of a drug, choosing a compatible fluid. Great care needs to be taken when using intravenous infusion devices to administer cytotoxic drugs peripherally, particularly vesicants, and especially with children who are too young to verbalise their discomfort. It is essential that agreed pressure alarms are set on infusion pumps when administering any fluids but especially solutions of cytotoxic drugs. Children receiving treatment for cancer are often immunocompromised and are therefore at greater risk of developing infections. It is important therefore that all venous access sites are observed carefully while a cannula is in situ and after removal, as the skin integrity has been broken and this is a potential site for infection to develop.

As with any intravenous drug preparation, aseptic technique is essential at all stages. Luer-lock syringes and fittings should always be used to prevent the possibility of the needle and syringe disconnecting and accidental spillage occurring.

Where practical, infusion bags should be attached to the lines away from the child, in the drug preparation area, in order to minimise contamination in the event of a bag being punctured. However, this is not always possible if attaching a bag to an existing infusion line. If the infusion bag is taken to the child on a tray and the procedure performed in the tray, at a low level, safety can be maintained. Under no circumstances should it be necessary to attach an infusion bag to a line while it is hanging from the 'drip stand'; doing so poses an unnecessary risk to the nurse and the child if the bag is accidentally punctured.

Extravasation

Extravasation is an inadvertent infiltration or leakage of intravenous fluids from the vein into the perivascular or surrounding subcutaneous tissues (Holmes, 1997). A vesicant can cause local tissue destruction both within and outside the venous system. The mechanism of how the damage occurs is uncertain but it is thought that the vesicant binds irreversibly to the subcutaneous tissue resulting in pain, oedema, erythema and tissue necrosis. This may be delayed from 48 hours to several weeks following the extravasation event (Jones & Coe, 2004). Data suggests that 0.5–6% of peripherally administered vesicant drugs result in extravasation (Chordas, 2005; Dougherty, 2005). Dougherty (2005) suggests that the incidence is higher in children; this may be because very young children cannot communicate pain in the same way as older children. The primary aim must be to prevent extravasation. Only appropriately trained staff should administer cytotoxic drugs and they should be aware of which drugs are vesicants (Table 3.2).

Table 3.2 Vesicant and irritant drugs

Vesicants	Irritants	Non-vesicants
Amsacrine	Carboplatin	L-asparaginase
Carmustine	Cisplatin	Bleomycin
		Cyclophosphamide
Dacarbazine	Etoposide	Cytarabine
Dactinomycin	Methotrexate	Ifosfamide
Daunorubicin	Irinotecan	Melphalan
Doxorubicin	Topotecan	Thiotepa
Epirubicin		
Idarubicin		
Mitozantrone		
Vinblastine		
Vincristine		
Vindesine		
Vinorelbine		

Source: Pinkerton *et al.* (2004)

Close observation of the site throughout administration is essential. Should extravasation occur, the first signs are usually tenderness or a burning, stinging pain, with induration, swelling or leaking at the injection site, followed by erythema. Close observation for these signs and symptoms should take place. Extravasation is not always immediately visible and therefore the monitoring of an administration site several hours or even days later is important to detect any adverse reactions. If extravasation has occurred, skin ulceration, blistering and necrosis may follow, leading to further problems, such as significant scarring around tendons, nerves and joints with possible contractures and loss of limb function. Necrosis and tissue ulceration may occur a considerable time after extravasation has taken place and in severe cases a plastic surgeon should be contacted as soon as possible when signs of skin deterioration occur.

There are a certain number of conflicting recommendations about the management of extravasation but a definite policy needs to be drawn up locally so that action can be taken immediately. All personnel who administer cytotoxic drugs must be aware of the policy and where appropriate an extravasation kit must be available at the time of administration.

There are some general principles that should apply to the management of extravasation and further refinement may be made at local level:

- Stop infusion/injection immediately, leaving the cannula or needle in place.
- Aspirate as much of the drug back as possible and draw back blood from the suspected infiltration site.
- Remove the cannula or needle.
- Take action to reduce localised skin damage.

Written documentation of the event must follow with all clinical details noted. The description of the affected site should be noted and should include diameter of the erythematous area and its appearance.

Liposuction and saline flush-out are two techniques used to remove extravasated material while conserving the overlying skin. Gault (1993) found that analysis of the flush-out material confirmed that the extravasated material was actually removed. Most of this study group (86%) healed without any soft tissue loss at all. The early referral to a plastic surgeon and treatment of extravasation injuries are therefore recommended.

Intrathecal route

Leukaemia, lymphoma and other malignant cells have the ability to penetrate into the central nervous system (CNS) and circulate within the cerebral spinal fluid (CSF). This means that some children require cytotoxic drugs intrathecally via a lumbar puncture, either as prophylactic or therapeutic treatment, as many of the drugs given by other routes are unable to cross the blood–brain barrier in sufficient concentrations. Drugs for intrathecal use must be reconstituted with preservative-free diluent to avoid neurotoxicity.

Administration of vinca alkaloids such as vincristine by the spinal route, rather than intravenously, invariably causes death or severe neurological damage. A total of 23 incidents of inadvertent administration of intrathecal vincristine are known to have occurred in the world. Thirteen of these incidents are known to have occurred in the UK (Sims, 2005). Patient safety is a key part of the government's clinical governance programme, which began with the publication of *An Organisation with a Memory* (Department of Health, 2001a). As a result, the government set a target to reduce the number of patients dying or being paralysed by maladministration of spinal injections to zero. Two influential reports influenced this target, these were:

- *The Prevention of Intrathecal Medication Errors* (DoH, 2001b);
- *The External Inquiry into the Adverse Incident that occurred at Queen's Medical Centre, Nottingham, 4 January 2001* (DoH, 2001c).

These reports stated that national guidance should be issued so that there would be uniform practice across the country. This should cover every step in the process of administering intrathecal chemotherapy. A health service circular was issued in 2001 (HSC/2001/022) (DoH, 2001e) and subsequently updated in 2003 (HSC/2003/010) (DoH, 2003). The key requirements are as follows:

- a written local policy covering all aspects of the national guidance;
- a register of all trained and competent staff;
- formal induction for all new staff;
- annual review of competence;
- a designated intrathecal prescription chart;
- a designated area for the administration of intrathecal injections;
- intrathecal chemotherapy should usually only be administered in working hours;

- explicit and universal labelling of intravenous vinca alkaloids;
- designated storage areas for intrathecal chemotherapy.

Surprisingly the requirements do not include a statement saying that vinca alkaloids should not be administered on the same day as intrathecal medicines. However, protocols have been altered to ensure that this does not happen (Hollis, 2002; Medical Research Council, 2006).

In the UK, performing a lumbar puncture is usually a doctor's role. Accessing the central nervous system (CNS) must be conducted as a sterile procedure to minimise the risk of introducing infection. Before the cytotoxic drugs are injected, a few drops of cerebral spinal fluid (CSF) are taken and later tested for the presence of malignant cells and for infection. An Ommaya reservoir may be employed to administer intraventricular chemotherapy in order to facilitate prolonged CNS-directed therapy for recurrent, refractory or chronic CNS disease. These reservoirs function in much the same way as implantable venous access ports, with a resealable membrane placed under the scalp. This is attached to a catheter that passes through a hole in the skull and leads to the lateral ventricle of the brain. Although a surgical procedure is required to place the reservoir and catheter, many individuals have benefited from the relief these devices offer in avoiding the distressing effects of repeated lumbar punctures, particularly if access is very difficult due to spinal abnormality, or in children who develop a CSF leak from repeated puncturing of the meninges, or who experience severe headaches following the procedure.

Recent recommendations state that it is preferable for the child to lie flat for at least one hour after the intrathecal procedure; this allows for better ventricular distribution of the intrathecal chemotherapy (Medical Research Council, 2006). This can prove to be challenging in younger children and units with limited space. Children experience post-lumbar puncture headaches only rarely in comparison to adults, the incidence and severity increasing throughout adolescence. Teenagers and younger children who have previously experienced headaches are advised to lie flat for at least two hours following a lumbar puncture, although each individual will usually discover the 'optimum' duration of lying horizontally by trial and error. Adequate analgesia and a quiet environment with dimmed lights can reduce the pain experienced.

Most children find the experience of a lumbar puncture extremely distressing and in the UK it is common practice to administer a light general anaesthetic to help them through this procedure. Efforts are made to find the most effective, yet practical anaesthetic approach for each oncology unit. Entonox® by inhalation can be used for older children to bring about relief of pain during a lumbar puncture. This is self-administered 'on demand' and can be very effective if the child is taught correct use and given support and supervision throughout the procedure. Children can also benefit from distraction strategies, and relaxation techniques may help them to manage this procedure under local anaesthetic.

The intramuscular and subcutaneous routes

Vesicant drugs are never given by this route. If at all possible, drugs are administered via alternative routes. The major exception is preparations of L-asparaginase which carries a high risk of anaphylaxis when given intravenously. The current protocol for treatment of acute lymphoblastic leukaemia requires that all patients are given intramuscular injections of pegylated L-asparaginase (Medical Research Council, 2006). The Royal College of Paediatricians and Child Health issued a position statement on the administration of intramuscular injections in children (RCPCH, 2002). Although this was made with reference to the administration of vaccines, it sets out some useful standards. It is recommended that all injections are given into the anterolateral thigh, in infants, and the deltoid muscle in older children. The needle should be a minimum of 5/8 of an inch long and over 1 inch in children over 5 years. It is recommended that no more than 2mls of the drug is given in one site (Medical Research Council, 2006). Ethyl chloride spray or a local anaesthetic cream can be applied locally to the area to numb it, but it has been found that topical anaesthesia is not very effective as only the peripheral nerve endings are numbed, whereas the pain from the injection is usually from the fluid entering the subcutaneous layer of tissue. Many of the children receiving intramuscular injections will be thrombocytopenic and there is some debate surrounding whether a platelet transfusion is necessary to support the procedure. General opinion is that pressure on the injection site is usually sufficient (Medical Research Council, 2006).

References

Boddy AV (2004) 'Chapter 8 – Cancer chemotherapy and mechanisms of resistance' *in*: Pinkerton, R, Plowman PN & Pieters R (eds) *Paediatric Oncology* (3rd edn). London: Arnold, pp. 142–168

Boyer H & Whiles L (2004) 'Nurse led assessment of children receiving chemotherapy' *Paediatric Nursing* 16(5): 26–27

Chordas C (2005) 'Chapter 8 – Chemotherapy' *in*: Tomlinson D & Kline N (eds) *Pediatric Oncology Nursing*. Berlin: Springer, pp. 162–192

Control of Substances Hazardous to Health Regulations (2002) London: HSE

Department of Health (1989) *The Children Act*. London: DoH

Department of Health (2000) *The Cancer Plan*. London: DoH

Department of Health (2001a) *An Organisation with a Memory*. London: DoH

Department of Health (2001b) *The Prevention of Intrathecal Medication Errors*. London: DoH

Department of Health (2001c) *The External Inquiry into the Adverse Incident that Occurred at Queen's Medical Centre, Nottingham, 4th January 2001*. London: DoH

Department of Health (2001d) *HSC/2001/023 Good Practice in Consent: Achieving the NHS Plan Commitment to Patient-centred Consent Practice*. London: DoH

Department of Health (2001e) *HSC/2001/022 National Guidance on the Safe Administration of Intrathecal Chemotherapy*. London: DoH

Department of Health (2003) *HSC/2003/010 Updated National Guidance on the Safe Administration of Intrathecal Chemotherapy*. London: DoH

Department of Health (2004) *Manual of Cancer Service Standards*. London: DoH

Dougherty L (2005) 'Chapter 10 – Intravenous management' *in*: Brighton D & Wood M (eds) *Cancer Chemotherapy*, London: Elsevier, pp. 93–108

Edwards J, Devine T & Soanes L (2005) 'Chapter 35 – Chemotherapy in childhood cancer' *in*: Brighton D & Wood M (eds) *Cancer Chemotherapy*. London: Elsevier, pp. 247–272

Gault DT (1993) 'Extravasation injuries' *British Journal of Plastic Surgery 46*: 91–96

Health and Safety Executive (2003) *Safe Handling of Cytotoxic Drugs*. London: DoH

Health and Safety at Work Act (1994) London: The Stationery Office

Health and Safety at Work Regulations (1999) London: The Stationery Office

Hollis R (2002) 'Accidental intrathecal administration of chemotherapy agents' *Cancer Nursing Practice 1*(1): 8–9

Holmes S (1997) *Cancer Chemotherapy: A Guide for Practice*. London: UK Asset Books, Ltd

Jones L & Coe P (2004) 'Extravasation' *European Journal of Oncology Nursing 8*: 355–358

Legge S (2005) 'Chapter 12 – Protracted venous infusion of chemotherapy (ambulatory chemotherapy)' *in*: Brighton D & Wood M (eds) *Cancer Chemotherapy*. London: Elsevier

Lilleyman JS & Lennard L (1996) 'Non compliance with oral chemotherapy in childhood leukaemia' *British Medical Journal 313*: 1219–1220

Lomath A (2005) 'Chapter 4 – Quality assurance' *in*: Brighton D & Wood M (eds) *Cancer Chemotherapy* London: Elsevier, pp. 43–48

Medical Research Council Working Party on Leukaemia in Children (2006) *UK Acute Lymphoblastic Leukaemia (ALL) Trial, UKALL 2003* (updated 2004, 2005). London: MRC

National Health Service (2002) *Guidelines for the Safe Handling and Administration of Cytotoxic Chemotherapy* (2nd edn). Edinburgh: NHS, Scotland

Oncology Nursing Society (2004) *Safe Handling of Hazardous Drugs*. Pittsburgh: National Guideline Clearinghouse

Personal Protective Equipment at Work Regulations (1992) London: HSE

Pinkerton R, Plowman PN & Pieters R (eds) *Paediatric Oncology* (3rd edn). London: Arnold

Power LA (2004) *New Approaches to Safe Handling of Hazardous Drugs*. Pittsburgh, PA: Oncology Nursing Society

Royal College of Nursing (2005) *Competencies: An Integrated Competency Framework for Training Programmes in the Safe Administration of Chemotherapy to Children and Young People*. London: RCN

Royal College of Paediatrics and Child Health (2002) *Position Statement on Injection Technique*. London: RCPCH

Sharkey I, Boddy AV, Wallace H, Mycroft J, Hollis R & Picton S (2001) 'Body surface area estimation in children using weight alone' *British Journal of Cancer 85*: 23–28

Sims J (2005) 'Chapter 3 – Risk management' *in*: Brighton D & Wood M (eds) *Cancer Chemotherapy*. London: Elsevier, pp. 31–42

Singleton LC & Connor TH (1999) 'An evaluation of the permeability of chemotherapy gloves to three cancer chemotherapy drugs' *Oncology Nursing Forum* 22(9): 1491–1496

United Nations Commission on Human Rights (1989) *The Convention on the Rights of the Child*. Geneva: United Nations

4 Side Effects of Chemotherapy

Karen Selwood

Introduction

The effects of antineoplastic agents on normal cells are described as the side effects of therapy. It is the cells which have a rapid mitotic rate, such as bone marrow, gastrointestinal mucosa, gonads and hair follicles, that are most vulnerable to these side effects. In addition, some chemotherapy drugs may have a direct effect on organ(s) in the body and cause toxicity over time. In parallel with the widespread cellular/tissue damage that results in site-specific side effects, the child undergoing chemotherapy may also experience generalised effects, such as fatigue, anorexia, taste changes, nausea and vomiting, and pain. In order to ensure effective care of these children, nurses need to be knowledgeable about both the treatment and side effects; they should have skills in assessment, technical expertise and be able to support the child and family emotionally throughout the course of treatment. Symptom management and psychosocial support must be well integrated. Most side effects are responsive to nursing interventions which will ultimately have an effect on the comfort, safety and quality of life of the child. In addition, effective nursing intervention can reduce recovery times, prevent serious complications and reduce prolonged hospitalisation.

Nurses have an important part to play in the prevention, detection and management of side effects of chemotherapy. Assessment is the first step, preceding planning, intervention and evaluation in the process of providing individual nursing care; with the care plan reflecting the physiological and emotional aspects of care, within a multidisciplinary framework. Assessment consists of the collection of data from a number of different sources: observation, measurement, communication and records (Casey, 1995a). Analysis of these data can then be expressed as a problem, need or a nursing diagnosis, resulting in the identification of the responses of the child and the family concerning nursing care as well as their need for information, support and teaching (Casey, 1995b).

It is essential to involve the child and the family in all aspects of care. However, parents and other family members can only take on the role of active care-givers if they have been fully prepared and feel supported in this new and seemingly complex environment. Knowledge about treatment and side effects is necessary to ensure the active participation of family members in decision-making about treatment plans, for example, timing of drug administration or monitoring of the child's side effects. Information needs to be open and honest and may need to be repeated. Families undergoing

Cancer in Children and Young People   Edited by Faith Gibson and Louise Soanes
© 2008 John Wiley & Sons, Ltd

the stress of coping with a child with cancer often do not assimilate the facts on first hearing. Teaching and reinforcement need to be a continuous process using the child's treatment protocol and highlighting the anticipated side effects. Written information does not replace verbal communication as the family may have previous experiences, both positive and negative, that need to be discussed and taken into consideration. Ongoing support and education are crucial (Evans, 1993) to enable the family to make informed decisions about care of the child and their part in it (Casey, 1995b). Promoting a realistic view is the best option as this will foster trust in which a partnership between the parents and health-care professionals will develop (Chanock *et al.*, 2006).

The play specialist has an important role in facilitating the child's understanding of chemotherapy as well as assessing their coping and adaptive mechanisms. Play specialists make use of various types of play depending on the child's needs, age and understanding to provide information about hospitalisation and to teach new information (Webster, 2000); 'even very young children are able to understand the nature and implications of their disease and treatment' (Faulkner *et al.*, 1995, p. 4). For older children and teenagers there are many published books and resources available that can facilitate understanding, possibly building on projects undertaken at school. Approaches to preparation should be individualised, to encompass cognitive abilities that may not always reflect age. Cultural issues, past experiences, coping abilities and physiological status also need to be taken into consideration (Vessey & Mahon, 1990). Parents are directly involved with the play specialist in preparing their child for chemotherapy since they know the child's strengths and fears as well as patterns of communication better than anyone else (Lansdown & Goldman, 1988).

Siblings also benefit from open and honest information that is clear and age-appropriate. Involvement in the care of the sick child and an understanding of treatment may help to resolve the strain of separation and fantasies about the hospitalised child (von Essen & Enskär, 2003). Play specialists will have an important part to play, alongside 'sibling groups' (Simms *et al.*, 2002), in providing information and offering an opportunity for siblings to express their feelings and ask questions of people other than family members.

The side effects of chemotherapy can occur any time during and after treatment. Site-specific side effects will be discussed in detail and, where accompanied by general effects of chemotherapy, are highlighted. Overall, the discussion that follows aims to provide a description of practice, where possible, supported by evidence from a combination of clinical practice, research and other published literature.

Gastrointestinal tract

Mucositis

Mucositis is a general term that refers to an inflammation of the mucous membranes throughout the gastrointestinal tract and is further specified according to location (Keefe *et al.*, 2004). When occurring in the oral cavity, it is referred to as stomatitis, in the oesophagus as oesophagitis. Generalised mucositis of the intestinal tract is characterised by proctitis, diarrhoea and abdominal pain. In practice, however, the terms mucositis and stomatitis are often used interchangeably (Phillips, 2005).

Stomatitis

This occurs due to damage and destruction of epithelial cells usually 5–7 days post-administration of chemotherapy. Therapy affects the oral epithelial cells both directly and indirectly; directly by interfering with actual cell production, maturation and replacement; indirectly due to bone marrow depression, where neutropenia and thrombocytopenia increase risks from bleeding and infection. Figure 4.1 illustrates the pathophysiology of stomatitis.

The prevalence of patients experiencing oral problems ranges from 30–75 % depending on treatment type (Dodd *et al.*, 2000; Fulton *et al.*, 2002) although there is limited evidence relating to children. The agents considered to be the most stomatoxic are the antimitotic antibiotics and the antimetabolites, as well as some of the alkylating agents, particularly in higher doses (Brown

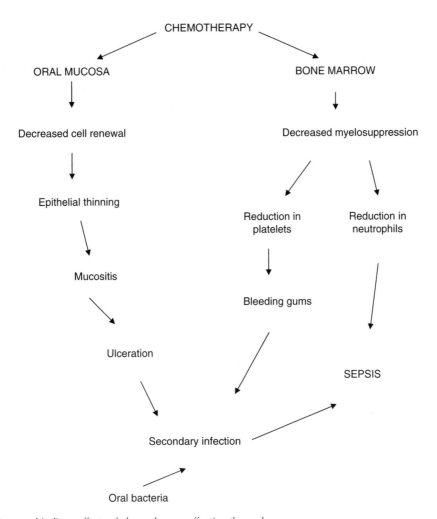

Figure 4.1   Direct and indirect effects of chemotherapy affecting the oral mucosa.

& Wingate, 2004). Their effects may be increased when used in combination.

- *Clinical features* – pain, swelling, xerostomia, inflammation, ulceration, desquamation of mucosa (gums and palate), dry and cracked lips, bleeding.
- *Management* – the principal objective of oral hygiene is to maintain the mouth in good condition, i.e. comfortable, clean, moist and free of infection and to minimise or prevent oral complications (Table 4.1).

The nurse has an important role in maintaining oral hygiene, either directly (by providing oral care) or indirectly (by providing advice

Table 4.1   Aims of oral hygiene

- Achieve and maintain a healthy and clean oral cavity
- Prevent the build-up of plaque on oral surfaces, thus helping to prevent dental caries
- Keep the oral mucosa moist
- Maintain mucosal integrity and promote healing
- Prevent infection
- Prevent broken or chapped lips
- Promote patient dignity, comfort and well-being
- Maintain oral function

Sources: Gibson & Nelson (2000), Glenny (2006).

and opportunities to provide self-care) (Torrance, 1990), or family care, thus contributing to the overall comfort of the child and subsequent improved quality of life. There is certainly no dispute that regular oral care is essential in reducing the detrimental effects of a compromised oral cavity; damage caused by cancer treatments cannot be avoided but oral care may prevent infections that cause further damage to the oral tissue. Many authors, however, suggest that oral care regimes are often based on tradition, anecdote and subjective evaluation (Thurgood 1994; Campbell *et al.*, 1995; Moore, 1995) citing limited published nurs-

ing research as the reason for this. However, it has also been suggested that even where there is research supporting practice, this may be ignored resulting in a theory–practice gap (Peate, 1993). Nurses must be accountable for the care they provide and, therefore, research on oral care must be utilised to inform their practice, as indiscriminate oral care not only causes physical problems but may also have psychological ramifications. Nurses have a pivotal role in deciding which form of mouth care to provide, including which tools

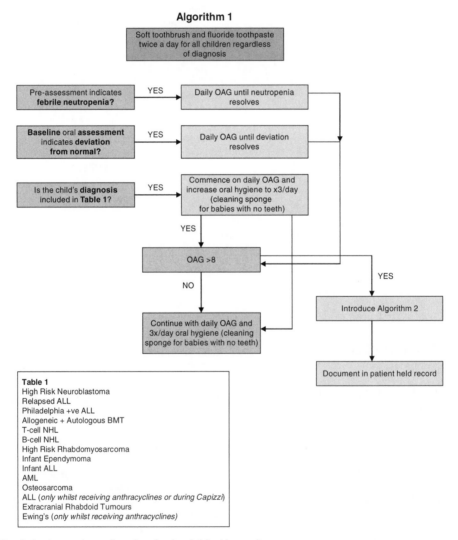

Figure 4.2   Prophylactic mouthcare flowchart for the child with a malignancy.
Source: Developed by the mouth care working party at Great Ormond Street Hospital for Children NHS Trust (October 2007). © Copyright GOSH.

Algorithm 2

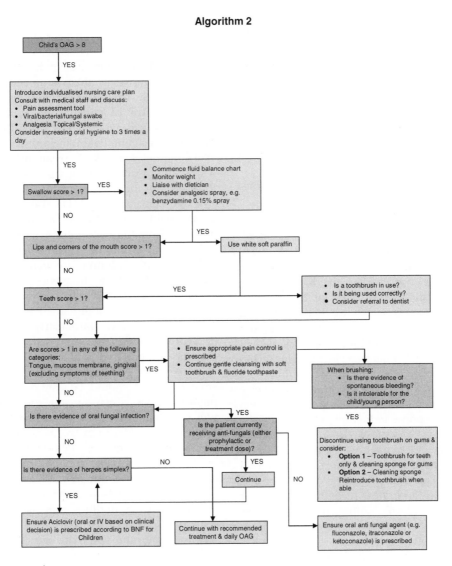

Figure 4.2   (Continued)

or solution to use and the frequency with which care is carried out (Krishnasamy, 1995). They therefore need knowledge and understanding in order to initiate appropriate oral care; care that is based on a sound scientific rationale. Decision-making may be facilitated by use of two algorithms that provide a step-by-step approach to the selection of appropriate oral care. One such framework has been introduced within a unit (Figure 4.2) and has the benefits of:

- ensuring that all children receive appropriate oral care;
- recommending practice that is based on current research;
- decreasing conflicting information and advice given to parents as well as other members of the health-care team;
- increasing confidence and competence of nursing staff in their decision-making process.

(Gibson & Nelson, 2000)

An accurate assessment is vital for effective oral care. Ideally the first assessment should be completed by a dentist but nurses may need to undertake this and liaise effectively with their dental colleagues. Prompt treatment of any dental disease may reduce oral infections (Collard & Hunter, 2001).

A thorough assessment is required to:

- provide baseline data of the teeth and gingival mucosa;
- predict, prevent or minimise oral complications;
- plan effective care;
- evaluate nursing interventions.

(Bryant, 2003)

The oral assessment tool of Eilers *et al.* (1988) has been successfully adapted (with the authors' permission) for use in the paediatric setting (Gibson & Nelson, 2000) The tool divides oral status into eight areas, which are then subdivided into three categories according to the presence or absence of symptoms (Table 4.2). Assessment represents the vital 'first step' in planning effective care (Campbell *et al.*, 1995); nursing intervention introduced to prevent, minimise or reverse changes in the oral cavity can then be individualised and the response to therapy monitored.

There is a great deal of conflicting information regarding which oral care regime is the most appropriate; although a recent evidence-based review of the literature pertaining to children has been undertaken and offers recommendations for practice (Glenny, 2006). Without clear guidance, nurses are uncertain as to which oral care regimes they should follow.

Kennedy and Diamond (1997) conclude that the toothbrush is most effective; a small-headed, soft, multi-tufted, nylon-bristled toothbrush is efficient at removing plaque and debris. Use of a toothbrush is recommended irrespective of platelet count, although in cases of severe stomatitis the child may not tolerate its use. In this situation, to minimise trauma, a foam stick may be introduced. Foam sticks are ineffective at removing plaque (Pearson, 1996) and therefore their use should be temporary: however, they may be the most appropriate tool to use with babies.

There is a general consensus that the use of fluoridated toothpaste is essential as it strengthens tooth enamel and decreases the risk of dental caries

(Glenny, 2006). There is less agreement about the use of a prophylactic antibacterial mouthwash. The benefits of their use, such as decreased plaque and mucosal inflammation, are not disputed (Galbraith *et al.*, 1991), however, there is no conclusion as to which mouthwash is the best one to use (Table 4.3).

Some groups of patients are at more risk of candidiasis and will benefit from the use of a preventative agent. Following a systematic review, Worthington *et al.* (2003) recommend the use of drugs fully absorbed (fluconazole, ketoconazole and itraconazole) and those partially absorbed (miconazole and clotrimoxazole). He also concludes there is little evidence to support the use of drugs not absorbed from the gastrointestinal tract.

There are, as yet, no research-based guidelines indicating the optimum frequency of oral care regimes and yet the frequency of intervention is likely to be the key to success (Beck, 1992). Normal oral care should involve cleaning teeth at least twice a day, particularly after meals and at bedtime. Frequency may alter according to oral assessment and will be increased if there is evidence of oral stomatitis. In cases of severe stomatitis care should be continued during the night, otherwise any progress made during the day will be negated. Moisturisers should be applied frequently in order to maintain comfort and lubricate the lips and mucosa. Petroleum jelly seems to be the most acceptable method of preventing dry and cracked lips (Campbell, 1987).

The choice of tools or agents used should reflect current research findings but also consider the individual needs of the child; there are occasions when an optimum oral hygiene regime may need to be sacrificed when balanced against the child's general comfort. Alterations in comfort from oral complications range from mild (from cracked lips) to severe (due to prolonged stomatitis) resulting in difficulties in eating and talking. It is important to assess the amount of pain the child is experiencing to ensure that adequate pain relief is given either topical or systemically. Oral hygiene becomes very painful and will only intensify the problem. Topical mouthwashes provide local relief but their action is short-lived and they can also desensitise the mouth.

Care needs to be taken with hot foods or drinks (Lever *et al.*, 1987). The use of anaesthetic mouthwashes in children under the age of 12 years is not

Table 4.2 Oral Assessment Guide for Children and Young People

Category	Method of assessment	1	2	3
Swallow	Ask the child to swallow or observe the swallowing process. Ask the parent if there are any notable changes.	Normal. Without difficulty	Difficulty in swallowing	Unable to swallow at all. Pooling, dribbling of secretions
Lips and corner of mouth	Observe appearance of tissue	Normal. Smooth, pink and moist	Dry, cracked or swollen	Ulcerated or bleeding
Tongue	Observe the appearance of the tongue using a pen-torch to illuminate the oral cavity	Normal. Firm without fissures (cracking or splitting) or prominent papilla. Pink and moist	Coated or loss of papillae with a shiny appearance with or without redness and/or oral *Candida*	Ulcerated, sloughing or cracked
Saliva	Observe consistency and quality of saliva	Normal. Thin and watery	Excess amount of saliva, drooling	Thick, ropy or absent
Mucous membrane	Observe the appearance of tissue using a pen-torch to illuminate the oral cavity	Normal. Pink and moist	Reddened or coated without ulceration and/or oral *Candida*	Ulceration and sloughing, with or without bleeding
Gingivae	Observe the appearance of tissue using a pen-torch to illuminate the oral cavity	Normal. Pink or coral with a stippled (dotted) surface. Gum margins tight and well defined, no swelling.	Oedematous with or without redness, smooth	Spontaneous bleeding
Teeth (If no teeth score 1)	Observe the appearance of teeth using a pen-torch to illuminate the oral cavity	Normal. Clean and no debris	Plaque or debris in localised areas	Plaque or debris generalised along gum line
Voice	Talk and listen to the child. Ask the parent if there are any notable changes	Normal tone and quality when talking or crying	Deeper or raspy	Difficult to talk, cry or not talking at all

NB if score >8 introduce pain assessment instrument
Source: Oral assessment guide Adapted from Eilers *et al.* (1988) by the Mouth Care Working Party at Great Ormond Street Hospital for Children NHS Trust (2005).
Copyright GOSH (2005)

Table 4.3 Recommendations for oral care

At diagnosis and during treatment	<ul><li>Brush teeth well twice a day using fluoride toothpaste and soft toothbrush.</li><li>While in-patient, oral assessment using OAG and score recorded. Frequency of assessment determined by individual need.</li><li>Use the oral assessment tool. If score >8, this means increased risk of oral complications.</li><li>Use of additional aids e.g. floss, fluoride tablets and electric toothbrushes – by recommendation of dental team only. Chlorhexidine is not recommended unless unable to brush teeth, clean mouth with oral sponges moistened with water or diluted chlorhexidine.</li></ul>

Source: Glenny (2006).

recommended without supervision as there is the potential for young children to swallow the mouthwash, resulting in problems with swallowing. Either oral analgesia or intravenous/subcutaneous opiates may be necessary and there should be a low threshold before commencing this pain management. The use of a pain assessment tool can help decide on the appropriate analgesia and its subsequent effectiveness. Good pain control will enable the child to perform adequate mouth care and hopefully maintain a good oral intake, all of which will assist in the healing process.

Most children are familiar with their parents helping them with oral care. However, parents may find having to cope with performing mouth care on their child an additional stress, particularly when the child may be experiencing pain or discomfort related to oral complications. Nursing staff can offer support and advice to children and parents at the beginning of treatment and reinforced at regular intervals. This should be both verbal and written. The child may be familiar with a toothbrush but not other oral care regimes that may need to be introduced while in hospital. Alongside the parents, the play specialist would be involved in preparing the child. Allowing the child to handle mouth care products, in a non-threatening environment, by practising on either a favourite toy, their parent or a nurse, may help to reduce anxiety and increase compliance: creativity and imagination taking central roles.

Preparation for teenagers is also important. They need information relating to the drugs in their protocol that may result in oral problems and when they are most likely to occur. Advice regarding the oral care regime is required with the teenager being given the responsibility to undertake this care independently, thus maintaining some control. Support and encouragement may be necessary to ensure compliance, particularly when pain and discomfort are discouraging factors.

The role of the nurse is to facilitate self-care and family-centred care, as well as educating, advising or referring children for more specialised dental assessment or treatment; maximising opportunities presented for health promotion.

Before discharge, parents need to be aware of their continued role in maintaining a normal hygiene regime for the child. Written information is useful and should identify further problems that may be experienced (e.g. oral thrush) and indicate the action needed to be taken. Most children will not need to continue the use of anti-bacterials or antifungals while at home, however, a written record of their regime is useful should they need to be admitted to their shared-care hospital.

Taste alteration

There are 10,000 taste buds situated on the tongue and oropharynx and these have a high cell turnover which can be damaged by chemotherapy. This, with the effect on salivary glands, results in taste alteration and possibly xerostomia (dry mouth). The effect varies in individuals depending on treatment received and is unique to the person experiencing the changes. This effect can also be influenced by antibiotic therapy, nausea and vomiting, oral stomatitis or infection. It can also be related to the disease process (Sherry, 2002). It can occur during chemotherapy administration, last a few hours, several days or even months (Rhodes et al., 1994). Offering a variety of sweets, e.g. mints during administration of certain drugs may help mask some symptoms.

- *Clinical features* – the child may complain of experiencing different tastes, these may be bitter or metallic, especially with vincristine, carmustine, dacarbazine, cisplatin or cyclophosphamide, or it may seem that everything tastes of cardboard, sawdust or may have no taste at all (Rhodes et al., 1994; Comeau et al., 2001). Some children develop an increased threshold for sweet foods; in contrast, some children develop a complete aversion to some foods and this may contribute to a loss of appetite and anorexia. Such aversions may also be a learned response, associating symptoms, disease and treatment (Mattes, 1994). Occasionally, the taste alteration may cause the child to feel nauseous and vomit, especially if it occurs when a particular drug is being administered.
- *Management* – the family should be made aware of this potential problem in order to help adjustment to what they may perceive as the child being fussy. The family should be encouraged to experiment with different foods, cooked in a variety of ways, in an attempt to tempt the child.

Serving foods warm will intensify the taste and the use of gravies or sauces will increase the moisture level thus facilitating swallowing if the child's mouth is dry. In addition, by establishing what foods the child likes/dislikes, diet can be planned to maintain adequate nutritional intake. However, the fact that such likes and dislikes may alter through the course of treatment will need to be highlighted. Children often develop a liking for very odd foods, often with strong tastes (for example, pickled onions, salt and vinegar crisps and spicy foods).

A dietician should be involved to offer support and advice to the family and nursing staff during this time as it is essential to maintain optimal nutrition. It is essential to stress that this will be a transient problem and should revert back to normal when the treatment is completed. Parents have reported that taste changes appear to be cyclical, depending on the treatment the child is receiving (Wall & Gabriel, 1983). Some parents may find this extremely frustrating, especially if the child changes his or her mind frequently about what food is wanted, and tempting the child to eat can be made even more of a problem. Maintaining oral care is essential to help offset the taste, keep the mouth clean from debris and maintain moisture level.

Nausea and vomiting

Chemotherapy-induced nausea and vomiting are considered to be among the most adverse of the side effects (De Boer-Dennert et al., 1997), causing much distress to the child and the family (Hockenberry-Eaton & Benner, 1990). Despite new developments in the use of pharmaceutical agents and evidence of a wider use of behavioural techniques aimed at controlling these distressing symptoms, nausea and vomiting remain significant problems for some children (Roila et al., 1998). Incidence and severity are related to the emetogenic potential of the drug. Although 'league tables' exist (Table 4.4), there are other variables, such as anxiety and stress, which may contribute to the child's overall experience. The potential to induce vomiting is a complex interaction between the chemotherapeutic agent given, the dosage, how it

Table 4.4 Emetic potential of common cytotoxic agents

Low	Moderate	High
bleomycin	amsacrine	cisplatin
busulphan	carboplatin	cyclophosphamide*
etoposide*	cytarabine*	dactinomycin
5-fluoroucil	daunorubicin	melphalan
methotrexate	doxorubicin	dacarbazine
mercaptopurine	mitozantrone	
thioguanine	ifosfamide*	
vincristine		

Note: *dose-related.
Source: Bender et al. (2002).

is administered and the child's response. It is well known that individuals vary considerably in their response to cytotoxic agents (Hogan, 1990) and that susceptibility in children varies (Ward, 1988), but what appears to be consistent is the degree to which these symptoms distress children (Tyc et al., 1997).

The physiology of nausea and vomiting has been well reviewed elsewhere (Andrews & Davis, 1993) and therefore only a summary will be provided here. Vomiting is believed to be controlled by the vomiting centre, which is localised in the lateral reticular formation of the medulla oblongata near the respiratory centre. The vomiting centre may be triggered by a number of pathways (Figure 4.3) including:

- via the chemoreceptor trigger zone (CTZ). This is situated in the area postrema in the floor of the fourth ventricle. This is a highly vascular area of the brain, emetic substances circulating in the blood or cerebrospinal fluid (CSF) stimulate the receptors of the CTZ which in turn stimulate the vomiting centre. Mechanisms of CTZ communications with the vomiting centre are not fully understood.
- via the afferent vagal and visceral nerves. These stimulate the vomiting centre in response to gastrointestinal irritation, distension or delayed gastric emptying.
- via the cerebral cortex and limbic system. These areas are stimulated by all the senses (particularly smell and taste), anxiety, pain and increased intracranial pressure. This stimulation is thought to have a direct effect on the vomiting centre and does not involve the CTZ.

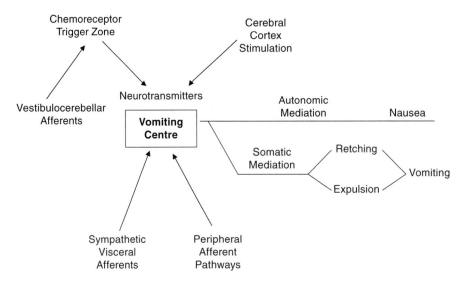

Figure 4.3   The physiology of nausea and vomiting.
Source: Yasko (1985).

This source of stimuli may be responsible for anticipatory nausea and vomiting.

- via the vestibulocerebellar afferents. These afferents are stimulated by rapidly changing body motions, with signals from the labyrinth of the inner ear. They are thought to play a minor role.
- via the sympathetic visceral pathway. Afferents from the gastro-intestinal tract, heart and kidneys may be stimulated as a result of inflammation, obstruction or distension.

The most likely explanation for chemotherapy-associated nausea and vomiting is that treatment causes a release of 5-HT (serotonin) from the enterochromaffin cells of the gut mucosa (Antonarakis & Hain, 2004). The 5-HT then activates vagal afferent nerve terminals to initiate vomiting and it may also enter the systemic circulation via the portal vein where hepatic afferent neurones can be activated (Hawthorn, 1995). However, it is likely that there is more than one process involving more than one transmitter (Dupuis & Nathan, 2003).

Anticipatory nausea and vomiting is more complex and is thought to result from stimulation received by the vomiting centre from the cerebral cortex and the limbic system (Yasko, 1985). It is described as a classic conditioned response during which previously neutral stimuli provide the thoughts, images or reminders that become the stimulus to recall the previous experience of chemotherapy administration (Montgomery et al., 1998), a process illustrated in Figure 4.4.

- *Clinical features* – nausea, retching and vomiting, frequently described in tandem. However, they are three separate problems that may occur in sequence, separately or in combination. The symptoms may lead to dehydration, metabolic abnormalities, poor nutritional intake with resulting weight loss and deterioration in the general condition of the child (Bender et al., 2002). A disruption of normal childhood activities may result. The child may also suffer from emotional and psychological stress associated with the vomiting which can lead to non-compliance and refusal of treatment, especially in teenagers (Pendergrass, 1998).
- *Management* – the goal is to minimise the direct effect of treatment and to facilitate the early recovery of the child; the distress of the symptom has far-reaching consequences not only for the child but for the parents, other family members, nursing and medical staff. It is suggested that if successful antiemetic therapy is achieved during the first course of chemotherapy, then nausea and vomiting may be avoided

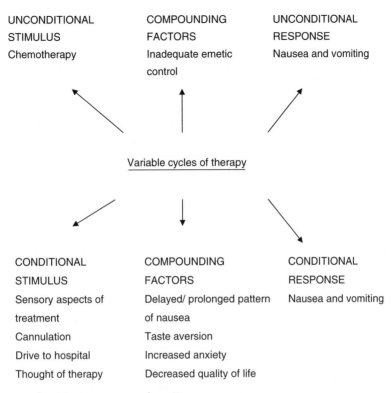

Figure 4.4   Development of anticipatory nausea and vomiting.
Source: Hogan (1990).

and, in practice, this appears to be the case (Tyc et al., 1997). At any age children can develop learned behaviours. A negative experience with the first course of chemotherapy may result in behaviour that is difficult to reverse (Dupuis et al., 1999). Children, especially teenagers, may develop anticipatory vomiting before or during the administration of chemotherapy if adequate control is not achieved (Dolgin et al., 1985). Non-pharmacological methods of controlling nausea may need to be explored with the family as these can assist in controlling emesis. The foundation for symptom control is an understanding of the various pharmacological and non-pharmacological interventions that are available (Keller, 1995). However, the effectiveness of interventions is rarely observed and documented methodically and this has resulted in a failure for ongoing management of these symptoms to inform 'best practice' within the variety of clinical situations. Added to this is the subjectiveness of the experience that often

complicates research studies and produces difficult situations in symptom management.

Nursing management commences with assessment and this will begin by identifying the child's previous experience of nausea or vomiting, highlighting actions that have been successful in the past. Parameters then to be considered in assessing symptoms are the frequency, duration and intensity and degree of distress experienced by the child (Bender et al., 2002). Assessment could significantly influence the choice of interventions and therefore enable the nurse to decrease the direct effects of treatment (Hockenberry-Eaton & Benner, 1990). It should be an ongoing process that begins with initial contact and continues throughout subsequent admissions (Bender et al., 2002). Overall, assessment should enable care to be planned and delivered more effectively as the nurse has information that relates to an individual child and his response to treatment. Various rating scales have been used in research studies (Rhodes & McDaniel,

1999; Rhodes *et al.*, 2000), however, their universal use in practice has yet to be seen, although studies have shown that children as young as five years of age can use a rating scale (Zeltzer *et al.*, 1988). In comparison, there is literature supporting the complex nature of the ability of children to self-report their symptoms, particularly in the younger age group (Abu-Saad, 1993; Gibson, 1994). Studies are needed that will result in a reliable and valid instrument to assess nausea and vomiting, qualitatively and quantitatively, as well as incorporating ease of use.

It is essential to include the child and the family when planning antiemetic intervention and with knowledge gained through teaching, the parents can be instrumental in instigating interventions and undertaking non-pharmacological approaches.

Pharmacological interventions

The administration of prophylactic antiemetics before, during and after chemotherapy should follow an antiemetic protocol or guidelines which indicate the emetic potential of the drugs with corresponding chemotherapeutic agents to be used, allowing for the individual needs of the child (Dupuis & Nathan, 2003; Schell, 2003). Strict attention to a protocol will ensure effective management as knowledge of the antiemetic potential of individual drugs will be utilised more fully. As nausea and vomiting can be a result of different stimuli, a combination of agents which are synergistic may be required to achieve control.

Antiemetics are used to block the pathway to the vomiting centre. The vomiting centre contains many muscarinic, cholinergic and histamine H_1-receptors; the CTZ is rich in dopamine receptors. The CTZ responds to chemical stimuli through the activation of dopamine or serotonin receptors. The majority of currently available antiemetics are dopamine receptor antagonists, even if they have other properties (Hawthorn, 1995). Recent studies have identified other agents, those capable of antagonising 5-hydroxytryptamine (5-HT serotonin), thought to be more important in controlling emesis. For classification of antiemetics, see Table 4.5.

It is a general rule that it is easier to prevent emesis from occurring rather than to control it once it has started (Hawthorn, 1995). Where the symptom is predicted, the child and the family should be informed and antiemetics given prophylactically; the timing of this will depend on the route of administration and the latency of the chemotherapeutic agent. For example, the onset and duration of emesis following cisplatin are 1–72 hours, compared to cyclophosphamide, which is 8–24 hours (Hawthorn, 1995). Antiemetics given the night before chemotherapy, particularly nabilone, may alleviate anticipatory symptoms.

It is inappropriate to prescribe antiemetics 'as required', nevertheless their successful administration will depend on the nurse caring for the child having appropriate knowledge. The antiemetic(s) prescribed will depend on:

- the emetic potential of all the chemotherapy agents to be given during the course of treatment;
- the child's previous response (if this is a subsequent course of treatment);
- the experience of the nurse gained previously in caring for children receiving particular chemotherapy regimes;
- knowledge of the action of the various antiemetics;
- the side effect profile (in some cases an antiemetic may be chosen for its sedative effect).

The route of administration will need to be decided. The intravenous route is often considered to be the most effective as it may be the only one available in a child who is vomiting. In some cases oral administration may be selected; oral ondansetron is as effective as the intravenous formulation (Cohen *et al.*, 1996). Some children like the choice but, with respect to cost, the oral route should be chosen.

Assessment of antiemetic intervention is essential to monitor effectiveness. In a child who continues to vomit, alternative antiemetics may be chosen or a 'cocktail' of agents may be effective. The pharmacist should be involved to provide advice and support; pharmacists may also be called upon in the search for information about current studies of new antiemetics or different approaches to antiemetics currently in use.

Table 4.5 Classification of antiemetics

Drugs	Site of action	Mode	Side effects
Substituted benzamides Metoclopromide	at low doses it antagonises dopamine receptors, but at high doses it is a 5-HT$_3$ receptor antagonist	IV Oral	sedation diarrhoea extrapyramidal reactions
5-HT$_3$ blockers Ondansetron Granisteron Tropisetron	binds to type 3 serotonin antagonist receptor 5-HT$_3$ in the gastrointestinal tract and central nervous system		headache dizziness constipation
Antihistamines Cyclizine Promethazine	antagonise the action of histamine at the H$_1$-receptor, poor as a single agent	IV Oral	sedation dizziness constipation
Corticosteroids Dexamethasone	unknown, may act by blocking prostaglandin	IV Oral	vomiting anal itching when given too quickly
Substituted butyrophenone Domperidone	antagonist of dopamine receptors, also acts at peripheral sites and does not readily cross the blood – brain barrier; has direct action on gastric motility	Oral Suppository	
Phenothiazines Chlorpromazine Prochloperazine Levomeprazine	dopamine receptor antagonist block in the CTZ	IV Oral	sedation dry mouth hypotension extrapyramidal reaction
Cannaboloids Nabilone	action unknown, relates to central nervous system depression, may also have as anti-opoid activity	Oral	drowsiness euphoria hypotension
Benzodiazepine Lorazepam Diazepam	may work by blocking cortical pathways to the vomiting centre, therefore may be useful in anticipatory vomiting	IV Oral	drowsiness amnesia

Source: Goodin & Cunningham (2002), Dupuis & Nathan (2003), Antonarakis & Hain (2004).

Extrapyramidal reactions

Antiemetics that work by blocking or antagonising dopamine receptors have the potential to cause extrapyramidal side effects. They result from excessive cholinergic activity in the extrapyramidal tract of the nervous system as a result of unintentional blockade of the post-synaptic dopamine receptors by the antiemetic drug, resulting in a disturbance of normal dopaminergic transmission causing an inability to coordinate voluntary movement, alterations in muscle tone and the occurrence of involuntary movements (Hawthorn, 1991). The child may experience varying effects: general restlessness and muscle tremor (irritable legs 'that want to keep walking'); limb dystonia (may resemble a seizure); opisthotonus (muscle spasm causing the back to be arched and the head retracted, with the muscles of the neck and back very rigid); or oculogyric crisis (rolling of the eyes together with laryngeal spasm that can result in respiratory distress). The effect is more common in children (Terrin et al., 1984), particularly in higher doses, with an increased risk related to metoclopramide (Graham-Pole et al., 1986).

This side effect can be managed by either concurrent administration of procyclidine or, following a reaction, the effect can be reversed with intravenous benztropine. However, the rate of incidence and the distressing nature of this side effect for the child and their parents have resulted in antiemetics that have extrapyramidal reactions in their side effect profile becoming unpopular in practice.

Non-pharmacological interventions

Alternative or complementary methods of controlling nausea and vomiting can be explored, to be used independently or in conjunction with antiemetics. Behavioural approaches include:

- hypnosis (Marchioro *et al.*, 2000);
- progressive muscle relaxation (Arakawa, 1997; Morrow & Roscoe, 1998);
- relaxation with guided imagery (Kwekkeboom *et al.*, 1998; Van Fleet, 2000);
- systemic desensitisation (Morrow & Roscoe, 1998).

Successful use of these techniques with children will be related to their involvement and their feelings of gaining control over a situation in which they may previously have felt helpless (Van Fleet, 2000). Non-pharmacological interventions may be more relevant for teenagers and be successful in managing anticipatory symptoms, and as a conditioned response, they may be more responsive to psychological intervention (Eckert, 2001).

In younger children simple techniques of distraction using storytelling may be useful, making the most of children's imagination and magical thinking. Providing different activities, such as play and education, can offer structure and focus the child on something other than the treatment. Also, acupressure wrist bands have shown some benefit in adults (Shin *et al.*, 2004) and children (Ming *et al.*, 2002). An understanding of complementary methods and an awareness of those members of the multidisciplinary team who can advise, assist or teach these skills (such as psychologists, play specialists and teachers) are essential.

Ongoing assessment is necessary in order to evaluate the various interventions and to anticipate further problems. Parents can be relied on to report their child's symptoms accurately (Gibson, 1994) and will take on the role of 'time keeper' by prompting the nurse caring for the child in advance of the antiemetic being due. The parents can also be involved in recording fluid intake and output, while also encouraging the child to continue with oral fluids and diet.

In the situation of the child who continues to vomit and is unable to tolerate oral intake, it may be necessary to introduce intravenous fluids to prevent dehydration and electrolyte imbalance. The dietician may also become involved to advise on maintaining adequate calorie and protein intake.

The overall distress caused by these symptoms can be minimised by adopting a sensitive approach; maintaining a constant supply of vomit bowls and providing privacy when children are vomiting. Oral care is essential, and rinsing the mouth should be encouraged after each episode of vomiting. This process will remove debris from the mouth as well as provide general comfort in terms of taste and oral freshness. The play specialist and ward teacher may need to be involved to provide gentle activities for those children not wanting to 'face the noise' of the playroom. The use of favourite tapes and the involvement of family members in reading stories may provide some distraction when the child may be feeling 'just awful'.

Before discharge after chemotherapy, some preparation is necessary, and antiemetics should be continued. If they need to be given intravenously the parents need to have been taught this skill and to feel confident to undertake this role. Written information should be provided to complement that given verbally (Price, 2003). Community nursing teams must be made aware of the child's planned discharge in order to provide support and care as necessary.

The family should also be aware of the potential problems from delayed or continued vomiting and should be given advice about fluid hydration and the reasons for re-admission. An understanding that it may also take time to re-establish a normal eating pattern after chemotherapy may provide reassurance for a family worrying that the child is still not eating. In addition, the family needs to be aware that a constant feeling of nausea or continuous vomiting is not normal and assistance should be sought if this is a problem.

Anorexia/weight loss

Anorexia is a loss of appetite which usually occurs as a result of the child's condition or treatment. Other factors that may contribute to this symptom are:

- nausea and vomiting;
- mucositis and/or stomatitis;
- altered taste;
- constipation;
- diarrhoea associated with typhlitis or other infections;

- pain;
- fatigue;
- metabolic disturbances.

In addition, an emotional response to being diagnosed and treated for a life-threatening illness may result in psychological factors that will need to be considered; depression can often be accompanied by a reluctance to eat. Children may be unable to differentiate between disease, treatment and side effects, thus contributing to their unwillingness to eat (Cunningham & Bell, 2000).

Nutritional status has a prognostic effect upon outcome (Andreyev *et al.*, 1998; Cunningham & Bell, 2000). Studies have indicated that adequate nutrition is essential, as children who are well nourished are better able to resist infection and tolerate treatment (den Broeder *et al.*, 2000). Weight loss can be a symptom of anorexia or present independently, related to infection, increased metabolism, eating problems or any one of the problems identified in relation to anorexia. Although several factors may play a part, the basic problem is often one of lack of intake of food.

- *Clinical features* – loss of appetite, lack of desire to eat, reduced calorie and protein intake, lack of energy, muscle wasting and low albumin, and weight loss.
- *Management* – assessment of anorexia is difficult as it involves the subjective experience of how the child is feeling and an objective measurement of food intake. A range of assessment techniques is available and includes physical examination, biochemical investigations, dietary history and dietary assessment (Nitenberg & Raynard, 2000; Brown, 2002).

Initial assessment is required to identify any underlying cause that may be exacerbating the anorexia or weight loss, as well as providing a baseline of the child's nutritional status, eating habits (that acknowledge cultural influences) and any problems perceived by the family. Ongoing assessment includes regular monitoring of weight in addition to recording intake and output. The frequency of weighing may vary but most centres record two or three times a week and thereby avoid weighing too often, as in the case of minimal weight gain the child may become despondent and more depressed, contributing further to the anorexia. Weight loss may be one of the few indications that the child is not receiving an adequate diet and therefore other methods of ensuring an adequate nutritional intake may need to be considered.

Children need good nutrition to maintain their normal growth and development. The goals of nutritional support are to maintain this need as well as to prevent nutritional depletion and to meet the needs of an increasing demand for nutrients during treatment (Bryant, 2003). When planning the management of symptoms consider the following:

- Identify children at risk.
- Undertake clinical assessment, including dietary history.
- Involve the multidisciplinary team.
- Introduce a nutritional care plan.
- Identify realistic goals.
- Involve the child and the family in all stages through ongoing education and participation in care.

The child should be encouraged to eat by being offered small, frequent meals of appetising foods. Identifying favourite foods and establishing a pattern of intake may be helpful. Well-balanced and nutritional meals should be offered but this may be difficult as children seem to crave certain foods, such as hamburgers and crisps, and at times this is all they will eat. Encouraging food and drinks that have lots of calories in them (not low sugar, low fat foods) and adding things like butter and cream to meals helps increase the calories. Encouraging the children in the ward to eat their meals together at a table fosters social interaction with others and provides some routine to the day. Allowing teenagers to eat later in the evenings may encourage food intake but this will rely on flexible kitchen arrangements. Some centres have cooking facilities in the ward area where the family can prepare meals for their child allowing them to have 'home-cooked food' within the ward environment. Some may also have their own chef or cook based on the wards who will provide individual nutritional meals for the child. If this is not possible, food can usually be brought in from home. It is important that mealtimes do not become a battle between the child and their parents. Some children may see this as a way of manipulating their parents or rebelling against their treatment and thus feel that they are maintaining control. Similarly, parents may feel that this is one area in which they can affect the outcome and also have some control (Panzarella & Duncan, 1993). Explanation is preferable to coercion. Children require time to express their feelings and may need help in making sense of their experiences.

Nursing staff will need to be prepared to assist and encourage children to eat, especially if it is becoming stressful for parents. Younger children may be encouraged to eat if they are able to feed themselves or 'pretend play' with food in the play room. Cooking can be encouraged as a school activity, if the child feels up to cooking, with the food being consumed following the activity. This gives some control back to the child, particularly in this area of their treatment.

Dieticians must be involved from the beginning of the child's hospitalisation at the time of prevention and not just intervention. They can offer support and advice, consult with the family regarding food selection, supplements and alternative means of nutritional support; oral steroids may be recommended to increase the child's appetite. Providing favourite foods and encouraging a child to eat can be an expensive process for some families who may require financial assistance.

Enteral or parenteral feeding is indicated when the child is unable to meet nutritional needs by mouth. Enteral feeding, via a nasogastric tube, can increase nutritional uptake if tolerated well and the gut is working adequately. It also preserves the integrity of the intestinal mucosa by keeping it functional (Nitenberg & Raynard, 2000). When considered alongside other interventions, nasogastric feeding may be dismissed as being psychologically traumatic for the child (Holden *et al.*, 1997), but it has been shown to be accepted by children and tolerated well, with nutritional benefits (den Broeder *et al.*, 2000). If nursing staff are negative about the use of enteral feeding, this attitude may be conveyed to the child and the family and result in poor compliance. Preparation for insertion of the tube is essential and will involve the skills of the nurse, parent and play specialist. Preparation time needs to be sufficient without increasing levels of anxiety. Adequate time needs to be allowed for parenteral feeding, providing time for the child

to express any worries and question the procedure. Equipment stored for this purpose can be used for the child to feel the tube and play with the syringes. Long-term access for enteral feeding may be needed for some children and this can be achieved by a gastrostomy usually placed while the child is anaesthetised. These have been shown to be effective in maintaining nutritional status and may be better accepted than a nasogastric tube (Matthew *et al.*, 1996).

Enteral products can be either complete meal replacements that will require digestion, or constitute elemental diets which require minimal or no enzymatic activity prior to absorption (Irwin, 1986). The dietician is responsible for calculating calorie requirements and for balancing fluid needs. The feed is introduced gradually and tolerance assessed daily. Feeding can be given via bolus feeds or overnight via a feeding pump. If given via a bolus, the child should be encouraged to eat a meal first and then receive the enteral feed as a 'top-up'. This allows mealtimes to be maintained and the child to attempt to eat normally. Overnight feeds allow the child to eat normally during the day while providing extra calories at night. If weight loss or anorexia continues to be a problem, then enteral feeding may be continued at home, following the parents' agreement and a comprehensive teaching programme.

Long-term use of enteral feeding in infants can lead to problems with sucking, eating and speech development (Johnson, 2001). Involvement of the speech therapist can help to alleviate these potential problems.

Enteral feeding is cheaper and less invasive than parenteral nutrition. However, the choice of feeding will be determined by other factors such as:

- nutritional requirements;
- degree of nutritional debilitation;
- disease process;
- timing in relation to treatment;
- a functioning gut;
- resources available.

(Rust *et al.*, 2000)

Total Parenteral Nutrition (TPN) may be indicated and be given via a central venous access device or very occasionally a peripheral line. A central venous access device is preferred as administration of high glucose concentrations is required for children to obtain sufficient calories (Han-Markey, 2000). In addition to glucose, TPN contains water, fats, carbohydrates, electrolytes, vitamins and minerals; in some cases the fat (lipid) component is given separately (Glynn, 2001). It is not without risks and these include fluid overload, metabolic, vascular and septic episodes in some patients (Glynn, 2001). Initially, daily monitoring of serum glucose is necessary and once stable, following a period of TPN administration, this may become less frequent. Lipids may affect liver function and this must be checked regularly. Nursing observation will include recording intake and output, daily urine testing for glucose and regular recording of weight.

Parenteral feeding is an expensive therapy to use and ideally must be managed by a nutrition team (Fawcett, 1995). Other methods, such as enteral feeding, may need to be considered before it is implemented, especially if the gut is functioning. Several days are needed to build up to full-strength parenteral nutrition for the child to obtain maximum calories from it, and for the metabolic adaptation of infused nutrients (Glynn, 2001). Infusion pumps are used to ensure a constant rate is delivered. Once established, TPN is infused over varying time periods with the ultimate aim of allowing the child some freedom from the restraining infusion lines. During the administration of parenteral nutrition the child should continue to be offered oral fluid and food to allow oral stimulation. The involvement of a psychologist may be beneficial in offering advice on ways to encourage the child to eat.

In summary, when planning interventions the following should be considered:

- Identify the child's favourite foods.
- Offer small, frequent meals.
- Encourage dietary supplements.
- Maintain assessment and involvement of the dietician.
- Manage the side effects of chemotherapy (e.g. nausea and vomiting) effectively.
- Consider enteral feeding early.
- Introduce TPN where appropriate.

Some children are very reluctant to eat while they are in hospital as they associate the ward environment with unpleasant treatments and experiences. Before discharge, the family can be reassured that eating will probably resume once the child is back at home. As part of a planned discharge, paediatric community teams need to be informed in advance of the child's discharge so that follow-up care can be arranged. Visits can be planned to provide ongoing support and encouragement to the child and the parents.

Cachexia

This is a syndrome of progressive wasting associated with anorexia and metabolic alterations (Capra *et al.*, 2001). It appears to progress with the disease and may result in profound loss in body weight and muscle tissue and a decrease in both functional status and quality of life (Grant & Rivera, 1995). It is thought to result from an imbalance between the energy needed by the body versus the energy available due to reduced intake alongside biochemical alterations (Nitenberg & Raynard, 2000).

Lindsey (1986) suggests that children who are at critical growth periods and receiving aggressive anticancer therapies are even more vulnerable to developing cachexia. Its cause is unknown, but there are several hypotheses:

- reduced oral intake and anorexia resulting from the malignancy or treatment (Picton, 1998; Nitenberg & Raynard, 2000);
- impaired digestion and absorption (Nitenberg & Raynard, 2000);
- increased energy expenditure despite a decreased calorie intake, leading to progressive wasting (Tisdale, 1997);
- alterations in carbohydrate metabolism, including decreased glucose tolerance and normal or increased fasting blood glucose. Glucose uptake by the tumour is increased and varies with the size of the tumour (Tisdale, 1997);
- tumour–host competition for nutrients, with the aggressive tumour winning over the host (Bozzetti *et al.*, 1999);
- abnormal lipid metabolism with depletion of fat reserves (Keller, 1993).

Cachexia cannot be explained as a result of starvation alone, but as part of a much more complex metabolic disorder (Theologides, 1979), with the tumour itself clearly inducing profound nutritional problems (Ward, 2001). Children most at risk are those who are nutritionally compromised at diagnosis; those who have a large tumour burden, particularly of the abdomen; or those requiring intensive chemotherapy (Foley *et al.*, 1993).

- *Clinical features* – weight loss, anorexia, early satiety, weakness, muscle atrophy, fatigue, impaired immune function, anaemia, decreased motor and mental skills, decreased attention and concentration abilities, muscle wasting and loss of body fat. It eventually leads to asthenia and emaciation (Lindsey, 1986).
- *Management* – this begins with an assessment which will highlight any contributory factors that may have a role to play, for example, taste changes, anorexia, psychological or emotional responses. It also includes a diet and weight loss history and this information will influence the planning of individual interventions. Nutritional support is required to meet the minimal calorie and protein requirements. The child's appetite needs to be increased and weight gain established. However, reversal of the effects depends largely on eradication of the cancer and prevention of the common side effects of treatment that have a debilitating effect. In some cases, despite increased calorie intake, the child may still fail to gain weight.

Nutritional support can be given orally, intravenously, or enterally; methods used alone as well as in combination. Aggressive use of total parenteral nutrition may be advocated allowing the body to cope with the chemotherapy (Wesdrop *et al.*, 1983). The issue of altered body image also needs to be addressed as this may also have implications for the child who is unable to eat (Sutton, 1988).

Diarrhoea

Diarrhoea is defined as an abnormal increase in stool liquidity caused by an impairment of absorption, secretion and rapid movement of faecal matter through the intestine (Hogan, 1998). The mucosal epithelial cells (villi and microvilli) lining the intestines are characterised by rapid cell division and if they are not replaced, the mucosal cells atrophy and become inflamed. The villi and microvilli shorten and become eroded and the inflamed mucosa produces large amounts of mucus which stimulates accelerated peristalsis. Malabsorption is also common. This is due not only to the diarrhoea but also to the direct effect on the absorptive surface of the intestinal lining. The villi and microvilli are responsible for both digestion and absorption of food; when damaged, absorption of nutrients, water and electrolytes does not occur (Barton Burke *et al.*, 1991), thus compromising nutritional status.

The cause of diarrhoea may be multifactorial, related to anxiety, a change in diet, use of nutritional supplements, medication (frequent antibiotics), infection, site of tumour and chemotherapy (particularly cisplatinum, cytarabine and irontecan) (Hogan, 1998; Cope, 2001). It can be very distressing and debilitating to the child, and cause them embarrassment, weight loss and potential electrolyte imbalance.

- *Clinical features* – frequent loose stools (which can be mucousy, bloody and on occasions contain sections of bowel mucosa), abdominal cramps, pain, flatus and rectal excoriation. This may lead to dehydration, fatigue, electrolyte imbalance, weight loss and malnutrition, and can also result in typhlitis.
- *Management* – an assessment of the child's normal bowel habits is vital so that the 'abnormal' can be recognised promptly. Accurate records of intake and output are maintained, noting number, amount, consistency and colour of stools. An increase in stools alone may not be a true indicator, it is more important to note an alteration to the child's normal habit. Identifying the cause can be difficult due to the range of possible contributory factors. A review of current drugs and the child's dietary history should be considered. Specimens should be sent to the laboratory for investigations virology, microscopy, culture and sensitivity and any infection treated.

Pseudomembranous colitis is a rare complication of antibiotic treatment which is characterised by proliferation of the bacterium, *Clostridium difficile*, in the colon, leading to diarrhoea (Andrejak *et al.*, 1996). Antibiotics (vancomycin and metronidazole) are used for the treatment of this specific problem (Thielman & Guerrant, 2004). Cryptosporidium can also cause diarrhoea in the immunocompromised child. This can be transmitted from person to person through ingestion of contaminated water or food (Juranek, 1995). This can be treated with the administration of spiramycin. Antidiarrhoeals are not recommended when an infection is present as the toxins would fail to be excreted although they may be of benefit especially if the diarrhoea is related to chemotherapy. Loperamide (an opioid) decreases intestinal motility and may be of benefit (Stern & Ippoliti, 2003). Administration of an antispasmodic agent, such as hyoscine-N-butyl bromide (Buscopan), may help to relieve the pain resulting from abdominal cramps.

Fluid balance charts should be maintained, weight recorded (frequency will depend on the severity of clinical symptoms) and observations made for signs of dehydration and electrolyte imbalance which should be treated promptly with intravenous fluids and electrolytes as needed. Early and effective interventions are necessary and short-term use of parenteral feeding may be required. Diarrhoea can also lead to the breakdown of skin and thus may increase the risk of opportunistic infections. Good general hygiene should be reinforced, teaching strict handwashing technique (Gould, 1995) when handling stools, as well as ensuring that the rectal area is kept clean and dry and applying barrier creams as required to help prevent excoriation. Daily examination of the area enables observation to see there are no signs of local infection, tissue breakdown or anal fissures. Infection in this area can occur easily in the immunocompromised child and can be the cause of much pain and distress. Pain can be relieved with the use of topical anaesthetic gels (lignocaine) alongside any systemic analgesics that may be required.

The importance of reporting episodes of diarrhoea must be stressed to the child and the family to ensure prompt treatment. The parents can be involved in keeping accurate records of intake and output; weighing nappies and disposing of bedpans. The child and the family need to be encouraged to discuss any problems with nursing staff without feeling embarrassed. For the child, unpredictable bouts of diarrhoea may result in a feeling of loss of control and they may choose to withdraw from social activities with other children (Aitken, 1992).

Diarrhoea can interfere with the activities and general lifestyle of the child and family, requiring support and understanding (Hogan, 1998).

Constipation

Constipation is defined as a decrease in the frequency of the passage of hard stool caused by either a complete or incomplete action of the bowels. There is a tendency for dry stools to accumulate in the descending colon where fluid absorption continues, thus dehydrating the stool even further (Cope, 2001). Considerable discomfort may be experienced from straining and may result in anal tears which may become infected, leading to abscess formation.

Constipation divides into three categories: primary, resulting from external factors, such as a lack of exercise, poor diet lacking in fibre and the failure to allow sufficient time for defecation (with children in hospital a lack of privacy resulting in embarrassment can also be a cause); secondary, resulting from pathological changes, such as spinal cord compression, intestinal obstruction or electrolyte imbalance; or iatrogenic, following administration of medications, such as opioids, vinca alkaloids (as a result of autonomic neuropathy) and antiemetics such as ondansetron (Smith, 2001).

- *Clinical features* – passage of irregular, infrequent hard stools usually accompanied by pain and discomfort. There may be nausea, abdominal distension with decreased bowel sounds and a decreased appetite.
- *Management* – prevention is the best management of constipation. Educating the child and the family on the causes and prevention is vital. Dietary advice regarding a nutritional well-balanced diet with plenty of fibre and fluids should be stressed but may not always be possible with a child who is unable to eat. Exercise should be encouraged as this appears to stimulate the bowel and may be beneficial in helping prevent constipation although this can be difficult if the child is debilitated. Ensuring that the child has privacy even from his or her parents when using the toilet or bedpan may help them to maintain normal bowel habits. It is important to acknowledge the child's embarrassment and be sensitive to individual needs.

Assessment of normal bowel habits is vital, as is the identification of any of the risks that may predispose the child to constipation. Ideally an assessment tool would be of benefit, however, there is not a validated tool available in paediatric oncology at the moment. The family needs to be encouraged to report any signs of constipation, such as irregular bowel actions, abdominal pain or a decreased appetite so that early interventions can be commenced if needed. Children and especially teenagers need to understand the importance of discussing their bowel habits and informing parents or nursing staff when they are experiencing difficulties. Some teenagers may find this difficult, although they may have developed a good relationship with one member of staff and may be encouraged to confide in them.

Accurate records need to be kept of the number and consistency of stools as well as dietary intake. Observation would include inspection of the anal area as well as noting any complaints of abdominal pain and difficulties with bowel movements.

If necessary, stool softeners/laxatives should be administered and their effectiveness monitored. These should be given prophylactically with the administration of opioids or vinca alkaloids (sometimes it is necessary to use both softeners and stimulants depending on the cause and the severity of the problem). Ongoing assessment is required in order to regulate symptoms and avoid diarrhoea. Very occasionally, suppositories or enemas are required but these should be used with great care in the neutropenic child as there is a risk of trauma to the anal area resulting in anal fissures, infection and bleeding which can be a particular problem in the child who is thrombocytopenic. Some units do not use suppositories or enemas for this reason.

Trauma caused by the child straining to pass a constipated stool can be relieved with topical anaesthetic (lignocaine) applied to the rectal area.

Typhlitis

This is a necrotising colitis which is usually localised in the caecum and commonly occurs in association with prolonged neutropenia and broad-spectrum antimicrobial therapy. Bacterial invasion of the mucosa of the bowel may progress from inflammation to full thickness infarction and perforation. It occurs most frequently from *Clostridium septicum* and Gram-negative organisms, especially *Pseudomonas aeruginosa* (Gorbach, 1998; Gorschluter *et al.*, 2001) (Figure 4.5).

- *Clinical features* – pain, usually in the right lower quadrant that can be 'colicky' or constant, pyrexia, neutropenia, ascites, altered bowel habits, nausea and vomiting. Shock can occur.
- *Management* – symptoms are identified through close observation and an understanding of this complication and the associated risk factors. Imaging of the abdomen particularly ultrasound or CT scan which shows thickening of the bowel wall has been of benefit to establish appropriate diagnosis (Schlatter *et al.*, 2002). The extent of thickening is also thought to relate to the prognosis of the patient (Cartoni *et al.*, 2001).

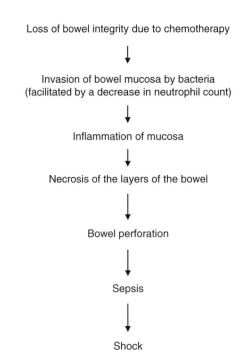

Figure 4.5 Pathological process of typhlitis.

Initial management is usually medical and consists of the following:

- nil by mouth;
- nasogastric tube;
- broad-spectrum antibiotics;
- intravenous fluids and electrolytes if required;
- pain relief.

Surgical resection of the necrotic bowel may be indicated if there is persistent gastrointestinal bleeding, perforation or deterioration in the child's overall condition (Jain *et al.*, 2000; Schlatter *et al.*, 2002). In the past, there has been some discrepancy concerning the role of granulocyte colony stimulating factors (G-CSF) in the treatment of typhlitis. Vlasveld *et al.* (1990) hypothesised that G-CSF may augment typhlitis by stimulating cytokines and thus potentially bacterial toxins, making the situation worse. However, in more recent literature, G-CSF has successfully been used to hasten neutrophil recovery with antibiotics in children with typhlitis (Gomez *et al.*, 1998; Picardi *et al.*, 1999; Sayfan *et al.*, 1999; Schlatter *et al.*, 2002).

Typhlitis can be a major complication of chemotherapy and it can have considerable mortality but this can vary from less than 20 % to as high as 45 % (Gomez *et al.*, 1998; Jain *et al.*, 2000; Cartoni *et al.*, 2001). Nursing care needs to be supportive, to monitor changes in the child and their response to the treatment; and to work closely with medical colleagues in giving optimum care to the child. The family will be under considerable stress in coping with the child's malignancy as well as a serious complication and will need support and information to help them to deal with this. Awareness of the needs of the child is vital. Both the child and the family will need frequent explanations and to be involved in care as appropriate, to enable them to cope with this illness and its complications (Kinrade, 1988; King, 2002).

Haematological problems

Chemotherapy destroys or damages the stem cells in the bone marrow. This results in neutropenia, thrombocytopenia and anaemia (see Table 4.6 for normal blood cell values in infancy and childhood). The point at which this occurs following chemotherapy depends on the lifespan of the circulating cells.

Anaemia

Anaemia is a reduction in the concentration of haemoglobin due to the number of circulating red cells (Montague, 2005). The lifespan of red blood cells is 120 days.

- *Clinical features* – pallor, fatigue, dizziness, dyspnoea, headache, sweating, irritability, tachycardia, tachypnoea or anorexia. Some younger children are able to adapt with minimal symptoms but if they feel cold or are reluctant to eat, this may be a sign of anaemia. It can also impact on the child's quality of life limiting the activities they can participate in. Adolescents, specifically, can experience potentially debilitating symptoms such as fatigue, dyspnoea and weakness with the resulting decrease in activity impacting quality of life.
- *Management* – transfusion of red blood cells is a supportive intervention which may be used when the child's haemoglobin falls below 7 g/dl, or if they are symptomatic.

If blood transfusions are carried out electively, it makes it easier for the transfusion service to provide specific requirements and avoids the need for 'emergency bloods'. Cross-matching of blood is important to help to prevent reactions. Many units transfuse cytomegalovirus (CMV) negative blood products to prevent CMV infection in the immunocompromised child although all blood is now leucodepleted at source, which will also help reduce the transmission of CMV. Occasionally, children are found to be CMV positive, in which case it is not required. Leucodepletion is also thought to reduce the potential risk of Creutzfeldt-Jakob disease (vCJD).

Packed cells are normally used for children. This allows the required concentration of red cells to be given in smaller volumes which may help prevent circulatory overload. The child should be monitored closely during transfusions for allergic reactions.

Febrile reactions

In the case of non-haemolytic febrile transfusion reactions (NHFTR), antibodies in the child's

Table 4.6 Normal blood count values in childhood

Age	Hb (g/dl)	WBC ($\times 10/l$)	Neutrophils ($\times 10/l$)	Lymphocytes ($\times 10/l$)	Monocytes ($\times 10/l$)
Birth	14.9–23.7	10–26	2.7–14.4	2.0–7.3	1–1.9
2 weeks	13.4–19.8	6–21	1.8–5.4	2.8–7.3	0.1–1.7
2 months	9.4–13.0	6–18	1.2–7.5	3–13.5	0.1–1.7
6 months	11.1–14.1	6–17.5	1.0–8.5	4–13.5	0.2–1.2
1 year	11.3–14.1	6–17.5	1.5–8.5	4–10.5	0.2–1.2
2–6 years	11.5–13.5	5–17	1.5–8.5	1.5–9.5	0.2–1.2
6–12 years	11.5–15.5	4.5–14.5	1.5–8.0	1.5–7	0.2–1.0
12–18 years	12.0–16.0	4.5–13	1.8–8.0	1.2–6.5	0.2–0.8

Source: Adapted from Hinchliffe (1992).

plasma react against transfused leukocytes in the blood and this tends to occur after multiple transfusions (Higgins, 2000).

- *Clinical features* – shivering (usually 30–60 minutes after the transfusion is commenced), tachycardia, fever.
- *Management* – the transfusion should be slowed or stopped and paracetamol given. The child's condition should be monitored and the child should be kept warm.
- *Prevention* – administering paracetamol before the transfusion may help alleviate this reaction. As blood is also leukocyte depleted, this should help prevent NHFTR (Gibson *et al.*, 2004).

Allergic reactions

In this case, the child has antibodies which react with proteins in the transfused blood components (Higgins, 2000).

- *Clinical features* – urticaria and itching within minutes of transfusion.
- *Management* – transfusions should be slowed and chlorpheniramine given. If no further symptoms, the transfusion should be continued. If repeated reactions, chlorpheniramine should be given 30 minutes before the transfusion and the child should be watched very carefully. Children receiving treatment for cancer are often on regular steroid treatment. It is therefore best to avoid giving steroids at other times as much as possible. It seems that a simple antipyretic is now thought to be as effective as

hydrocortisone and, in some cases, chlorpheniramine (McClelland, 1996).

For the management of anaphylaxis, see Chapter 5.

In cases of severe anaemia, blood may need to be administered over a longer time span than usual so as not to compromise the cardiovascular system. It is important to remember, however, that blood can stay out of the fridge for a maximum of four hours.

Some children and families find the concept of blood transfusion difficult. They may be aware of the potential risks associated with blood-borne diseases, such as HIV, hepatitis B and vCJD and the impact on their child. Reassurance about testing and about how the blood is prepared is therefore vital. In some cases families prefer the bag to be covered while blood is infusing as it seems to give them more confidence, especially if they do not like the sight of blood.

Erythropoesis-stimulating factors may also be used. Erythropoietin (EPO) is an endogenous growth factor that controls the body's response to anaemia by regulating the proliferation, maturation and differentiation of red blood cells (Spivak, 1994). Recombinant human EPO is now available and it has been shown to be a safe and effective treatment for anaemia in paediatrics, however, the evidence is limited and more clinical trials are needed (Porter *et al.*, 1996; León *et al.*, 1998; Feusner & Hastings, 2002). It is also perceived as expensive, however, blood shortages often occur and donors are decreasing so other forms of correcting anaemia will need to be considered in the future. The use of EPO may also help in families who are Jehovah's Witnesses. At the moment the child usually becomes a ward of court to allow life-saving measures to be taken if necessary such as blood product transfusion. The use of EPO to correct or prevent anaemia may alleviate the need for blood transfusions and the controversy this may bring (Estrin *et al.*, 1997).

Thrombocytopenia

After chemotherapy, the number of circulating platelets falls with the associated risk of bleeding. Platelets have a short lifespan, lasting between 8 and 11 days (Lowis *et al.*, 2004).

- *Clinical features* – petechiae, purpura, bruising, bleeding (especially from the nose and gums) and menorrhagia.
- *Management* – the prevention of bleeding is important and the child and the family should be taught how to observe for signs of low platelets in which case they might need to have their blood count checked. Prevention of trauma to susceptible areas is helpful, for example, the use of a soft toothbrush or foam sticks for mouth care will help lessen trauma to the gums. It may be necessary to discourage children from activities such as roller blading until their platelet count recovers. The use of progesterone may be recommended in young women with menorrhagia to suppress menstrual bleeding.

Transfusion of platelets may be necessary to sustain the child until his own platelet production recovers, but this will depend on local policy. Some units will only transfuse platelets if the child is symptomatic or about to undergo an invasive procedure but, in general, in the absence of bleeding, platelets are given if the blood count is less than $10' 10^9/l$. In some cases, because transfused platelets have a short lifespan, they are given routinely before a procedure, e.g. a lumbar puncture to ensure that there is an adequate number of platelets circulating.

If the child receives platelets and has a fever, infection, hepatosplenomegaly, antiplatelet antibodies or alloimmunisation, their effectiveness may be decreased (British Committee for Standards in Haematology, 2003). As with blood transfusions,

there is the potential for reactions and this increases the more transfusions the child receives. The symptoms of a platelet reaction are the same as for a blood transfusion (see under 'Anaemia'). Anaphylactic shock may also occur (see Chapter 5).

To minimise damage, platelets should be filtered and administered 'free-flowing', unless a peristaltic infusion pump is used. There has been some controversy about the use of infusion pumps and a study carried out by Norville *et al.* (1994) found that a peristaltic pump is acceptable because it does not negatively affect platelet recovery. This is a useful study as it is clearly safer and more accurate to use a pump.

Neutropenia

Neutropenia remains a major cause of morbidity in children with cancer (Hann *et al.*, 1997). The cytotoxic effect of chemotherapy increases the child's vulnerability to infection because there is a reduction in circulating white cells. This impairment to the host's defences results in an increase both in the incidence and in the severity of infection (Reigle & Dienger, 2003).

It is important that the child and the family understand how to minimise infection and know the signs to look for. Parents should be advised to check the child's temperature at regular intervals and to telephone the hospital if he is febrile. Individual centres have different guidance but usually this is one temperature above 38.5°C or two temperatures of 38°C on two separate occasions, usually one hour apart. Although it is important to stress from the outset that parents should be vigilant, it must be remembered that most bacterial infections that the child develops will be from his own skin or gut. The vulnerable areas that parents need to watch are the peri-anal area, the mouth and central venous access device sites.

At the same time, the child should lead as normal a life as possible, so a balance must be negotiated. Parents often worry about the child catching infections from school, but the risk of catching bacterial infections is minimal and unless they are unwell children do not necessarily need to stay away from school even when they are neutropenic. It must be stressed, however, that parents must be contactable by the school. School teachers may worry about the child, because they rarely see children with cancer. Paediatric oncology outreach nurse specialists provide a valuable service in that they are able to visit schools to make teachers aware of the potential risks to the child but will also encourage teachers to allow the child to mix with their friends without being over-protective (Larcombe et al., 1990).

Advice regarding the use of paracetamol or other antipyretics at home is vital and should be discouraged until antibiotic treatment is under way as this may mask a temperature. If pain relief is required, an alternative, such as codeine, will need to be found.

- *Clinical features* – fever may be the only sign of infection in the neutropenic child, although some children (especially infants) may present with no temperature but may have tachycardia and poor perfusion. Other signs and symptoms indicating an inflammatory response, such as erythema, swelling or pain, are absent because there are no neutrophils to contribute to pus formation (Freifeld et al., 1997).
- *Management* – children should be treated for an infection with antibiotics on presentation with a fever as there is a risk of the infection progressing rapidly and leading to septic shock (Barber, 2001; Hughes et al., 2002). Before this, a septic screen should be performed. This will include the following:

  - central line blood cultures (and sometimes peripheral);
  - urine sample;
  - stool sample (if diarrhoea is present);
  - swabs from any potentially infected area;
  - chest X-ray (if the child has respiratory symptoms).

Antibiotic therapy should be commenced within 30–60 minutes of presentation (Pizzo, 1999). A variety of antibiotic combinations are used in individual centres depending on local policy and local drug resistance patterns. This can be the use of one, two or three antibiotics to ensure that the 'cover' is adequate prior to the availability of blood culture results. The duration of the course of antibiotic therapy depends on the nature of the infection, the neutrophil count and the

child's response (Barber, 2001). Often antibiotics are stopped when the child has been afebrile for 48 hours unless they have positive blood cultures when they will be treated according to the microorganism cultured.

Monitoring of vital signs should take a high priority in acutely unwell neutropenic children as they are at risk of septic shock not just on admission but throughout their stay when neutropenic. Accurate recording assists in evaluating the response to antibiotics. Once antibiotics have been commenced, paracetamol can be administered to help alleviate the temperature. It is clear that substitution of oral for intravenous drugs could be beneficial to the child and family and this is being developed in some units. Usually there is a stratification of high- or low-risk patients.

General criteria for low-risk patients

- clinically well;
- no associated comorbidity;
- low-risk protocols e.g. ALL on maintenance;
- access to a telephone and not living too far away from emergency facilities.

The child would also need to be able to take and tolerate oral medication (Vidal et al., 2004).

Some parents and teenagers are taught to give intravenous antibiotics at home through a central venous access device, and with the support of paediatric oncology outreach nurse specialists this can be a successful way to promote early discharge with associated advantages for the family. A study by Hooker (1996) looked at the safety and desirability of home administration of intravenous drugs and found that few clinical problems were encountered and that parents welcomed this initiative. Wiernikowski et al. (1991) found that such a programme can be cost-effective in terms of saving bed spaces. At the same time, parents should not be persuaded to take their child home for this purpose.

Most centres now emphasise the need to avoid foods which are likely to be contaminated with bacteria, such as re-heated foods or soft cheeses, unless in the case of bone marrow transplant patients when guidelines are much stricter (see Chapter 8 for more details). Isolation of neutropenic patients certainly varies from one unit to another. In some cases, children are nursed in a single room with or without filtered air while others are nursed on an open ward. There appears to be no conclusive evidence which will benefit the child most (Mank & van der Lelie, 2003), but the psychological disadvantage of isolating children must clearly be considered. One solution to the problem is to isolate children being nursed on a general medical ward but this is not necessary on a paediatric oncology ward unless the child is likely to infect others.

The use of G-CSF for neutropenic children is now established practice in paediatric oncology when there is an overwhelming infection. It is, however, an expensive drug and its use does need to be justified. G-CSF can reduce the severity and duration of neutropenia and may allow chemotherapy to be given in higher doses and at more frequent intervals (Reigle & Dienger, 2003). It is given either intravenously or subcutaneously but if it is given subcutaneously a higher leucocyte count is seen (Lieschke et al., 1990). There is also some evidence that if it is given prophylactically following chemotherapy, the rate of febrile neutropenia is reduced (Sung et al., 2004), however, not all children will develop a febrile neutropenia and therefore it may not be a cost-effective management of these children.

In the past, leukocyte transfusions have been used for neutropenic children with documented infections that are not responding to treatment but they are not recommended for routine use (Bishton & Chopra, 2004). The use of leukocyte transfusions is now limited, due to the increasing use of G-CSF, as they can increase the risk of reactions to blood products although there may be an occasional situation when they would still be used, e.g. prolonged unresponsive febrile neutropenia (Catalano et al., 1997).

Children who present with a fever but are not neutropenic need to be investigated as to the cause and treated appropriately with antibiotics and analgesia. They are usually assessed on the oncology unit if they are undergoing treatment to ensure that there is no underlying problem such as an infected central venous access device.

Several hospitals may be involved in the care of the child with cancer and liaison is vital to ensure all information is available and the same policies are followed when the child is neutropenic. Paediatric oncology outreach nurse specialists have a crucial role here in maintaining continuity and support, and in promoting shared care.

Prophylaxis

There is some controversy about the use of drugs as prophylaxis for endogenous infections in the neutropenic child and some units will elect not to use any prophylaxis as the use of antimicrobials may encourage resistance (Rogers, 1995). However, they may be used with patients who are undergoing treatment which may lead to a prolonged neutropenic episode (Shelton, 2003). Regimes vary according to local policy and may include oral non-absorbed agents, such as neomycin, colistin and nystatin, and systemically absorbed co-trimoxazole and fluroquinolines, such as ciprofloxacin. Rogers (1995) suggests that each of these regimes is beneficial in reducing bacterial infections due to Gram-negative rods (e.g. Escherichia coli, Proteus) because the intestinal flora is decreased. This may explain the emergence of resistant Gram-positive bacteria as a cause of sepsis in neutropenic patients. There are, however, no antibiotics which can provide cover for these pathogens and which can be given safely throughout neutropenia.

There is a variety of agents used in the prophylaxis of fungal infections. Nystatin and oral amphotercin B are used which suppress colonising yeasts in the intestinal tract but are not absorbed and therefore offer no systemic protection against fungal infections (Rogers, 1995). Fluconazole, itraconazole and ketoconazole are often used and although they reduce the risk of candida, they do not reduce the risk of aspergilliosis (Bohme et al., 1999). If the child is to receive prophylactic drugs during the neutropenic phase of his illness, the issue of compliance should be addressed. The child and the family should understand why they are receiving the drugs and how they should be given.

Other attempts to reduce the risk of infection in neutropenic children include the use of a sterile diet and protective isolation. Evidence on the effectiveness of these measures is limited. Moody et al. (2002) found lack of evidence for a neutropenic diet and suggested there also were deficiencies in vitamins and minerals for some children. Further work is required in this area to establish further evidence.

The compromised immune system

The child undergoing treatment with chemotherapy will often have lymphocytes in their blood but their function will be impaired and the immune system will not fight infections adequately. They are therefore at risk of many opportunistic infections.

Pneumocystis carinii pneumonia (PCP)

Pneumocystis carinii is a fungal organism which can become an opportunistic infection causing pneumonia. Many chemotherapy protocols aim to prevent the development of PCP with the use of prophylactic cotrimoxazole, although bone marrow suppression and hypersensitivity may limit its use (Neville *et al.*, 2002). If this is the case, either oral dapsone or nebulised pentamadine may be used (Wilkin & Feinberg, 1999). The incidence has reduced with the use of various prophylaxis but it is still seen.

- *Clinical features* – may be subtle, such as pyrexia, dyspnoea, non-productive cough. There is a characteristic chest X-ray which shows diffuse ground-glass interstitial or perihilar infiltrates appearing as a white mottled area (Bastow, 2000).
- *Management* – initial treatment is with high-dose cotrimoxazole although this has some unpleasant side effects including vomiting and headache. High-dose steroids may also be administered to reduce infection-associated inflammation and increase oxygenation (Collin & Ramphal, 1998). If the child does not respond within 72 hours, other agents such as intravenous pentamidine may be considered (Neville *et al.*, 2002).

Viral infections

Viral infections can be potentially fatal in the immunocompromised child, and the family must be aware of the danger of contact with these diseases.

Varicella

Varicella (chickenpox) is an acute and highly infectious disease which is common during childhood. It is spread by direct contact or droplet infection and the incidence is at its peak from March to May. The incubation period is between 10 and 21 days. The characteristic vesicles usually cover most of the body, although in mild cases may be less easy to find. The infectious period is one to two days before the rash appears and until the vesicles are dry (around 21 days). This time may be prolonged in immunosuppressed children, however, and can be as long as 28 days.

Varicella can cause serious problems for the immunocompromised child as it carries the risk of dissemination of the virus to the lungs, brain, liver or skin (Rogers, 1995). The child's antibody status should always be checked at diagnosis. If they are not immune, such children should receive passive immunisation with *Varicella zoster* immune globulin (VZIG) within seven days of contact with the disease (Salisbury & Begg, 1996). VZIG may not prevent the child developing the illness but it may reduce its severity (Weinstock *et al.*, 2004). If a second exposure to the disease occurs after three weeks, VZIG will need to be repeated (Salisbury & Begg, 1996). It is extremely important to isolate the infected child should he need to visit hospital, and, where possible, to keep visits to a minimum. Some units do not use VZIG but if the child has been in contact with chickenpox, a course of prophylactic aciclovir is administered instead and has been shown to be as effective (Weinstock *et al.*, 2004). If the child develops chickenpox, he is then treated with acyclovir and nursed in strict isolation, if hospitalised (Hockenberry & Kline, 2002). Very few children die from chickenpox since acyclovir has become available (Atra *et al.*, 1993).

Shingles is a reactivation of the varicella zoster virus – the child must have had chickenpox in the past and they cannot 'catch' shingles although a child who has not had chickenpox can catch chickenpox from someone with shingles and will need prophylactic management.

- *Clinical features* – may be vague and the child may experience numbness, tingling, itching or pain before the rash resembling chickenpox appears. The distribution of the rash usually follows a single nerve path called a dermatome (Zamula, 2001).
- *Management* – this needs to be treated in the same way as chickenpox.

Although the family must be aware of the potential dangers of chickenpox, they must not become over-protective. The child should be encouraged to attend school and teachers need to be aware of the potential problems and inform the family if there is chickenpox in the class or school.

Herpes simplex

Most Herpes simplex infections are due to HSV type 1 which manifests as oropharyngitis, cold sores or generalised sepsis. Clinically, the lesions appear as clear vesicle eruptions in clusters on an erythematous base but may be nondescript and atypical in appearance. HSV type 2 infection more commonly involves the genital area. Treatment is with oral or intravenous acyclovir (Whitley and Roizman, 2001). If it is used orally, large doses are required to maintain high levels as only 20–30 % of the drug is absorbed. It also has a half-life of 3–3.5 hours which means the drug needs to be given every 4–6 hours (Whitley, 2002).

Measles

Measles is an acute viral disease and is transmitted by droplet infection. The introduction of the measles, mumps, rubella (MMR) vaccination programme in 1988 reduced the incidence of measles which was (up until that time) a major cause of mortality in children with cancer. Recent controversies over the safety of the immunisation and links with autism have reduced the uptake of this vaccination and could lead to an increased incidence of measles in the general population. The risk, although still minimal, is still present and measles in the immunocompromised child can lead to pneumonia and encephalitis.

- *Clinical features* – there is normally a prodomal period which lasts 2–4 days before the rash

appears: fever, conjunctivitis, malaise and cold. Koplik's spots appear in the mouth and a maculopapular rash which initially starts at the hairline and progress down the body. The incubation period is between 6 to 19 days (Richardson *et al.*, 2001). Measles is highly infectious from the prodromal period until four days after the appearance of the rash which usually takes 2–4 days to appear (Salisbury & Begg, 1996).

- *Management* – passive immunisation with human immunoglobulin (HIG) should be given within six days of exposure to the disease and if given within 72 hours the virus can be completely prevented from infecting the individual (Stalkup, 2002).

Immunisation

Live vaccines, such as measles, polio, rubella and BCG, are contraindicated in immunocompromised children because there is a risk of them developing the infection (Albano & Pizzo, 1988). Other immunisations, such as tetanus, diphtheria and pertussis, are not contraindicated but the response is often poor and it is best to delay them until at least six months after treatment is complete (Royal College of Paediatrics and Child Health, 2002). This includes any that may have been missed and in some cases, children may need total revaccination. Their antibody status should be reviewed at this point. The influenza vaccine is recommended annually for all patients, family members and close contacts or carers (Royal College of Paediatrics and Child Health, 2002).

Siblings should continue with their immunisation programme while their immunocompromised brother or sister is receiving treatment to minimise the risk of infecting the child with the natural disease. There is no risk of vaccine strain spread; however, the inactivated preparation of the polio vaccine (IPV) should be used to prevent cross-infection from the oral–faecal route.

Cutaneous side effects

Alopecia

Chemotherapy destroys the rapidly dividing epithelial cells of the hair follicle reducing hair growth on the body and causing alopecia. The degree of hair loss depends upon the dose, the route and the nature of the treatment as well as the child's health prior to treatment (Randall & Ream, 2005). Crounse van Scott (1960) found that at any given time 90% of human hair follicles are in the dividing phases of the cell cycle and are therefore susceptible to the effects of chemotherapy. Hair loss can be extremely distressing for both the parents and the child and can have a severe effect on body image.

All body hair may be affected and hair loss usually begins 1–2 weeks after commencing chemotherapy with regrowth 1–2 weeks after the final course of treatment. It is more severe with drugs that have a long half-life of active metabolites, such as doxorubicin, the nitrosoureas and cyclophosphamide. Preparation and advice to the child and the family are very important and should include referral to wig specialists at an early stage so that they may be matched to the original colour style and hair texture. Many children cope well with a variety of hats and caps that are popular today.

There is very little that can be done to prevent alopecia. Scalp cooling has been tried in adults and it is thought to inhibit cellular uptake of a drug that is temperature-dependent but there are inconsistencies in the method, length of time involved and how much hair is eventually retained (Massey, 2004). Scalp cooling is more effective when certain drugs are used, for example, daunorubicin (David & Speechley, 1987; Noble-Adams, 1998) and more recently the taxane group of drugs (Christodoulou *et al.*, 2002). There are concerns that because hypothermia decreases the drug concentration to the scalp, it may become a sanctuary for micrometastatic malignant cells (Barton Burke *et al.*, 1991) although Protiere *et al.* (2002) have evaluated this risk and found it to be minimal. There are contraindications to the use of scalp cooling in that it requires specific skills which are time-consuming, and, more importantly, it can be unpleasant for the child.

Skin

The child may have problems with their skin, particularly after high-dose cytarabine, which causes rashes that may be an irritant and blister.

The following guidelines should be observed:

- Pay careful attention to skin hygiene to ensure that it is kept clean and free from irritation.
- Apply moisturising cream as skin often becomes dry during chemotherapy.
- Act promptly when rashes or abnormalities are seen.
- Ensure that the child wears total sunblock when outside because the skin becomes more sensitive to sunlight during chemotherapy.

Nephrotoxicity

Certain chemotherapy drugs, e.g. Cispatinum and methotrexate, can cause direct damage to the renal cells. To try and prevent problems it is vital the children have adequate hydration and an adequate urine output in relation to the fluid administered.

- *Clinical features* – this is usually first seen in a deterioration of the renal function tests such as GFR. Alterations may also be seen in the child's renal profile.
- *Management* – once the renal function begins to deteriorate, chemotherapy dosages may need to be reduced, another chemotherapy agent may be used or the drug may be completely omitted. There also needs to be care with other nephrotoxic agents, e.g. aminoglycoside antibiotics, as they may not be excreted adequately and can also exacerbate any damage.

Haemorrhagic cystitis

This occurs in 5–10% of patients receiving cyclophosphamide and in 20–40% of patients receiving ifosfamide (West, 1997). It can occur immediately, during or after administration, but can also occur months, possibly years later. The toxicity appears to be dose-related and happens when toxic metabolites, in particular acrolein, come into contact with the bladder wall. Mesna is oxidised in the plasma to a stable form then excreted by the kidneys where it is re-activated in the kidney tubules as needed. This then reacts with the metabolites in the urine to reduce or eliminate the toxic effects of these drugs in the bladder without interfering with the anti-tumour effect of the drugs (Russo, 2000).

- *Clinical features* – haematuria (varying from microscopic to macroscopic), pain, dysuria.
- *Management* – adequate pre- and post-dose hydration is essential to prevent haemorrhagic cystitis, with concurrent mesna in susceptible patients or those receiving high doses. Mesna must be in the bladder before cyclophosphamide or ifosfamide is administered and given after the last dose to be most effective (Russo, 2000). An accurate input and output chart needs to be maintained with all urine being tested for blood and results documented. If haemorrhagic cystitis occurs, the chemotherapy should be stopped and hydration only given to dilute the urinary concentration of the toxin (West, 1997). Pain relief is important and a large bore catheter may need to be passed to enable the child to pass the clots or to allow bladder irrigation if required. Ideally the platelets should be kept above $10^9/l$ to help decrease blood loss. Occasionally the bladder goes into spasm, and medication, such as oxybutinin, may be required to relieve it. Surgery may be required for an endoscopy, evacuation of clots and possible cauterisation of bleeding points. This can be a traumatic experience for the child and family and they will need ongoing support and information.

Cardiac problems

These problems are associated with the anthracycline drugs. Within 24 hours of administration the child can develop acute arrhythmias, conduction abnormalities and decreased left ventricular function, but these are usually transient problems (Balis *et al.*, 1996). Some children, however, will develop problems with the minimal amount of treatment. Most cardiac problems seem to be long term and are seen after treatment has ceased, characterised by myocardial cell loss and replacement fibrosis (Keefe, 2000). However, the anthracyclines appear to be less cardiotoxic when given as an infusion rather than a bolus.

- *Management* – prevention and early detection of problems are essential. The more chemotherapy given, the increased potential for problems. It is important to record cumulative

doses and no more than $550mg/m^2$ should be given. During treatment and follow-up, cardiac echocardiograms should be performed to observe either left ventricular ejection fraction or fractional shortening as these can indicate potential cardiac problems.

The development of chelating agents (ICRF-187) administered concurrently may block the cardiotoxic effects of the anthracyclines. There is some evidence that ICRF-187 protects against doxorubicin-induced cardiotoxicity in the short term (Venturini *et al.*, 1996; Wexler *et al.*, 1996; Lopez *et al.*, 1998), however, it may have limitations due to its potential side effects and possible interference with anti-tumour activity (van Dalen *et al.*, 2005). There is a need for more studies to establish its efficacy and potential side effects.

Another potential drug which may reduce cardiotoxic toxicity is liposomal doxorubicin. This was designed to reduce the cardiotoxicity of doxorubicin while preserving anti-tumour efficacy. Batist *et al.* (2001) have shown that there was a reduction in cardiotoxicity when used with cyclophosphamide but there has been limited research in paediatrics.

Respiratory problems

Respiratory problems relate to chemotherapy regimens that include bleomycin, methotrexate, cyclophosphamide, carmustine (BCNU) or lomustine (CCNU). Bleomycin is the most common cause of fibrosis. Initially, there is a decrease in type I pneumocytes and an increase and redistribution of type II pneumocytes into the alveolar spaces, leading to pneumonitis. The alveolar septas become thickened and decrease in number, with an increase in the amount of collagen secreted by the interstitial fibroblasts. The use of concomitant radiotherapy with bleomycin may exacerbate the problem as does exposure to high-inspired oxygen concentrations which may be a problem for anaesthetics (Limper, 2004).

Prevention or early recognition can be established by performing lung function tests and subsequent withholding of the drug. Once the drug is stopped, there is usually recovery.

- *Clinical features* – dyspnoea, nonproductive cough and fever which may occur weeks to years after chemotherapy.

The child and family need to be aware of these potential problems and of the symptoms they are looking for especially in later life with the use of anaesthetics.

Neurological problems

These are seen with the neurotoxic chemotherapy drugs, especially vincristine, cisplatin and Paclitaxel (Postma & Heimans, 2000). The vinca alkoids bind to microtubules and provide a conduit for neurotransmission along the nerve axons and thus there is the potential for problems along these axons. The effect from these and paclitaxel tends to occur while the child is receiving chemotherapy and usually resolves on a reduction or completion of therapy. Cisplatin-induced neuropathy, however, occurs after cumulative doses and may worsen once treatment has stopped, leading to an impact on quality of life (Siegal & Haim, 1990). The use of high-dose regimens and various combinations of chemotherapy using more than one neurotoxic drug may increase these problems in the future.

- *Clinical features* – loss of deep tendon reflexes, pain in legs, unable to put foot on ground, walking on toes, drop foot, motor weakness, numbness, tingling fingers, jaw pain and constipation.
- *Management* – families need to be aware of the potential problem, so they can report symptoms at the earliest opportunity and receive appropriate support and advice. Analgesia may be required for pain and they may need input from the physiotherapy department. The doses of chemotherapy may need to be decreased or omitted depending on the severity. Ongoing physiotherapy and rehabilitation may be required.

Hearing

Hearing problems are related to the chemotherapy drug cisplatin (and to a lesser extent carbo-

platin). The loss is usually irreversible and affects high frequency sounds initially (Reddel *et al.*, 1982; Bertolini *et al.*, 2004) and it increases significantly with cumulative doses although it can begin soon after the first dose (Bergeron *et al.*, 2005). There is a need for routine assessment of hearing before and during treatment as they can show deterioration in hearing and subsequent modification in the child's treatment. Ideally otoacoustic emissions (OAE) which are low levels of acoustic energy should be measured in response to auditory stimulation as they tend to change prior to pure-tone thresholds and problems may be picked up earlier (Plinkert & Krober, 1991; Cevette *et al.*, 2000).

Fatigue

Fatigue has been recognised for a while as a prevalent and distressing symptom of cancer and its treatment in adults (Stone *et al.*, 2003). In children and young people there has been increasing recognition but there still needs to be a substantial amount of research to establish the impact and management of this distressing symptom. There also needs to be an increased awareness by healthcare professionals of this phenomenon so they are able to recognise and offer help to families.

Hockenberry-Eaton *et al.* (1999, p. 9) define fatigue in children as 'a profound sense of being tired, or having difficulty with movement such as arms and legs, or opening eyes which is influenced by environmental, personal/social and treatment related factors and can result in difficulties with play, concentration and negative motions (most typically anger and sadness)'. A study by Gibson *et al.* (2005) found adolescents explaining symptoms as absolute and complete exhaustion, preventing normal activity, and leaving them weak, inactive and unmotivated.

Symptoms can include tiredness, lethargy, poor sleep, not feeling rested even after sleeping in excess of 8 hours, lack of concentration and mental fatigue (Gibson *et al.*, 2005). It can occur during and after treatment and last for many years postchemotherapy, having an impact on the child's or young person's quality of life. It can also foster a dependence on other family members as they need assistance to perform daily activities.

Individuals often find various ways of coping and this can include changing their sleep pattern, physical activity, social activities/interactions with friends and family, correction of anaemia and some complementary therapies.

Nurses need to have an awareness of fatigue and the impact it can have on the child's and family's life. Part of a nursing assessment should include asking about the impact of treatment of their life away from the hospital and how they are able to socialise with their peers. This may help recognise potential problems and help plan interventions to try and alleviate them. If possible, this should be backed up by written information. This is an area where more work is needed to establish the way children and families can be supported through this distressing symptom of their disease and treatment.

Conclusion

The care of the child undergoing chemotherapy is both challenging and rewarding for the paediatric oncology nurse. Knowledge of the actual and the potential side effects of treatment ensures that the nurse is able to assess, manage and evaluate care. The oncology nurse also needs to develop a mature and professional approach to care, in order to be able to offer appropriate advice and support to families.

References

Abu-Saad H (1993) 'Pediatric pain management: an intervention study' paper presented at Royal College of Nursing 1st International Conference in Paediatric Medicine, Cambridge, 2–4 September

Aitken TJ (1992) 'Gastrointestinal manifestations in the child with cancer' Journal of Pediatric Oncology Nursing 9(3): 25–29

Albano EA & Pizzo PA (1988) 'Infectious complications in childhood acute leukaemias' The Pediatric Clinics of North America 35(4): 873–901

Andrejak M, Lafon B, Decoq G, Chetaille E, Dupas JL & Ducroix JP (1996) 'Antibiotic associated pseudomembranous colitis: retrospective study of 48 cases diagnosed by colonoscopy' Therapie 51(1): 81–86

Andrews PLR & Davis CJ (1993) 'The mechanisms of emesis induced by anti-cancer therapies' in: Andres PLR & Sanger G (eds) Emesis in Anti-Cancer Therapy: Mechanisms and Treatment. London: Chapman & Hall

Andreyev HJN, Norman AR, Oates J & Cunningham D (1998) 'Why do patients with weight loss have a worse outcome when undergoing chemotherapy for gastrointestinal malignancies?' European Journal of Cancer 34(4): 503–509

Antonarakis ES & Hain RDW (2004) 'Nausea and vomiting associated with cancer chemotherapy: drug management in theory and practice' Archives of Disease in Childhood 89(9): 877–880

Arakawa S (1997) 'Relaxation to reduce nausea, vomiting, and anxiety induced by chemotherapy in Japanese patients' Cancer Nursing 20(5): 342–349

Atra A, Richards S & Chessels JM (1993) 'Remission death in acute lymphoblastic leukaemia: a changing pattern' Archives of Diseases in Childhood 69(5): 550–554

Balis FM, Poplack DG & Horowitz ME (1996) 'Randomized trial of the cardioprotective agent ICRF-187 in pediatric sarcoma patients treated with doxorubicin' Journal of Clinical Oncology 14(2): 362–372

Barber FD (2001) 'Management of fever in neutropenic patients with cancer' Nursing Clinics of North America 36(4): 631–644

Barton Burke M, Wilkes GM, Berg D, Bean CK & Ingwerson KI (1991) Cancer Chemotherapy: A Nursing Process Approach. Boston: Jones and Bartlett Publishers Inc

Bastow V (2000) 'Identifying and treating PCP' Nursing Times 96(37): 19–20

Batist G, Ramakrishnam G, Rao CS, Chandrasekharan A, Gutheil J, Guthrie T, Shah P, Khojasteh A, Nair MK, Hoelzer K, Tkaczuk K, Park YC & Lee LW (2001) 'Reduced cardiotoxicity and preserved antitumor efficacy of liposome-encapsulated doxorubicin and cyclophosphamide compared with conventional doxorubicin and cyclophosphamide in a randomized, multicenter trial of metastatic breast cancer' Journal of Clinical Oncology 19(5): 1444–1454

Beck SL (1992) 'Prevention and management of oral complications in the cancer patient' Current Issues in Cancer Nursing Practice Updates 1(6): 1–12

Bender CM, McDaniel RW, Murphy-Ende K, Pickett M, Rittenberg CN, Rogers MP, Schneider SM & Schwartz RN (2002) 'Chemotherapy-induced nausea and vomiting' Clinical Journal of Oncology Nursing 6(2): 94–102

Bergeron C, Dubourg L, Chastagner P, Mechinaud F, Plouvier E, Desfachelles AS, Dusol F, Bautard B, Edan C, Plantaz D, Froehlich P & Rubie H (2005) 'Long-term renal and hearing toxicity of carboplatin in infants treated for localized and unresectable neuroblastoma: results of the SFOP MBL90 Study' Pediatric Blood and Cancer 45(1): 32–36

Bertoloni P, Lassalle M, Mercier G, Raquin MA, Izzi G, Corradini N & Hartmann, P (2004) 'Platinum compound related ototoxicity in children' Journal of Pediatric Hematology Oncology 26(10): 649–655

Bishton M & Chopra R (2004) 'The role of granulocyte transfusions in neutropaenic patients' *British Journal of Haematology* 127(5): 501–508

Bohme A, Kartthaus M & Hoelzer D (1999) 'Antifungal prophylaxis in neutropenic patients with haematological malignancies: Is there a real benefit?' *Chemotherapy* 45(3): 224–232

Bozzetti F, Gavazzi C, Marianin L & Crippa F (1999) 'Artificial nutrition in cancer patients: which route, what composition?' *World Journal of Surgery* 23(6): 577–583

British Committee for Standards in Haematology (2003) 'Guidelines for the use of platelet transfusion' *British Journal of Haematology* 122(1): 10–23

Brown CG & Wingate J (2004) 'Clinical consequences of oral mucositis' *Seminars in Oncology Nursing* 20(1): 16–21

Brown JK (2002) 'A systematic review of the evidence on symptom management of cancer-related anorexia and cachexia' *Oncology Nursing Forum* 29(3): 517–530

Bryant R (2003) 'Managing side effects of childhood cancer treatment' *Journal of Pediatric Nursing* 18(2): 113–125

Campbell SJ (1987) 'Mouthcare in cancer patients' *Nursing Times* 83(29): 59–60

Campbell ST, Evans MA & MacTavish F (1995) *Guidelines for Mouthcare*. London: The Paediatric Oncology Nursing Forum, Royal College of Nursing

Capra S, Ferguson M & Ried K (2001) 'Cancer: impact of nutrition intervention outcome – nutrition issues for patients' *Nutrition* 17(9): 769–772

Cartoni C, Dragoni F, Micozzi A, Pescarmona E, Mecarocci S, Chirletti P, Petti MC, Meloni G & Mandelli F (2001) 'Neutropenic enterocolitis in patients with acute leukaemia: prognostic significance of bowel wall thickening detected by ultrasonography' *Journal of Clinical Oncology* 19(3): 756–761

Casey A (1995a) 'Nursing assessment and communication' *in*: Campbell S & Glasper EA (eds) *Whaley and Wong's Children's Nursing*. London: CV Mosby

Casey A (1995b) 'Partnership nursing: influences on involvement of informal carers' *Journal of Advanced Nursing* 22(6): 1058–1062

Catalano L, Fiontana R, Scarpato N, Picardi, M, Rocco S & Rotoli B (1997) 'Combined treatment with amphotercin B and granulocyte transfusion from G-CSF-stimulated donors in an aplastic patient with invasive aspergilliosis undergoing bone marrow transplantation' *Haematological* 87(1): 71–72

Cevette MJ, Drew D, Webb TM & Marion MS (2000) 'Cisplatin ototoxicity, increased DPOAE amplitudes and magnesium deficiency' *Journal of the American Academy of Audiology* 11(6): 323–310

Chanock SJ, Kundra V, Johnson FL & Singer, MD (2006) 'The other side of the bed: what caregivers can learn from listening to patients and their families' *in*: Pizzo PA & Poplack DG (eds) *Principles and Practice of Pediatric Oncology* (5th edn) Philadelphia: Lippincott, Williams & Wilkins, pp. 1446–1465

Christodoulou C, Klouvas G, Efstathiou Zervakis D, Papazachariou E, Plyta M & Sharlos DV (2002) 'Effectiveness of the MSC cold cap system in the prevention of chemotherapy induced alopecia' *Oncology* 62(2): 97–102

Cohen LF, Barlow JE, Macgrath IT, Poplack DG & Collins JM (1996) 'Pharmacokinetics and clinical monitoring' *in*: Chabner BA & Longo DL (eds) *Cancer Chemotherapy and Biotherapy*. Philadelphia: Lippincott-Raven

Collard MM & Hunter ML (2001) 'Oral and dental care in acute lymphoblastic leukaemia: a survey of United Kingdom Children's Cancer Study Group Centres' *International Journal of Paediatric Dentistry* 11(5): 347–351

Collin BA & Ramphal R (1998) 'Pneumonia in the compromised host including cancer patients and transplant patients' *Infectious Disease Clinics of North America* 12(3): 781–805

Comeau TB, Epstein JB & Migas C (2001) 'Taste and smell dysfunction in patients receiving chemotherapy: a review of current knowledge' *Supportive Care Cancer* 9(8): 575–580

Cope DG (2001) 'Management of chemotherapy-induced diarrhoea and constipation' *Nursing Clinics of North America* 36(4): 695–707

Crounse van Scott (1960) cited in Price B (ed.) (1990) *Body Image: Nursing Concepts and Care*. London: Prentice Hall

Cunningham RS & Bell R (2000) 'Nutrition in cancer: an overview' *Seminars in Oncology Nursing* 16(2): 90–98

David J & Speechley V (1987) 'Scalp cooling to prevent alopecia' *Nursing Times* 83(32): 36–37

De Boer-Dennert M, de-Wit R, Schmitz PI, Djontono J, Beurden V, Stoter G & Verweij J (1997) 'Patient perceptions of the side-effects of chemotherapy: the influence of 5HT3 antagonists' *British Journal of Cancer* 76(8): 1055–1061

Den Broeder E, Lippins RJJ, van't Hof M, Tolboom JJ, Sengers RC & Staveren WA (2000) 'Association between the change in nutritional status in response to tube feeding and the occurrence of infections in children with solid tumour' *Pediatric Hematology Oncology* 17(7): 567–575

Dodd MJ, Miaskowski C, Dibble SL, Paul SM, MacPhail L, Greenspan D & Shiba G (2000) 'Factors influencing oral mucositis in patients receiving chemotherapy' *Cancer Practice* 8(6): 291–297

Dolgin MJ, Katz ER, McGinty K & Siegal SE (1985) 'Anticipatory nausea and vomiting in pediatric cancer patients' *Pediatrics* 75(3): 547–552

Dupuis LL, Lau R & Greenberg ML (1999) 'Effectiveness of strategies for the prevention of acute antineoplastic-induced nausea and vomiting in children with acute lymphoblastic leukaemia' *Canadian Journal of Hospital Pharmacy* 52: 350–361

Dupuis LL & Nathan PC (2003) 'Options for the prevention and management of acute chemotherapy-induced nausea and vomiting in children' *Paediatric Drugs* 5(9): 597–613

Eckert RM (2001) 'Understanding anticipatory nausea' *Oncology Nursing Forum* 28(10): 1553–1558

Eilers J, Berger AM & Petersen MC (1988) 'Development, testing, and application of the oral assessment guide' *Oncology Nursing Forum* 15(3): 325–330

Estrin JT, Ford PA, Henry DA, Stradden AP & Mason BA (1997) 'Erythropoetin permits high dose chemotherapy with peripheral stem-cell transplant for Jehovah's Witness' *American Journal of Hematology* 55(1): 51–52

Evans M (1993) 'Paediatric oncology' *in*: Glasper EA & Tucker A (eds) *Advances in Child Health Nursing*. London: Scutari Press

Faulkner A, Peace G & O'Keefe G (1995) *When a Child Has Cancer*. London: Chapman & Hall

Fawcett H (1995) 'Nutritional support for hospital patients' *Nursing Standard* 9(48): 25–28

Feusner J & Hastings C (2002) 'Recombinant human erythropoietin in pediatric oncology: a review' *Medical and Pediatric Oncology* 39(4); 463–468

Foley GV, Hochtrain D & Hardin Mooney K (1993) *Nursing Care of the Child with Cancer*. Philadelphia: WB Saunders

Freifeld AG, Walsh TJ & Pizzo PP (1997) 'Infections in the cancer patient' *in*: DeVita VT, Hellman S & Rosenberg S (eds) *Cancer: Principles and Practice of Oncology* (5th edn). Philadelphia: Lippincott Raven, pp. 2659–2704

Fulton J S, Middleton GJ & McPhail JT (2002) 'Management of oral complications' *Seminars in Oncology Nursing* 18(1): 28–35

Galbraith I, Bailey D, Kelly L, Rehn K, Spear S, Steinle G, Vaughan G & Wehange S (1991) 'Treatment for alteration in oral mucosa related to chemotherapy' *Paediatric Nursing* 17(3): 233–237

Gibson BES, Todd A, Roberts I, Pamphilon D, Rodeck C, Bolton-Maggs P, Burbin G, Duguid J, Boulton F, Cohen H, Smith N, McClelland DBL, Rowley M & Turner G (2004) 'Transfusion guidelines for neonates and older children' *British Journal of Haematology* 124(4): 433–453

Gibson F (1994) 'The phenomena of chemotherapy – associated nausea and vomiting examined in relation to the ability of children to use a self-report instrument' unpublished MSc dissertation, University of Surrey

Gibson F, Mulhall AB, Richardson A, Edwards JL, Ream E & Sepion BJ (2005) 'A phenomenological study of fatigue in adolescents receiving treatment for cancer' *Oncology Nursing Forum* 32(3): 651–660

Gibson F & Nelson W (2000) 'Mouth care for children with cancer' *Paediatric Nursing* 12(1): 18–22

Glenny A (2006) *Mouth Care for Children and Young People with Cancer: Evidence-based Guidelines*. London: UKCCSG-PONF Mouth Care Group

Glynn R (2001) 'Parenteral nutrition' *in*: Shaw V & Lawson M (eds) *Clinical Paediatric Dietetics* (2nd edn). Oxford: Blackwell Science, pp. 43–52

Gomez L, Martino R & Rolston KV (1998) 'Neutropaenic enterocolitis: spectrum of the disease and comparison of definite and possible causes' *Clinical Infectious Diseases* 27(4): 695–699

Goodin S & Cunningham R (2002) '5-HT3 receptor antagonists for the treatment of nausea and vomiting: a reappraisal of their side-effect profile' *The Oncologist* 7(5): 424–436

Gorbach SL (1998) 'Neutropaenic enterocolitis' *Clinical Infectious Diseases* 27(4): 700–701

Gorschluter M, Glasmacher A, Hahn C, Leutner C, Marklein G, Remig J, Schmidt-Wolf IGH & Sauerbruch T (2001) 'Severe abdominal infections in neutropaenic patients' *Cancer Investigation* 19(7): 669–677

Gould D (1995) 'Hand decontamination: nurses; opinions and practices' *Nursing Times* 91(17): 42–45

Graham-Pole J, Weare J, Engel S, Gardner R, Mehta P & Gross S (1986) 'Antiemetics in children receiving cancer chemotherapy: a double blind prospective randomized study comparing metoclopromide with chlorpromazine' *Journal of Clinical Oncology* 4(7): 1110–1113

Grant MM & Rivera LM (1995) 'Anorexia, cachexia and dysphagia: the symptoms experience' *Seminars in Oncology Nursing* 11(4): 266–271

Han-Markey T (2000) 'Nutritional considerations in pediatric oncology' *Seminars in Oncology Nursing* 16(2):146–151

Hann I, Viscoli C, Paesmans M, Gaya H & Glausner M (1997) 'A comparison of outcome from febrile neutropenic episodes in children compared with adults: results from four EORTC studies' *British Journal of Haematology* 99(3): 580–588

Hawthorn J (1991) 'The management of nausea and vomiting induced by chemotherapy and radiotherapy: a comprehensive guide for nurses' *European Journal of Cancer* 1(1): 23–26

Hawthorn J (1995) *Understanding the Management of Nausea and Vomiting*. Oxford: Blackwell Science

Higgins C (2000) 'The risks associated with blood and blood transfusion' *British Journal of Nursing* 9(2): 2281–2290

Hinchliffe RF (1992) 'Reference values' *in*: Lilleyman JS & Hann IM (eds) *Paediatric Haematology*. Singapore: Churchill Livingstone, pp. 1–28

Hockenberry MJ & Kline NE (2002) 'Nursing support of the child with cancer' *in*: Pizzo PA & Poplack DG (eds) *Principles and Practice of Pediatric Oncology* (4th edn). Philadelphia: Lippincott, Williams & Wilkins, pp. 1333–1350

Hockenberry-Eaton M & Benner A (1990) 'Patterns of nausea and vomiting in children: nursing assessment and intervention' *Oncology Nurses Forum* 17(14):575–584

Hockenberry-Eaton M, Hinds P, O'Neill J.B, Alcoser P, Bottomley S, Kline NE, Euell K, Howard V & Gattuso J (1999) 'Developing a conceptual model for fatigue in children' *European Journal of Oncology Nursing* 3(1): 5–13

Hogan CM (1990) 'Advances in the management of nausea and vomiting' *Nursing Clinics of North America* 25(2): 475–497

Hogan CM (1998) 'The nurse's role in diarrhoea management' *Oncology Nursing Forum* 25(5): 879–886

Holden CE, MacDonald A, Ward M, Ford K, Patchell C, Handy D, Chell M, Brown GB & Booth, IW (1997) 'Psychological preparation for nasogastric feeding in children' *British Journal of Nursing* 6(7): 376–381, 384–385

Hooker L (1996) 'An evaluation of parent-administered home intravenous drug therapy (abstract)' *Medical & Pediatric Oncology* 27(4): 274

Hughes WT, Armstrong D & Bodey GP (2002) 'Guidelines for the use of antimicrobial agents in the neutropenic patient with cancer' *Clinical Infectious Diseases* 34: 730–751

Irwin MM (1986) 'Enteral and parenteral nutrition support' *Seminars in Oncology Nursing* 21(1): 44–54

Jain Y, Arya LS & Kataria R (2000) 'Neutropenic enterocolitis in children with acute lymphoblastic leukaemia' *Pediatric Hematology and Oncology* 17(1): 99–103

Johnson T (2001) 'Enteral feeding' *in*: Shaw V & Lawson M *Clinical Paediatric Dietetics* (2nd edn). Oxford: Blackwell, pp. 31–42

Juranek DD (1995) 'Cryptosporidiosis: sources of infection and guidelines for prevention' *Clinical Infectious Diseases* 21(supplement 1): 57–61

Keefe DL (2000) 'Cardivascular emergencies in the cancer patient' *Seminars in Oncology Nursing* 27(3): 244–255

Keefe D, Gibson RJ & Hayer JM (2004) 'Gastrointestinal mucositis' *Seminars in Oncology Nursing* 20(1): 36–37

Keller U (1993) 'Pathophysiology of cancer cachexia' *Supportive Cancer Care* 1(6): 290–294

Keller VE (1995) 'Management of nausea and vomiting in children' *Journal of Pediatric Nursing* 10(5): 280–286

Kennedy L & Diamond J (1997) 'Assessment and management of chemotherapy-induced mucositis in children' *Journal of Pediatric Oncology Nursing* 14(3): 164–174

King N (2002) 'Nursing care of the child with neutropaenic enterocolitis' *Journal of Pediatric Oncology Nursing* 19(6): 198–204

Kinrade LC (1988) 'Typhlitis: a complication of neutropenia' *Pediatric Nursing* 14(4): 291–295

Krishnasamy M (1995) 'The nurse's role in oral care' *European Journal of Palliative Care* (supplement 1): 8–9

Kwekkeboom K, Huseby-Moore K & Ward SW (1998) 'Imaging ability and effective use of guided imagery' *Research in Nursing and Health* 21(3): 189–198

Lansdown R & Goldman A (1988) 'The psychological care of children with malignant disease' *Journal of Child Psychology and Psychiatry* 29(5): 555–567

Larcombe IJ, Walker J, Charleton A, Meller A, Morris Jones P & Mott M G (1990) 'Impact of childhood cancer on return to normal schooling' *British Medical Journal* 301(6744): 169–171

León P, Jiménez M, Barona P & Sierrrasesúmaga L (1998) 'Recombinant erythropoietin and cancer anaemia' *Medical and Pediatric Oncology* 30: 110–116

Lever SA, Dupuis LL & Chan HS (1987) 'Comparative evaluation of benzydamine oral rinse in children with antineoplastic-induced stomatitis' *Drug Intelligence and Clinical Pharmacology* 21(4): 359–361

Lieschke GJ, Maher D, O'Conner M, Green M, Sheridan W, Rallings M, Bonnem E, Burgess A W *et al.* (1990) 'Phase 1 study of intravenously administered GM-CSF and comparison with subcutaneous administration' *Cancer Research* 50(3): 606–614

Limper AH (2004) 'Chemotherapy-induced lung disease' *Clinics in Chest Medicine* 25(1): 53–64

Lindsey AM (1986) 'Cancer cachexia; effects of the disease and its treatment' *Seminars in Oncology Nursing* 2(1): 19–29

Lopez M, Vici P, Di Lauro L, Conti F, Paoletti G, Ferraironi A, Sciuto R, Fiannarelli D & Maini C (1998) 'Randomised prospective clinical trial of high-dose epirubicin and dexrazoxane in patients with advanced breast cancer and soft tissue sarcomas' *Journal of Clinical Oncology* 16(1): 86–92

Lowis SP, Goulden N & Oakhill A (2004) 'Acute complications' *in*: Pinkerton R, Plowman PN & Pieters R (eds) *Paediatric Oncology* (3rd edn). London: Arnold

Mank A & van der Lelie H (2003) 'Is there still an indication for nursing patients with prolonged neutropenia in protective isolation? An evidence-based nursing and medical study of 4 years experience for nursing patients with neutropenia without isolation' *European Journal of Oncology Nursing* 7(1): 17–23

Marchioro G, Azzarello G, Viviani F, Barbato F, Pavanetto M, Rosetti F, Pappagallo GL & Vinante O (2000) 'Hypnosis in the treatment of anticipatory nausea and vomiting in patients receiving cancer chemotherapy' *Oncology* 59(2): 100–104

Massey CS (2004) 'A multicentre study to determine the efficacy and patient acceptability of the Paxman Scalp Cooler to prevent hair loss in patients receiving chemotherapy' *European Journal of Oncology Nursing* 8(2): 121–130

Mattes RD (1994) 'Prevention of food aversions in cancer patients during treatment' *Nutrition and Cancer* 21(1): 13–24

Matthew P, Bowman L, Williams R, Jones D, Rao B, Schropp K, Warren B, Klyce MK, Whitington G & Hudson M (1996) 'Complications and effectiveness of gastrostomy feedings in pediatric cancer patients' *Journal of Pediatric Hematology/Oncology* 18(1): 81–85

McClelland B (1996) *Handbook of Transfusion Medicine* (2nd edn). London: HMSO

Ming J, Kuo BI, Lin J & Lin L (2002) 'The efficacy of acupressure to prevent nausea and vomiting in post-operative patients' *Journal of Advanced Nursing* 39(4): 343–351

Montague SE (2005) 'The blood' *in*: Montague SE, Watson R & Herbert RA (eds) *Physiology for Nursing* (3rd edn). Barcelona: Elsevier, pp. 335–382

Montgomery GH, Tomoyasu N, Bovbjerg DH, Andrykowski MA, Currie VE, Jacobsen PB & Redd WH (1998) 'Patients' pre-treatment expectations of chemotherapy-related nausea are an independent prediction of anticipatory nausea' *Annals of Behavioural Medicine* 20(2): 104–108

Moody K, Charlson ME & Finlay J (2002) 'The neutropenic diet: what's the evidence?' *Journal of Pediatric Hematology/Oncology* 24(9): 717–721

Moore J (1995) 'Assessment of nurse administered oral hygiene' *Nursing Times* 91(9): 40–41

Morrow GR & Roscoe JA (1998) 'Anticipatory nausea and vomiting, models, mechanisms and management' *in*: Dicato MA (ed.) *Cancer Treatment-induced Emesis*. London: Martin Dunitz Ltd, pp. 149–166

Neville K, Renbarger J & Dreyer Z (2002) 'Pneumonia in the immunocompromised pediatric cancer patient' *Seminars in Respiratory Infections* 17(1): 21–32

Nitenberg G & Raynard B (2000) 'Nutritional support of the cancer patient: issues and dilemmas' *Critical Reviews in Oncology/Hematology* 34(3): 137–168

Noble-Adams R (1998) 'Scalp cooling: a critical examination' *Nursing Practice in New Zealand* 13(3): 35–43

Norville R, Hinds P, Wilmas J, Fairclough D, Fischl S & Kunkel K (1994) 'Platelet count, morphology, and corrected count increment in children with cancer: in vitro and in vivo studies' *Oncology Nursing Forum* 21(10): 1669–1673

Panzarella C & Duncan J (1993) 'Nursing management of physical care needs' *in*: Foley GV, Fochtman D & Mooney KH (eds) *Nursing Care of the Child with Cancer* (2nd edn). Philadelphia: WB Saunders

Pearson LS (1996) 'A comparison of the ability of foam sticks and toothbrushes to remove dental plaque: implications for nursing practice' *Journal of Advanced Nursing* 23(1): 62–69

Peate I (1993) 'Nurse-administered oral hygiene in the hospitalised patient' *British Journal of Nursing* 2(9): 249–262

Pendergrass KB (1998) 'Options in the treatment of chemotherapy-induced emesis' *Cancer Practice* 6(5): 276–281

Phillips K (2005) 'Maintaining nutritional status during chemotherapy' *Cancer Nursing Practice* 4(7): 14–19

Picardi M, Selleri C, Camera A, Catalano L & Rotoli B (1999) 'Early detection by ultrasound scan of severe post-chemotherapy gut complications in patients with acute leukaemia' *Haematologica* 84(3): 222–225

Picton SV (1998) 'Aspects of altered metabolism in children with cancer' *International Journal of Cancer* 11(supplement): 62–64

Pizzo PA (1999) 'Current concepts: fever in immunocompromised patients' *New England Journal of Medicine* 341(12): 893–900

Plinkert PK & Krober S (1991) 'Early detection of cisplatin induced ototoxicity using evoked otoacoustic emissions' *Laryngorhinootologie* 70(9): 457–462

Porter JC, Leahey A, Polise K, Bunin G & Manno CS (1996) 'Recombinant human erythropoietin reduces the need for erythrocyte and platelet transfusions in pediatric patients with sarcoma: a randomized double-blind, placebo-controlled trial' *The Journal of Pediatrics* 129(5): 656–660

Postma TJ & Heimans JJ (2000) 'Grading of chemotherapy-induced peripheral neuropathy' *Annals of Oncology* 11(5): 509–513

Price J (2003) 'Information needs of the child with cancer and their family' *Cancer Nursing Practice* 2(7): 35–38

Protiere C, Evans K, Camerlo J, d'Ingrado MP, Macquart-Moulin G, Viens P, Maraninichi D & Genre D (2002) 'Efficacy and tolerance of a scalp cooling system for the prevention of hair loss and the experience of breast cancer patients treated by adjuvant chemotherapy' *Supportive Care in Cancer* 10(7): 529–537

Randall J & Ream E (2005) 'Hair loss with chemotherapy: at a loss over its management?' *European Journal of Cancer Care* 14(3): 223–231

Reddel RR, Kefford RF, Grant JM, Coates AS, Fox RM & Tattersall MH (1982) 'Ototoxicity in patients receiving cisplatin: importance of dose and method of drug administration' *Cancer Treat Rep* 66: 19–23

Reigle BS & Dienger MJ (2003) 'Sepsis and treatment-induced immunosuppression in the patient with cancer' *Critical Care Nursing Clinics of North America* 15(1): 109–118

Rhodes VA & McDaniel RW (1999) 'The index of nausea, vomiting and retching: a new format of the index of nausea, vomiting and retching' *Oncology Nursing Forum* 26(5): 889–894

Rhodes VA, McDaniel RW, Hanson B, Markway E & Johnson M (1994) 'Sensory perception of patients on selected antineoplastic chemotherapy protocols' *Cancer Nursing* 17(1): 45–51

Rhodes VA, McDaniel RW, Homan SS, Johnson M & Madsen R (2000) 'An instrument to measure symptom experience: symptom occurrence and symptom distress' *Cancer Nursing* 23(1): 49–54

Richardson M, Ellman D, Maguire M, Simpson J & Nicholl A (2001) 'Evidence base of incubation periods, periods of infectiousness and exclusion policies for schools and preschools' *Pediatric Infectious Disease Journal* 20(4): 380–391

Rogers TR (1995) 'Infectious complications of treatment' *Baillière's Clinical Paediatrics* 3(4): 683–698

Roila F, Aapro M & Stewart A (1998) 'Optimal selection of antiemetics in children receiving cancer chemotherapy' *Supportive Care in Cancer* 6(3): 215–220

Royal College of Paediatrics and Child Health (2002) *Immunisation of the Immunocompromised Child: Best Practice Statement*. London: RCPCH

Russo P (2000) 'Urologic emergencies in the cancer patient' *Seminars in Oncology,* 27(3): 284–298

Rust DM, Simpson JK & Lister J (2000) 'Nutritional issues in patients with severe neutropenia' *Seminars in Oncology Nursing* 16(2): 152–162

Salisbury DM & Begg NJ (1996) *Immunisation Against Infectious Diseases*. London: HMSO

Sayfan J, Shoavi O, Koltan L & Benyamin N (1999) 'Acute abdomen caused by neutropenic enterocolitis: surgeon's dilemma' *European Journal of Surgery* 165(5): 502–504

Schell FM (2003) 'Chemotherapy-induced nausea and vomiting: the importance of acute antiemetic control' *The Oncologist* 8(2): 187–198

Schlatter M, Snyder K & Fryer D (2002) 'Successful nonoperative management of typhlitis in pediatric oncology patients' *Journal of Pediatric Surgery* 37(8): 1151–1155

Shelton BK (2003) 'Evidence-based care for the neutropenic patient with leukemia' *Seminars in Oncology Nursing* 19(2): 133–141

Sherry VW (2002) 'Taste alteration among patients with cancer' *Clinical Journal of Oncology Nursing* 6(2): 73–77

Shin YH, Kim TI, Shin MS & Juan H (2004) 'Effect of acupressure on nausea and vomiting during chemotherapy cycle for Korean postoperative cancer patients' *Cancer Nursing* 27(4): 267–274

Siegal T & Haim N (1990) 'Cisplatin-induced peripheral neuropathy: frequent off-therapy deterioration, demyelinating syndromes and muscle cramps' *Cancer* 66(6): 1117–1123

Sieve R & Betcher D (1994) 'Pentamidine' *Journal of Paediatric Oncology Nursing* 11(2): 85–87

Simms S, Hart N, Veves J & Ward F (2002) 'Sibling support in childhood cancer' *Paediatric Nursing* 14(7): 2–22

Smith S (2001) 'Evidence based management of constipation in the oncology patient' *European Journal of Oncology Nursing* 5(1): 18–25

Spivak JL (1994) 'Recombinant erythropoietin and the anaemia of cancer' *Blood* 84(40): 997–1004

Stalkup JR (2002) 'A review of the measles virus' *Dermatologic Clinics* 20(2): 209–215

Stern J & Ippoliti C (2003) 'Management of acute cancer treatment-induced diarrhoea' *Seminars in Oncology Nursing* 19(4): 11–16

Stone M (1993) 'Lending an ear to the unheard: the role of support groups for siblings with cancer' *Child Health* 1(2): 54–58

Stone P, Ream, E, Richardson A, Thomas H, Andrews P, Campbell P, Dawson T, Edwards J, Goldie T, Hammick M, Kearney N, Lean M, Rapley D, Smith AG, Teague C & Young A (2003) 'Cancer-related fatigue – a difference of opinion? Results of a multi-centre survey of healthcare professionals, patients and caregivers' *European Journal of Cancer Care* 12(1): 20–27

Sung L, Nathan PC, Lange B, Beyene J & Buchanan GR (2004) 'Prophylactic granulocyte colony-stimulating factor and granulocyte-macrophage colony-stimulating factor decrease febrile neutropenia after chemotherapy in children with cancer: a meta-analysis of randomized controlled trials' *Journal of Clinical Oncology* 22(16): 3350–3356

Sutton A (1988) 'Cancer cachexia' *Nursing Times* 84(3): 65–66

Terrin BN, McWilliams NB & Maurer HM (1984) 'Side effects of metoclopromide as an antiemetic in childhood cancer therapy' *Journal of Pediatrics* 104(1): 138–140

Theologides A (1979) 'Cancer cachexia' *Cancer* 43(3): 2004–2012

Thielman NM & Guerrant RL (2004) 'Acute infectious diarrhoea' *New England Journal of Medicine* 350(1): 38–47

Thurgood G (1994) 'Nurse maintenance of oral hygiene' *British Journal of Nursing* 3(7): 332–353

Tisdale MJ (1997) 'Cancer cachexia: metabolic alterations and clinical manifestations' *Nutrition* 13(1): 1–7

Torrance C (1990) 'Oral hygiene' *Surgical Nurse* 3(4): 16–20

Tyc VL, Mulhern RK, Raymond K & Bieberich AA (1997) 'Anticipatory nausea and vomiting in pediatric cancer patients: an analysis of conditioning and coping variables' *Journal of Developmental and Behavioural Pediatrics* 18(1): 27–33

van Dalen EC, Caron HN, Dickinson HO & Kremer LCM (2005) 'Cardioprotective interventions for cancer patients receiving anthracyclines' The Cochrane Database of Systematic Reviews, Issue 1

van Fleet S (2000) 'Relaxation and imagery for symptom management: improving patient assessment and individualizing treatment' *Oncology Nursing Forum* 27(3): 501–510

Venturini M, Michelotti A, Del Maestro L, Gallo L, Carnino F, Garrone O, Tibaldi C, Molea N, Bellina RC, Pronzato P, Cyrus P, Vinke J, Testore F, Guelfi M, Lionetto R, Bruzzi P, Conte PF & Rosso R (1996) 'Multicenter randomised controlled clinical trial to evaluate cardioprotection of dexrazane versus no cardioprotection in women receiving epirubicin chemotherapy for advanced breast cancer' *Journal of Clinical Oncology* 14(12): 3112–3120

Vessey JA & Mahon MM (1990) 'Therapeutic play and the hospitalised child' *Journal of Pediatric Nursing* 5(5): 328–333

Vidal L, Paul M, Ben-Dor I, Soares-Weiser K & Leibovici L (2004) 'Oral versus intravenous antibiotic treatment for febrile neutropaenia in cancer patients' The Cochrane Database of Systematic Reviews (online), 4

Vlasveld LT, Ten-Bok K, Hunink WW & Rodenhuis S (1990) 'Neutropenic enterocolitis in a patient with ovarian cancer after treatment with high dose carboplatin and granulocyte macrophage colony stimulating factor (GM-CSF)' *Netherlands Journal of Medicine* 37(3–4): 156–161

von Essen L & Enskär K (2003) 'Important aspects of care and assistance for siblings of children treated for cancer' *Cancer Nursing* 26(3): 203–210

Wall DT & Gabriel LA (1983) 'Alterations of taste in children with leukaemia' *Cancer Nursing* 6(6): 447–452

Ward E (2001) 'Nutritional support: leukaemias, lymphomas and solid tumours' *in*: Shaw V & Lawson M (eds) *Clinical Paediatric Dietetics* (2nd edn). Oxford: Blackwell Science, pp. 351–360

Ward P (1988) 'Antiemesis' *in*: Oakhill A (ed.) *The Supportive Care of the Child with Cancer*. London: Wright

Webster A (2000) 'The facilitating role of the play specialist' *Paediatric Nursing* 12(7): 24–25

Weinstock DM, Boeckh M, Boulad F, Eagan JA, Fraser VJ, Henderson DK, Perl TM, Yokoe D & Sepkowitz KA (2004) 'Postexposure prophylaxis against varicella-zoster virus infection among recipients of hematopoietic stem cell transplant: unresolved issues' *Infection Control and Hospital Epidemiology* 25(7): 603–608

Wesdrop RI, Krause R & Van-Meyenfeldt M (1983) 'Cancer cachexia and its nutritional implications' *British Journal of Surgery* 70(6): 352–355

West NJ (1997) 'Prevention and treatment of hemorrhagic cystitis' *Pharmacotherapy* 17(4): 696–706

Wexler LH, Andrich MP, Venzon D, Berg SL, Weaver-McClure L, Chen CC, Dilsizian V, Avila N, Jarosinski P, Balis FM, Poplack DG & Horowitz ME (1996) 'Randomized trial of the cardioprotective agent ICRF-187 in pediatric sarcoma patients treated with doxorubicin' *Journal of Clinical Oncology* 14(2): 362–372

Whitley RJ (2002) 'Herpes simplex virus infection' *Seminars in Pediatric Infectious Diseases* 13(1): 5–11

Whitley RJ & Roizman B (2001) 'Herpes simplex virus infections' *The Lancet* 357(9267): 1513–1518

Wiernikowski J, Rothney M, Dawson S & Andrew M (1991) 'Evaluation of a home intravenous antibiotic program in pediatric oncology' *American Journal of Pediatric Haematology/Oncology* 13(2): 144–147

Wilkin A & Feinberg JD (1999) 'Pneumocystis carinii pneumonia: a clinical review' *American Family Physician* 60(6): 1699–1708, 1713–1714

Worthington HV, Clarkson JE & Eden OB (2003) 'Interventions for preventing oral candidiasis for patients with cancer receiving treatment' (Cochrane Review) *in*: The Cochrane Library, Issue 1, Oxford: Update Software

Yasko JM (1985) 'Holistic management of nausea and vomiting caused by chemotherapy' *Topics in Clinical Nursing* 7(1): 26–38

Zamula E (2001) 'Shingles: an unwelcome encore' *FDA Consumer* 35(3): 21–25

Zeltzer LK, LeBaron S, Richie M, Reed D, Schoolfield J, & Prihoda TJ (1988) 'Can children understand and use a rating scale to quantify somatic symptoms? Assessment of nausea and vomiting as a model' *Journal of Consulting and Clinical Psychology* 56(4): 567–572

5 Oncological Emergencies

Karen Selwood

Introduction

Emergencies can happen at any time during a child's presentation, diagnosis and ongoing treatment for a malignancy. The nurse needs to be observant for changes in the child's condition and have an understanding of the potential problems they may encounter. Prompt early detection of any problem can help improve the outcome from the emergency encountered. This chapter will address some of the common emergencies relating to or resulting from treatment with chemotherapy.

Septic shock

This is one of the commonest causes of treatment-related mortality in childhood cancer. It is a specific clinical syndrome which is characterised by systemic sepsis with evidence of circulatory insufficiency and inadequate tissue perfusion (Tan, 2002). The mechanism begins with the proliferation of micro-organisms at an infection source which then invade the bloodstream and stimulate both endotoxins and exotoxins. These then have a profound influence on the physiological

mechanisms of the heart, other organs and vasculature (Annane et al., 2005) (Figure 5.1).

Early diagnosis and intervention are essential to pre-empt septic shock, but it can develop from any infectious disease. The onset can be sudden with no previous signs or symptoms and the child may present in a collapsed state. The most common organisms to cause septic shock are Gram-negative ones, such as Pseudomonas, Klebsiella or *Escherichia coli* (Edwards, 2001; Tan, 2002). Any proven Gram-negative infection should be treated with great caution. Gram-positive shock has increased, however, due to the increased use of central and indwelling lines (Tan, 2002).

- *Clinical features* – raised pulse and respiration rate; hypotension or a falling blood pressure; fever, chills; decreased tissue perfusion with pallor, clammy skin and cool extremities; mental confusion, apprehension; and oliguria. In addition, there may be a current history of skin, urinary or gastrointestinal infection or the child may recently have had surgery.
- *Management* – treatment is aimed at optimising perfusion of the critical vascular beds, particularly the kidneys, as there can be a risk of renal failure. The underlying cause needs to be established and treated (Tan, 2002). Therefore,

Cancer in Children and Young People   Edited by Faith Gibson and Louise Soanes
© 2008 John Wiley & Sons, Ltd

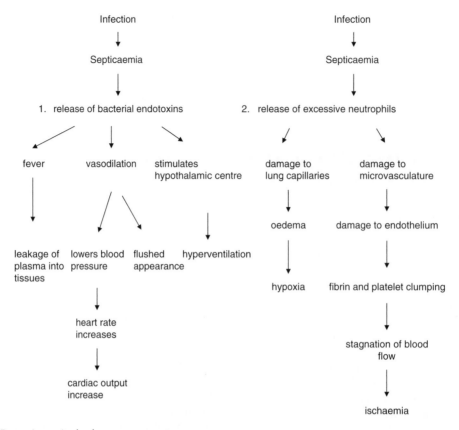

Figure 5.1   Events in septic shock: a two-stage process.

a full septic screen is performed and broad-spectrum antibiotics need to be commenced promptly.

Supportive care involves the use of oxygen therapy to maintain adequate oxygenation to all organs; correction of hypovolaemia with blood, plasma and fluids as required; and antipyretics to control the temperature (Bench, 2004). Close observation of the child is vital as his or her condition can deteriorate quickly, requiring further support with intubation and ventilation.

Nursing care comprises:

- ensuring there is reliable venous access;
- observing the child's general condition carefully;
- administering all medications and supportive measures promptly;
- monitoring temperature, pulse, respiration;
- taking blood pressure frequently;

- monitoring urine output;
- supporting the child and the family during this critical time;
- keeping the parents informed of what is happening to their child and of the child's general condition in an open, honest and supportive manner. Parents will need the opportunity to be involved in care as they feel able and have the opportunity to voice their anxieties.

The general outcome of septic shock usually relates to early recognition and speedy intervention especially in relation to administration of antibiotics (Natsch et al., 2000; Larché et al., 2003).

Home care

A child can deteriorate very quickly with overwhelming sepsis. It is therefore necessary to stress to families the importance of observing the neutropenic child at home for any fever. Parents should also be made aware that they may need to seek help promptly if they are unhappy about the child's general condition, as infection can occur without fever. Paediatric oncology outreach nurse specialists and community children's nurses have an important part to play in reinforcing the information parents receive from their oncology centres.

Written and verbal advice to families on going home after chemotherapy should include the following:

- Take the child's temperature regularly.
- Observe respiratory rate.
- Note if the child's skin colour changes.
- Note if the child is lethargic or off-colour.

- Ring the hospital for advice on any of the above.
- Call an ambulance if the child collapses.

Disseminated intravascular coagulation (DIC)

Disseminated intravascular coagulation (DIC) can be a confusing syndrome because there are several reasons for its occurrence. It is characterised by coagulation and haemorrhage occurring simultaneously (Figure 5.2).

The management of DIC is particularly challenging when children have leukaemia because of the abnormalities in blood formation which are already present. In fact, children with leukaemia may present with features of DIC without actually having the syndrome. This syndrome occurs when the coagulation process is abnormally activated (Table 5.1).

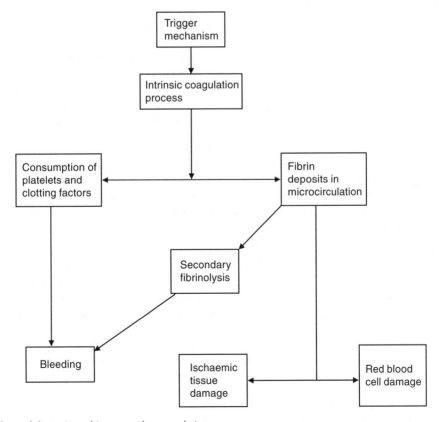

Figure 5.2   Effects of disseminated intravascular coagulation.
Source: Whaley & Wong (1987).

Table 5.1 DIC: Laboratory findings.

	Normal	In DIC
Platelets	150–450,000	decreased
Prothrombin time (PT)	10.5–12.9 sec	prolonged
Partial thrombin time (PTT)*	24.3–36.3 sec	prolonged
Fibrinogen	200–440 mg/100 ml	<150 mg/100 ml
FDP	>10	<40
Haemoglobin (Hb)	>40	decreased

Note: *A raised PTT, decreased platelet count and decreased fibrinogen is generally indicative of DIC.
Source: Adapted from Kurtz (1993).

There is over-activity in four main areas:

1. Extensive thrombus formation in greater amounts than can be neutralised by the body. There is conversion of fibrinogen to fibrin and aggregation and destruction of platelets.
2. Fibrinolysis with destruction of clotting factors and associated haemorrhage.
3. Decreased macrophage clearing function, limiting the removal of activated clotting factors so that obstruction and eventual necrosis of tissue occur.
4. Damage and haemolysis of red blood cells.

DIC is a cluster of symptoms, not a disease and is associated with an underlying condition such as infection, sepsis or newly diagnosed or relapsing acute non-lymphoblastic leukaemia, particularly promyelocytic leukaemia. It occurs less frequently in disseminated neuroblastoma and other metastatic solid tumours. It has been reported that up to 90% of patients with acute promyelocytic leukaemia (APML) have haemorrhagic complications secondary to DIC (Kwaan *et al.*, 2001). DIC can also be associated with transfusions or drug reactions and haemorrhage. It is therefore important to know whether the child has any allergies.

- *Clinical features* – oozing at surface injuries; petechiae, purpura; variable degrees of haemorrhage from multiple sites; and variable degrees of circulatory failure and shock.
- *Management* – the primary management is treatment of the underlying cause and supportive

therapy (Mammen, 2000; Gobel, 2002a). Venous access (usually in the form of a central line) is essential to treat these children as they may require supportive therapy quickly.

Supportive therapy includes broad-spectrum antibiotics; platelets and fresh frozen plasma (if the child has mucosal or internal bleeding); and red cell transfusions to correct anaemia (DeSancho & Rand, 2001). The use of coagulation factors is not recommended as they may be contaminated with activated coagulation factors which may precipitate thrombosis (Levi & Ten Cate, 1999).

The child's prognosis depends on the severity of the DIC and the prognosis of the underlying disease. Close observation of these children is essential, looking for signs of further haemorrhage. Nursing care includes:

- monitoring for an increased thready pulse and decreased blood pressure;
- observing for petechiae (especially in less obvious places such as under the arms);
- discouraging the child from picking their nose or blowing it too hard;
- packing nasal passages if epistaxis occurs;
- avoiding all venepunctures if possible and applying firm pressure if they become essential;
- encouraging gentle mouthcare to avoid trauma to the gums by use of a soft toothbrush or foam sticks;
- avoiding rectal drugs;
- providing psychological care and support (symptoms can be frightening, especially for younger children);
- taking blood samples to monitor U&Es.

Heparin has been used for the treatment of DIC in children but its usefulness has been debated. It may be suggested for use in patients with a thrombotic tendency to prevent the formation of thrombus but a delicate balance is required to prevent unnecessary haemorrhage (Bick, 1998; DeSancho & Rand, 2001). The use of all-trans retinoic acid (ATRA) for patients with APML initiates cell differentiation and appears to have some effect on the potential problems of DIC especially if administered before initiating treatment (Tallman *et al.*, 2002), although there is also some evidence that the continued use of ATRA can improve overall outcome of APML patients (de Botton *et al.*, 2004).

Anaphylaxis

This is a severe life-threatening antigen–antibody response resulting from exposure to a foreign substance, an allergen. Antibodies are produced and attach themselves to the mast cells which remain in the body. Ingestion of subsequent allergens causes a reaction with the mast cells which can lead to a rapid, complex series of events from the mediators released in the body. A reaction occurs which may be exacerbated after each exposure to the allergen (Zanotti & Markman, 2001). It can be extremely frightening for the child and the family as well as the nursing staff.

Anaphylaxis is often associated with specific drugs in paediatric oncology – asparaginase, etoposide, tenoposide and cisplatin. It can also occur during or after transfusion of blood products or administration of antibiotics (most commonly with second or subsequent doses of antibiotics). It can occur very quickly and the child's condition deteriorates rapidly. It can also occur if a child has a specific food allergy.

- *Clinical features* – symptoms of systemic shock (see 'Septic shock' on p. 73), urticaria, itching, paroxysmal coughing, dyspnoea, wheezing, cyanosis, vomiting and anxiety.
- *Management* – removal of the causative agent is vital, therefore stop the transfusion or drug. Maintain venous access, administer oxygen therapy, give drugs as prescribed (e.g. adrenaline, chlorpheniramine), give salbutamol by nebuliser and get expert advice (Chamberlain, 1999).

All staff working within paediatric oncology should be aware of the potential for children to have an anaphylactic reaction to chemotherapy and be aware of local policy on how to deal with this situation. It is essential that all staff are aware of the exact location of appropriate drugs so that they are readily available. Some centres will call the arrest team if such an episode occurs, to ensure that medical assistance arrives promptly but this may not always apply. A record should be kept of reactions, including the cause and the treatment used.

Anaphylaxis is not usually dose-related but an increased frequency of allergic reactions is seen with cumulative doses, high doses, intra-venous administration and single-drug administration (Gobel, 2005).

Asparaginase should be given intramuscularly or subcutaneously in an effort to avoid reactions but the child may still suffer a delayed reaction. Some protocols do advocate the use of intravenous asparaginase and care should be given when it is administered this way. It is recommended that the child remains on the ward or in clinic for at least one hour post-administration so that they can be observed for any late reaction. It is for this reason that asparaginase is not given in the community setting but should always be administered in hospital with resuscitation facilities available.

If the child suffers a mild reaction to a drug, it should be fully documented so that if the drug is given in the future all staff are made aware. The decision may be to administer hydrocortisone and chlorpheniramine 'cover' or avoid further administration of the allergen. The family should be made aware of the drug which caused the reaction, so that they can ensure it is avoided in the future if appropriate. The family should be given instructions as to what to do in an emergency (see 'Septic shock' on p. 73).

Acute tumour lysis syndrome (ATLS)

Acute tumour lysis syndrome (ATLS) is a potentially fatal metabolic complication that occurs as a result of the rapid release of intracellular metabolites (uric acid, potassium, phosphate) from the destruction (lysis) of malignant cells in quantities that exceed the excretory capacity of the kidneys with the initiation of treatment (Jeha, 2001). The metabolic abnormalities that occur are hyperuricaemia (usually in the early phase), hyperkalaemia and hyperphosphataemia with resultant hypocalcaemia; all of which may occur in isolation or in combination (Baeksgaard & Sørensen, 2003). Complications typically manifest within 12–72 hours of the start of chemotherapy (Rheingold & Lange, 2002). The signs and symptoms observed will be directly related to the metabolic changes that are occurring (Figure 5.3). ATLS occurs most commonly in patients who have a large tumour cell burden that is also extremely sensitive to chemotherapeutic agents, for example, B cell lymphoma, T cell leukaemias/lymphomas

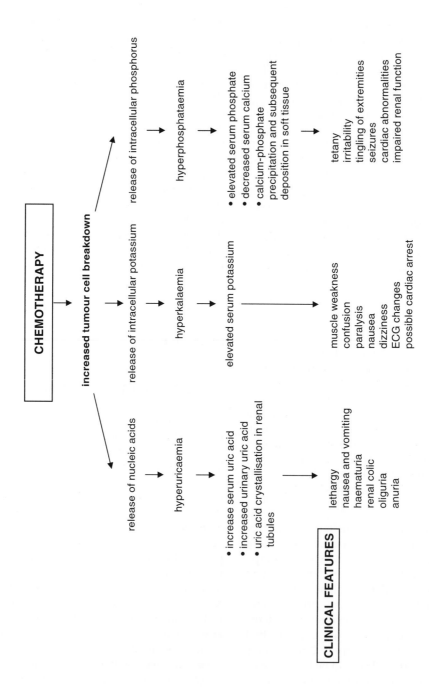

Figure 5.3 Sequence of events in acute tumour lysis syndrome (ATLS).

and children presenting with a high white cell count at diagnosis. It may also occur in children presenting with evidence of renal infiltration at diagnosis. Although rare, this complication has been reported with other solid tumours (Jeha, 2001; Baeksgaard & Sørensen, 2003).

Prevention of ATLS is the main aim; adequate prehydration and regular metabolic evaluation being two of the most important features. Before commencing chemotherapy the child's renal function will be established and a baseline blood pressure and weight recorded. Vigorous hyperhydration is essential and this needs to commence at least 12–24 hours prior to chemotherapy although it must be remembered that this can promote cell lysis. Administration of allopurinol or recombinant urate oxidase also commences at this time to promote the breakdown of uric acid and thus reduce urate precipitation in the renal tubules. A renal ultrasound may be performed to assess whether there are any infiltrates or problems (such as renal enlargement) that may compromise renal function once treatment has commenced.

Liaison with other medical teams that may be involved in the child's care is important, especially the renal service who may provide not only advice regarding management but also haemodialysis; prior knowledge of the child could save time at a later stage. If the child has an extremely high white cell count, leukopheresis may be considered to attempt to lower the white cell count before chemotherapy treatment commences. Although leukopheresis is now rare, it has been shown to prevent severe ATLS in some patients (Maurer et al., 1988), but others have found that in some patients the white cell count only alters by about 30% (Cuttner et al., 1983). Leukopheresis, therefore, could benefit some patients and should be considered as a method to reduce the white cell count if the facility is available (Porcu et al., 2000). Any child who has the potential to develop ATLS should only commence treatment when adequate medical cover is available; commencing chemotherapy in the early hours of the morning ensures that any major problems expected would then hopefully occur later in the day.

Once treatment has started, it is vital to maintain an accurate fluid balance, record weight twice daily and blood pressure at least four hourly, undertake frequent monitoring of urea, electrolytes (in particular, potassium, magnesium and urate), calcium and phosphate, and take action upon any abnormalities (Jeha, 2001). The frequency of monitoring the urea and electrolytes will depend on the previous results, but may be undertaken every 4–6 hours (this may vary within different units). Urine output greater than 3 ml/kg/hr is essential, with frusemide being used to achieve this if oral intake is poor. Cardiac monitoring may be introduced to observe for peaked T waves and dysarhythmias associated with hyperkalaemia.

In relation to the overall management it may take time to organise the insertion of a central venous access device, as well as organise haemodialysis. It is for this reason that some units have introduced indicators, such as:

- absolute indications for haemodialysis: potassium greater than 5 mmol/l; and/or phosphate greater than 2.5 mmol/l; pulmonary oedema; and anuria (ensuring that the bladder is empty, catheterising the child if needed);
- relative indications for haemodialysis: rapid rise in potassium, phosphate or urate; oliguria unresponsive to frusemide; urea greater than 15 mmol/l or creatinine greater than 150 mmol/l.

Medical management requires consideration and correction of each chemical imbalance, thus each metabolic abnormality will be addressed individually.

Hyperuricaemia

Uric acid is the end-product of the metabolism of purines, which are the building blocks of DNA and RNA; the purine bases, xanthine and hypoxanthine, are converted to uric acid by the enzyme, xanthine oxidase. The kidneys eliminate the greatest percentage of uric acid from the body with a small amount being eliminated within the faeces. The normal blood value is 0.1–0.45 mmol/l.

Urinary pH and urinary uric acid concentration are the main factors affecting uric acid solubility in the renal tubules; prolonged dehydration may be an exacerbating factor (Stucky, 1993). Uric acid is insoluble in body fluids and therefore small increases above normal blood value may result in uric acid precipitation. The child's urine needs to be alkaline to aid solubility and excretion. If the urine is acidic and there is excessive uric acid circulating due to the breakdown of tumour cells, deposits of uric acid crystals can occur in the kidneys, ureters and bladder leading to renal failure (Jones *et al.*, 1995). The resulting oliguric renal failure is known as uric acid nephropathy and is potentially life-threatening (Jeha, 2001).

- *Clinical features* – lethargy, nausea and vomiting, haematuria, renal colic, oliguria, anuria (Jones *et al.*, 1995; Jeha, 2001).
- *Management* – aim to decrease uric acid production and increase the solubility of uric acid in the urine. Intravenous hydration commenced prior to chemotherapy is usually calculated at three times maintenance hydration. This will aid the kidneys to excrete the uric acid. Concurrent administration of the drug allopurinol will help decrease uric acid levels as allopurinol inhibits the enzyme xanthine oxidase which is necessary for the production of uric acid, however, it does not reduce the level of uric acid that is already present (Jeha, 2001). Recombinant urate oxidase is also being used to reduce the level of uric acid although there is a small risk of anaphylaxis. It works by catalysing the conversion of uric acid into allatonin which is easily excreted in the urine with less potential for precipitation (Jeha, 2001). Blood samples of children who are on recombinant urate oxidase need to be kept on ice immediately after collection, during transport and before analysis as there continues to be a breakdown of the uric acid in the sample and results will be incorrect (Lim *et al.*, 2003). Maintaining an alkaline urine may also help excrete the uric acid, however, there is some debate as to whether sodium bicarbonate should be included in the hydration fluid as it may enhance the deposition of calcium phosphate or xanthine precipitation in the renal tubules (Flombaum, 2000; Baeksgaard & Sørensen, 2003). Ten Harkel *et al.* (1998) suggest only using sodium bicarbonate hydration when plasma levels of uric acid are increased and discontinuing once normal. Overall, alkalisation of urine is not recommended if the fluid input is adequate (Flombaum, 2000).

If the child develops renal failure, dialysis will be necessary, preferably haemodialysis as this achieves a more rapid reduction of plasma uric acid and prompt correction of any other electrolyte abnormalities (Jeha, 2001). Within some units the insertion of a rigid dialysis catheter is selected as a precaution at the start of prehydration. These lines are more rigid and have a wider bore; thus are more suitable for haemodialysis than other types of central venous access devices.

Hyperkalaemia

Normally 98 % of the body's potassium is intracellular. However, with ATLS, intracellular potassium is released as the tumour cells are destroyed, causing an elevation in serum potassium (Cantril & Haylock, 2004). Dehydration and acidosis may accentuate the problem as both result in extracellular shifts of potassium. In addition, as the kidneys play an important role in maintaining potassium balance, uric acid nephropathy or calcium deposits will affect the excretion of potassium and therefore exacerbate hyperkalaemia. Normal blood value for potassium is 3.5–5.0 mmol/l.

- *Clinical features* – muscle weakness, cramps, confusion, paralysis, nausea, dizziness, ECG abnormalities (elevated T waves, prolonged PR, QRS and ST segments and arrhythmias) and possible cardiac arrest (Cairo & Bishop, 2004).
- *Management* – includes decreasing potassium intake, facilitating the shift of extracellular potassium and aiding excretion. In the presence of hyperkalaemia, intravenous hydration fluids, containing no added potassium, will need to be increased. Urine output may need to be maintained by use of frusemide. In theory, the child should not be given any foods containing potassium (such as bananas, fruit juices, malted drinks, Marmite, potato crisps, chocolate and milk). In practice, however, this is rarely an issue due to a general poor oral intake.

Close monitoring of electrolyte levels during treatment induction is essential. If the potassium level is increasing then the administration of a potassium binding resin, such as 'Kayexalate' (sodium polystyrene sulfonate), may be indicated (Jeha,

2001; Gobel, 2002b). This can be given orally or rectally. However, as it is unpalatable to swallow, either a nasogastric tube may need to be passed or the rectal route selected. Once it is mixed, it becomes quite thick and may need further dilution to administer via the nasogastric tube or to be given rectally.

Occasionally calcium gluconate or glucose and insulin may also be given intravenously to help shift the extracellular potassium back into the cells, consequently reducing serum levels, improving myocardial function and restoring a normal ECG (Flombaum, 2000). Patterson and Klopovich (1987) suggest that the child has a cardiac monitor if there are significant ECG changes, however, nursing staff need to be able to recognise abnormalities promptly for this to be of benefit. Salbutamol (either intravenously or nebulised) has also been used to lower potassium by shifting the extracellular potassium back into the cells (McClure *et al.*, 1994). However, Mahoney *et al.* (2005) recognise that the combination of nebulised or inhaled salbutamol and IV insulin and glucose may be most effective if the hyperkalaemia is severe. If the serum potassium continues to rise, then haemodialysis would be indicated. In some units haemodialysis is introduced as a first-line measure.

Hyperphosphataemia and hypocalcaemia

Hyperphosphataemia results from the release of intracellular phosphate into the blood during ATLS. This then interacts with the extracellular calcium causing a precipitation of calcium salts and subsequent hypocalcaemia (Jones *et al.*, 1995). Calcium phosphate crystals precipitate in the microvascular and renal tubules which can lead to tissue damage and hypocalcaemia. Hypocalcaemia results from hyperphosphataemia and the inverse relationship between calcium and phosphate (Jones *et al.*, 1995; Cantril & Haylock, 2004).

Normal blood values are:

calcium – infant 1.75–3 mmol/l, child 2–2.6 mmol/l;
phosphate – at 1 year 1.23–2.1 mmol/l, at 2–5 years 1.13–2.20 mmol/l, above 5 years 0.97–1.45 mmol/l.

- *Clinical features* – usually asymptomatic from hyperphosphataemia, symptoms are related to the resulting hypocalcaemia; numbness, tingling of extremities, irritability, muscle cramping and seizures, cardiac abnormalities (prolonged QT interval) and impaired renal function (Altman, 2001). On physical examination carpopedal spasm and a positive Chvostek or Trousseau's sign may be evident (Stucky, 1993).

- *Management* – in theory, an increase in phosphate intake needs to be avoided by excluding food items such as bran, hard cheeses, nuts, dried fruit and vegetables. In practice (due to general poor oral intake) this is rarely followed. Administration of aluminium hydroxide orally will enhance excretion of phosphate in the stool but it can also precipitate constipation, and this should be avoided if possible. If they are used, laxatives should also be prescribed at the same time. Correction of the high phosphate should increase the hypocalcaemia. It can be corrected by intravenous calcium gluconate but is avoided if possible as it can lead to metastatic calcifications (Flombaum, 2000).

Nursing implications of ATLS

Nursing staff need to be aware of the children who may develop ATLS. Preventative measures can be taken as recommended, with the child observed closely. Any abnormalities that do occur need to be reported promptly and action should be taken to prevent further complications. During this time the family is going to be under considerable stress, initially from the diagnosis and treatment and then from the possible complications. Frequent explanations should be provided on what is happening, how it is being managed and the expected outcome. Preparation should incorporate the possibility of the child being transferred to another unit, such as a renal or intensive care unit. Although such a transfer is usually temporary, none the less, it will increase the overall anxiety of the family. They will need support from all members of the multidisciplinary team to help them through this difficult period. The child will also be anxious and frightened and will need support and reassurance. During this time the child will need close observation, numerous blood tests and some unpleasant procedures. Full explanations of all of this will help the child and the family to deal with this situation.

Spinal cord compression

Spinal cord compression can occur at any time but is often seen at diagnosis, usually relating to neuroblastoma, Ewing's sarcoma, non-Hodgkin's lymphoma (NHL), Hodgkin's disease or at relapse (Lewis *et al.*, 1986). Prolonged compression will cause irreversible neurological damage with paralysis, sensory loss and sphincter incompetence and is therefore treated as an emergency (Kelly & Lange, 1997; Osowski, 2002). It usually occurs from epidural compression from extension of a paravertabral tumour through the intervertebral foramina (Prasad & Schiff, 2005).

- *Clinical features* – back pain (localised or radiating), weakness, sensory loss, incontinence secondary to sphincter disturbance although this is usually a late sign, paralysis.
- *Management* – diagnosis is confirmed by an MRI scan which needs to include the whole spine to exclude potential multiple areas of compression (Bucholtz, 1999). If there is rapid dysfunction, then immediate treatment is required as the prognosis depends on the severity at diagnosis and the duration of symptoms and time to diagnosis. The initial aim of treatment is to relieve pain and to try and maintain or restore neurological function. Often intravenous steroids are administered initially to reduce oedema while the need for appropriate treatment in the form of radiotherapy, surgery or chemotherapy is considered (Bucholtz, 1999). Radiation therapy is often used to treat compression (see Part 4). Surgery is considered if the tumour is not chemotherapy- or radiotherapy-sensitive (Flounders & Ott, 2003) or may be used to debulk the tumour while waiting for further treatment. Chemotherapy has an effect on certain tumours, particularly neuroblastoma, NHL, Hodgkin's disease and Ewing's sarcoma (Sanderson *et al.*, 1989; Geetha *et al.*, 1999).

Families will find this a frightening and difficult time. It is important to keep them informed and involved in their child's care and treatment. Special attention will be required to the skin, and close monitoring of the child's bladder and bowel function. Any changes in function and mobility should be recorded to allow subtle changes to be noted and if necessary acted upon (Flounders & Ott, 2003). Assistance may need to be given if the child is mobile to ensure they can do so safely and this will need the assistance of physiotherapists to assess and plan their ongoing needs. If and when mobility returns there will need to be a period of rehabilitation and possibly adaption to limited mobility and the changes that will bring to their life.

Conclusion

The treatment and prognosis for children with cancer continue to change and challenge nurses in their everyday practice. Early recognition of any abnormalities, especially any which if acted upon quickly may improve the outcome for the child, is vital.

References

Altman A (2001) 'Acute tumor lysis syndrome' *Seminars in Oncology* 28(2 supplement): 3–8

Annane D, Bellissant E. & Cavaillon J. (2005) 'Septic shock' *The Lancet* 365(9453): 63–78

Baeksgaard L & Sørensen JB (2003) 'Acute tumor lysis syndrome in solid tumors – a case report and review of the literature' *Cancer Chemotherapy Pharmacology* 51(3): 187–192

Bench S (2004) 'Clinical skills: assessing and treating shock: a nursing perspective' *British Journal of Nursing* 13(12): 715–721

Bick RL (1998) 'Disseminated intravascular coagulation: objective clinical and laboratory diagnosis, treatment and assessment of therapeutic response' *Seminars in Thrombosis and Hemostasis* 22(1): 69–88

Bucholtz JD (1999) 'Metastatic epidural spinal cord compression' *Seminars in Oncology Nursing* 15(3): 150–159

Cairo MS & Bishop M (2004) 'Tumour lysis syndrome: new therapeutic strategies and classification' *British Journal of Haematology* 127(1): 3–11

Cantril CA & Haylock PJ (2004) 'Tumor lysis syndrome' *American Journal of Nursing* 104(4): 49–52

Chamberlain B (1999) 'Emergency medical treatment of anaphylactic reactions: Project Team of the Resuscitation Council UK' *Journal of Accident and Emergency Medicine* 16(4): 243–247

Cuttner J, Holland JF, Norton L, Ambinder E, Button G & Meyer RJ (1983) 'Therapeutic leukopheresis for hyperleukocytosis in acute myelocytic leukaemia' *Medical and Pediatric Oncology* 11(2): 76–78

de Botton S, Coiteux V, Chevret S, Rayon C, Vilmer E, Sanz M, de La Serna J, Philippe N, Baruchel A, Leverger G, Robert A, San Miguel J, Conde E, Sotto JJ, Bordessoule D, Fegueux N, Fey M, Parry A, Chomienne C, Degos L & Fenaux P (2004) 'Outcome of childhood acute promyelocytic leukaemia with All-Trans-Retinoic-acid and chemotherapy' *Journal of Clinical Oncology* 22(8): 1404–1412

DeSancho MT & Rand J.H (2001) 'Bleeding and thrombotic complications in critically ill patients with cancer' *Critical Care Clinics* 17(3): 599–622

Edwards S (2001) 'Shock: types, classifications and explorations of their physiological effects' *Emergency Nurse* 9(2): 29–38

Flombaum CD (2000) 'Metabolic emergencies in the cancer patient' *Seminars in Oncology* 27(3): 322–334

Flounders JA & Ott BB (2003) 'Continuing education: oncology emergency modules: spinal cord compression' *Oncology Nursing Forum* 30(1). Online exclusive

Geetha N, Hussain BM, Ratheesan K, Ramachandran K, Chandralekha B & Nair MK (1999) 'Intraspinal leukaemia with cord compression' *Medical and Pediatric Oncology* 33(2): 132–133

Gobel BH (2002a) 'Disseminated intravascular coagulation in cancer: providing quality care' *Topics in Advanced Practice Nursing, eJournal* 2(4)

Gobel BH (2002b) 'Management of tumor lysis syndrome: prevention and management' *Seminars in Oncology Nursing* 18(3): 12–16

Gobel BH (2005) 'Chemotherapy-induced hypersensitivity reactions' *Oncology Nursing Forum.* 2(5): 1027–1035

Jeha S (2001) 'Tumor lysis syndrome' *Seminars in Hematology* 38(4): 4–8

Jones DP, Mahoud H & Cheney RW (1995) 'Tumor lysis syndrome: pathogenesis and management' *Pediatric Nephrology* 9(2): 206–212

Kelly KM & Lange B (1997) 'Oncologic emergencies' *Pediatric Clinics of North America* 44: 809–830

Kurtz A (1993) 'Disseminated intravascular coagulation with leukaemia patients' *Cancer Nursing.* 16(6): 456–463

Kwaan HC, Wang J. & Boggio LN (2001) 'Abnormalities in hemostasis in acute promyelocytic leukaemia' *Hematological Oncology* 20(1): 33–41

Larché J, Azoulay E,. Fieux F, Mesnard, L, Moreau, D, Thiery, G, Darmon, M, Le Gall, J & Schlemmer, B (2003) 'Improved survival of critically ill cancer patients with septic shock' *Intensive Care Medicine* 29(10): 1688–1695

Levi, M & Ten Cate H (1999) 'Disseminated intravascular coagulation' *New England Journal of Medicine* 341(8): 586

Lewis DW, Packer RJ, Raney B, Rak IW, Belasco J & Lange B (1986) 'Incidence, presentation and outcome of spinal cord disease in children with systemic cancer' *Pediatrics* 78(3): 438–443

Lim E, Bennett P & Beilby J (2003) 'Sample preparation in patients receiving uric acid oxidase (rasburicase) therapy' *Clinical Chemistry* 49(8): 14–17

Mahoney BA, Smith WAD, Lo DS, Tsoi K, Tonelli M & Clase CM (2005) 'Emergency interventions for hyperkalaemia' *The Cochrane Library* (Oxford), No. 4

Mammen EF (2000) 'Disseminated intravascular coagulation' *Clinical Laboratory Science* 13(4): 239–249

Maurer HS, Steinherz PG, Gaynon PS, Finklestein JZ, Sather HN, Reaman GH, Bleyer WA & Hammond GD (1988) 'Management of hyperleukocytosis in childhood with acute lymphoblastic leukaemia' *Journal of Clinical Oncology* 6(9): 1425–1432

McClure RJ, Prasad VK & Brocklebank JT (1994) 'Treatment of hyperkalaemia using intravenous and nebulised salbutamol' *Archives of Disease in Childhood* 70(2): 126–128

Natsch S, Kullberg BJ, Meis JF & van der Meer JW (2000) 'Earlier initiation of antibiotic treatment for severe infections after interventions to improve the organization and specific guidelines in the emergency department' *Archives of Internal Medicine* 160(9): 1317–1320

Osowski M (2002) 'Spinal cord compression: an obstructive oncologic emergency' *Topics in Advanced Practice Nursing eJournal* 2(4)

Patterson KL & Klopovich P (1987) 'Metabolic emergencies in pediatric oncology: the acute tumor lysis syndrome' *JAPON* 4(3/4): 19–24

Porcu P, Cripe LD, Ng EW, Bhatia S, Danielson CM, Orazi A & McCarthy LJ (2000) 'Hyperleukocytic leukemias and leukostasis: a review of pathophysiology, clinical presentation and management' *Leukaemia and Lymphoma* 39(1–2): 1–18

Prasad D & Schiff D (2005) 'Malignant spinal-cord compression' *Lancet Oncology* 6(1): 15–24

Rheingold SR & Lange BJ (2002) 'Oncologic emergencies' in: Pizzo PA & Poplack DG (eds) *Principles and Practice of Pediatric Oncology* (4th edn). Philadelphia: Lippincott, Williams & Wilkins

Sanderson IR, Pritchard J, Marsh HT (1989) 'Chemotherapy as the initial treatment of spinal neuroblastoma' *Journal of Neurosurgery* 10(5): 73

Stucky LA (1993) 'Acute tumour lysis syndrome; assessment and nursing implications' *Oncology Nursing Forum* 20(1): 49–57

Tallman MS, Nabhan C, Feusner JH. & Rowe JM (2002) 'Acute promyelocytic leukaemia: evolving therapeutic strategies' *Blood* 99(3): 759–767

Tan SJ (2002) 'Recognition and treatment of oncologic emergencies' *Journal of Infusion Nursing* 25(3): 182–188

Ten Harkel ADJ, Kist-Van Holthe JE, Van Weel M & Van der Vorst MMJ (1998) 'Alkalinization and the tumor lysis syndrome' *Medical and Pediatric Oncology* 31(1): 27–28

Whaley LF & Wong DL (1987) *Nursing Care of Infants and Children* (3rd edn). St Louis, MO@ CV Mosby

Zanotti KM & Markman M (2001) 'Prevention and management of antineoplastic-induced hypersensitivity reactions' *Drug Safety* 24(10): 767–779

6 Future Trends

Karen Selwood

Introduction

Developments in chemotherapy treatment have been matched by progress in nursing practice in response to the needs of children and their families. Intensive, multiple-drug chemotherapy schedules have drastically improved the prognosis of most childhood malignancies, but have increased the toxicities experienced by children receiving treatment. Knowledge of the potential side effects of chemotherapy regimes, in both the short and long term, has enabled the design of strategies aimed at prevention and monitoring, and the provision of appropriate treatment and support. This has meant that more children survive the potentially lethal effects of cytotoxic treatment and thereby have the best possible chance of surviving their cancer.

As new treatments are developed, paediatric oncology nurses face fresh demands upon their practice. If nurses are to be able to meet the needs of future patients, they must be involved in discussions about the care those patients may require. All aspects of paediatric nursing practice, patient and family care, research, the management of services, and professional education, must meet the challenges presented by treatment innovations if the achievements of the past are to be sustained into the future.

Rapidly advancing scientific knowledge of specific tumour types, the genetic basis of cancers, the behaviour of normal and malignant cells and the exact mechanisms by which chemotherapy agents exert their cytotoxic effect are increasingly influencing treatment developments. As more is known about prognostic indicators of specific tumour types and presentations, drug treatments are becoming more 'tailored' to the needs of individuals.

Treatment strategies continue to be developed with two interrelated aims:

1. to increase survival from tumours where classic agents have had limited therapeutic impact;
2. to limit the toxicities of treatment (Lashford, 2004).

The ideal cancer therapy would be one that was capable of eradicating all malignant cells while causing no harm to the patient. As yet, this is not available, and treatment developments are attempting to improve the efficacy of existing drugs, alongside development of new agents and innovative approaches to therapy. This chapter explores future possibilities for progress in treatment for childhood cancer, based on current treatment trends and research activities, and discusses the possible implications of these for nursing practice.

Treatment strategies

Historically, the major breakthroughs in cancer treatment occurred when the existing treatment modalities were, in their turn, introduced. By refining their use, alone and in combination, their effectiveness has increased. Two-thirds of children with cancer are now cured, and advances in the treatment of the still-incurable minority are likely to be on a smaller scale than previously. It is possible that the limits of existing modalities have been reached and that further refinements in their application will make small steps, rather than giant leaps forward. Research into new chemotherapy agents and strategies to optimise the use of existing drugs continues, but for those malignancies that are proving largely incurable despite contemporary therapies, perhaps entirely different approaches are required, rather than new drugs. Increased scientific understanding of cellular biology and the genetic basis of malignant transformation paves the way for novel treatment approaches. Some exploit the natural control and defence mechanisms of the body, whereas others seek to alter the DNA within cancer cells to therapeutic advantage. Understanding of how cancer cells survive, thrive and metastasise has enabled research to focus on creating targeted therapies to try and minimise harmful side effects. Some of them will be briefly discussed here.

Targeted approaches

Antibodies are normally produced by B lymphocytes in response to an antigenic stimuli that have an ability to bind to tumour antigens with high specificity and selectivity (Weiner, 1999). Increased knowledge of tumour biology and anti-tumour properties of antibodies resulted in the development of monoclonal antibodies. To obtain monoclonal antibodies there is a need to immunise an animal (usually a mouse) and then obtain immune cells from its spleen and fuse the cell with a cancer cell to make them immortal, i.e.

they will grow and divide indefinitely (Sanders, 2002). The tumour of the fused cells is called a hybridoma and these cells secrete monoclonal antibodies. This allows the production of substantial quantities of highly purified material suitable for clinical use (Weiner, 1999). Monoclonal antibodies are now being designed which recognise specific antigens, alter activity of the targeted antigen, recruit immune cells to destroy the cells and initiate apoptosis (Gemmill & Smith Idell, 2003).

Cancer cells secrete growth factors which enable their continued division and evasion of cell death (apoptosis). These factors are essential to the cell's ability to obtain a blood supply, proliferate, thrive and metastasise and include vascular endothelial growth factor (VEGF), epidermal growth factor (EGF) and its receptor (EGFR) (Capriotti, 2005). In cancer cells these appear to be overexpressed and serve as potential targets for treatment (Nam & Parang, 2003). Proteasome, a molecular complex that has a role in cell metabolism and regulates cell death, is also thought to be an appropriate target as this will block proliferation and induce self-destruction of the cancer cell (Mitchell, 2003).

Vascular endothelial growth factor (VEGF)

VEGF is necessary for the development of new blood vessels (angiogenesis) needed for tumour growth and in the majority of solid tumours there is an increased expression (Meisheid, 2005). Genetic mutations such as the loss of the tumour suppressor gene function (see p. 87) can cause a decrease in angiogenesis inhibitors and enhance VEGF secretion (Muehlbauer, 2003). Monoclonal antibodies can target the VEGF to prevent tumour receptor binding to epithelial cells stopping the processs of angiogenesis (Yarbo et al., 2005). Without new blood vessels the tumour's growth is halted. Bevacizumub (Avastatin) is a monoclonal antibody directed against VEGF and used in trials for renal cell carcinoma, non-small cell lung cancer and metastatic breast cancer.

Epidermal growth factor receptor (EGFR)

EGFR is a gycoprotien on the outside of the cell membrane that is expressed in cells of epithelial origin. It is overexpressed in several tumours including head and neck, pancreatic, colon, breast. This can indicate poor prognosis, increased reoccurrence and decreased survival (Woodburn, 1999). As EGFR is increased in tumour cells and is involved in the signalling pathways that regulate cell division, repair, and survival, then if it is inhibited, tumour growth may be halted (Meisheid, 2005).

About 30% of women with breast cancer overexpress the HER2 gene located on chromosome 17q21, which is related to a poor prognosis (Sanders, 2002). Trastuzamub (Herceptin) is a monoclonal antibody which targets the epitome on the extracellar domain of the HER2 and blocks the receptor which inhibits the growth (Weiner, 1999). As it is able to target specific cells and is also selective about the cells it interacts with, it also has minimal side effects (Stebbing et al., 2000).

Tyrosine kinase inhibitors

EGFR has components both outside and inside cells. The intracellular element contains a signal transduction enzyme known as tyrosine kinase. There has been development of EGFR tyrosine inhibitors which are small molecule compounds that compete or interact with adenosine triphosphate binding sites. Gefitinib is an EGFR-tyrosine kinase inhibitor which blocks signal transduction and results in decreased angiogenesis, increased apoptosis and fewer tendencies for invasion and metastatic potential and has been used in advanced non-small cell lung cancer (Yarbo et al., 2005).

Bcr-Abl is a gene present on the Philadelphia chromosome and is a tyrosine kinase oncogene that is uniquely causative to chronic myeloid leukaemia. Imatinib mesylate (Glivac) is a non-EGFR tyrosine kinase inhibitor that blocks the binding site of tyrosine kinase which then prevents the transmission of signals needed for cellular proliferation (Meisheid, 2005). This has been used in trials for the treatment of Philadelphia-positive chronic myeloid leukaemia with some success (Gale, 2003).

Proteasome

Proteasome is a macromolecular complex within all cells essential for metabolism. Inhibition of proteasome activity causes cell growth inhibition and cell death and, although not well understood, apoptosis shows tumour cell selectivity (Veal & Newell, 2004). Bortezomib is a proteasome inhibitor which has been developed and shown to be effective in refractory multiple myeloma (Richardson et al., 2003). Further work is ongoing and in particular it is also enhances the apoptotic effect of conventional chemotherapy agents (ironetecan, doxorubicin) and radiotherapy which may have implications for future practice (Mitchell, 2003).

The ongoing research into the targeted therapies in adults may provide opportunities to discover more effective treatments for paediatric malignancies in the future, however, there needs to be more research to support their use in practice (Smith, 2006).

Gene therapy

Gene therapy is the process of transferring selected genes into a host with the hope of halting or curing a disease (Robertson & Fritz, 1996). It was initially seen as a way to treat genetic disorders but now covers a wide range of diseases including cancer. It can be used to destroy cancer by correcting a genetic defect, manipulating genes or both (Rieger, 2001).

A number of mutant oncogenes and fusion transcripts have been identified in childhood cancers that have an impact on the malignant process but often there are multiple abnormalities. Correction of these abnormalities is difficult as correction of a single deficit may leave multiple pre-malignant cells still in situ leading only to a transient benefit (Brenner, 2002).

Another approach is to neutralise transdominant malignant genes by destroying the function of an expressed gene (Brenner, 2002). Ribozymes may be used to destroy transcripts from the unwanted host cell DNA sequence while leaving the messenger RNA originating from the transgene (Brenner, 2002). Sometimes these can be delivered at the same time as a corrective gene or they may be chemically modified and administered as a drug. At the moment there is still limited use in practice.

Genes are transferred into the patient via a vector (carrier) which can be a DNA injection or chemicals, e.g. liposome encapsulation, or viral. Viruses are used as they have an innate ability to insert genetic material into the cytoplasm or genome of a host cell (Chester & Hull, 2002). A virus that is commonly used as a vector is adenovirus which is genetically modified to prevent infection of other cells. Trials in adults are under way in liver, head and neck and prostate cancer using adenovirus vectors for the gene therapy (Chester & Hull, 2002).

Tumour vaccines

Vaccination involves the administration of an agent that stimulates the immune system to react against the foreign substances (antigens) of the vaccine. It is expected that the person will then develop immunity so subsequent exposure to the antigen will initiate an immune response to destroy the antigen (Muehlbauer & Schwartzentruber, 2003). The aim of a cancer vaccine is to mobilise the immune system to attack the cancer cells by targeting and destroying tumour-associated antigens which are present on tumour cells. However, the tumour-associated antigens must be recognised as foreign by the immune system and then the immune system needs to respond to the antigen by a proliferation of T cells. These T cells should then find the tumour expressing the same antigen and destroy it (Muehlbauer & Schwartzentruber, 2003).

Clinical trials have been undertaken for a variety of conditions including melanoma, renal cell carcinoma, B cell lymphoma, Hodgkin's lymphoma and chronic myeloid leukaemia (Dermime et al., 2002). In malignant melanomas the vaccines aim to increase specific cellular and humoral responses (T and B cell responses), enhance dendritic cells' capacity to prevent antigens to T cells, thus promoting immune response and promote resistance to local immunosuppressive factors secreted in melanomas (Demierre et al., 2005a). There have been no large randomised trials to demonstrate an overall survival advantage but the use of vaccine trials is offered to patients in the United States of America as part of the melanoma guidelines (NCCN, 2006). Vaccines have relatively few side effects (fatigue and local inflammatory skin reactions) compared to conventional chemotherapy (Demierre et al., 2005b). There has been little research in paediatrics but this may be an area where further advances may come in the future.

Hormone therapy

Growth of 70–80% of all breast cancers are stimulated by oestrogen and respond well to treatment that interferes with or blocks the production of oestrogen (Cancer Research UK, 2005). Tamoxifen, which blocks oestrogen receptors within each cancer cell, thereby preventing circulating oestrogens from stimulating their growth, has been used for many years although it has stimulatory effects and may lead to endometrial carcinoma in a small number of people (Harmer, 2005). Aromatase inhibitors, a new class of hormone treatment, work by blocking the conversion of the enzyme aromatase, found in fatty tissue, which is the main source of oestrogen in the post-menopausal women whose ovaries have stopped functioning. With less oestrogen available the growth of oestrogen-sensitive cancer cells is slowed down or stopped and tumour size may reduce (Harmer, 2005). This specifically has a use in post-menopausal hormone-sensitive breast cancer. At the moment there is no evidence that hormone therapies will have a use in paediatrics, however, this may change in the future.

Combination therapy

The future of chemotherapy and radiotherapy may be improved by the addition of any of the above therapies. Many of the targeted therapies require a longer treatment period before a true response can be seen. The combination of conventional treatment and target-based therapy may allow the initial tumour burden to be reduced while waiting for the effect of the targeted treatment (Nam & Parang, 2003). It may also allow optimal therapy as they have different mechanisms of action. This is another area where research is being undertaken and may impact the way care is delivered in the future.

New treatments for cancer – the nurse's role

Research into new therapies is a prerequisite for advances in treatment, but presents many challenges. Participation in trials of investigational treatments may be offered when all known therapeutic options have been exhausted, when efforts are usually directed at symptom control and providing emotional support for families who are facing the death of their child. Conducting research within the context of palliative care is challenging (Ling & Penn, 1995), and can create tensions within the multidisciplinary team, as some people perceive any research involving dying patients as exploitative (Thorpe, 1992). Conflicts may also arise in relation to what course of action is considered to be in the best interests of the child if the parents make decisions that nurses disagree with (Akers & Bell, 1994). Nurses involved in trials of potential new treatments play a pivotal role in the ethical conduct of the research, and often bear the brunt of such conflicts (Cogliano-Shutta, 1986). Working with families participating in investigational drug trials requires knowledge, open communication, sensitivity and organisational skills in order to meet the needs of the terminally ill child and his family while fulfilling the rigorous requirements of clinical research.

Rieger (2001) describes the multifaceted role of nurses working in clinical trials as: patient and family education, direct caregiving, accurate implementation of study procedures and data collection. The research nurse is in a unique position, working with families, medical staff, trial coordinators (often from the pharmaceutical industry) and other nursing teams. The needs and perceptions of these groups may be disparate; the research nurse must maintain good working relationships with all parties while working effectively and ethically.

The families of terminally ill children are vulnerable, and their desire to avoid or delay their child's death may make them susceptible to suggestions that a new treatment strategy may hold a last hope of cure. It is vital, therefore, that full and frank discussion regarding what is offered by trial participation takes place, and that they are not pressured into making a decision. The role of the research nurse as advocate for families is critical (Ocker & Plank, 2000) to ensure that, whatever decision is made, when the child eventually dies, it is not regretted.

Consent to trial participation must be freely given and informed, and families must be reassured that a decision not to participate, or to withdraw, may be made at any time without having to give a reason, and without fear of prejudice regarding their child's future care (British Paediatric Association, 1992). Clearly written information about the nature of the trial, the alternatives that exist, what participation will involve, and the possible benefits to the child and to society should be given in addition to verbal discussion (Hendrick, 1997). Booklets concerning the conduct of clinical trials have been produced for adult patients, and may prove useful for parents and teenage patients (BACUP, 2004). The consent of competent minors and the assent of younger children to undergo new therapies should be sought, and reconfirmed throughout the trial, based on information that is appropriate to their age, understanding, previous experience and concerns (Terry & Campbell, 2001).

Withdrawal of children from new agent studies, due to deteriorating health, toxicity or the wishes of the family, is a difficult and emotionally charged event. The family may have perceived, despite explicit and honest discussion prior to and during the trial, that the new drug offered a final hope, which has now faded. It is important to stress here that participation in research trials does not preclude excellent symptom management or the process of psychological support in preparation for the child's eventual death, and by ensuring that the child and family have enjoyed the continued support and input from the hospital and community nursing teams throughout the trial, the transition to palliative care may be eased.

References

Akers JA & Bell SK (1994) 'Should children be used as research subjects?' Nursing Forum 29(3): 28–33

BACUP (2004) www.cancerbacup.org (accessed March 2006)

Brenner MK (2002) 'Gene transfer and the treatment of pediatric malignancy' in: Pizzo PA & Poplack DG (eds) Principles and Practice of Pediatric Oncology (4th edn). Philadelphia: Lippincott, Williams & Wilkins

British Paediatric Association (1992) Guidelines for the Ethical Conduct of Medical Research Involving Children. London: British Paediatric Association

Cancer Research UK (2005) www.cancerresearchuk.org. Accessed March 2006

Capriotti T (2005) 'New oncology strategy: molecular targeting of cancer cells' *Dermatology Nursing* 17(3): 181–185

Chester M & Hull D (2002) 'The role of the gene therapy nurse in cancer care' *Cancer Nursing Practice* 1(8): 25–29

Cogliano-Shutta NA (1986) 'Pediatric phase 1 clinical trials: ethical issues and nursing considerations' *Oncology Nurses Forum* 13(2): 29–32

Demierre M, Alten & Brown R (2005a) 'New treatments for melanoma' *Dermatology Nursing* 17(4): 287–296

Demierre M, Swetter SM & Sondak VK (2005b) 'Vaccine therapy of melanoma: an update' *Current Cancer Therapy Reviews* 1(2): 115–125

Dermime S, Armstrong A, Hawkins RE & Stern PL (2002) 'Cancer vaccines and immunotherapy' *British Medical Bulletin* 62(1): 149–162

Gale DM (2003) 'Molecular targets in cancer therapy' *Seminars in Oncology Nursing* 19(3): 193–205

Gemmill R & Smith Idell C (2003) 'Biological advances for new treatment approaches' *Seminars in Oncology Nursing* 19(3): 162–168

Gill D (2004) 'Ethical principles and operational guidelines for good clinical practice in paediatric research: recommendations of the Ethics Working Group of the Confederation of European Specialists in Paediatrics (CESP)' *European Journal of Pediatrics* 163(2): 53–57

Harmer V (2005) 'Breast cancer: new treatments, new strategies' *British Journal of Nursing* 14(16): 844–845

Hendrick J (1997) *Legal Aspects of Child Health Care* London: Chapman & Hall

Lashford LS (2004) 'Novel approaches to therapy' *in*: Pinkerton R, Plowman PN & Pieters R (eds) *Paediatric Oncology* (3rd edn). London: Arnold, pp. 573–582

Ling J & Penn K (1995) The challenge of conducting clinical trials in palliative care' *International Journal of Palliative Nursing* 1(1): 31–34

McIntosh N, Bates P, Brykczynska G, Dunstan G, Goldman A, Harvey D, Larcher V, McCrae D, McKinnon A, Patton M, Saunders J & Shelley P (2000) 'Guidelines for the ethical conduct of medical research involving children' *Archives of Disease in Childhood* 82(2): 177–182

Meisheid A (2005) 'Targeted therapies in the treatment of cancer' *The Journal of Continuing Education in Nursing* 36(5): 191–193

Mitchell BS (2003) 'The proteasome – an emerging therapeutic target in cancer' *The New England Journal of Medicine* 348(26): 2597–2598

Muehlbauer PM (2003) 'Anti-angiogenesis in cancer therapy' *Seminars in Oncology Nursing* 19(3): 180–192

Muehlbauer PM & Schwartzentruber DJ (2003) 'Cancer vaccines' *Seminars in Oncology Nursing* 19(3): 206–216

Nam NH & Parang K (2003) 'Current targets for anticancer drug discovery' *Current Drug Targets* 4(2): 159–179

NCCN (2006) National Comprehensive Cancer Network. Melanoma version 1. Available at: www.nccn.org.

Ocker BM & Plank DMP (2000) 'The research nurse role in a clinic-based oncology research setting' *Cancer Nursing* 23(4): 286–292

Richardson PG, Barlogie B, Berenson J, Singhal S, Jagannath S, Irwin D, Rajkumar SV, Srkalovic G, Alsina M, Alexanian R, Siegel D, Orlowski RZ, Kuter D, Limentani SA, Lee S, Hideshima T, Esseltine DL, Kauffman M, Adams J, Schenkein DP & Anderson KC (2003) 'A phase 2 study of bortezomib in relapsed, refractory myeloma' *The New England Journal of Medicine* 348(26): 2609–2617

Rieger PT (2001) 'The role of oncology nurses in gene therapy' *Lancet Oncology* 2(4): 233–238

Robertson P & Fritz JB (1996) 'Gene targeting approaches to the autonomic nervous system' *Journal of Autonomic Nervous System* 61(1): 1–5

Sanders A (2002) 'Developments in breast cancer care' *Cancer Nursing Practice* 1(1): 22–25

Smith MA (2006) 'Evolving molecularly targeted therapies and biotherapeutics' *in*: Pizzo PA & Poplack DG (eds) *Principles and Practice of Pediatric Oncology* (5th edn). Philadelphia: Lippincott, Williams & Wilkins, pp. 366–404

Stebbing J, Copson E & O'Reilly S (2000) 'Herceptin (trastuzamab) in advanced breast cancer' *Cancer Treatment Reviews* 26(4): 287–290

Terry L & Campbell A (2001) 'Focus on children's nursing. Are we listening to children's views about their treatment?' *British Journal of Nursing* 10(6): 384–390

Thorpe G (1992) 'Experiments on the dying' *in*: Williams CJ (ed.) *Introducing New Treatments for Cancer: Practical, Ethical and Legal Problems*. Chichester: John Wiley & Sons, Ltd

Veal GJ & Newell D (2004) 'Recent advances in cancer chemotherapy' *in*: Pinkerton R, Plowman PN & Pieters R (eds) *Pediatric Oncology* (3rd edn). London: Arnold, pp. 583–608

Weiner LM (1999) 'An overview of monoclonal antibody therapy in cancer' *Seminars in Oncology* 26(4 supplement 12): 41–50

Woodburn J (1999) 'The epidermal growth receptor and its inhibition on cancer therapy' *Pharmacology and Therapeutics* 82(2–3): 241–250

Yarbo C, Frogge M & Goodman M (2005) *Cancer Nursing: Principles and Practice* (6th edn). Boston: Jones and Bartlett

Part 2

Haematopoietic Stem Cell Transplantation

Commentary

Haematopoietic Stem Cell Transplantation

Helen Webster

It has been a great pleasure to review the bone marrow transplant Part of the second edition of this textbook. First, it has to be pointed out that anyone working within the area of paediatric oncology will be familiar with the first edition, known in many units as 'The Red Book'. This excellent resource has been well used both as a reference guide for those in day-to-day clinical practice and as a more formal reference source for nurses undertaking academic studies.

Paediatric oncology is one area within health care where all nurses benefit from being well informed and educated. This could be said of all areas of nursing, however, it is well understood that caring for children within the Stem Cell Transplant (SCT) setting has added stresses and strains to the already present pressures of working within the National Health Service. This book not only addresses the clinical aspects of caring for a child undergoing SCT but also the complex emotional and ethical issues that SCT nurses face on a daily basis.

The SCT section provides nurses with a comprehensive background to transplant. It clearly explains the transplant process and the growth in the science and supportive care: the path taken to our present state in the twenty-first century. This excellent nursing care guidance is presented in a user-friendly style facilitated by the inclusion of diagrams and tables. Part 2 will be a valuable resource for nursing staff already experienced in paediatric oncology and a good starting point for new members to the team.

The collection of stem cells is clearly and comprehensively discussed in Chapter 9, explaining the rationale behind the decision to collect bone marrow or peripheral blood stem cells. This chapter briefly mentions umbilical cord stem cell collection, outlining the process of collection and the advantages and disadvantages of choosing cord blood as the source of cells. However, it omits to include the collection of directed umbilical cord blood. Some transplant centres recommend the collection and storage of umbilical cord stem cells from siblings born into a family where there is known genetic disease amenable to stem cell transplant. Umbilical cord stem cells can also be stored from a sibling of a child with an acquired disease who may require stem cell transplant in the future (Hows, 2001). As with many areas within health care, financial considerations have a significant bearing on practice; the collection and storage of cord blood are costly. Careful consideration within each unit as how best to manage and support the increasing requests from families for cord blood collections needs to be given. It would be interesting for further work to be carried out in this field looking at the use of collected directed cord stem

Cancer in Children and Young People   Edited by Faith Gibson and Louise Soanes
© 2008 John Wiley & Sons, Ltd

cells in comparison to the use of unrelated cord blood, and the associated cost implications.

Chapters 7 and 8 outline the background of SCT but the main focus of Part 2 is the management of children undergoing transplant – protective isolation and the associated complications. What stands out without question in these two chapters is the focus on nursing care. Many books written with the title of 'Nursing' have an enormous amount of medical, biological information and are often tempted away from the basis of the book, that of a guide for nursing. However, the authors in Part 2 have maintained the emphasis on nursing the patient through transplant, not the physiology behind the procedure. This is not to say that the disease process is not clearly explained, but the practicalities of nursing a child in this situation are the main focus. This approach is what makes this book such a valuable resource for paediatric oncology settings.

Overall, the chapters are well referenced throughout although some of the references might be considered old, particularly Skinhoj *et al.* (1987), referring to HEPA/LAF filtration in combination with the use of skin and gut decontamination, now some 20 years old. However, it is important to point out that no new significant evidence has come to light since this research was carried out. The inclusion of this study clearly highlights that not all 'old research' is out-dated, and some just stands the test of time.

Nutrition has always been an important issue for children undergoing SCT, it is well recognised that this is one aspect of caring that the family can have some control over. However, with the need for a safe, clean diet, some of this control has been taken away, and the authors approach this topic with sensitivity and, more importantly, common sense. The chapter is well referenced, including Sahdev and Botwinick (2004), which is a significant piece of research in paediatric SCT, which does, as the authors suggest, need to be the focus of further study.

The infection screening section is, however, limited and omits to address the problem of children (usually older children) who choose to have a shower daily. There is some evidence that supports no risk of line infection from contact with water, such as showering and swimming as long as a waterproof occlusive dressing is used to protect the exit site (Bravery, in press).

The effects of isolation on the child and family are often overlooked, so it is refreshing to see this has been given considerable attention. As we are all aware, the internet is becoming a significant part of all our lives. Children are introduced to computers as early as pre-school, and using e-mail and the internet is often part of a child's daily routine, providing a source of both communication and entertainment. The installation of suitable IT equipment could be an enormous support for a family, especially with the invention of video messaging, thus families can keep in touch with extended family and friends who may live some distance from the centre. The use of a webcam for transplant families has been a great success in a unit in the north-west of England, although the idea of being watched when carrying out nursing procedures or interacting with the patient was initially a concern for nursing staff, in reality, families only use the webcam facility in private. The benefits are twofold, not only can the family at home see the hospitalised child but the parent in hospital can see how the rest of the family at home are managing. Hopefully this simply installed device can go some way to addressing parents' anxieties about hospitalisation, as described by Darbyshire (1994).

The chapter on complications of stem cell transplant (Chapter 11) is perhaps the most comprehensive of all the chapters in terms of physiology and clinical management. However, the authors continue to keep the nursing focus throughout. The information is presented in a clear format, again with the use of helpful diagrams and bullet points. For example, the list of signs and symptoms and the nursing considerations divide up this chapter and therefore make it easier for the reader to comprehend, especially if a novice to stem cell transplant. For the more advanced or experienced reader, there are some very useful references to research in progress that could guide the reader to investigate the topic further and possibly influence practice, for example, the development of cytomegalovirus-specific cytotoxic T cells.

Chapter 12 deals with discharge planning and psychological issues for the family post-stem cell transplant and raises some thought-provoking issues, where not only the family has to readjust to getting back to normal and maybe returning to work but also forming new relationships with local nursing and medical teams. This chapter is comprehensive in the descriptions of the extent to which the family have to adjust. This chapter should be recommended to all nurses caring for a child in the transplant setting as the process of discharge requires an enormous amount of time and effort. Chapter 13 discusses the topic of staff support.

The final chapter (Chapter 14) looks at further developments, predominantly gene therapy. Although overall this area of transplant is relatively new, the work as described is encouraging and exciting. Once again, while clearly explaining the process and science behind gene therapy, the authors include very relevant aspects of nursing care including parental support. The final sub-heading for this chapter is 'The Future'; this discusses some interesting topics to consider for further research which hopefully would motivate any reader to explore the topics in more depth.

Part 2 on the stem cell transplant procedure is an excellent piece of well-researched, clearly presented work. The approach throughout is holistic, often raising issues that may be overlooked by many practitioners in this area. The whole text flows well, each chapter giving a good background to the subject and focusing on nursing care and parental support. Throughout, the authors give sound common-sense suggestions, particularly in relation to communication within the multidisciplinary team. The comment that stands out without

doubt is 'health care professionals recognising that they are an expert not the expert'. This comment is a perfect example of the theme of this Part. The traditional roles of the nurse and doctor are less defined now, but this book supports both roles, giving each a comprehensive understanding of the clinical and emotional battles for the child and the family facing stem cell transplant. This second edition of 'The Red Book' will be tattered very soon through constant use.

References

Bravery K (in press) 'Paediatric intravenous therapy in practice' in: Dougherty L & Lamb J (in press) Intravenous Therapy in Nursing Practice (2nd edn). Oxford: Blackwell Publishing

Darbyshire P (1994) Living in Hospital with a Sick Child: The Experience of Parents and Children. London: Chapman & Hall

Hows JM (2001) 'Status of umbilical cord blood transplant and banking' Annual Review Med. 57: 403–417

Sahdev I & Botwinick MA (2004) 'Nutrition for the child undergoing stem cell transplantation' in: Mehta P (ed.) Pediatric Stem Cell Transplantation. Boston: Jones and Bartlett, pp. 69–85

Skinhoj JP, Jacobsen N, Hoiby N, Faber, V & the Copenhagen Bone Marrow Transplant Group (1987) 'Strict protective isolation in allogeneic bone marrow transplantation: effect on infectious complications, fever and graft versus host disease' Scandinavian Journal of Infectious Diseases 19(1): 91–96

7 Background to the Haematopoietic Stem Cell Transplant (HSCT) Procedure

Nikki Bennett-Rees and Sian Hopkins

History

In 1891, bone marrow, in the form of an oral preparation, was given to treat patients with leukaemia and disorders where there was a known defective blood formation (Quine, 1896). This treatment appeared to have little effect on the patient. However, minimal changes in treatments were made over the following decades.

In 1937, Shretzenmayr (cited in Treleaven & Barrett, 1993) treated patients with intramuscular preparations of bone marrow. This was the first time the technique of transferring live cells into a patient had been attempted, and with fair effect. However, two years later Osgood et al. (1939) infused bone marrow cells intravenously and, in 1940, there were reports of bone marrow being injected into the intramedullary space (Santos, 1983). Unfortunately, these first two attempts at the use of therapeutic doses of bone marrow in patients with aplastic anaemia were unsuccessful.

As a result of the discovery of atomic energy and the release of the atomic bomb in the mid-1940s, there was a revival in research into the effects of an intensive dose of irradiation on the bone marrow of survivors in Hiroshima and Nagasaki. Pioneering work carried out by Jacobson et al. (1950) and Lorenz et al. (1952) was the forerunner of today's successful bone marrow transplants. In 1950, the work of Jacobson et al. demonstrated that mice whose spleens (a haematopoietic organ for a mouse) had been shielded from lethal doses of irradiation, could recover. Their work continued to demonstrate that infused bone marrow cells could also provide protection against death. Lorenz et al. (1952) went on to prove beyond doubt that normal bone marrow function could be restored to lethally irradiated mice and guinea-pigs by infusing bone marrow cells.

With the knowledge that engraftment of bone marrow cells was a possibility, clinicians made several attempts in the late 1950s and 1960s to treat a variety of human disorders. Clinicians were presented with numerous difficulties because most of these experimental transplants were carried out on patients with end-stage disease. Consequently, patients died either before engraftment could be established or from a 'secondary disease' (Barnes et al., 1962). This is now recognised as 'graft versus host disease' (GVHD). In addition to these problems, there was the lack of treatment for life-threatening viral or fungal infections.

During the 1960s, progress in developing effective treatments was slow and only approximately

Cancer in Children and Young People   Edited by Faith Gibson and Louise Soanes
© 2008 John Wiley & Sons, Ltd

10 % of patients receiving allogeneic bone marrow transplant showed clinical improvement (Pegg, 1966). However, the work of Thomas *et al.* (1957) on preventing GVHD, and that of Terasaki and McLelland (1964) on the human leukocyte antigens (HLA) system, pushed the role of bone marrow transplant (BMT) into a new era. There was now increasing success in the treatment of patients with aplastic anaemia and leukaemia. Meanwhile work carried out in Holland by De Koning *et al.* (1969) led to the successful treatment of infants with severe combined immunodeficiency syndromes (SCID), until then, a fatal disorder. In fact, as Morgan (1993) reports, the first successful HLA-matched sibling transplants were performed in 1968, on two children with primary immunodeficiency disorders.

By the end of the 1970s progress was such that BMT became a treatment modality, which had a measurable success rate for diseases such as SCID, severe aplastic anaemia and leukaemia. The 1980s saw a vast increase in the number of BMT centres worldwide. Data banks were set up and the number and range of diseases treated by BMT expanded. In the paediatric setting, children with haemoglobinopathies, such as sickle cell disease and thalassaemia (Borgna-Pignatti, 1992), and a variety of ultimately lethal metabolic disorders (Vellodi *et al.*, 1992; Peters & Steward, 2003) were able to undergo transplant successfully using HLA compatible siblings.

During the 1990s there continued to be further developments in the field of BMT:

- improvement in the technology of HLA typing enabling more children in whom there is no matched sibling donor to receive bone marrow from a matched, or mismatched unrelated donor.
- the expanded use of prophylactic drug therapy both before and during the transplant period;
- the continued development of efficacious antiviral and anti-fungal therapy, thus reducing both morbidity and mortality;
- the development and increased use of cytokines and growth factors therefore enhancing both haematological and immunological reconstitution;
- the ability to successfully HLA type, harvest, cryo-preserve and use umbilical cord blood

from newborn infants as a stem cell source for transplantation;

- the development of gene transfer in the autologous setting for the treatment of children with genetic disorders (Jenkins *et al.*, 1994);
- the development of successful mobilisation, collection of allogeneic and infusion of allogeneic and autologous peripheral blood stem cells (Gray & Shea, 1994; Walker *et al.*, 1994; Vaux, 1996);
- the development of reduced intensity non-myeloablative conditioning (RIC) has enabled SCT in children who already have organ dysfunction prior to or at the time of transplantation (Amrolia *et al.*, 2000).

Table 7.1 highlights the main advantages and disadvantages in terms of availability, cost and accessibility of collecting cells from various sources. In addition, it shows the difference in rates of engraftment/GVHD risk, rejection and most importantly speed of immune reconstitution.

Types of transplant

A stem cell transplant involves harvesting bone marrow, peripheral blood stem cells or umbilical cord blood stem cells from a donor and then transfusing (or grafting) these cells into the recipient. There are three different types of transplant:

1. *Autologous marrow/stem cells* – these cells are harvested from the patient (i.e. self) prior to receiving dose-escalating intensive myeloablative therapy. Autologous cells are generally used in children with a malignancy such as a solid tumour, very occasionally, acute myeloid leukaemia (AML) and in those children with a rheumatological disorder. In addition, autologous cells are being used for children undergoing gene therapy. The advantage of an autologous transplant is the lack of GVHD. The disadvantage is the risk of tumour cells being present in the harvested marrow; also there will be no graft versus leukaemia (GVL) effect (an advantage discussed in detail on p. 159).

2. *Allogeneic marrow/peripheral stem cells/umbilical cord cells* – these cells are harvested from another person who may be related or unrelated, matched or mismatched. Ideally, the

Table 7.1 Advantage and disadvantage of allogeneic stem cells

Donor	Unrelated bone marrow	Unrelated cord blood	Haploidentical family PBSC
Availability	10/10 = 50 % 9/10 = 80 % Ethnic minority = 20 %	> 5/6 = 45 % >4/6 90 %	>90 %
Access (Re-access)	Slow (possible)	Fast (no)	Immediate (no)
Cost	High	Moderate	Low
Rejection Risk	Low	High	Moderate
Engraftment	Moderate	Slow	Fast
GvHD Risk	Moderate	Low	Low
Immune Reconstitution	Moderate	Slow	Very slow

Table 7.2 PBSCT: a brief history

1909	Documented existence of haematopoietic stem cells by Alexander Maximow (cited by Korbling & Fleidner, 1996)
1962	Stem cells identified in circulating blood
1965	Flow cell separator introduced (Freireich *et al.*, 1965)
1980s	Autologous blood stem cell transplants used for adult patients with chronic myeloid leukaemia (CML) (Goldman *et al.*, 1988)
1985	Peripheral stem cells shown to reconstitute haematopoietic function in humans (Kessinger *et al.*, 1986)
1988	Use of cytokines to mobilise stem cells into peripheral circulation
1996	Peripheral stem cells mobilised with growth factors have widely replaced autologous BMT

donor would be an HLA-identical sibling. Where there is no suitable matched donor, a parent may be used i.e. a haplo-identical donor.

3. *Syngeneic marrow/peripheral stem cells/umbilical cord cells* – these cells are harvested from an identical twin. These transplants are ideal in children with an acquired bone marrow failure, such as aplastic anaemia, as both the donor and recipient are identical in every aspect and there will be no risk of the recipient developing GVHD.

The use of peripheral blood stem cells (PBSC) in both the autologous and allogeneic setting has become common practice (Table 7.2). In addition, successful engraftment using umbilical cord stem cells both in the sibling and unrelated donor setting has become another source of stem cells (Wagner *et al.*, 1992; Gluckman *et al.*, 1997). In the child, where a suitable donor remains impossible to find, the use of haplo-identical PBSC continues to be an option. The donor in the haplo setting is usually a parent, but could be a sibling, whose HLA typing matches half the child's HLA type. While it may

be technically possible to use a young sibling as a haplo-identical donor, many centres would argue about the ethics of using underage siblings in such a high-risk procedure.

Diseases for which haematopoietic stem cell transplant is a treatment modality

For a child with a malignancy, the aim of treatment is to eradicate the malignancy and then 'rescue' the child from the life-threatening effects of the myeloablative therapy (Table 7.3). For the child with leukaemia, there may be an additional GVL effect from allogeneic stem cell transplant. Cells used for transplant can be bone marrow, peripheral blood stem cells or umbilical cord cells and can be autologous, allogeneic, matched or mismatched.

For a child with a non-malignant disorder, such as bone marrow failure or bone marrow dysfunction, or who requires replacement of a missing enzyme in an otherwise healthy bone marrow, the

Table 7.3   Malignant diseases for which stem cell transplant is a treatment modality

Leukaemia
>   Acute lymphoblastic leukaemia
>   Acute myeloid leukaemia
>   Chronic myeloid leukaemia
>   Juvenile myelo-monocytic leukaemia
>   Myelodysplastic syndrome

Lymphomas
>   Non-Hodgkin's lymphoma
>   Hodgkin's disease

Solid tumours*
>   Brain tumours
>   Ewing's sarcoma
>   Primitive neuroectodermal tumour
>   Retinoblastoma
>   Rhabdomyosarcoma

Others
>   Haemophagocytic lymphohistiocytosis (HLH)

Note: *Cells used are usually autologous bone marrow or PBSC.

Table 7.4   Non-malignant diseases for which stem cell transplant is a modality

Acquired marrow failure
>   Severe aplastic anaemia

Congenital marrow failure
>   Fanconi's anaemia
>   Kostman's syndrome
>   Diamond-Blackman anaemia
>   Schwachman's syndrome

Genetic/metabolic disorders
>   Hurler's syndrome
>   Maroteaux–Lamy syndrome
>   Adreno-leukodystrophy
>   Osteopetrosis

Haemoglobinopathies
>   Thalassaemia major
>   Sickle cell disease

Immune disorders
>   Severe combined immune deficiency
>   X linked lymphoproliferative disorder
>   Wiskott-Aldrich syndrome
>   MHC class II deficiency
>   CD 40 Ligand deficiency
>   Chronic Granulomatous disease
>   Undefined severe immune deficiencies

Rheumatology disorders
>   Juvenile idiopathic arthritis

aim is to remove the malfunctioning marrow and replace the system with healthy cells, thus restoring a normal functioning haematopoietic system (Table 7.4). Cells for transplant are used from bone marrow/peripheral stem cells/umbilical cord cells and are allogeneic, either matched or mismatched.

The successful outcome of SCT depends on a variety of factors, such as:

- ability of the underlying malignancy to go into remission pre-SCT;
- amount of previous therapy (such as chemotherapy, blood transfusions or enzyme replacement therapy) the child has undergone;
- tissue-matching of donor;
- age and sex of donor and recipient.

As this field of medicine is continually evolving, so the results of long-term survival will change. Table 7.5 provides a current summary of long-term survival.

Tissue typing

Tissue typing is a key process in the pre-transplant phase. It is the basis by which the most suitable donor for transplant is chosen. Blood is taken from the patient, parents and siblings to establish HLA type and determine matches within the family group. Failure to find a match within the immediate family will necessitate extending the search to the extended family members and/or unrelated donors on national and international registries.

Tissue type refers to a series of polymorphic proteins found on the surface of almost every cell in the body. These proteins are known as human leukocyte antigens (HLA) and are involved in the cell-to-cell interaction of the immune system. Tissue type is, in simple terms, a list of these antigens carried on the surface of cells (Ord, 1995). In SCT, the donor is chosen according to the similarity of their HLA in relation to the patient's HLA (Figure 7.1). The HLA system is a major determinant in the success of SCT (Welte, 1994). Before its introduction in the 1960s, the results of allogeneic BMT were very poor. At the time of introducing HLA, enthusiasm for BMT was falling and the future of the speciality was in doubt. Today

Table 7.5 Survival outcomes for children undergoing stem cell transplant

Disease	Transplant	Long-term survival (%)
Malignant disease		
ALL (1st CR)	allogeneic	40
AML (1st CR)	allogeneic	50
AML (2nd CR)	allogeneic	20–50
AML (2nd CR)	autologous	40
Myelodysplasia	allogeneic	60–70
Neuroblastoma stage IV	autologous	30
Non-malignant disease		
Aplastic anaemia	allogeneic (non-transfused)	80
Aplastic anaemia	allogeneic (multiple transfusions)	70
SCIDS/CID	allogeneic (sibling)	90
SCIDS/CID	allogeneic (haploidentical)	50
SCIDS/CID	allogeneic (unrelated donor)	70
Thalassaemia major	allogeneic (sibling)	70–75
Inborn errors of metabolism	allogeneic	Early studies show good results for some hereditary metabolic diseases

Notes: ALL = acute lymphoblastic leukaemia; AML = acute myeloid leukaemia; SCIDS = severe combined immune deficiency syndrome; CID = combined immune deficiency; CR = complete remission.
Sources: Fischer *et al.*, 1990; Lucarelli *et al.*, 1990; Chessells *et al.*, 1992; Barrett *et al.*, 1994; Nesbit *et al.*, 1994.

its impact and development in the field of BMT are well known. It is, however, only 38 years since the first BMT using HLA matching was carried out (Treleaven & Barrett, 1993).

There are over 90 separate HLA antigens that can form 26 million combinations. Despite this, some tissue types are fairly common and yet others may occur only once in a million individuals. Individuals inherit their HLA antigens from their parents in a Mendelian inheritance in the same way that eye colour is inherited (Welte, 1994). Certain tissue types are found in certain ethnic and racial groups and a matched unrelated donor is more likely to be found for patients from their own racial background. HLA genes are found on the short arm of chromosome 6. Individuals inherit two sets of antigens: a paternal haplotype and a maternal haplotype (Figure 7.1). There are two groups of antigens. Class I antigens (of which at least 17 have been identified) are expressed not only in leukocytes but also in most nucleated cells in the body cells (HLA-A, HLA-B and HLA-C are the ones of prime concern in SCT). In contrast, Class II antigens are only expressed in a limited range of cells (B lymphocytes, macrophages, endothelial and dendritic cells except in the placenta and central nervous system (CNS)). These are known as the HLA-D region and have been mapped into five distinct sub-regions: DN, DO, DP, DQ and DR. In SCT, the HLA-DR is the most important of the Class II antigens (Roitt & Male, 1996).

The function of the HLA system

The most important role of the HLA system is reactivity with foreign antigens. The antigen is processed by being presented to macrophages and scrutinised by a T cell receptor, which then initiates the appropriate T cell response in order to rid the body of invading antigens. There are some T cells, however, which are capable of responding directly to cells bearing foreign HLA, without prior processing. Methods of identifying the number of these circulating T cells, such as cytotoxic T cell precursor assay (CTLP) and mixed lymphocyte culture (MLC) are a useful adjunct to choosing a suitable donor. A high CTLP frequency

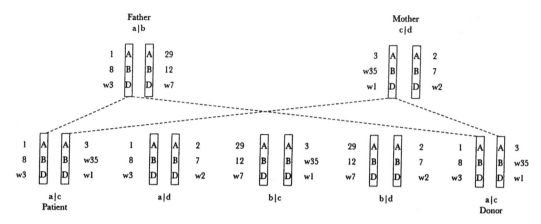

Figure 7.1　Possible combinations of human leukocyte antigens (HLA).

is an indicator that a donor may induce GVHD if used in transplant.

As well as the major histocompatibility antigens, there are so-called minor histocompatibility (mH) loci that encode molecules in recognition and rejection. Despite their name, these mH loci are strongly implicated in GVHD, particularly in the setting of HLA-matched related SCT (Reiser & Martelli, 1995). Minor histocompatible differences are not routinely assessed in SCT donor recipient pairs. In the future, matching mH may further reduce the incidence of GVHD, but in transplants for leukaemia such minor histocompatibility can be an advantage in the production of the GVL effect (Vogelsgang & Hess, 1994).

ABO blood typing

ABO-incompatible marrow grafting can be accomplished with little of the haemolytic transfusion reactions seen in the past. This is due to improved techniques to remove red blood cells from the marrow, but if un-manipulated marrow is to be used, then, as with normal blood transfusions, haemolytic transfusion reactions will occur. Appropriate blood products need to be compatible with both the donor and recipient in the early stages of the transplant. The patient and the family should be informed that following SCT the patient's ABO blood type will convert to that of the donor, and that the time taken for this varies.

Adult unrelated donors

The birth rate in the industrialised world has been falling for many years. At present the average number of children in a family is 1.9. This has meant that only 30% of patients needing a SCT have a suitable donor within their immediate or extended family (Vowels *et al.*, 1991). The failure to find a donor within the family group leads to the search for compatible stem cells from an unrelated donor. Currently, the use of children as non-related donors does not occur, for ethical and moral reasons discussed in Chapter 8 in relation to sibling donors. Adult donors used for unrelated transplants volunteer to donate their stem cells and are required to register with one of the bone marrow registries that exist throughout the world.

Donor panels

Donor panels arose as a result of the growing need for a centralised unrelated bone marrow registry in the 1970s. This need was recognised following the failure to find suitable donors for individuals in a variety of countries at this time. In the UK, the case of Anthony Nolan, a small boy with Wiskott Aldrich Syndrome, and the unsuccessful search for a donor in 1974 led to the formation of the Anthony Nolan Bone Marrow Registry now known as the Anthony Nolan Bone Marrow Trust (ANBMT www.anthonynolan.org.uk). Alongside the ANBMT are two further registries within the

UK, the Welsh panel and the Bristol Bone Marrow Transplant Registry (BBMTR). Similar registries exist in many countries worldwide. In addition, umbilical cord banks have been set up and grown worldwide. Within the UK at present there is one cord blood bank centre. These registries provide information that may lead to the identification of a suitable donor for patients in both national and international bone marrow units. Through this collaboration, the pool of potential donors for those patients for whom a sibling donor cannot be found on a national register has widened. The people on the registries are volunteers who have agreed to enter details of their HLA status onto a central register. Initially, details of their relevant medical and social history are recorded and a sample of blood taken to determine their Class I antigens. Details of these are added to a database and held until required or the donor becomes too old to donate. A bone marrow transplant unit approaches the registry with details of patients requiring a donor. At this stage, further matching of Class II antigens identifies potential donors and further tissue typing is undertaken to elicit the most suitable donors. Those identified as being the most likely potential donors are then screened for suitability, using a lengthy selection process which can take months, and assesses both physical and mental suitability to donate marrow or stem cells.

Selection of adult unrelated donors

Due to the complexity of human major histocompatibility, approximately 50% of transplants are carried out as a result of volunteered matched unrelated donors. Although the aim of HLA typing in SCT is to select the donor with the closest possible match, this may not necessarily identify the most suitable donor. Other factors that come into play in donor selection are listed below (see also Figure 7.2).

- donor age;
- donor/recipient gender;
- cytomegalovirus (CMV) status;
- ethnic group;
- physical and mental health;.
- ABO matching.

Donor choice

1. Matched sibling donor or phenotypic matched donor or fully matched related cord blood[#]
2. 10/10 molecular match unrelated donor or 6/6 matched unrelated cord blood[#]
3. 1 allelic mismatched unrelated donor or 5/6 matched family donor < 2/6 mismatched unrelated cord blood[#]
4. 2 allelic mismatched unrelated donor or 2 allelic mismatched family donor

Notes: # with neutrophil count dose greater than 3.7×10^7/kg recipient weight

Options 3 and 4 should only be considered in poor risk patients for whom alternative treatment is unavailable or has failed.

Stem Cell Source

1. MSD*; BM is preferred to PBSC
2. MUD*; BM is preferred to PBSC
3. MMUD/MMF; PBSC are preferred to BM

Notes: *Adult sibling and related donors should be allowed a choice after non-directive counselling by a physician independent of the transplant unit.

Donor preference

Patient	Donor
Male	Male preferred to female
Female	Male preferred to female

CMV status	
Positive	Positive donor in preference to a negative donor
Negative	Negative donor in preference to a positive donor
Age	Younger donors are preferred to older donors
ABO	Aim for a match in heavily pre-transfused patients

Figure 7.2   CCLG BMT Group donor selection guidelines.

The age at which volunteers can donate their marrow/stem cells varies from country to country. At present the minimum age in the UK for joining a register is 18 years and the maximum is 40. The maximum age at which a potential donor can donate marrow/stem cells recommended by the ANBMT is 56 years (this relatively young upper age limit is due to the increased risk of a general anaesthetic in older donors). However, the upper age limit is higher in donors who are able to give PBSCs. Ideally, the donor and recipient should be of the same sex, and this is due to the risk of GVHD, which is higher in female-to-male transplants. Male donors are generally preferred to avoid sensitisation by pregnancy.

The CMV and Epstein Barr Virus (EBV) status of donors is of paramount importance. Ideally, where possible, the CMV status of the donor and recipient should be matched to reduce the chance of post-transplant viral reactivation and disease. Likewise, blood product support during and after the transplant episode is important, if the recipient and donor are both CMV negative, then CMV negative blood and platelet support must be given. However, if either the donor or recipient is CMV positive, then the recipient could receive unscreened products. Donors are also screened for HIV and hepatitis B and C antibodies.

The ethnic group is also of prime concern in SCT, as a matched donor is more likely to be found among the recipient's own ethnic group. The majority of unrelated donor volunteers are Caucasian and this has led to a shortage of potential donors from ethnic populations. Added to this, some ethnic groups have cultural and religious objections to the donation of marrow or stem cells.

There is also a shortage of male donors, which may compound the above situation, as the incidence of many of the conditions requiring SCT in children is higher in males or has an X-linked inheritance, Wiskott Aldrich Syndrome being one example. Campaigns to recruit from ethnic groups and to encourage male donors to come forward are frequently undertaken by registries in order to raise awareness and recruit more suitable candidates for donation.

ABO compatibility might take on greater significance in the future. In heavily transfused patients such as those with Fanconi's anaemia, thalassaemia or severe aplastic anaemia, the aim would be to have an ABO-compatible donor to reduce the risk of rejection.

Evaluation of the unrelated adult donor

Donors are required to complete a detailed medical questionnaire before entry to the registry. The physical criteria for donation include stringent assessment of the donor as suitable for general anaesthetic. Exclusion includes previous medical history of respiratory disease, cerebrovascular

disease, current pregnancy and back problems. Exclusion from donation on these grounds is due to the potential risk to the donor as a result of the anaesthetic or the process of marrow/stem cell collection. Once admitted to the registry the potential donor waits to be called forward to donate their marrow/stem cells (this may take many years). Each registry has its own limits as to how many times a person may donate their marrow/stem cells. Adult unrelated donors may donate to two separate recipients with a gap of one year between donations. Agreement to donate more than twice is extremely rare due to the increased risk to the donor of repeated anaesthetics. However, a collection of T cells from the donor may be collected in the case of pending rejection four to six weeks after the initial collection of marrow/stem cells (Anthony Nolan Bone Marrow Trust, 1996).

Once called for donation, the donor will not only be assessed physically but also psychologically for suitability to donate. During this early physical and psychological assessment written consent is sought from the donor to proceed with preparation to donate; although not legally binding, consent is sought on moral and ethical grounds. Assessment of the donor's perceptions and attitudes towards transplant may uncover distortions in the donor's concepts of the procedure. Many donors have no previous experience of hospital and may have misconceptions of what the procedure entails. Education about the donation process and potential complications following donation and general anaesthetic are given (donors who are not fully confident in their decision to donate are encouraged to withdraw as soon as possible from the selection process). It is also explained that should the recipient of the marrow/stem cells die or face serious complications as a result of the transplant, the donor is not responsible.

Personal information about the recipient is given only on request and disclosure of personal details is kept to a minimum (gender, age-group and country in which the transplant is to take place). Strict confidentiality between the two parties is maintained and contact discouraged throughout the pre- and immediate transplant period. This ensures that the privacy of both the donor and recipient is maintained (Cleaver, 1993).

Receiving a gift of such magnitude as bone marrow/stem cells without thanking the donor is difficult for many families. In such cases cards and small gifts may be passed on through the registry to the donor at the time of the transplant. Sometimes the donor and recipient may meet or make contact months after the transplant has taken place. Again, the registries offer support and advice in these situations, to protect both parties from over-involvement by the other and to offer support for the emotional response such a meeting may produce. The preparation of the related adult donor does not involve the support and services of the bone marrow registry and is coordinated by the BMT centre caring for the child. The physical preparation is similar to that already described.

Umbilical cord blood (UCB) donors

In the past decade UCB transplants have become more of an optional source of cells for transplantation in children, with either genetic or malignant disease. Initial success was with sibling transplants, and with this success worldwide cord blood banks were set up for the future use of unrelated donor allogeneic cord blood transplants. The parents of the newborn baby donating the cord blood hand over all rights to the collected blood, which is stored anonymously, for use by transplant centres worldwide, to date, there have been over 3,000 such transplants (Wall, 2004). Some advantages of UCB over donor stem cells/marrow is that all information regarding the cells is available at the time of the donor search, thereby reducing the time to transplant. Furthermore, there is a low level of viral contamination with CMV or EBV (the two most significant clinically important transplant-related viruses). Also it has been noted that less GVHD occurs, therefore allowing a greater mismatched donor to be used (4/6 HLA). For children with rare immune types or those from ethnic minorities, a UCB transplant could be a more viable option (Wall, 2004).

References

Amrolia P, Gaspar B, Hassan A, *et al.* (2000) 'Non-myeloablative stem cell transplantation for congenital immunodeficiency' *Blood* 96: 1239–1246

Anthony Nolan Bone Marrow Trust (1996) *A Guide for Potential Bone Marrow Donors* Information sheet for potential donors. www.anthonynolan.org.uk.

Barnes DW, Loutit JF & Micklem HS (1962) 'Secondary disease of radiation chimeras; a syndrome due to lymphoid aplasia' *Annals of the New York Academy of Science 99*: 374–385

Barrett J, Horowitz MM & Pollock BH (1994) 'Bone marrow transplants from HLA-identical siblings as compared with chemotherapy for children with acute lymphoblastic leukaemia in a second remission' *New England Journal of Medicine 331*(19): 1253–1258

Borgna-Pignatti C (1992) 'Bone marrow transplantation for the haemoglobinopathies' *in*: Treleaven J & Barrett J (eds) *Bone Marrow Transplantation in Practice*. London: Churchill Livingstone, pp. 151–159

Chessells JM, Bailey CC, Wheeler K & Richards SM (1992) 'Bone marrow transplantation for high-risk childhood lymphoblastic leukaemia in first remission: experience in MRC UKALL X' *The Lancet 340*: 565–568

Cleaver S (1993) 'The Anthony Nolan Bone Marrow Research Centre and other matching registries' *in*: Treleaven J & Barrett J (eds) *Bone Marrow Transplantation in Practice*. London: Churchill Livingstone, pp. 361–366

De Koning J, Van Bekkum D, Dicke K, Dooren L, Radl J & Van-Rood K (1969) 'Transplantation of bone marrow cells and foetal thymus in an infant with lymphopenic immunological deficiency' *The Lancet 1*(608): 1223–1227

Fischer A, Landais P, Friedrich W, Morgan G, Gerritsen B, Fasth A, Porta F, Griscelli C, Goldman S, Levinsky R & Vossen J (1990) 'European experience of bone marrow transplantations for severe combined immunodeficiency' *The Lancet 2*(8515): 850–854

Freireich EJ, Judson G & Levin RH (1965) 'Separation and collection of leukocytes' *Cancer Research 25*(9): 1516–1520

Gluckman E, Broxmeyer H & Auerbach AD (1997) 'Hematological reconstitution in a patient with Fanconi's anaemia by means of umbilical cord blood from a HLA identical sibling' *New England Journal of Medicine 321*(17): 1174–1187

Goldman JM, Ciale RP, Horrowitz MM, Biggs SC, Chapman E & Gluckman E (1988) 'Bone marrow transplant in CML chronic phase: increased risk for relapse associated with T-cell depletion' *Annals of Internal Medicine 108*(6): 806–814

Gray T & Shea T (1994) 'Current status of peripheral blood progenitor cell transplantation' *Seminars in Oncology 21*(5) (suppl. 12): 93–101

Jacobson L, O'Simmons EL, Marks EK, Marks E, Robson M, Bethard W & Gaston E (1950) 'The role of the spleen in radiation injury and recovery' *Journal of Laboratory and Clinical Medicine 35*(5): 746–751

Jenkins J, Wheeler V & Albright L (1994) 'Gene therapy for cancer' *Cancer Nursing* 17(6): 447–456

Kessinger A, Armitage JO, Landmark JD & Weisenburger DD (1986) 'Reconstitution of human hematopoietic function with autologous cryopreserved circulating stem cells' *Experimental Hematology* 14(3): 192–196

Korbling M & Fleidner TM (1996) 'The evolution of clinical peripheral blood stem cell transplantation' *Bone Marrow Transplantation* 17(2): S4–S11

Lorenz E, Congdon CC & Uphoff D (1952) 'Modification of acute radiation injury in mice and guinea pigs by bone marrow injections' *Radiology* 58(6): 863–877

Lucarelli G, Galimberti M, Polchi P, Angelucci E, Baronciani D, Giardini C, Politi P, Durazzi SM, Muretto P & Alberinin F (1990) 'Bone marrow transplantation in patients with thalassaemia' *New England Journal of Medicine* 322(7): 417–421

Morgan G (1993) 'Bone marrow transplantation for immunodeficiency syndromes' *in*: Treleaven J & Barrett J (eds) *Bone Marrow Transplantation in Practice*. London: Churchill Livingstone, pp. 119–136

Nesbit Jr, ME, Buckley JD, Feig SA, Jacobsen L, Simmons, E, Marks E, Robson M, Bethard W & Gaston E (1994) 'Chemotherapy for induction of remission of childhood acute myeloid leukaemia followed by marrow transplantation or multiagent chemotherapy: a report from the Children's Cancer Group' *Journal of Clinical Oncology* 12(1): 127–135

Ord J (1996) 'Introduction to HKLA typing' personal communication

Osgood EE, Riddle MC & Mathews T J (1939) 'Aplastic anemia treated with daily transfusions and intravenous marrow' *Annals of Internal Medicine* 13(2): 357–356

Pegg DE (1966) 'Allogeneic bone marrow transplantation in man' *in*: Pegg DE (ed.) *Bone Marrow Transplantation*. London: Lloyd-Luke Medical Books Ltd

Peters C & Steward CG (2003) 'Haematopoetic cell transplantation for inherited metabolic diseases: an overview of outcomes and practice guidelines' *Bone Marrow Transplant* 31: 229–239

Quine WE (1896) 'The remedial application of bone marrow' *Journal of the American Medical Association* 26(19): 1012–1013

Reiser Y & Martelli M (1995) 'Bone marrow transplantation across HLA barriers by increasing the number of transplanted cells' *Immunology Today* 16(9): 437–440

Roitt I & Male D (1996) 'Introduction to the immune system' *in*: Roitt I, Brostoff J & Male D (eds) *Immunology* (4th edn). London: Mosby

Santos GW (1983) 'History of bone marrow transplantation' *Clinical Haematology* 12(3): 611–639

Terasaki PI & McLelland JD (1964) 'Microdroplet assay of human serum cytotoxins' *Nature* 204(4962): 998–1000

Thomas E, Lochte HL, Wan Ching LW & Ferrebee, J (1957) 'Intravenous infusion of bone marrow in patients receiving radiation and chemotherapy' *New England Journal of Medicine* 257(11): 491

Treleaven J & Barrett J (1993) 'Introduction to bone marrow transplantation' *in*: Treleaven J & Barrett J (eds) *Bone Marrow Transplantation in Practice*. London: Churchill Livingstone, pp. 3–10

Vaux Z (1996) 'Peripheral stem cell transplants in children' *Paediatric Nursing* 8(2): 20–22

Vellodi A, Comba, L & McCathy D (1992) 'Bone marrow transplantation for unborn errors of metabolism' *in*: Treleaven J & Barrett J (eds) *Bone Marrow Transplantation in Practice*. London: Churchill Livingstone, pp. 161–176

Vogelsgang G & Hess A (1994) 'Graft versus host disease: new directions for a persistent problem' *Blood* 84(7): 2061–2067

Vowels MR, Tang TL, Mameghan H, Honeyman M & Russell S (1991) 'Bone marrow transplantation in children using closely matched related and unrelated donors' *Bone Marrow Transplantation* 8(2): 87–92

Wagner JE, Broxmeyer HE, Byrd RL, *et al.* (1992) 'Transplantation of umbilical cord blood after myeloablative therapy: analysis of engraftment' *Blood* 79: 1874–1881

Walker F, Roethke SK & Martin G (1994) 'An overview of the rationale, process and nursing implications of peripheral blood stem cell transplantation' *Cancer Nursing* 17(2): 141–148

Wall D (2004) 'Umbilical cord blood transplantation' *in*: Mehta P (ed.) *Paediatric Stem Cell Transplantation*. Boston: Jones & Bartlett, pp. 337–351

Welte, K (1994) 'Matched unrelated donors' *Seminars in Oncology Nursing* 10(1): 20–27

8 Preparation for Bone Marrow Transplant

Nikki Bennett-Rees, Sian Hopkins and Joanna Stone

The family

While stem cell transplantation (SCT) becomes the accepted form of treatment for an increasing range of childhood disorders, the needs of families will differ greatly depending upon the child's underlying disease and hence hospital experience. For the family whose child has a malignancy, the progression to a SCT may be the natural course of events or it may be the last hope for cure, following either a relapse or a disease refractory to treatment. Such families have experienced chemotherapy and maybe even radiotherapy. There will be aspects of SCT which will be very new to them; however, if the oncology unit is attached to the transplant unit, the families will know their surroundings and staff. If the transplant unit is in a referral centre, these families will have to leave behind everything which has been familiar and supportive during previous treatments.

For the family whose child has SCID or severe aplastic anaemia (SAA), there may be either little or no hope of cure without a SCT. Such children may have had varying experiences ranging from long intensive hospitalisation to minimal inpatient treatment. Children with metabolic disorders may also have had minimal hospital admissions, but without a SCT may suffer progressive deterioration, making their quality of life untenable (Peters & Steward, 2003).

The life expectancy for children with haemoglobinopathies has increased dramatically over the years. Thus, parents have a difficult decision to make when balancing the chance of potential cure versus acute and long-term side effects of SCT (Borgna-Pignatti, 1992). No matter how much information and knowledge the family already has, there is still a great deal of information to be given and discussed at the first consultation. Specific information will include the child's need for a transplant; long-term outlook with or without the transplant and problems that might be faced during and after transplant. Following this initial consultation the parents should receive a letter detailing all the issues which were discussed. In addition, at the first consultation, it is essential that a SCT nurse, as well as the unit psychologist, is present (Table 8.1). This serves to build up a relationship between the family and extended team as well as ensuring that continuity of information is given. In future, meetings with either the nurse or psychologist will be able to provide further answers to queries.

The possibility of parents feeling confused, frightened and shocked is not uncommon (Haberman, 1988). It is therefore essential that,

Table 8.1 Summary of the role of the nurse in giving information before stem cell transplant

Be included in the initial family/consultant meeting
Have the ability to assess the family's understanding
Be consistent in giving information appropriate to the family's understanding
Be able to discuss levels of family involvement in the care of their child
Be available to answer questions in the coming weeks
Be able to support the above with written information
Maintain support of the family.

following this consultation, the transplant nurse has the time to go through what has been discussed, step by step with the parents. The nurse is in an ideal position to further this discussion with the family, as he or she will be caring for both children and families undergoing SCT, and thus will be able to answer a wide range of questions. It is the role of the transplant nurse to deliver information and support which is individualised for each family, ensuring that the information given is both accurate and paced appropriately (Downs, 1994). In families for whom English is not the first language or whose 'medical' knowledge of English is limited, it is essential to make use of an interpreter at this meeting, preferably one who is attached to the hospital services. Experience has shown that using a family member as an interpreter (especially if a sibling) places too great a burden on that person; ultimately, it can become questionable whether all the information is relayed accurately. While the interpreter is present, it is important to find out if the family follows any cultural routines or has special dietary needs to ensure that these can be met.

For families who are new to the area, a visit to the transplant unit following the meeting will help to allay some of their fears of the unknown. It is often a time when, to relieve the anxieties of the day, toys and activities for the child can be discussed. It may be useful to give parents a taped copy of the first meeting as this will enable them to go through relevant information in the safety of their home (Hogbin, 1989). In addition, a specifically designed information book about transplant, which includes treatments, side effects, restrictions and daily routines of the unit, will enhance the family's knowledge and understanding. An added

advantage of the book and/or tape is that the extended family, who may not be allowed to visit, can feel involved in what is going to happen. Before admission, the family and the child may have further appointments at the hospital. These visits offer an ideal opportunity to consolidate family knowledge, answer problems as they arise and give the family time to revisit the unit, thus making it more familiar. Some families may find it beneficial to meet another family going through the SCT process. If possible, this can be arranged in conjunction with the family to meet some of the ward and other relevant support staff.

On admission to the unit, usually the day prior to commencing conditioning therapy, most information is given by the nursing staff. It is essential to confirm what the family's and the child's knowledge of the forthcoming treatment is and to establish what their immediate needs are. Once the family has adjusted to the new environment, the forthcoming treatment can be discussed and the child's care planned. This time before transplant is enormously stressful for parents. On top of the worry about the 'sick' child, there will be worry about the safety of their 'healthy' child donor. In the case of the donor being unrelated, the added worry concerns the donor's fitness or, indeed, whether he or she might change their mind. Keeping the parents well informed through each day of conditioning helps to reduce their anxiety. The length of the conditioning regimen and the timing of moving the child into isolation will dictate how much additional information needs to be given in the first few days. Parents should be given a copy of their child's conditioning protocol. This can then be used to guide the parents' questions through each stage as well as explaining each of the individual drugs and their side effects. In addition, parents will need to understand and learn about the isolation technique. This will vary between units but will range from the way to enter the room, to making a snack for their child.

Clear and consistent explanations of the procedures ahead form an important part of the process of consent for transplant. Truly informed consent is both difficult and time-consuming to achieve but is a useful tool for building a more equitable relationship with parents and children. In some units the task of obtaining consent for the transplant procedure has evolved into a collaboration between senior medical and nursing staff thereby giving families a more comprehensive picture of what may lie ahead.

Negotiation

Generally, once the stem cells have been transfused, parents feel less stressed and are able to take in much more information. As soon as the time is right for the parents, discussion as to how much involvement they are either able or willing to offer, should be negotiated. Research provides overwhelming evidence of the benefit of parental involvement (Gibson, 1989; Taylor & O'Connor, 1989; Cleary, 1992). Thus, for the child to receive optimum care, he should be nursed in an environment which actively promotes the practice of parental involvement (Casey, 1988). Nurses need both to recognise and to value the expertise that the family brings to their sick child, yet it must be taken into account that not all families will either want, or indeed be able, to participate in their child's care (Casey, 1988). However, whatever the level of parental involvement, for parents to be effective in their child's care, they need appropriate teaching and support. Furthermore, to create a truly effective partnership with nurses, care for the child's needs must be negotiated between the child, the parents and the nurse, and then evaluated. Some parents will be expert carers in terms of their child's 'medical' needs, able to perform tasks ranging from giving oral medicines to intravenous medications and caring for the central line. Others will be novices in dealing with a hospitalised child. Whatever the contribution to the child's care, it must be valued and regarded positively. For the child, the parent's sheer presence acts both as a support and as a buffer against the unknown.

Thus, from admission through to discharge, the daily planning of the child's care will enable parents to be involved in the 'nursing care' in which they feel able to participate. Confusion regarding role negotiation is often the source of conflict between clinical staff and parents, ultimately leading to substandard care for the child (Coyne, 1995; Lee, 2004). Much of the confusion can be eliminated by clear negotiation on a shift-by-shift basis. If this does not happen, staff may be unable to appreciate that parents may have days when they feel unable to give their child's care or, alternatively, wish to undertake additional roles.

Support

Both during the time leading up to SCT and during hospitalisation it is crucially important to provide support for parents. This can be given in many ways, but two of the most fundamental are staff providing detailed and accurate information and staff being freely available to parents. The sharing of care between staff and parents and acceptance by staff that parents have unique knowledge of their child's needs empower parents who may find themselves in an alien environment.

Support can also be offered at a very practical level. For example, some parents may find the financial burden extremely heavy while one or both is taking time off work, sometimes for an extended period. In addition to loss of earnings, extra expenses may be incurred, such as extra child care for siblings, travel costs and accommodation fees. Funds may be available through, for example, the CLIC Sargent Fund for families whose child has leukaemia or cancer. For other families, there are some charitable organisations which may help with travel expenses and holidays for siblings and families, especially at discharge. At another level, offering simple stress-reducing therapies, such as massage and aromatherapy, on the unit allows parents some relaxation which again acts as a support. Finally, recognising the need for parents to have time out together, while their child is cared for by a member of staff, is perhaps one of the simplest forms of support.

Each person's need for support is unique, whether it is emotional, financial, practical or indeed a combination of all these things. The experienced SCT team should be able to recognise this and ensure that support is ongoing. If parents are well supported, they, in turn, will be able to support their child. The overall effect of this will help ensure a good atmosphere in the ward, which has a direct result on the well-being of the child (Pot Mees, 1989).

Preparation of children

No matter what role a child plays in the transplant procedure (i.e. as donor, recipient or sibling), each will have individual needs and concerns. In order for these to be met, the preparation required should be both age- and developmentally appropriate to that child. This is particularly important for children where the recipient of bone marrow does not have a malignant disorder and consequently 'bone marrow' and 'bone marrow transplant' are entirely new words and/or concepts. Examples of misconceptions can vary from confusing bone marrow with the 'marrow bone' which comes in tins and is fed to dogs, to the child who thought his brother was having a 'bow and arrow' transplant! Another 'experienced' child, having undergone many surgical procedures for multiple abnormalities, none the less thought that his umbilical cord cell transplant meant that his 'belly button' was going to be cut open to give blood in. Words and procedures which are common everyday experiences to SCT staff are totally new and often bewildering to many adults, let alone children.

Ideally, preparation of children should be a shared family experience rather than an individual procedure, with family members being facilitated in the continuous process of information-giving, questioning and support. Research indicates that shared preparation enables family members to better understand the experiences and feelings each undergoes and they are therefore able to identify their role in supporting each other. For some families, however, this may be neither practically nor emotionally possible. The need or desire for some individual preparation should be respected and provided in addition to family preparation.

Psychological preparation of a child undergoing transplant

The child who is to undergo a SCT may be a baby with no outside experiences; a child who has had a previously uneventful life and now needs a transplant to cure an acute illness; or a child who has had years of treatment. The needs of each child will be unique. The preparation will be based on their actual knowledge, and at a level appropriate and individualised to their needs.

The key to successful preparation is to reduce the anxiety that results from lack of knowledge. The play specialist will be able to discover the appropriate emphasis and extent of preparation the child will need pre-SCT. This preparation will be determined in the main by the child's age, development, knowledge and previous hospital experiences, but the child's need to know and consequent ability to cope with stress have to be balanced with the parents' wishes. Parents may not wish their child to be told about certain procedures or issues and staff must always respect this. For example, questions from the child may range from length of stay/isolation, to procedures such as insertion of NG tubes or finger pricks or to the more complex issues surrounding death and dying. Staff should indicate to parents, however, that if the child asks a direct or specific question an honest answer will have to be given. It is a delicate area, needing sensitive handling for all parties.

For the younger age group, preparation involving therapeutic play sessions using 'models' (e.g. teddy bears) with a variety of Hickman® lines, peripheral lines, nasogastric tubes in situ proves very successful. The child is able to give medicines either by mouth or by one of the lines, take blood samples and change dressings, in the hope that new and possibly painful procedures will be learnt and coping strategies acquired. For the older child, preparation includes the use of books showing what various treatments look like, and handling equipment such as Hickman® lines, syringes or needles as well as giving accurate information. This should help the child to formulate questions, and encourage an understanding of why and how certain procedures will happen. Essential for all children is the ability to build up a trusting relationship with the play specialist and nursing staff. Without this trust, it can be difficult for the child to believe that he or she is being told the truth and that there are no hidden surprises.

For the teenager undergoing SCT the whole procedure can become exceptionally stressful. In addition to the causes of stress described earlier, there may be additional ones linked particularly to adolescence:

- sperm banking;
- awareness and resentment at loss of independence and control;
- consequent dependence on parents and nursing staff;
- concern about alteration in body image;
- concerns about changes to 'sexual' identity.

This last stress factor involves reactions to future loss of fertility and the repercussions not only of having someone else's blood in one's system but also possibly the blood of someone of the opposite sex (Wiley *et al.*, 1984; Futerman & Wellisch, 1990). In the ideal setting, teenagers should have their transplant in units which are able to provide adequate physical and emotional care to meet their special needs. Where this is not possible, access and referral to approriate specialists become important.

The general nursing preparation for the child receiving the transplant will need to take into account age, development, experience and need (Table 8.2). Bearing this in mind, the methods and details of nursing will consequently vary for each child. The following general issues, however, will need full explanations of what to expect and how to cope with them.

Table 8.2 General preparation of children for hospitalisation for stem cell transplant

---

For previously non-hospitalised children
  Central line insertion
  Central line dressing
  Nasogastric tube
  Gastrostomy tube
  Mouth care
  Hair loss
  Concordance with oral medication
  Finger pricks
  Isolation
  Altered body image
For children with experience of hospitalisation
  New environment
  New staff
  New method of nursing
  Nasogastric tube
  Gastrostomy tube
  Finger pricks
  Isolation
  Altered body image

Physical preparation of the child

Physical preparation of the child before SCT will show slight variations between clinical units. The most frequent pre-SCT evaluations are highlighted here. Much of the physical preparation is undertaken on an outpatient basis. Information is needed to assess the child's health and disease status before being deemed fit enough for the transplant to proceed. This also serves as a baseline for measurement of the child's future growth and development following the transplant. The process also monitors the effects of conditioning regimens and treatment in the long term. The coordination of physical preparation is usually undertaken by a transplant coordinator, often a nursing role. The physical and psychological preparation, if coordinated by the same person, can allow a seamless preparation period for the child and family. During this time, the coordinator can introduce members of the multidisciplinary team with whom the child is likely to come into contact at a later date. The child and family can also familiarise themselves with the hospital, its routines and staff over this period of time. It offers an opportunity for questions and concerns to be raised and dealt with as they arise. Information overload is a threat during this time, and support through open telephone access to the coordinator and clear written information will be needed to support the plethora of information given to the family. The presence of a third party, a named nurse or coordinator, at interviews and new investigations can offer support to the family and can help in the later clarification of information.

Physical preparation can be stressful and time-consuming. Fear that one of the many investigations will reveal an obstacle to the transplant or indicate disease recurrence or progression is reported by many parents at this time. Support for the family is vital in a period of intense physical and psychological activity. In order to save time and reduce travelling for the family, many of the physical investigations should take place on one day. Follow-up calls by the coordinator to the family after such days can help the family to feel supported and allow the opportunity to discuss issues raised. The stress of such days should not be under-estimated. In response to this, some units are now offering separate days on which to address issues of psychological preparation for the child, the family and, if applicable, sibling donors.

Physical preparation of the child for stem cell transplant includes the procedures shown in Table 8.3.

Fertility issues

The issue of fertility warrants further discussion in this chapter as children who have undergone previous chemotherapy may regain some fertility, with boys retaining spermatogenesis and girls possibly retaining a small degree of functioning ova (Sanders *et al.*, 1996). Before the start of the conditioning regimen it may be possible to collect semen from older boys and thus retain the hope of fatherhood for them. For girls, cryopreservation of ovarian tissue is a possibility although this sadly remains elusive in clinical practice despite improving techniques (Grundy *et al.*, 2001).

It is the use of conditioning regimens in SCT that will render the child sterile. The most likely causes of such sterility are total body irradiation (TBI) and the use of cyclophosphamide. It has been shown that 90 % of males who received TBI are permanently azoospermatic (Sanders *et al.*, 1989). In adult patients it has been suggested that sperm may be

Table 8.3 Physical preparation of the child for SCT

Medical history and physical examination

- Previous treatment history
- Diagnosis treatment history
- Identification of other medical problems
- Transfusion history
- Allergy and immunisation history
- Psychological and neurophysiological assessment

Histocompatibility

- Confirmation of HLA and MLC testing and selection of donor
- Transfusion support planning
- Determination of markers for engraftment (allogeneic patients)

Major organ assessment

- Full blood count, differential and platelets
- Electrolyte assessment
- Hepatitis screening
- Viral assessment (CMV, Herpes simplex, Varicella zoster, Epstein Barr)
- Pulmonary function
- Cardiac evaluation (ECG, echocardiogram)
- Glomerular filtration rate (GFR)
- Chest X-ray
- Nutritional evaluation
- Dental evaluation (teeth with evidence of caries should be extracted before the insertion of new central lines and should not be undertaken at the same time; this is due to the release of pathogens from the affected teeth which may be released into the peripheral circulation and may colonise the newly inserted line)

Tumour/disease evaluation
Central line insertion
PEG gastrostomy insertion
Sperm banking
Cryopreservation of ovarian tissue
Back-up bone marrow harvest
From child (this is collected and stored in case the donated marrow in allogeneic bone marrow transplant fails to engraft and the child needs 'rescuing' from the ablative therapy of conditioning regimens)

collected up to 30 days after the commencement of conditioning chemotherapy. The rationale for this time being that the life expectancy of mature sperm in the epididymis is 30 days so, in theory, these sperm will have matured before the onset of chemotherapy. This extra time may be vital in adolescent boys in the preparation time for the collection of sperm. In girls, the damage to ova is more devastating as females are born with a finite number of ova and, once damaged, there is no opportunity for regeneration (Sanders *et al.*, 1996). By the age of 14 most boys have entered puberty and may be able to masturbate and ejaculate. However, raising this subject will require great tact and diplomacy at a time of family stress (Williams & Wilson, 1989). Discussion of sperm banking will need the following areas to be taken into consideration: information, privacy, confidentiality, support and follow-up (Hopkins, 1991). Discussion with the young man will need to include why sperm collection is necessary and this may be difficult for the family to instigate. Discussion of a young son's sexuality at any time is difficult for families; during preparation for SCT with stress already at a high level, it may be impossible. After discussion with the parents and the young man, a male nurse or doctor may be chosen to talk in private about the issue of sperm donation. This includes concerns about masturbation (which in some religions may be a sensitive issue, for example, the Roman Catholic and Jewish faiths). Masturbation still has a stigma attached to it in western society (Hopkins, 1991). Information as to how the sperm is collected and stored should be discussed, with attention being paid to the amount of information given. The ability and comfort of the young man to comprehend what is discussed should be clues as to the length of such sessions.

Centres vary in their time limits of sperm storage. Ten years is the average time and this means that although provision for fatherhood has been made, even this has a limit. This will have implications for the future for the young man involved in deciding when to have a family. Arrangements for longer storage will need to be considered according to age at donation and will require negotiation with the local sperm bank.

For some boys who undergo SCT, the issue of sperm banking does not arise due to their age. Taking an early morning urine sample will show if there is any sperm present. Should there be no sperm, it would be pointless for the young boy to try producing a sample. However, parents should be informed of their child's future infertility and the effect this may have on the family should not be under-estimated. Although at the time of preparation for SCT the prime concern of the parents is the potential cure of their child, issues such as loss of future grandchildren may have future implications for some families (Heiney, 1989).

Following preparation and the decision about sperm donation by the young man, even with guidance and support, the collection of the sperm may still be difficult to achieve. Masturbation, even in a secluded room within the hospital with sexual stimuli from magazines, may be impossible (Hopkins, 1991). The specimen can be collected at home, but needs to be stored within four hours, making this option difficult. In the event of failure to obtain a specimen, psychological support and information on other options available will be needed by the young man. If collection is successful, he will need information as to how to recover the sperm at a later stage, and details should be given about the length of storage time (Kaempfer *et al.*, 1983).

For girls, this situation is further complicated by the current lack of technology with which to collect and preserve ova successfully. Experimental advances in the collection of ova or sections of ovaries have yet to prove successful in the clinical setting, but there have been calls for further ethically sound research in this area (Grundy *et al.*, 2001). But, for those young women faced with infertility as a result of conditioning regimens of SCT, counselling and advice, by trained infertility counsellors, in order to make clear future options should be offered prior to the preparation for transplant. Recent research (Sanders *et al.*, 1996) indicates that 5 % of prepubertal girls receiving TBI or high-dose chemotherapy prior to transplant developed normal gonadal function.

Conditioning regimens

Prior to stem cells being transfused, the child will undergo a preparative conditioning regimen. Conditioning regimens vary according to the child's diagnosis, age, type of transplant and any additional research therapies which may be introduced. The rationale behind conditioning therapy is:

- to treat any residual disease;
- to make 'space' for the donor cells to grow;
- to immunosuppress the child in order to decrease the risk of graft rejection, in the allogeneic setting.

To achieve these three goals the regimens may be:

- *full conditioning*: comprising a myeloablative combination of high-dose IV chemotherapy and high-dose oral chemotherapy with or without total body irradiation (TBI);
- *reduced intensity conditioning (RIC)*: a number of non-myeloablative or RIC regimens are used. One such regimen, a combination of IV fludarabine and melphalan, is now widely used in children who are physiologically unable to tolerate the expected toxicities of conventional ablative conditioning due to significant organ damage pre-transplant;
- *minimal intensity conditioning*: a combination of IV fludarabine, a single fraction of TBI with or without YTH 24.5/54.2 anti-CD 45 antibodies, may be given for those children unable to tolerate the RIC.

The RIC was initially designed for children unable to tolerate full myeloblative treatment due to significant organ damage, such as compromised airways or severely damaged lungs or gastrointestinal (GI) tract, as a result of either infection or previous toxic therapies. It is now also widely used in children with immunology disorders where full ablative therapy is not needed in order to cure their disease (Amrolia *et al.*, 2000; Veys *et al.*, 2005). It is hoped that future research will show that less myeloablative therapies will result in low levels of transplant-related morbidity (TRM) and reduce long-term late effects. Clearly the risk of using non-myeloablative regimens in the malignant setting is one of relapse where lingering malignant cells are not sufficiently destroyed by the conditioning chemotherapy (Veys & Rao, 2004). Further immunosuppression may be required, particularly with the use of either unrelated or haploidentical donors and this is usually achieved using antithymic globulin (ATG)

or more commonly a monoclonal antibody such as Alemtuzumab (Campath 1H). Table 8.4 outlines the most common combinations of therapies used.

Table 8.4 The most common combinations of therapy used in conditioning regimens

Drug therapy	Type of stem cell transplant	Disease
High-dose melphalan +/− Oral/IV busulphan	Autograft	Solid tumours
Oral/IV busulphan + IV cyclophosphamide	Allogeneic	Children less than 2 years old and /or with a non-malignant disease
IV cyclophosphamide + TBI	Allogeneic	Children more than 2 years old with some malignant diseases such as AML, CML and MDS, non-TBI regimens are now favoured
Oral/IV busulphan + IV cyclophosphamide + IV melphalan	Allogeneic	Children with JMML and other paediatric myelodysplasias
IV fluodarabine + IV alemtuzumab + IV melphalan	Allogeneic	Children with some immunology or metabolic disorders

Due to the large doses of treatment used, any combination of the therapies in Table 8.4 will result in the child having some degree of nausea and vomiting. Vomiting can range from mild to severe. It is clear that the use of a $5HT_3$ inhibitor such as ondansetron is effective in any antiemetic protocol. Combining this with dexamethasone seems to elicit an enhanced antiemetic effect (Dick *et al.*, 1995). On a few occasions, a third antiemetic such as cyclizine or metoclopramide may need to be considered. Although there is little documented research, experience has shown that babies and young children appear to tolerate conditioning very well and are less likely to vomit, but the degree of nausea they experience is unknown. It therefore seems reasonable to administer at least a single-agent antiemetic such as ondansetron, on a regular basis regardless of the perceived degree of nausea and/or vomiting. This should continue through the conditioning regimen. However, while it is clear that a $5HT_3$ inhibitor is highly effective as a chemotherapy-related antiemetic, the causes of emetogenicity are multiple in transplant. Therefore, beyond the conditioning period, a structured and systematic approach using a cascading protocol of different antiemetics is called for rather than relying on polypharmacy where 'we throw everything' at the problem (Gibson & Hopkins, 2005). If the child's nausea and vomiting are well controlled from the outset, anticipatory nausea and vomiting may be averted and both the parents and the child will feel more in control and better able to cope. This, in turn, will have a direct effect on staff morale.

In addition to the nausea and vomiting and the well-documented general side effects of chemotherapy, the conditioning drugs have specific side effects. Cyclophosphamide when given in high doses can cause haemorrhagic cystitis, although both busulphan and etoposide are also implicated. This is caused by a metabolite of the drug acrolein, which is toxic to the bladder lining. To counteract this, the child is given hyperhydration. Nursing staff need to measure the child's input/output accurately to ensure that retention of fluid, containing mesna, which reacts with the acrolein and reduces its urothelial toxicity, is not occurring. The child's urinary output must be tested for blood, the presence of which indicates further hydration and/or mesna is required. Continent children should be encouraged to void every couple of hours to minimise bladder toxicity, while nappy-wearing children need changing frequently to minimise contact between skin and excreted cyclophosphamide. For children wearing nappies, the safest way of testing for blood is to place a cotton wool ball into each nappy. The wet cotton wool can then be squeezed on to the multistix. Of note, the presence of excreted mesna in the urine will cause a false positive of ketones on urinalysis, due to the mesna in the urine reacting with the ketone pad on all brands of urine-testing strips.

It must be noted that occasionally late-onset haemorrhagic cystitis may occur after engraftment, therefore it is important that urine output is always observed and tested, while the child is in hospital. Treatment for haemorrhagic cystitis may include hyperhydration, bladder irrigation and maintaining a high platelet count. Some success has been found with the short-term use of oestrogen although the mechanism for this is unclear. Late-onset haemorrhagic cystitis may have a viral cause such as adenovirus, CMV or BK virus.

Busulphan is a drug which is available as an oral or an IV preparation. It has been shown to be as effective as TBI when combined with high-dose cyclophosphamide (Lucarelli *et al.*, 1985) in children without a malignancy or those under 2 years of age who are undergoing rapid development and are therefore saved from additional side effects of radiotherapy. If taken orally, it is essential that the child is able to take and absorb the busulphan tablets and if there is any doubt about the child's ability to take the dose, a nasogastric tube must be passed for the duration of the drug to ensure the correct dose is absorbed. For some parents, this can be extremely distressing. If the issue of passing the tube is approached appropriately and the safety measures for the child, parents and staff are discussed the night before commencing the administration of busulphan, stress levels can be reduced.

Research studies have shown that oral busulphan is significantly better absorbed if given on an empty stomach. The best regimen is for the child to be nil by mouth two hours pre- and a half-hour post-dose. To achieve this, negotiation of dosing times, within either a 12-hourly or 6-hourly schedule, which suit the child and the parents is essential to ensure concordance. Extended nil by mouth times can clearly cause some degree of distress for both the child and the parent. It appears that busulphan is of a moderate emetogenicity. Therefore, it may be preferable to give an antiemetic such as ondansetron prior to each dose, particularly with oral preparations, to avoid having to calculate the amount of busulphan lost in vomit.

The main side effect of busulphan is that some children may suffer seizures. On account of the small chance of seizures occurring it is advisable for the child to remain in the unit for the duration of the course of busulphan. Again, experience shows that seizures are more likely to occur in older children, or in children who have had previous CNS problems, such as seizures or febrile convulsions. On account of this, it may be a good policy to give anticonvulsants to high-risk children for a period of time surrounding the busulphan course. The decision to give anticonvulsants is based on an individual clinical need alongside unit policy. Busulphan also causes alteration in skin colour. This is particularly notice-able in non-Caucasian children, and on the scrotum of Caucasian boys. For some parents this causes concern, however, the skin colouring should return to normal several months post-SCT. A later side effect associated with high busulphan levels is the occurrence of veno-occlusive disease (VOD) (Bear-man, 1995). Nurses play a significant role in the early detection of VOD by commencing twice-daily weight and girth measurements at the start of the busulphan therapy.

Fludarabine, while being highly immunosup-pressive, is a generally well-tolerated cytotoxic drug with a low emetogenicity. Given as a short infusion over several consecutive days, a transient and self-resolving rise in creatinine in some chil-dren seems to be the only immediate side effect, according to anectodal reports.

Melphalan carries a degree of renal toxicity, requiring concurrent hyperhydration. It carries a high emetic potential, requiring appropriate antiemetic interventions as well as a degree of generalised gut toxicity frequently causing mucosi-tis and diarrhoea, both of which can range from mild to severe.

Total body irradiation (TBI) is the most effec-tive treatment in reaching sanctuary sites (i.e. the CNS and testes) in children with a haematologi-cal malignancy. It is also the single most effective immunosuppressant therapy. The unpleasant side effects seen when TBI was given as a single dose have been greatly decreased since the introduction of fractionated TBI over 6–8 doses. Most children tolerate the treatment well and an oral dose of ondansetron before treatment is usually sufficient.

Alemtuzumab (Campath 1H) is a drug that may be used in clinical units where children receive unrelated or haploidentical donor marrow, or stem cells. A monoclonal antibody is used to eradicate recipient lymphocytes, thereby reducing the risk of rejection. However, it also exerts a degree of T cell depletion on the donated stem cells, thereby reducing the risk of GVHD (Graft Versus Host Disease). Generally given over five days, the most toxic effects occur on day 1, when there is greatest activity following breakdown of the lymphocytes. The main side effects are hyperpyrexia, tachycar-dia, headache and nausea.

If a pre-medication of IV pethidine, chlor-phenanine, methylprednisolone and metoclopra-mide as well as paracetamol is given 1.5 hours pre-alemtuzumab, the toxic effects are reduced. In some centres administering the methylpred-nisolone up to 12 hours prior to the alemtuzumab seems to further reduce the risk of a severe reac-tion. The paracetamol must be continued 4-hourly during the infusion to ensure maximum comfort is achieved. On day 1, the alemtuzumab should be infused slowly over 8 hours. If this regimen of pre-medication and infusion is well tolerated, on the subsequent days the alemtuzumab can be infused as fast as tolerated, but no faster than over 2 hours. In addition, if the drug is well toler-ated, the pre-medication can be weaned down so that by days 3–4, the child may not need any pre-medication.

At the start of the conditioning regimen, it is the nurse's responsibility to both teach and explain to the parents the safety aspects of caring for a child receiving chemotherapy. This will include the wearing of vinyl gloves when changing nappies, helping with bedpans and urine bottles or vomit bowls. The length of time recommended for the use of gloves is seven days following the last dose of chemotherapy. However, universal precau-tions would include the wearing of gloves when in contact with any body fluids at any time. No matter which regimen is used, the two most important aspects for nurses are:

- to be aware of actual and potential side effects and thus be able to act effectively on that knowledge;
- to be able to support both the child and parents.

For parents whose child is undergoing chemother-apy for the first time, this is a new and frightening experience. Similarly, for parents whose child is receiving radiotherapy for the first time, the fear of TBI may be overwhelming and a point of no return, where they need to continue with the transplant. Preparation for the conditioning period by rele-vant members of the health care team is therefore crucial.

Preparation of a sibling donor

Sibling donor preparation begins once the choice of donor has been established. It may be that informed consent from the child has not yet been dealt with because up until this point the parents will have given consent on behalf of the donor. In the first instance the parents, with the help if necessary of the unit staff, will need to discuss with the child, or children, the need to have a blood sample taken. Preparation should include practical issues such as blood taking and understanding the need for repeated blood tests. The donor is a 'well' child and may have no understanding of the need to be in hospital having needles and medicine. There may be children who fear the truth has not been told. At the same time the donor should be prepared (if old enough and with parental consent) for wider issues, such as the patient developing severe GVHD, rejecting the marrow or dying. These negative aspects can have a huge impact on the donor and may result in the need for ongoing support, possibly from outside the family. The unit psychologist may well be the best person to provide continuity of support and long-term follow-up of the donor. Preparation of the donor prior to admission must aim to allow them to accept that whatever the outcome is, it is not their responsibility. None the less, this must be balanced with the hope that the healthy marrow will enable the sibling to undergo transplant safely with a positive outcome.

Once the admission date for the donor is established, being able to address any other worries is essential. These may range from physical concerns to emotional fears, depending upon the age and development of the child. Physical worries may arise from repeated blood tests, anaesthesia and the anticipation of post-procedural pain from aspiration sites. The emotional fears in the young child may include those of separation from family and home even though only for a short time, to the fear of having a Hickman line or becoming bald like the other children on the unit. For the older child the fear of the bone marrow not being good enough may be a huge burden. In addition, the donor may not want to go through with the procedure and may be feeling guilty and frustrated (Freund & Siegel, 1986; Lwin, 2000; Parmar et al., 2003). Some of these fears may be lessened by being made to feel special and important during the period of the donor admission. As the donor is generally an inpatient for only 48 hours, good preparation is clearly essential. The donor should have a clear understanding of what bone marrow/stem cells

are, where they come from, and also how they should expect to feel and look on return to the ward from the harvest. Being able to address some of the deeper issues surrounding the fears of the older donor may be difficult to achieve in such a short time span.

During the inpatient time the donor is often made to feel very special and receives a good deal of attention from their parents. Once discharged, however, both the parents may become deeply involved in the care of the child receiving the SCT. If the donor is the only sibling, the feelings of isolation will increase as he or she is shut out of the sibling's room and away from the attention of their parents. The sibling donor needs to be given a gentle and tactful explanation as to why it is not possible to go into the isolation room. If this child is to remain a frequent visitor to the unit, continued work and involvement with the play specialist will be beneficial (Rollins, 1990).

Ethical use of sibling donors

Thirty per cent of donated stem cells used in SCT come from family members. Of this, a large proportion comes from siblings. In adult transplants the sibling donor is often an adult too, and is therefore able to understand what is required, give a degree of informed consent and understand the implications of donating cells. However, when the sibling donor is a child, the situation becomes more complex, particularly from an ethical stance. Ethics is a branch of moral philosophy, which aims to enquire into the rights/wrongs of human actions. It calls professionals to consider everyday actions and judgements but is not an examination of what is 'legal'. Ethical theories describe the world as it ought to be, rather than as it is. This is not to say that ethics is purely an academic ideal: ethical theories provide a framework, which may contextualise principles of clinical activity. This framework can provide a basis from which to examine and clarify values and beliefs in practice and begin to understand the reasons behind them (Richardson & Webber, 1995). The use of ethics in conjunction with moral theory can offer the experience of examining what has gone before, evaluating events and aiding decision-making processes for the future (Brykczynska, 1990).

An awareness of these issues in an area of medicine such as SCT where new and experimental treatments are undertaken in an effort to prevent a child from dying is fundamental. Of all the members of the multidisciplinary team, nurses often have the greatest contact with families. They spend longer periods of time with them and intense relationships with the child and immediate family can form. Indeed, it may be the nurse who first identifies and confronts the ethical and moral dilemmas related to bone marrow transplant. How they then deal with these issues in support of the family will in many cases have an effect on the final outcome of the situation. If nurses wish to have a voice that is heard in the growing debate surrounding paediatric SCT, and hope to be part of the decision-making process in the future, they first need to examine and be comfortable with their own beliefs and values.

Two of the most common ethical issues that confront nurses in paediatric SCT are informed consent and the rights of donors, particularly donors who are children. Ethically, the removal of bone marrow from consenting adults for someone else's benefit is generally permitted because it supports the principle of respecting autonomous choice for individuals choosing to donate and the risks and harms do not contravene public policy. Tissue donation is seen as a socially admirable act that provides hope of a huge improvement in the quality of life of the recipient (Mumford, 1998). Brykczynska (1990) states that society expects organs and tissues to be donated without concern for the donor. The adult is able to make an autonomous decision to act altruistically with the knowledge that the outcome of transplantation is not always good, but that their marrow may offer a chance of survival in an otherwise potentially life-threatening situation. Indeed, the high potential benefits to the recipient and the relatively low risks to the donor may make refusals to donate morally questionable (McFall v Shrimp, 1978). Nevertheless, to force a bone marrow donation would harm the ethical values of individual autonomy, privacy and bodily integrity (Mersel & Roth, 1978). After all, the cost of the gift of donating cells can be high and has been identified as a process that is not without psychological and emotional implications (Kinrade, 1987; Pot Mees, 1989).

Fundamental to the donor in acceptance of bone marrow donation is respect for the autonomy of the individual concerned. There is an absolute requirement for the donor to provide informed consent to the procedure. Briefly, informed consent involves a two-part process. First, the patient consenting to treatment should be fully informed and understand the benefits and risks of treatment. This information also needs to include the identification and discussion of alternatives available to this proposed treatment. The second part of the process involves the explicit giving of consent: this should not be assumed through lack of dissent. The health-care professional giving this information should not use their power or influence to coerce the potential donor in this decision-making process.

There has been concern about the ability of those to donate to give truly free and voluntary consent (Caplan, 1993). It has been argued that it is simply not possible for the living donor, even when competent, to give legitimate consent. There may be the problem of health-care professionals providing objective information when they are responsible for advocating simultaneously for the recipient and the donor, although this can easily be overcome by using separate teams. Furthermore, there is the concern that family members are vulnerable to an extraordinary pressure to 'volunteer' to donate for fear of being blamed for failing to help. However, this pressure may be legitimate in that it is formed as a result of the mutual obligations that exist between family members (Patenaude et al., 1986). It is highly probable that the process of donating bone marrow to save the life of a family member would be saturated with feelings of pressure, from the ill relative, other family members and internally by the donor. But this does not seem to be a significant objection to prevent all bone marrow donations. However, it does highlight the need for health-care professionals to be cautious when accepting the consent of a relative to be harvested, to ensure that the donor is not acting merely because of coercion, but has a genuine desire to donate.

What, though, if the donor is below the legal age of adulthood, as is often the case, when the recipient is a child? Does he have the right to informed consent and, if so, is it afforded to him by adults acting on his behalf? Does he also have the right of dissent, that is, does he have the right to say 'No' at any point during the time before the marrow is collected if he feels has not been fully informed? The moral position is less clear when considering the position of children who are unable to give their consent and exercise their autonomy. An attempt to save a life is clearly a morally commendable thing to do that is applauded by society. When it is discovered that a child within the family is a match for the sick child requiring an SCT, the news is greeted with relief and joy. A potential lifesaver has been found close at hand and often the transplant procedure commences without further ado. But what of the rights of the sibling donor? Children may be unable to demonstrate the necessary understanding to provide their consent, to such an extent that the issue of child autonomy is much more complicated. The moral defence of altruism is no longer relevant, as to force someone to act altruistically somewhat defeats the nature of gift giving. Furthermore, gift giving is not as simple as it may appear. It involves a three-stage process of giving, receiving and repaying (Mauss, 1967, cited in Brykczynska, 1990). In donating marrow or peripheral stem cells, there is no exchange of gifts but just one person giving to another. In receiving cells from a sibling, a child can never adequately repay such a gift, yet how does he or she know when that debt has been repaid? For the child who donates, more than a donation of marrow/cells is involved. Indeed, the survival and future functioning of a family are included. Giving such a gift is accompanied by feelings of responsibility for both the recipient's life and possibly death. A young child is rarely in a position to refuse offering such a gift to a sick sibling and so the question arises, when does the responsibility stop?

The moral implications of the use of children as bone marrow donors can be explored using two theories that are particularly prevalent in contemporary medical ethics: deontology and utilitarianism. The predominant deontological theory is that proposed by Immanuel Kant whose ultimate moral principle was to 'act so that you treat humanity, whether in your own person or in that of another, always as an end and never as a means only' (Kant, 1997). Kant's idea implies that we must never use people to achieve our purposes, regardless of how good the purposes may be. With regards to children being used as donors of bone marrow, it would appear that we are in danger of violating this principle. It could be claimed that the child is being used merely as a means – their body parts are removed from them in order to benefit another. For individuals with this strong viewpoint, bone marrow donation by children who lack the autonomy to decide for themselves may be morally impermissible.

For the utilitarian, morality requires that in deciding what to do we should act so as to bring about the greatest amount of happiness for all those affected (Rachels, 1999). The child who survives, his parents, siblings, friends and relatives will all be made happier if the bone marrow transplant is successful. In this context, utilitarianism would support bone marrow donation by minors. Month (1996) uses this argument and states that the donor sibling is, in effect, saving the family from the trauma of losing one of its members, stating that the loss of a sibling is potentially more harmful than the physical risks of donation even when the sibling is too young to have formed an emotional bond with the recipient. His evidence is based on psychological research relating to children whose siblings have died rather than sibling donors of SCT, so can parallels be drawn? However, adopting a utilitarian philosophy cannot fully answer the problems encountered in bone marrow transplantation. Primarily, we need to consider what the effect will be if clinicians allow the procedure and it fails. There is a very slight chance that the donor will die during anaesthetic, and the parents will face the possible death of two of their children. More probable is the possibility that the recipient will die during transplantation. The family subsequently will be surrounded by unhappiness, and there is a possibility that the sibling donor will be damaged by the consequences of donating. Research has shown that the child may feel guilt that he could not save his sibling and develop a low sense of self-worth related to feeling that his bone marrow was inadequate (Mahon & Page, 1995).

With regards to the negative effects on the donor, it has been proposed that with appropriate information and support, the impact on the child can be reduced and even if the transplant is unsuccessful, the donor can be left with positive feelings from the experience of giving and sharing. Furthermore, even if the transplanted child dies, the parents may gain some comfort in the knowledge that they did all that they could to save their child (Savulescu, 1996). Additionally, a major problem with adopting the utilitarian approach is that if we are saying that it is justifiable to harvest a minor for the benefit of his sibling because it maximises happiness, why stop there? Why not harvest all children for the benefit of any member of society? Donating to an unrelated individual who may die without the transplant will increase overall happiness along the same lines. Furthermore, one of the main components of utilitarianism is the idea of impartiality (Mill, 1972). In determining the happiness that is caused, no one's happiness or unhappiness is more important than anyone else's. Adopting such a principle means that we should ignore the significance of family relationships. Surely most people would question whether it was justifiable to subject a child to harm to save the life of a person whom he did not know? This is not even a risk that we impose on consenting adults, so it surely cannot be the guiding principle in the care of children. For any moral justification for children donating their bone marrow to their siblings seems to be related in some way to the fact that it is their sibling, and not someone unknown to them. Whether or not it is morally acceptable to use a child as a bone marrow donor can be seen to be somewhat controversial when applying the traditional principles of contemporary medical ethics. Why then is bone marrow transplantation between children a procedure that has become so readily accepted? The importance of the relationship between family members has been examined to see whether parents are justified in allowing their healthy child to be used as a bone marrow donor (Friedman Ross, 1993).

The nature of the problem of bone marrow donation between siblings is whether it is right to place a healthy child at risk for the benefit of an ill child (Dwyer & Vig, 1995). Parents are called upon to settle the conflict between the interests of their two children. They are deprived of the opportunity to take the course of action that serves the best interests of each of their children and are faced with the challenge of resolving a situation where there are competing claims that cannot simultaneously be met. Such conflict is common in everyday family life, where parents are frequently expected to balance the interests of one child against those

of another. In such instances, parents are required to solve the conflict by responding to the children's competing needs, taking into account the difference in the urgency of each child's claims. As a result of this process, parents frequently deprive their children of rights and exercise their authority over their children in ways that would be unacceptable in other contexts. The evolutionary development of parents' rights to raise their children as they consider best is based on the assumption that they have natural affections for their children and a shared interest in promoting each member of the family's well-being.

The relationship of the family is seen therefore as a moral one rather than a biological one (Schoeman, 1980). Within the family the child is dependent upon the adult for emotional and material needs and the adult is dependent on the child for a unique form of intimacy. This intimate relationship is suggested as the primary reason why adults choose to become parents (Schoeman, 1980). Consequently, parents have a responsibility to provide opportunities for their children to develop identity, character and meaning (Schoeman, 1985). Society predominately considers that it is in the child's best interests to live in his or her own family and so we give the family some flexibility to allow them to flourish as a functioning, integrated unit. Thus the family is awarded rights of privacy and family autonomy. To foster intimacy and trust, the family requires considerable privacy. This right to privacy means that parents are entitled to raise their children without the scrutiny of others in society, except in exceptional circumstances. Families require a wide degree of autonomy to promote the relationship between the child and the parent that is essential for the child's moral development.

It is the concept of 'family autonomy' that has been suggested as forming the moral justification for bone marrow transplantation between children (Friedman Ross, 1993). The decision to allow one child to donate tissue to a sibling is seen as morally permissible provided there is an ongoing intimate relationship between the parents and the child. Schoeman (1980) proposes that important ends are served by allowing parents the right to decide important issues for their family members, even if this is in conflict with the interest of the individual family members. The concept of family autonomy provides the parents with the freedom to consider using their healthy child as a bone marrow donor for their sick child, to promote the well-being and functioning of their whole family and to instil in the child the ability to consider the wider implications of his actions on others. Interference in family autonomy should be limited to situations where the family's actions will cause the child harm or neglect. Hence, the right to privacy and family autonomy is not absolute. Nevertheless serving the interests of a family cannot always be at the expense of an individual's self-interests. Friedman Ross (1993) believes that family autonomy is constrained by the principle of respect for persons, but not respect for the rights of the person. She suggests that with regards to children, we show respect for him or her as a person by acting so that we promote conditions that will help them to achieve the capacity to act autonomously. She refers to the Aristotelian concept of flourishing, and subsequently concludes that parents can allow their children to be donors so long as they do not reduce the child's ability to act autonomously and they promote the child's capacity to flourish in other ways. If the donation is inconsistent with respecting the child as a person, parents should be prevented from allowing it to proceed. The ascertainable wishes of the child should be considered.

The role of the nurse in the ethical debate surrounding sibling donors is complex. Appropriate education regarding the issues involved in marrow donation is a key factor in informed consent (Downs, 1994). The nurse can be seen as the family's advocate in providing for, assessing and supporting the family and the child in his decision to donate marrow. The sibling donor will for a short while be a patient afforded the same rights as his sick sibling in accordance with the Children Act (Department of Health, 1989; Scottish Office, 1995; Department of Health and Social Services, 1995). If a sibling donor should disclose doubts about donating marrow to his sibling, the ethical and moral duty of the nurse is to the sibling donor. Should the child receiving the marrow die, the nurse has a duty to understand the needs of the donor and the family by coordinating care and identifying families at risk.

Nurses need to be aware of the current ethical decisions concerning paediatric SCT if they are to support the family in their time of stress and reach a decision regarding the use of one child to help another. In addition to the nurse using her skills in communication, if she is to act as an advocate for the child and family, she needs to be clear, in her own mind, about the value of helping the child to reach informed consent. Nurses should formulate and be comfortable with their own ethical opinions and be happy to act on them (Vogel-Smith, 1996). The support offered to the sibling donor incorporates the guidance of child psychologists and skilled play specialists, in sessions both as a family and as an individual; to ensure the child is fully informed of what donation entails, and that as an individual rather than as a child, they are happy with the decision to proceed.

Saviour siblings

A donor option, which has been highlighted in the press in recent times, is the choosing of an embryo, via in vitro fertilisation, which is both a tissue match and disease-free (in the case of the sick child having a genetic disorder) (Alby, 1992). The cord blood can then be used in an attempt to save the sick child. Ethicists believe that the concept of choosing a 'saviour sibling' could deprive the donor infant of the right to autonomy. In addition it could be argued that the child could be blamed for not succeeding in his 'mission', that is in the saving of his sibling's life (Cheema & Mehta, 2004). On the other hand there are debates that to choose a child/embryo for a specific reason can be more acceptable a reason than other causes for which babies may be born. Furthermore it might be argued that embryo selection for HLA matching to save a life is more justified than, say, choosing an embryo for gender selection. In the UK, the authorities (HEFA, the Human Embryonic Fertilisation Authority) have addressed the issues surrounding 'saviour siblings' with caution, and have a strict criteria for selecting embryos to be used as donors:

- The condition of the affected child must be serious or life-threatening.
- The embryos themselves must be at risk from the condition which the existing child is suffering.

- All other possibilities of treatment and sources of tissue for the affected child should have been explored.
- The technique should not be available where the intended recipient is a parent.
- Only cord blood should be taken.
- Appropriate counselling is a requirement.
- Embryos may not be genetically modified to provide a tissue match.

(Leather, 2003)

Preparation of non-donor siblings

Initially, all children in a family will have undergone blood tests to determine their tissue type and suitability to act as a donor. For the child who is not a 'match' various feelings may emerge. On the one hand, there may be great relief in not having to undergo any further tests. On the other, there may be feelings of guilt and anger at not being able to be included in the transplant process (Patenaude et al., 1979; Eiser, 1993). Furthermore, exclusion from the physical process means the exclusion of the 'healthy' children from their parents. In cases where both parents wish to be with their sick child, siblings are often sent to other family members. Visiting may then only occur at weekends when the children may only have minimal access to their parents. In the two different environments of hospital and alternative 'home', siblings may well feel a loss of control over what they can do, and restrictions not previously experienced may be placed upon them. The joy at being with their parents at the weekend may be lost if the parents are too worried or tired to provide the attention that is needed (Eiser, 1993).

With these issues in mind, the setting up of a sibling support group can prove enormously beneficial for all the siblings of children undergoing SCT. This special time given to siblings allows them to mix with other children in the same position, thus enabling them to share their feelings and act as a support to each other. In addition, it provides an outlet for possible feelings of frustration, guilt and anger (Patenaude et al., 1979; Kramer & Moore, 1983; Freund & Siegel, 1986). Although the play specialist has a key role in the preparation and ongoing emotional support of all the children, it is by no means exclusively his or her role. When the psychologist, ward nurses and the play specialist combine their skills and time to work together, the emotional needs of both the child undergoing SCT and the siblings will be met (Harding, 1996).

References

Alby N (1992) 'The child conceived to give life' Bone Marrow Transplant 9 (suppl. 1): 95–96

Amrolia P, Gaspar B, Hassan A, et al. (2000) 'Non-myeloablative stem cell transplantation for congenital immunodeficiency' Blood 96: 1239–1246

Bearman S (1995) 'The syndrome of hepatic veno-occlusive disease after marrow transplantation (Review article "Blood")' Journal of the American Society of Hematology 85(11): 3005–3020

Borgna-Pignatti C (1992) 'Bone marrow transplantation for the haemoglobinopathies' in: Treleaven J & Barrett J (eds) Bone Marrow Transplantation in Practice. London: Churchill Livingstone, pp. 151–159

Brykczynska G (1990) 'The gift of an organ' Paediatric Nursing October 12: 12

Caplan A (1993) 'Am I my brother's keeper?' Suffolk University Law Review 27(4): 1195–1208

Casey A (1988) 'A partnership with child and family' Senior Nurse 8(4): 8–9

Cheema P & Mehta P (2004) 'Ethical concerns' in: Mehta P (ed.) Paediatric Stem Cell Transplantation. Boston: Jones & Bartlett, pp. 91–99

Cleary J (1992) Caring for Children in Hospital: Parents and Nurses in Partnership. London: Scutari Press

Coyne I (1995) 'Parental participation in care' Journal of Advanced Nursing 21(4): 716–722

Department of Health (1989) The Children Act. London: HMSO

Department of Health and Social Services (1995) The Children (Northern Ireland) Order. Belfast: HMSO

Dick GS, Meller ST & Pinkerton CR (1995) 'Randomised comparison of ondansetron and metoclopramide plus dexamethasone for chemotherapy induced emesis' Archives of Disease in Childhood 73(3): 24–25

Downs S (1994) 'Clinical issues in bone marrow transplantation' Seminars in Oncology Nursing 10(1): 58–63

Dwyer J & Vig E (1995) 'Rethinking transplantation between siblings' Hastings Center Report 25(6): 7–12

Eiser C (1989) 'Psychological effects of chronic disease' Journal of Child Psychology 31(1): 85–98

Freund B & Siegel K (1986) 'Problems in transition following bone marrow transplantation: psychosocial aspects' American Journal of Orthopsychiatry 56(2): 244–252

Friedman Ross L (1993) 'Moral grounding for the participation of children as organ donors' *Journal of Law,
Medicine and Ethics* 21(2): 251–257

Futerman AD & Wellisch DK (1990) 'Psychodynamic
themes of bone marrow transplant - when I becomes
thou' *Haematology/Oncology Clinics of North America*
4(3): 699–709

Gibson F (1989) 'Parental involvement in bone marrow
transplant' *Paediatric Nursing* 1(7): 21–22

Gibson F & Hopkins S (2005) 'Feeling sick is horrible, and
being sick is very frightening . . . say Jasper and Polly
(Pearman, 1998)' *European Journal of Oncology Nursing*
9: 6–7

Grundy R, Larcher V, Gosden RG, Hewitt M, Leiper
A, Spoudeas HA, Walker D & Wallace WHB (2001)
'Fertility preservation for children treated for cancer
(2): ethics of consent for gamete storage and experimentation' *Archives of Diseases in Childhood* 84:
360–362

Haberman M (1988) 'Psychosocial aspects of bone
marrow transplantation' *Seminars in Oncology Nursing*
4(10): 251–254

Harding R (1996) 'Children with cancer: the needs of
siblings' *Professional Nurse* 11(9) 588–590

Heiney S (1989) 'Adolescents with cancer: sexual
and reproductive issues' *Cancer Nursing* 12(2):
95–101

Hogbin B (1989) 'Getting it taped: the bad news consultation with cancer patients' *British Journal of Hospital
Medicine* 41(4): 330–333

Hopkins M (1991) 'Sperm banking' *Nursing Times* 87(47):
38–40

Kaempfer S, Hoffman D & Willey F (1983) 'Sperm banking: a reproductive option in cancer therapy' *Cancer
Nursing* 6(1): 31–38

Kant I (1997) *Groundwork of the Metaphysics of Morals.*
Cambridge: Cambridge University Press

Kinrade LC (1987) 'Preparation of a donor for bone
marrow transplant harvest' *Procedure Cancer Nursing*
10(2): 77–81

Kramer R & Moore I (1983) 'Childhood cancer: meeting
the special needs of healthy siblings' *Cancer Nursing*
6(3): 213–217

Leather S (2003) 'Saviour siblings: is it right to create
a baby for the benefit of someone else?' unpublished Progress Educational Trust Debate, London,
16 October

Lee P (2004) 'Family involvement: are we asking too
much?' *Paediatric Nursing* 16(10): 37–41

Lucarelli G, Polchi P, Galimberti M, Izzc T, Delfini C,
Manna M, Agostinelli F, Baronciani D, Giorgi C,
Angelucci E, Giardini C, Politi P & Manenti F (1985)
'Marrow transplantation for thalassaemia following
busulphan and cyclophosphamide' *The Lancet (8442)*:
1355–1357

Lwin R (2000) 'Impact of paediatric bone marrow transplant on sibling donors and sibling relationship' PhD
thesis in progress and personal communication

Mahon M & Page M (1995) 'Child bereavement after
the death of a sibling' *Holistic Nurse Practitioner* 9(3):
15–26

Mersel A & Roth L (1978) 'Must a man be his cousin's
keeper?' *Hastings Center Report* 8(5): 5–7

Mill JS (1972) 'On liberty' *in:* Warnock M (ed.) *Utilitarianism.* Glasgow: Collins

Month S (1996) 'Preventing children from donating may
not be in their best interests' *British Medical Journal*
312(7025): 240

Mumford S (1998) 'Bone marrow donation: the law
in context' *Child and Family Law Quarterly* 10:
135–146

Parmar G, Wu JWY & Chan KW (2003) 'Bone marrow
donation in childhood: one donor's perspective'
Psycho-Oncology 12: 91–94

Patenaude A, Rappenport J & Smith B (1986) 'The physician's influence on informed consent for bone marrow
transplant' *Theoretical Medicine* 7: 165–179

Peters C & Steward CG (2003) 'Haematopoetic cell
transplantation for inherited metabolic diseases: an
overview of outcomes and practice guidelines' *Bone
Marrow Transplant* 31: 229–239

Pot Mees C (1989) *The Psychosocial Effects of Bone Marrow
Transplantation in Children.* Delft: Eburon

Rachels J (1999) *The Elements of Moral Philosophy.* New
York: Oxford University Press

Richardson J & Webber I (1995) *Ethical Issues in Child
Health Care.* London: CV Mosby

Rollins J (1990) 'Childhood cancer siblings draw and tell'
Paediatric Nursing 16(1): 21–35

Sanders J, Hawley J, Levy W, Gooley T, Buck-
ner C, Deeg H, Doney K, Storb R, Sullivan K,
Witherspoon, R & Appelbaum F (1996) 'Pregnancies following high-dose cyclophosphamide with or
without high-dose busulfan or total body irradiation and bone marrow transplantation' *Blood* 87(7)
3045–3052

Sanders J, Sullivan K, Witherspoon R, Doney K,
Ansetti C, Beatty P & Peterson F (1989) 'Long term
effects and quality of life in children and adults after
bone marrow transplantation' *Bone Marrow Transplantation* 4: 27–29

Savulescu P (1996) 'Substantial harm but substantial
benefit' *British Medical Journal* 312: 241–242

Schoeman F (1980) 'Rights of children, rights of parents
and the moral basis of the family' *Ethics* 91(1):
6–19

Schoeman F (1985) 'Parental discretion and children's
rights: background and implications for medical
decision-making' *Journal of Medicine and Philosophy* 10:
45–61

Scottish Office (1995) *Scotland's Children: A Brief Guide to The Children (Scotland) Act Scotland*. Edinburgh: Scottish Office

Taylor M & O'Connor P (1989) 'Resident parents and shorter hospital stay' *Archives of Disease in Children* 64(2): 274–276

Veys P & Rao K (2004) 'Advances in therapy: megatherapy allogeneic stem cell transplantation' *in*: Pinkerton R, Plowman PN & Pieters R (eds) *Paediatric Oncology* (3rd edn). London: Arnold, part 3A, pp. 513–517

Veys P, Rao K & Amrolia P (2005) 'Stem cell transplantation for congenital immunodeficiencies using reduced intensity conditioning' *Bone Marrow Transplant* 35: 543–547

Vogel Smith K (1996) 'Ethical decision-making by staff nurses' *Nursing Ethics* 3(1): 17–24

Wiley FM, Lindamood MM & Pfefferbaum-Levine B (1984) 'Donor-patient relationship in paediatric bone marrow transplantation' *Journal of Association of Pediatric Oncology Nurses* 1(3): 8–15

Williams HA & Wilson M (1989) 'Sexuality in children and adolescents with cancer: pediatric oncology nurses' attitudes and behaviors' *Journal of Pediatric Oncology Nursing* 6(4): 127–132

9 Collection and Infusion of Bone Marrow, Peripheral Blood Stem Cells and Umbilical Cord Cells

Nikki Bennett-Rees and Sian Hopkins

Collection of bone marrow

The method of collecting bone marrow from a donor is an individual procedure that varies from unit to unit. However, the principles remain the same for both adult and child donors and these are described below.

The donor is admitted to hospital the day before the bone marrow is collected. A routine preoperative physical evaluation is carried out in preparation for an anaesthetic and consent for the procedure obtained. The collection of bone marrow is undertaken in an operating theatre using a sterile technique and lasts 30–90 minutes. The donor is laid in the prone position to allow aspiration from the posterior iliac crests; in cases of poor collection from this site the patient may be turned and the anterior iliac crests and possibly the sternum used. Epidural anaesthetics have been used in bone marrow collections, though not in situations where marrow collection from the iliac crests is likely to be insufficient and the sternum used.

Two or three skin punctures are made at the chosen site of collection. The marrow is then aspirated in 5 ml aliquots using multiple penetrations with the aspiration needle being redirected to a new area of bone as needed. The aim of using only two or three skin incisions and stretching the skin across is to minimise scarring.

The collected marrow is then injected into a blood transfusion pack containing anticoagulant. The total amount of bone marrow aspirated varies in each case and is calculated during the procedure by measuring the number of nucleated cells in a sample of marrow and estimating the required amount of bone marrow needed to supply an adequate number of stem cells to ensure engraftment. The marrow is then filtered through a series of fine mesh filters in order to remove fat, bone and fibrin clots. If required within the next 72 hours, the marrow will be stored at 4°C. Longer periods of storage at this temperature result in stem cell death. If the marrow is to be transfused after this time (as in the case of autologous marrow and cord blood), then it will be cryopreserved (marrow from unrelated adult donors should not be cryopreserved except in extreme circumstances). For effective cryopreservation, the

Cancer in Children and Young People   Edited by Faith Gibson and Louise Soanes
© 2008 John Wiley & Sons, Ltd

cryopreservative, dimethylsulphoxide (DMSO), is introduced; this involves DMSO being added to the marrow, which is then frozen in liquid nitrogen, liquid nitrogen vapour or mechanical deep freezers.

The freezing process can have an adverse effect on the marrow. If frozen too quickly, damage to the stem cells may occur, ice crystals may form in the bags and the freezing process acting on different metabolic processes in the cell may cause disruption to the cell and result in cell-toxic metabolites forming. Large quantities of marrow may be divided into smaller bags in order to allow uniform freezing at a controlled rate; this is also valuable if one bag is rendered unusable in the freezing or thawing process as some marrow is still available for re-infusion. Marrow preserved in this way can be used up to five years following donation but the use of DMSO carries some risk for the patient; this is discussed in the section on transfusion of the marrow.

On completion of the harvest, up to a litre of bone marrow may have been aspirated from the adult donor (less from children). In preparation for this the donor may have given some of their own blood to replace that lost in the collection (autologous blood). This is preferred as it reduces the risk of transfusing white cell antibodies from a third party. Haemoglobin levels are assessed prior to discharge and the need for further transfusions are made on an individual basis.

On return to the ward from the operating theatre the donor will require the same post-operative care as any patient after a general anaesthetic. Other specific post-operative care involves assessing the puncture sites for haemorrhage. If haemorrhage occurs it is usually slight and can be controlled with the application of pressure dressings to the puncture sites. Donors should be made aware that the skin incisions will result in scarring, although small and not visible during everyday life. The dressings covering the puncture sites can be removed after a few days and left exposed if the wound is clean and dry.

Discomfort is the most commonly reported side effect of donating marrow. Following donation, physical discomfort from the puncture sites may require oral analgesia for a few days and slight stiffness may be experienced on walking up stairs and, for adults, driving is reported to be difficult.

Donors are advised to mobilise as soon as possible following donation, to prevent severe stiffness. For young children this is rarely a problem, though older patients whose bones are denser may find mobilising quite difficult initially. The donor is often fit enough to leave hospital the following day and rarely requires any further medical or nursing intervention. He or she may, however, feel a little lethargic as a result of the anaesthetic and should not return to work or school for a few days following the bone marrow collection. If the donor's haemoglobin is on the low side, they may receive an oral iron supplement to take until normal levels are restored.

On discharge from hospital, advice should be given on recognising the symptoms of complications that may need medical attention. Such problems may include persistent pain and signs of infection (discharge, pain and fever). Written documentation of the expected recovery time, signs and symptoms of complications and the telephone number of a person to contact, are useful and reinforce the verbal information given on discharge.

Complications of donation

The long-term sequelae of unrelated adult donors are not well documented. Most registries maintain contact and offer support to unrelated adult donors for a period of time after donation, this may be up to a year. Details of the welfare of the bone marrow recipient may be passed on in brief. In exceptional circumstances, the donor and the recipient may meet. In such cases both parties receive counselling to prepare for the emotional effects this may have. Complications following donation are very rare but reports exist of physical complications ranging from haematomas to persistent back problems and continuing pain from the aspiration sites.

Collection of peripheral blood stem cells (PBSC)

What are stem cells?

All blood cells are produced in the bone marrow and released into the peripheral bloodstream as required at various stages of maturity. Mature cells all originate from one cell type, known as the pluripotent stem cell. These are unlike other blood cells as they have the ability to replicate in unlimited numbers and can also differentiate into whichever mature cells are required (Walker *et al.*, 1994) (Figure 9.1). As shown in Figure 9.1, there are several lines of haematopoietic precursor cells arising from the pluripotent

stem cell. The cells, which are commonly counted at the time of harvest, are the colony-forming units, granulocyte–macrophage (CFU-GM) that are committed to the neutrophil line. Burst-forming units–erythrocyte (BFU-E) are another indicator of the presence of haematopoietic stem cells. There are, however, only 0.1% of CFU-GM cells circulating at any one time, although 98% are found in the bone marrow (Fliedner & Steinbach, 1988).

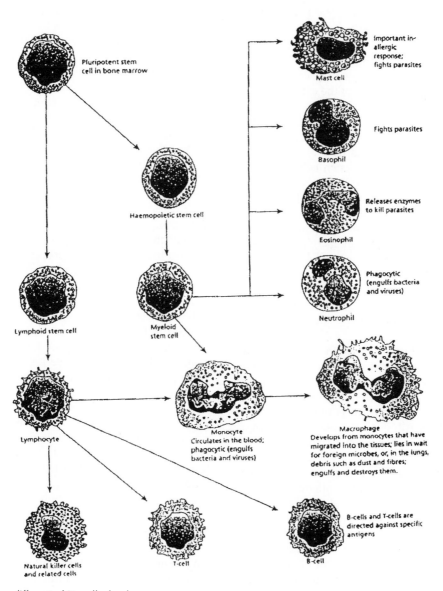

Figure 9.1   How different white cells develop.
Source: Roberts (1994).

In order to mobilise stem cells into the peripheral circulation it is necessary for the child to have a dose of non-stem-cell toxic chemotherapy, and a short course of daily colony-stimulating factors.

Mobilisation of PBSC in the autologous or allogeneic setting

The physical and psychological assessment of the child undergoing autologous PBSCT is similar to that previously mentioned. An important aspect is the indication of normal renal function; this will be required prior to the high-dose chemotherapy, as reduced renal function may cause complications due to the delayed excretion of the cytotoxic drugs used, especially melphalan.

Stem cells must first be mobilised from the bone marrow into the peripheral circulation in order to obtain a good yield. This is usually achieved by the administration of a non-stem cell toxic drug, such as IV cyclophosphamide, approximately 10 days before the harvest is anticipated. This induces a degree of myelosuppression, which, in turn, encourages new growth of the stem cell population. Given alone, this can increase the GFU-GM population by 10–18 times its previous level (Korbling, 1993) and BFU-E levels can increase eight-fold. With the addition of a haematopoietic growth factor, such as G-CSF, GM-CSF or IL-3, this can increase to as much as 370 times (Fliedner & Steinbach, 1988).

A daily injection of growth factor, usually G-CSF, is given subcutaneously for approximately 10 days commencing the day after the cyclophosphamide. There exists some discrepancy between units at present as to which is the most effective protocol to use. Although the dose of cyclophosphamide is relatively low, many units routinely give a dose of mesna and a minimum of four hours post-hydration to prevent the risk of haemorrhagic cystitis. An effective antiemetic, such as metoclopramide/ondansetron ± dexamethasone, is also recommended to prevent nausea and vomiting. The child will need to be in hospital as a day case, although some units prefer an overnight stay. The injection of growth factor can be a daunting prospect for the child and the family as up to this point, it has been possible to give most medicines either by mouth or painlessly through an existing central line. It must be explained fully that the most effective way of giving this particular drug is by subcutaneous injection; there is the advantage that the child can remain an outpatient or, even better, have the treatment at home.

There may be a family member willing to learn the technique of giving the injection but if this is not an option, it can usually be arranged for a paediatric community nurse or practice nurse to administer the G-CSF, thus keeping hospital visits to a minimum. Some children may prefer such procedures to be undertaken by nursing staff; and there are some who trust only themselves. One such patient refused to let anyone give him any of his injections. Instead, he preferred to practise on his favourite toys and an orange, and completed the full course with the help of some ethyl chloride spray. Each unit will have its own policy and regulations for the administration of injections at home. Often the first injection, if not the first two or three, will need to be given under supervision either in hospital, or at home.

For those parents who wish to give the injections, various booklets and videos available from drug companies, which produce growth factors, can enhance education given by nursing staff to support them in this role. Hospital play specialists are skilled in helping both parents and children with these procedures by the use of dolls or puppets in the play setting. Most families will opt to have injections given at home, and will indeed succeed in this, with support and education. The use of an ethyl chloride spray for the child over 5 years can be of considerable help, and EMLA or ametop cream is also thought to be of use in some cases, although there is some doubt about its anaesthetic effect below the skin. For some children, the use of EMLA cream has been seen to be of psychological benefit. Children may have an insuflon inserted, which should last for seven days, thus reducing the need to have daily needles, in order to give the GCSF.

Venous access

Approximately 8–10 days following cyclophosphamide administration, a full blood count should show a significant increase in the neutrophil population, indicating an appropriate time to commence the cell harvest (though approximately 10% of the general population will never mobilise enough stem cells, especially if they have received several intensive courses of chemotherapy prior to the stem cell harvest). In order to achieve the cell harvest, a temporary rigid double lumen leukopheresis line will be inserted under anaesthetic (Vaux, 1996), as the existing central venous line is unlikely to be sufficiently rigid or to have a wide enough bore to withdraw the required amount of blood volume without collapsing. The temporary line may be inserted into any of the following veins: subclavian, internal jugular or femoral. If a new line is necessary, the child must have a full explanation of why it is needed and be well prepared both for the line itself and a general anaesthetic.

The related or unrelated donor will have gone through the same stringent medical and psychological assessment and preparation as the donor of bone marrow. In order to mobilise the stem cells into the peripheral circulation the adult donor requires a five-day course of subcutaneous growth factor (GCSF) and the donor's GP or practice nurse usually gives this. However, in the case of a parent being the donor, it may be possible to give the injection on the ward where their child will be having treatment. The donor will require a daily full blood count to ensure that the total white cell count is rising. While in the neutropenic child GCSF seems to have few side effects, in the healthy adult reports of flu-like symptoms with joint pain are common. Usually a regular dose of paracetamol is sufficient to take the aches and pains away. For the adult donor venous access is usually through two wide-bore cannulas, one in each antecubital fossa to allow from one site the removing of blood and through the other arm the return of the cells which are not needed.

Stem cell collection

Although much of this can be achieved on an outpatient basis, it can be a frightening procedure if not fully understood especially as the cell separator machine is large. At a convenient time prior to the first collection, the child and the family should visit the department, see the machine and meet the nurse or technician who will be involved in the

harvesting process. It is sometimes helpful to see another patient connected to the machine as reinforcement of the explanation and reassurance that it really is a painless procedure. Ideally, a nurse and/or play specialist whom the child knows well, should stay with them for at least the first part of the collection until the child feels settled. In some hospitals, the machine may be transported to the child's bedside, which may help to reassure them, but in many units, the machine is in a separate department, which may be more unsettling. Once venous access is achieved, the stem cells can be collected using an apheresis process through a cell separator machine. This is often a COBE Spectra, which is the most suitable for use in small children. The machine removes blood from the child via the leukopheresis line, spinning it in a centrifuge. The machine will have been programmed to separate the blood into the different layers of red cells, white cells and platelets in the buffy coat, and plasma according to density. The buffy coat, containing the mononuclear cells, is then transferred into a collection bag while the remaining blood is returned to the patient. This process takes 2–4 hours to complete and it may be necessary to repeat it for 2–3 days, although one day is usually sufficient. It is necessary to prime the lines in the cell separator machine before commencing the collection process. A saline solution is usually used for this but for children weighing less than 30 kg, it is necessary to prime the machine with blood to prevent shock developing from the sudden loss of blood volume. The packed red cells used should be fully cross-matched, CMV-negative and leukodepleted (Vaux, 1996). To prevent blood in the collection tubing from clotting, an anticoagulant, acid citrate dextrose (ACD) or heparin, is added, a small amount of which will be received by the patient in the return line. The citrate inhibits normal coagulation by binding to ionised serum calcium and can therefore reduce blood calcium levels resulting in hypocalcaemia, also called citrate toxicity (Hooper & Santas, 1993; Purandare, 1994). The first signs of hypocalcaemia are often numbness or tingling of the peripheries, particularly the nose, ears, fingertips or toes (Walker et al., 1994). This effect is rapidly reversed at onset with the administration of IV calcium gluconate or calcium chloride. If it is not treated with the onset of symptoms, the child may complain of painful muscle spasms, particularly in the hands or feet which may lead to muscle twitching and convulsions (tetany). Cardiac arrhythmias may also be present. In some units, the donor/patient is encouraged to drink plenty of milk before and during the harvesting procedure to help boost the calcium levels in the blood, although this will only have a gradual and ongoing effect and will not help when levels are already low. When any of the above symptoms are noticed, the cell separator machine should be slowed down to a level tolerated by the patient.

Another side effect, which may be seen during this procedure, is hypovolaemia, particularly when the child is first connected to the machine. As previously mentioned, it is necessary to prime the lines with blood for low-weight children, and 0.9 % sodium chloride for older children or adult donors. Baseline observations of pulse and blood pressure should be recorded. The platelet count can drop significantly after apheresis as the platelets may stick to the apheresis machine and not be returned to the patient (Hooper & Santas, 1993). A baseline blood count should be taken prior to apheresis and a platelet transfusion may be required if the level is less than $50 \times 10^9/l$.

On completion of each collection, a blood sample is taken to ascertain the stem cell concentration. This is usually counted initially by the number of mononuclear cells or CD-34 antigen-positive cells, which gives an adequate indication of the number of stem cells in the collection (CD-34 antigen is found on the surface of early progenitor cells). Although CD-34 antigen-positive cells do not measure the pluripotent stem cell, a count greater than $5 \times 10^6/kg$ is said to be adequate for successful engraftment (Vaux, 1996). The number of mononuclear cells required for engraftment is thought to be in the range of $3–10^8/kg$ bodyweight (Vose et al., 1993).

Due to the length of time the procedure takes, it will be necessary for distraction therapy to be arranged to relieve the boredom for the child. This should be planned with the child in advance of the procedure. Some children may be quite content to watch a video or play computer games, but some will prefer interactive board games, which can be played with parents, the play specialist or a nurse as available (Hooper & Santas, 1993; Vaux, 1996). Following completion of the stem cell harvest the child may either be discharged home for a short

period or may continue immediately with the conditioning regimen and the re-infusion of cells. For the adult donor suitable books/videos/music or even work should be organised before being attached to the machine. Following the final collection (depending on the cell dose harvested, there may be collections on one or two days), the cannula will be removed and the patient discharged.

Should the conditioning therapy and re-infusion of cells occur within a few days, the harvested stem cells need only be refrigerated until the child is prepared for re-infusion. If the cells are to be re-infused at a later date, the cells require the addition of the cryopreservative, DMSO, and be stored frozen in liquid nitrogen at approximately $-200°C$ (Vose et al., 1993). Conditioning regimens vary according to the underlying disease and may be over one day, i.e. melphalan, or as long as six days, i.e. BEAM (BCNU, etoposide, melphalan and cytarabine). This will be one factor, which predetermines the need for cryopreservation of the stem cells prior to re-infusion.

There are significant differences between the use of peripheral stem cells and bone marrow cells for transplant purposes, as shown in Table 9.1.

Collection of umbilical cord blood cells

Worldwide there are many active public donor cord banks. Usually cord blood is collected from a 'volunteer' donor during or after the third stage of labour after the healthy infant has been delivered (i.e. cells are collected either before placental separation or the placenta is delivered). Opinions vary as to which of these two occasions allows for the greatest yield of cells. The collection of cells must be a painless procedure, which does not interfere with, or change the delivery of, the infant. The cord is clamped, cleaned and the umbilical vein is then cannulated and the sample collected into a blood transfusion bag containing an anticoagulant. The sample may then be stored in a refrigerator for a few days or frozen in DMSO (Apperley, 1994). Red cell depletion of the UCB is used in some units, but as the sample is often small (approximately 100 mls) this is not thought necessary by all units. Extensive screenings of both the donor mother and the cord cells are performed prior

Table 9.1   Comparison of stem cell and bone marrow harvesting

Peripheral stem cells	Bone marrow
Harvesting is painless.	Harvest site may cause discomfort.
General anaesthetic is required to insert rigid central venous access line.	General anaesthetic is required.
Can be collected with the child as an outpatient (in older children who can cope with collection using peripheral venous cannulation).	A short inpatient admission is necessary.
Stem cell collection may need to be carried out more than once, the sessions last 2–4 hours.	Bone marrow is harvested in one session, the session may take up to 2 hours.
Each stem cell collection requires laboratory time and cost; adequate storage space is essential.	Bone marrow can frequently be re- infused within 24 hours.
A suitable cell separator machine and trained nurse or a technician are required, allowing for the treatment of very small children needing specialist paediatric care.	A fully equipped and staffed operating theatre is required for a potential of 2 hours.

to any information being released to transplant centres. In addition to the screening carried out on other bone marrow/PBSC donors, the cord blood is also screened for:

- genetic screening, in particular, for familial inherited haematological/metabolic and immunological disorders;
- culture for bacterial or fungal contamination;
- total nucleated cell count with differential including mononuclear cell count and nucleated red blood cell quantitation (Wall, 2004).

The anonymity of the donor and family in cord blood banking means that there is only one chance to obtain cells. Therefore there is no chance of returning to the donor for extra cells in the case where the child either fails to engraft, or has low levels of engraftment. The units of collected cord cells are cryopreserved and at present may be stored for up to 10 years.

Issues surrounding umbilical cord banking

Cord blood banks have been set up and are successful in finding donors for children in whom other sources of stem cells have not been available. Donation of a child's cord cells to a national bank is an act of beneficence by the parent to society as a whole. In donating their child's cells parents sign away any later claims that they could use the cells, should the need arise, for the child who was the donor. Over the last few years there has been an increase in the number of private

cord blood banks who will collect, store and save cells, for a fee, in the event that the child may develop a disease requiring a stem cell transplant. With the advent of private cord banks there is the chance that fewer parents will donate to national banks thereby reducing the numbers of available cells for both children and adults needing stem cell transplants. As in many areas of medicine, there are both advantages and disadvantages in using umbilical cord blood stem cells (Table 9.2).

Bone marrow/stem cell infusion

Harvested cells will remain 'fresh' at room temperature for at least 72 hours but they should be infused as soon as both the cells and the recipient are ready. Delays from time of harvest to infusion occur if the donor is much older and larger than the recipient or has a different blood group. In either of these cases the marrow will be plasma-depleted and the red cells removed respectively. Alternatively, stem cells from an unrelated donor may undergo a degree of T cell depletion, however, this seems to be a technique, which is now seldom used.

The aim of T cell depletion of stem cells is to remove the cells responsible for causing transplant-related complications, especially GVHD. In removing all the T cells, however, the risk of graft rejection, or indeed the risk of leukaemia relapse, is increased.

Inevitably, the day on which the harvested cells are infused is one of mixed emotions for all the

Table 9.2 Advantages and disadvantages of the use of cord blood

Advantages	Disadvantages
Greater availability of stem cells from ethnic minority groups.	The donor initially will be unable to donate further cells.
Cord blood less likely to contain viruses.	Second transplants are impossible.
Shorter preparation time of patient.	Screening for all genetic disorders is impossible at birth.
Banked cord blood reduces the search time for a donor; practical financial implications are involved.	Little evidence of GvL is shown in UCBT, therefore its use in children with leukaemia is uncertain.

family. There may be a sense of relief that the cells have been safely harvested whether from a sibling or an unrelated donor, while there can be feelings of both optimism and trepidation about the actual infusion. If the cells have been freshly harvested from a sibling, parents will want to spend time with both the donor and the recipient and may experience a swing of emotions relating to the situation of each child. Although the harvested cells need to be infused as soon as possible, if it is from a sibling donor both parents and the donor may need to be given some time to gather themselves and prepare for the next stage of the infusion itself.

Once the cells arrive on the unit, the recipient, donor and parents appreciate being able to see the bag of cells before it is attached to the 'giving set'. However, seeing the cells can be something of an anticlimax as it looks like a normal bag of blood, or in the case where the red cells are removed, the cells are a yellowish colour and look like platelets. Nonetheless, it is not uncommon for the parents to take a photo of the donor holding the bag of cells, to record this achievement. In a recent case a mother had difficulty in pinpointing exactly why she took photographs, but felt that it marked 'a new beginning'.

If the cells have not undergone processing the child should not require any pre-medication. If there is an ABO incompatibility or a large volume of cells, the cells will have been red cell and/or plasma-depleted. A pre-medication of IV chlorphenamine may be given to ensure any risk of reaction due to the processing is reduced. Depending upon the volume of the cells to be infused, or the child's ability to cope with intravenous fluids, a diuretic may be necessary. Following this, the bag of cells can be infused. They can be attached to a standard blood-giving set and either set at a free-flow rate or infused via a pump to regulate the rate. Generally, the child will be 'specialled', this

will enable the nurse to record half-hourly readings of temperature, pulse, respiration and blood pressure, and to ensure there is no line blockage or leakage of cells due to a faulty infusion set. In addition, the nurse will be able to both support and act as a resource for the child and the parents during this emotional time. On completion of the infusion the bag should be washed through with 0.9 % IV sodium chloride to ensure that all the cells have been infused through the bag and central line. If the infusion has occurred uneventfully, the recordings of vital signs can return to four-hourly.

For patients who are to have bone marrow or stem cells (peripheral or umbilical cord), which have been harvested some time ago, both the procedure on the unit and the nursing implications are different. The bone marrow or stem cells will have been cryopreserved in DMSO and prior to infusion the preserved bags of marrow or stem cells need to be thawed at 40°C in a large water bath. Ideally, this process should take place on the unit in order that time is not wasted in transportation after the preserved bags have been thawed. Once the bags are thawed, each bag should be infused over 15 minutes.

Before thawing the marrow or stem cells, the child and parents must be prepared. Although cases of anaphylaxis, cardiac failure and arrhythmias have been documented, these are extremely rare. Most of the side effects or reactions occur as a result of the DMSO. These may include nausea, vomiting, abdominal cramps, headache, hypo- or hypertension. These side effects can be minimised by ensuring the child has a pre-medication of IV hydrocortisone, chlorphenamine, hyoscine-N-butylbromide and ondansetron/metoclopramide, 30 minutes prior to the infusion. In addition, some units recommend a regimen of hyper-hydration for several hours post-infusion. As the DMSO is broken down and excreted via the lungs, an overwhelming smell of 'garlicky-sweet corn' soon becomes apparent to everyone except the child who, instead, will have an extremely unpleasant taste in their mouth. Eating strong-flavoured sweets, such as mints or cherry drops, will help to lessen this taste and it is worth having a good supply ready, out of the wrapper, before infusing the marrow.

On completion of the infusion, especially following frozen bone marrow, the parents and the child need to be aware of the haemoglobinuria that can last up to 24 hours following the infusion so that they do not become worried about bloodstained urine. This is caused simply by the breakdown of old red blood cells. If the child feels well enough to drink, hyper-hydration can be continued orally to prevent small-clot retention blocking the renal tubules.

The infusion of defrosted cells is generally a quick procedure and the recording of observations during the procedure is half-hourly. The child's general condition will alert the nurse as to how they are coping with the DMSO. Regardless of whether the bone marrow or stem cells are fresh or preserved, allogeneic or autologous, the family will generally have mixed feelings after the infusion, as they may have done prior to it. Although they may experience relief that the cells have been infused safely and uneventfully, and the donor child, if there is one, is well, none the less they may turn their thoughts to the future and be concerned about what will happen next. Will, for example, the new cells engraft successfully or will there be added complications? Might the disease return despite the transplant? Such concerns may well be at the forefront of their minds and the nurse has a vitally important role at this stage in providing both emotional and physical support.

Once the cells have been infused, they begin to migrate to the empty marrow spaces. From the day of the infusion, i.e. day 0 to approximately 14 days post-infusion, the child is most vulnerable to infection. From day 10 onwards, circulating neutrophils start appearing and generally, by day 28, engraftment has occurred with a neutrophil count greater than $1.0 \times 10^9/l$. Thus, during the first two weeks post-infusion the child has no functioning immunity and the expert assessment and care given by the transplant nurse, with medical interventions, should prevent or lessen overwhelming complications.

References

Apperley JF (1994) 'Umbilical cord blood progenitor cell transplantation' *Bone Marrow Transplantation* 14(2): 187–196

Fliedner TM & Steinbach KH (1988) 'Repopulating potential of hematopoietic precursor cells' *Blood Cells* 14(2–3): 393–410

Hooper PJ & Santas EJ (1993) 'Peripheral blood stem cell transplantation' *Oncology Nurses Forum* 20(8): 1215–1221

Korbling M (1993) 'Some principles of blood stem cell transplantation' *Transfusion Science* 14(1): 61–64

Purandare L (1994) 'Therapeutic apheresis' *Professional Nurse* 9(9): 626–631

Vaux Z (1996) 'Peripheral stem cell transplants in children' *Paediatric Nursing* 8(2): 20–22

Vose JM, Armitage JO & Kessinger A (1993) 'High dose chemotherapy and autologous transplant with peripheral blood stem cells' *Oncology* 7(8): 23–29

Walker F, Roethke SK & Martin G (1994) 'An overview of the rationale, process and nursing implications of peripheral blood stem cell transplantation' *Cancer Nursing* 17(2): 141–148

Wall D (2004) 'Umbilical cord blood transplantation' *in*: Mehta P (ed.) *Paediatric Stem Cell Transplantation.* Boston: Jones & Bartlett, pp. 337–351

10

Protective Isolation
Nursing issues

Nikki Bennett-Rees and Sian Hopkins

Introduction

The consequences of life-threatening infections remain the major cause of morbidity and mortality in patients undergoing SCT. There are three distinct phases, depending upon the child's immune recovery, where they are at risk from the wide range of microbiological pathogens (Barnes, 1992a, b) (Figure 10.1).

- the neutropenic phase (days 0–21);
- the post-engraftment phase (days 28–100);
- the late phase (day 100 onwards).

Infections during the neutropenic phase are principally bacterial and/or fungal in origin. However, viral infections may also cause concurrent complications during this time. Common viruses during the neutropenic phase include reactivation of herpes simplex virus causing oropharyngeal mucositis, rotavirus, causing profuse diarrhoea, and respiratory syncytial virus (RSV) causing upper respiratory tract infection. While RSV may limit itself to a mild respiratory tract infection, it can lead to a devastating primary pneumonia that carries a high mortality rate of around 50 % despite

vigorous antiviral treatment with IV and nebulised ribavirin. RSV pneumonia is most common early in transplant pre-engraftment and tends to be seasonally confined to the spring and winter months. As well as carrying a high mortality risk, RSV is also highly contagious and can spread rapidly through a transplant unit. Because of this, many centres carry out an NPA (nasal pharyngeal aspirate) on admission. If RSV were detected at this stage, the procedure would be delayed if at all possible (Veys & Rao, 2004).

The child will be at most risk during the neutropenic phase, when a period of physical isolation is required. In order to prevent exposure to exogenous sources of infection, many SCT units advocate the use of laminar air flow (LAF) with or without the use of high-efficiency particulate air (HEPA) filtration. The use of these two systems should remove most bacterial and fungal spores from the air. For units in cities and where building work is ongoing, the use of LAF and HEPA filtration will have an effect on reducing the risk of infection with aspergillus (Fenelon, 1995). However, it should be noted that children might be harbouring pre-existing aspergillus spores on entry to the unit. Those particularly at risk

Cancer in Children and Young People   Edited by Faith Gibson and Louise Soanes
© 2008 John Wiley & Sons, Ltd

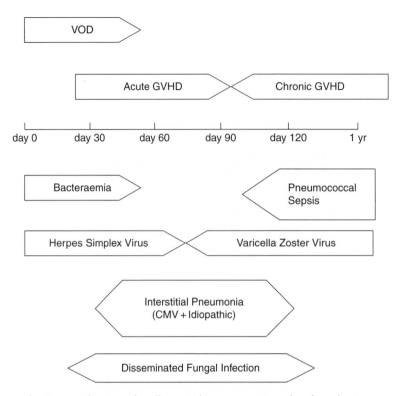

Figure 10.1 Sequence of major complications after allogeneic bone marrow transplant from day 0.
Source: Press, Schaller & Thomas, 1986, cited by Groenwald *et al.*, 1992.

are children who have suffered long periods of neutropenia and/or received prolonged courses of steroid therapy.

There is no evidence to show that LAF and HEPA filtration decreases the incidence of fever post-transplant or, indeed, the occurrence of acute GVHD. However, in units that combine LAF/HEPA filtration with skin and gut decontamination regimens, there appears to be a 'lower incidence of early infectious' problems (Skinhoj *et al.*, 1987).

Infection prophylaxis

The assessment and care needed to prevent infections during the neutropenic phase are a major concern for nurses. Infection prophylaxis is aimed at the prevention of fungal, viral and bacterial infections. Measures taken to prevent these three common types of infection in the child undergoing SCT include:

- use of an air filtration system such as LAF or HEPA;
- restricting the number of people allowed into the isolation room;
- encouraging the child to cooperate with oral medication, diet restrictions, mouth and skin care.

Although the environment may be protected by one or both of the filtration systems, there is a need for additional environmental measures. These will include a daily cleaning programme: it is sufficient to both 'damp dust' the surfaces and clean the floors using a new cloth and hot water with an appropriate detergent. Terminal cleaning need only be carried out on discharge or pre-admission of a child. Fresh flowers and plants must be avoided as both are sources of fungal and bacterial spores and their water is likely to harbour pseudomonas (Barnes, 1992a, b).

Protective isolation

The issue of what constitutes protective precautions varies widely between units, not only throughout the UK but also throughout 91 SCT centres in the USA (Poe *et al.*, 1994; Dunleavy, 1996). The type of precautions carried out will depend upon the physical amenities available and whether the unit is a dedicated SCT unit, as opposed to one that is integrated with another speciality. Exogenous infections come not only from airborne bacterial and fungal spores but are also transmitted on the hands and clothes of staff and parents (Barnes, 1992a, b). There are therefore some fundamental principles of protective precautions that must be adhered to regardless of unit specifications:

- scrupulous hand washing and drying (Laison & Lusk, 1985; Gould, 1991; Fenelon, 1995);
- use of a clean plastic apron on entering an isolation room; the apron must be changed when soiled (Pinkerton *et al.*, 1994; Fenelon, 1995).

These two simple but essential precautions lay down the basis for good practice in nursing the child undergoing BMT. Moreover in the modern climate of MRSA outbreaks, such measures should be part of everyday nursing practice in all areas and specialities. However, it should be noted that plastic aprons have been found to be heavily contaminated with bacteria and nurses should therefore not rely on aprons to protect their uniforms from contamination (Callaghan, 1998). In addition, water (which is a common carrier of pseudomonas) and food can transmit a multitude of infections with potentially serious implications for the child post-SCT (Barnes, 1992a, b; Fenelon, 1995). The micro-organisms most commonly responsible for food poisoning are salmonella, staphylococcus aureus and clostridium perfringens as well as Escherichia coli and campylobacter (Henry, 1997).

Certain foods have high microbial loads, such as uncooked foods: soft or raw eggs carry salmonella; soft cheeses carry listeria; spices carry bacteria and fungal spores; pepper is associated with aspergillus; unpeeled fruit and salad carry pseudomonas; E coli, klebsiella and hepatitis A have been isolated in watercress. Cooking with microwaves is also discouraged as research has shown that microwave ovens generate more Gram-positive bacteria than conventional ovens. Cook-chill foods should also be avoided as they are associated with both listeria and E coli (Henry, 1997; Sahdev & Botwinick, 2004). Perhaps the most effective way to protect the child is the use of oral antibiotics to ensure gut sterilisation and by offering a sterile diet. Unfortunately, once the food has been irradiated to render it sterile, it often tastes unpleasant. Efforts to tempt children to eat such unappetising food can lead to increasing stress for parents and the child. In a situation where the child is already reluctant to take oral medications, especially when they have severe mucositis, the pressure to take additional oral antibiotics is too great. Added to this is the risk of the child developing resistance to antibiotics. It is therefore recommended that it is sufficient for a transplant diet to be low microbial which basically involves food being well-cooked in hygienic conditions and for the child to finish eating it before it has become cold (Henry, 1997). As water is a known carrier of pseudomonas, it is good practice to provide the child with bottled sterile water or boiled tap water both for drinking and teeth cleaning although the use of tap water is controversial. Because mineral water is not subject to the same level of rigorous microbiological testing as tap water, it may carry higher levels of contamination and is therefore not recommended in transplant (Henry, 1997).

The more difficult infections to eliminate are the endogenous ones from the child's own skin and gut flora. As all children have a central line in situ, both the entrance site and the handling of the line present an ideal source for infection. In addition, with young children who explore with their fingers, the transference of infection from toys and scratched 'bottoms' to the mouth is a problem that appears to be irresolvable.

The restrictions necessary to care for the child under protective precautions must be both manageable and adhere to safe practice. It would be of great interest for a national working party to research this area and produce guidelines on the amount of protection needed by children undergoing allogeneic SCT. Thus, the implications for nursing children both pre- and during SCT will concern anticipating, reducing and treating infections before they become overwhelming.

In addition to protective isolation and a clean diet, the child's hospital room also needs to be kept, within reason, free from excessive numbers of toys, games, DVDs, as they often sit on the floor/surfaces and collect dust. It helps the child to have a system whereby toys and games can be rotated to lessen the boredom. Generally, toys and games should either be washable, such as Lego® and Duplo®, or nearly new, as with books and games. Soft toys that the child may need should also be new or (in the case of the favourite teddy) should be washed and tumble-dried: if the soft toy is placed inside a pillowcase when being tumble-dried, the rubber nose and glass eyes will remain intact.

Restrictions on visitors and staff will depend upon unit policy. Restrictions on the number of visitors allowed entering the room or, indeed, the unit may be in place, but also taken into account will be the age and health of visitors. It should be mandatory that no one enters the isolation room if they have a cold, sore throat, cough, have diarrhoea and/or vomiting, have a cold sore or conjunctivitis. It may be argued that wearing a mask will give protection to the child from the infected person, but greater safety is provided if people with such afflictions do not enter the room. None the less, there are units where the wearing of masks as part of the isolation precautions is the norm. Again, it may be argued that the benefit of wearing a mask is heavily outweighed by the detrimental effect on the well-being of the child. For example, in one unit the wearing of masks was abolished when a deaf child who could only lip-read was admitted for SCT.

There does not appear to be adequate data to determine absolutely whether siblings should be allowed to visit. It is believed that school-aged children are more likely to bring a variety of viral infections, including chickenpox, and therefore refusing school-age visitors entry to the isolation room appears to be a sound precaution. However, allowing children, especially the patient's siblings, into the unit to speak through an intercom link will both reduce the mystery of the SCT procedure and help to maintain the sibling relationship. The balance between the child's psychological needs and the increased risk of infection from a variety of people entering the room (or indeed the unit) needs to be carefully assessed in the formulation of the unit policy. Finally, whatever the unit policy, it should be adhered to in order to prevent inter-family friction if different 'rules' apply to different families.

Dietary restrictions

Most children undergoing SCT stop eating as a result of nausea and/or vomiting following conditioning therapy, mucositis, feeling generally unwell, or because eating can become an issue over which they can exercise control in a situation where otherwise they have little or none. Isolation and dietary restrictions can also play a part in inadequate intake (Sahdev & Botwinick, 2004). In addition, alterations in taste and smell (Hanigan & Walter, 1992) or the onset of GVHD can cause further nutritional problems. Furthermore, high-dose chemotherapy and/or radiation damage the gastrointestinal mucosa resulting in malabsorption (Sahdev & Botwinick, 2004). Effective nutrition therefore plays a vital role in the management of children undergoing stem cell transplantation and adequate nutritional support is vital both pre- and post-transplant to maintain target weight and, indeed, prevent weight loss. There is a belief that good nutrition may help to lessen the occurrence of severe acute GVHD and malnourishment is also associated with higher infection rates (Gauvreau et al., 1981; Sahdev & Botwinick, 2004). As discussed earlier, the type of oral diet, whether sterile or low microbial, will depend on the unit policy. Irrespective of the policy the child who is unable to maintain an adequate oral intake will require nutritional support.

Nutritional support can be achieved either via enteral tube feeding or through total parenteral nutrition (TPN) via a central line. Enteral feeding has a vital role to play in nutritional support, both pre- and post-transplant and in the recovery of the child post-engraftment. During the first three to four weeks post-transplant, when the child is at greatest risk of infection, bleeding, oesophageal/oral mucositis as well as nausea, vomiting and diarrhoea, the passing and use of a nasogastric tube may exacerbate these problems. In such situations nutritional support may be achieved with the use of TPN: it has been noted that this method is particularly beneficial for children under the age of 10 years (Souchon, 1992). However, TPN carries potential risk factors including infection and fluid overload and recent studies have suggested that good enteral nutrition using either nasogastric or gastrostomy feeding may be beneficial and more cost effective in transplant (Sahdev & Botwinick, 2004). Furthermore, maintaining a degree of gut motility, even at very low rates and volume of feed, seems to promote healing. Clearly insertion of either a nasogastric or gastrostomy tube must occur before either profound neutropenia or mucositis occurs and therefore should be discussed as part of the pre-transplant preparation. It should be noted that the insertion of nasogastric tubes could cause a great deal of distress to both parents and children so if long-term nutritional problems are anticipated, a gastrostomy may be the preferable alternative.

The aim should be for TPN to be concentrated and infused over 20 hours to enable the child, if well, to have a few hours 'off the lines'. As the child recovers and the mucositis resolves, so their appetite will slowly recover. Equally, as the child's oral intake improves, the TPN rates and length of infusion can be decreased, allowing the child more time 'off the lines'. Following consultation with the dietician, food and drinks can be fortified, if necessary, thus enabling a high calorie intake. By approximately six weeks post-SCT, most children will have recovered their sense of taste and, in addition, when the child is discharged home and resumes a family life and home cooking, diet and fluid intake appear to return to normal.

For the child who wants to eat, there are some dietary restrictions that will have been decided upon by the unit staff in conjunction with the microbiologist and dietician. Foods that are excluded are those with high microbial loads, as mentioned previously. For children who are able to continue to eat portions of food, they should be of the right size to enable them to finish what they are given. Sometimes this might mean very small portions served on a small plate. The advantage of having a diet-cook employed to prepare meals for children undergoing SCT is that it allows the children to have some choice and therefore control over their diet. The cook will be able to discuss with the children and parents the type of food and size of portion that will tempt them to eat. Many children appear to have an increased appetite in the evening and, in order to boost their calorie intake and satisfy their needs, it should be possible to make snacks for the child on the unit. Whatever the meal or snack, the child, especially if young, will often want to eat with their fingers. There is no harm in this as long as the hands are thoroughly washed and dried before eating.

Mouth care

To ensure that the mouth, skin and especially the perineum, are kept at their healthiest, frequent mouth and skin care regimes need to be commenced on admission. Before admission for SCT, at one of the outpatient sessions, the child will have had a full dental assessment to identify and correct any problems such as dental caries or teeth that may need extracting. If treatment is needed, antibiotic cover is given to prevent colonisation of the central line with dental organisms and treatment given as far from the transplant day as possible. During the inpatient period the aim of mouth care is prophylaxis. Mucositis, however (discussed further in Chapter 11), is almost a universal problem in patients undergoing SCT; mucositis appears to be more severe in patients who have been given methotrexate as part of GVHD prophylaxis.

To help prevent, or at least lessen, the impact of mucositis, the nurse's role is to ensure that thorough mouth care is carried out. While the child's gums remain healthy and the platelet count is adequate, the following regimen can be used. Teeth cleaning using a 'favourite' brand of fluoride toothpaste with a soft-headed baby toothbrush followed by a chlorhexidine-based mouthwash with or without a fully absorbed oral antifungal agent to follow (Beck, 1992). It is good practice to have a new toothbrush on a daily basis, and for the unit to provide these toothbrushes. In many units the use of a once daily dose of the anti-fungal drug itraconazole reduces the need to give another antifungal drug following mouth care. For babies with no teeth, or those children whose mouths are too painful for a toothbrush, the use of dental sponges soaked in chlorhexidine replaces the toothbrush. The use of chlorhexidine mouthwash as an agent that can reduce the severity of mucositis (Ferretti et al., 1987) is debatable with no evidence that it prevents candidiasis (UKCCSG-PONF, 2006).

Some researchers have found side effects, such as gingival bleeding and epithelial desquamation, to limit patient tolerance (Ainomo *et al.*, 1982). To help prevent dental caries, a once-daily dose of fluoride has been found to be beneficial (Gordon, 1983; Beck, 1992), particularly in those children drinking sterile water as opposed to tap water that contains fluoride. While there are national guidelines (UKCCSG-PONF, 2006) to mouth care post-chemotherapy (see Part 1), many transplant units have adapted these guidelines to suit the group of patients being treated.

Skin care

A daily bath or shower promotes skin care. Damp flannels and sponges encourage the growth of pseudomonas so the child must be given a new disposable washcloth at each bath time. The use of commercial bars or liquid soaps should be avoided as they can cause further drying of the skin, which is already affected by the chemo-radiotherapy used during conditioning. The use of antimicrobial soaps or lotions on the skin followed by the use of antibacterial creams to various parts of the body may be standard practice in some units. However, it is sufficient to ensure that the child is bathed daily and their skin kept moisturised to prevent drying. To prevent the skin from becoming dry, oil such as oilatum should be used in the bath, followed by the application of an unperfumed moisturiser, such as diprobase, once the skin is dry. While drying and then applying the cream, the parent and/or nurse will be able to observe the child for bruises, spots/rashes, scratches and the general healthiness of the skin. Particular attention must be given to children who still wear nappies to prevent breakdown of the skin in the nappy area. Nappies must be changed 1–2 hourly (especially during conditioning) to prevent excreted chemotherapy damaging the skin. With each nappy change the perineum can be cleaned using gauze swabs or a disposable cloth, and water, but if the area looks red and painful the use of oil (instead of water) for cleaning is more soothing. Once clean, an effective barrier cream, such as a mixture of metanium and white soft paraffin, must be applied. The use of sucralfate to any broken areas of skin on the perineum has

been shown to be effective in preventing further damage to the skin. The use of urine bags on children who have delicate or broken patches of skin should be avoided to prevent breakdown of the area. To collect a specimen of urine either place sterile cotton wool balls in the nappy or leave the nappy off and sit the child over a potty on the parent's or the nurse's lap and entertain the child until successful!

Infection screening

Specific care needs to be applied to the central line exit/entry site. This care generally comprises cleaning the site with an antiseptic solution, drying it and then re-dressing with a transparent permeable dressing, such as Opsite 3000®. This care should be maintained weekly unless the dressing is wet, is falling off or there is a problem with the entry/exit site looking infected (Maki, 1991).

Screening of stools and urine should be carried out once or twice per week. Swabs from the nose, throat and Hickman line exit site as well as any lesions on the lips, mouth or skin, should also be taken as indicated. Most children dislike having their nose and throat swabbed. If children are taught how to carry out the sampling, they can do their own at a time when they are ready. Alternatively, if the parents wish to take on this 'nursing' role for their child, they too can be taught and can undertake this procedure.

The effects of isolation

The protective precautions required in caring for a child undergoing SCT result in the parents and child being isolated from other members of their family and friends. In addition, the separation from previous support networks, including school friends, as well as the loss of freedom places a heavy burden on the whole family. It is therefore essential to work out strategies by which to lessen the impact of isolation.

To achieve a semblance of normal life, the isolation room should be furnished with a television, DVD player, radio/cassette player and telephone. These items alone will help family and friends to keep in contact with what is happening. Home-made videos and tapes from family and friends can often be a great source of support and amusement. Personal effects, such as photos, books and hobbies, for both the child and the parents are essential items, which must go into the isolation room. Precisely which items may be taken into the isolation room will depend on individual unit policy. Items such as letters, cards and postcards can be taken out of their envelopes and taken into the room. However, it is not uncommon for staff to misinterpret which items may potentially be seen as an infection risk to the child. If staff are unsure, the parents may be misinformed or, worse, may receive conflicting information.

For children of school age a daily visit from the unit schoolteacher will become routine. School sessions are planned around the child's ability to participate in a session. For babies, similar sessions with a physiotherapist or occupational therapist may be appropriate. This is particularly important in infants with SCID who may have had long periods of hospitalisation prior to SCT. The work of the physiotherapist/occupational therapist will help the infant to reach the normal developmental milestones (Sims, 2006).

In addition, the use of a play specialist/occupational therapist/music therapist/art therapist/activity worker plays a major role in ensuring that a 'normal' atmosphere is maintained for all children in isolation. For example, music therapy has been shown to meet a range of psychosocial needs that both the child and family experience during hospitalisation for SCT (O'Neill & Pavlicevic, 2003). A variety of activities provide play and stimulation to achieve developmental goals by ensuring that the physical, intellectual, language, emotional and social development of the child in isolation is maintained or enhanced. Physical development may be the most difficult to achieve due to the confines of space. Any activity which combines exercise and play, such as skittles, mini-snooker and basketball, gives both stimulation and enjoyment, thus helping to lessen the feelings of boredom and isolation. It is crucial for play specialists, activity workers and nursing staff to work well together and for nurses and doctors to avoid interrupting play/activity sessions with medical/nursing activities.

Children who are old enough can be encouraged to write letters to school friends, thus starting up a communication link, which keeps friends and family in touch. Parents, especially if one parent is the main resident carer, can also be encouraged to keep a diary of life in isolation. This will help them, when discharged, to re-live their feelings and describe to the family at home what happened each day. Some families also encourage siblings and other family members 'at home' to keep a similar concurrent diary. The respective experiences can then be joined and shared after discharge. For parents caring for their child in isolation, life can become a round of 'nursing', entertaining and washing clothes. To relieve this stress they should be encouraged to have 'time out', especially when the teacher, play therapist or nurse is with their child. Families who are able to take turns at being resident often appear less overwhelmed by the isolation. Although initially relieved from the restrictions of isolation and having to manage their sick child's day, the parents may remain anxious about their child when not with them (Darbyshire, 1994). Nonetheless, one of the main feelings for both children and parents in isolation is the loss of control. By negotiating the daily schedule for nursing, play, and education with the parent and child, and encouraging participation in care and planning, the family will be able to regain a degree of control. This, it is hoped, will at least lessen the feeling of helplessness in such a restrictive environment (Abramovitz & Senner, 1995).

References

Abramovitz L & Senner A (1995) 'Pediatric bone marrow transplantation update' Oncology Nursing Forum 22(1): 107–115

Ainomo J, Asikainen S & Paloheimo L (1982) 'Gingival bleeding after chlorhexidine mouth rinses' Journal of Clinical Periodontology 9(4): 337–345

Barnes R (1992a) 'Infections following bone marrow transplantation' in; Treleaven J & Barrett J (eds) Bone Marrow Transplantation in Practice. London: Churchill Livingstone, pp. 281–287

Barnes R (1992b) 'Treatment of bacterial, fungal and viral infections in hospital' in: Treleaven J & Barrett J (eds) Bone Marrow Transplantation in Practice. London: Churchill Livingstone, pp. 299–306

Beck S (1992) 'Prevention and management of oral complications in the cancer patient' in: Hubbard S,

Greene P & Knobf M (eds) *Current Issues in Cancer Nursing Practice Updates*. Pennsylvania: JB Lippincott

Callaghan I (1998) 'Bacterial contamination of nurses' uniform: a study' *Nursing Times* 13(1): 37–42

Darbyshire P (1994) *Living in Hospital with a Sick Child: The Experience of Parents and Children*. London: Chapman & Hall

Dunleavy R (1996) 'Isolation in BMT: a protection or a privation?' *British Journal of Nursing* 5(11): 663–668

Fenelon L (1995) 'Protective isolation: who needs it?' *Journal of Hospital Infection* (suppl.) 30: 181–222

Ferretti G, Ash R, Brown A, Largent B, Kaplan A & Lillich T (1987) 'Chlorhexidine for prophylaxis against oral infections and associated complications in patients receiving bone marrow transplantation' *Journal of American Dental Association* 114(4): 461–467

Gauvreau J, Lenssen P, Cheney C, Aker S, Hutchinson M & Barale K (1981) 'Nutritional management of patients with graft-versus-host disease' *Journal of the American Dietetic Association* 79(6): 673–675

Gordon H (1983) 'Fissure sealants' *in*: Murray JJ (ed.) *The Prevention of Renal Disease*. Oxford: Oxford University Press, pp. 175–187

Gould D (1991) 'Nurses' hands as vectors of hospital-acquired infection: a review' *Journal of Advanced Nursing* 16(10): 1216–1225

Groenwald SL, Hansen Frogge M, Goodman M & Henke Yarbo C (1992) *Treatment Modalities*. Boston: Jones & Bartlett

Hanigan M & Walter G (1992) 'Nutritional support for the child with cancer' *Journal of Pediatric Oncology Nursing* 9(3): 110–118

Henry L (1997) 'Immunocompromised patients and nutrition' *Professional Nurse* 12(9): 655–659

Laison E & Lusk E (1985) 'Evaluating hand washing technique' *Journal of Advanced Nursing* 10(6): 547–552

Maki DG (1991) 'Infection caused by intravascular devices: pathogenesis, strategies for prevention' *in*:

Maki DG (ed.) *Improving Catheter Site Care*. London: Royal Society of Medicine Services Limited

O'Neill N & Pavlicevic M (2003) 'What am I doing here? Exploring a role for music therapy with children undergoing bone marrow transplantation at Great Ormond Street Hospital, London' *British Journal of Music Therapy* 17(1): 8–16

Pinkerton CR, Cushing P & Sepion B (1994) 'Bone marrow transplantation' *in*: Pinkerton CR, Cushing P & Sepion B (eds) *Childhood Cancer Management*. London: Chapman & Hall, pp. 106–125

Poe S, Larson E, McGuire D & Krumm S (1994) 'A national survey of infection prevention practices on bone marrow transplant units' *Oncology Nursing Forum* 21(10): 1687–1694

Sahdev I & Botwinick MA (2004) 'Nutrition for the child undergoing stem cell transplantation' *in*: Mehta P (ed.) *Pediatric Stem Cell Transplantation*. Boston: Jones & Bartlett, pp. 69–85

Sims A (2006) 'The development of children under 5 years of age who have received a bone marrow transplant' in preparation

Skinhoj JP, Jacobsen N, Hoiby N, Faber, V and the Copenhagen Bone Marrow Transplant Group (1987) 'Strict protective isolation in allogeneic bone marrow transplantation: effect on infectious complications, fever and graft versus host disease' *Scandinavian Journal of Infectious Diseases* 19(1): 91–96

Souchon V (1992) 'Nutrition during bone marrow transplantation' *in*: Treleaven J & Barrett J (eds) *Bone Marrow Transplantation in Practice*. London: Churchill Livingstone, pp. 329–336

UKCCSG-PONF Mouthcare Group (2006) *Mouthcare for Children and Young People with Cancer: Evidence-based Guidlines*. Leicester: UKCCSG

Veys P & Rao K (2004) 'Advances in therapy: megatherapy allogeneic stem cell transplantation' *in*: Pinkerton R, Plowman PN & Pieters R (eds) *Paediatric Oncology* (3rd edn). London: Arnold, part 3A, pp. 513–517

11

Complications of Stem Cell Transplant

Nikki Bennett-Rees and Sian Hopkins

Introduction

The complications described here are those that most commonly occur in the transplant period, days 0–100, and therefore include the neutropenic and post-engraftment phases. Most occur as a direct result of the ablative chemotherapy and radiotherapy used in conditioning the child for transplant. Complications rarely occur in isolation and signs and symptoms often overlap. The nurse's role in the prevention, early detection and management of these complications is discussed as they are often called upon to coordinate the care of these acutely sick children while offering support and education to the child and family. Good management of these complications has a direct impact on the successful outcome of SCT.

Mucositis

One of the predictable side effects of SCT is mucositis. The use of high-dose chemotherapy agents, such as cyclophosphamide, melphalan and TBI, gives rise to widespread gastrointestinal mucosal damage. This damage may be further compounded by the use of methotrexate in the

prevention of GVHD. Stomatitis first occurs within 7–10 days of conditioning and may last for 14 days (Kanfer, 1993). It can cause pain, ulcerations leading to bleeding and infection, taste alterations, and xerostomia, which inevitably result in poor nutritional intake. This can have physical and psychological implications for the child. Xerostomia is often due to TBI; older children may find relief in sucking chips of ice or sucking ice-lollies or hard sweets. Small, frequent warm drinks are easier to swallow than ice-cold ones if stomatitis extends to the oesophagus, as will frequently be the case.

A quantitative assessment of the oral mucosa is necessary and provides documentation of the onset, severity and resolution of mucositis (Zerbe et al., 1983). An established oral assessment guide to ensure uniformity of assessment within the unit should be used (Gibson et al., 2006). Many of these exist (Beck, 1979; Eilers et al., 1988). These assessment guides use numerical and descriptive data to assess the level of stomatitis and the effect on the patient. In order to be successful the chosen model should be user-friendly and staff should be educated to ensure adherence and reliable use.

The loss of mucosal integrity can lead to infections both locally and systemically. Most units initiate prophylactic antifungal and antiviral agents; with the loss of the ability to swallow, these may temporarily need to be administered intravenously until the mucosa recovers, along with the establishment of white cell recovery approximately two weeks following bone marrow stem cell infusion. The treatment of mucositis aims to offer physical support to the patient and prevention of complications. The physical risks of stomatitis due to immunosuppression and infection account for some of the morbidity associated with SCT patients (Ezzone *et al.*, 1993) as the loss of the epithelial lining of the mucosa provides a portal of entry for micro-organisms into the systemic circulation and may result in life-threatening infections (Zerbe *et al.*, 1983).

Psychologically, the loss of comfort from thumb and dummy sucking can be distressing for small children and alternative methods of comfort may be sought by the child, such as holding the dummy, or alternative comfort measures found (attachment to soft toys). It is often the case that once the mucositis subsides the child reverts to the previous use of dummies and thumbs. Loss of verbal communication as the mouth becomes too sore to speak can be distressing for the school-aged child. Although alternative measures such as writing may be successful at first, as the child becomes weaker, these may be abandoned and the use of nods and shakes of the head for simple questions may be all that is tolerated. Loss of self-image due to inability to swallow saliva can distress the older child who may perceive dribbling and spitting into tissues embarrassing. The maintenance of privacy for the child in this instance is paramount.

For the child, pain is likely to be the worst symptom associated with an ulcerated mucosa of the gastrointestinal tract and this is often the first symptom reported by the child before the visible signs of mucosal damage appear. At first, pain often occurs with swallowing (due to mouth breathing) and speaking, progressing to continuous pain, often requiring the use of opiates to provide adequate analgesia.

As the mucositis progresses, gastrointestinal manifestations emerge. Again, pain is often the first indicator of mucosal ulceration and nausea, vomiting and diarrhoea commonly occur. Due to the severity and frequency of diarrhoea, peri-anal excoriation and ulceration can occur, especially in small children and babies who wear nappies. The older child will find frequent diarrhoea and the dependence on others for toileting embarrassing and involving altered perceptions of body image. The recently toilet-trained child may return to nappy-wearing in protest.

Treatment and nursing implications

Oral hygiene

Oral hygiene, although unable to prevent stomatitis, can help lessen its severity and prevent infection. The method, frequency and evaluation of oral hygiene will vary from unit to unit. Present practices are currently under review, and transplant centres may follow those recently developed in the paediatric oncology setting (see Chapter 10). However, because practice may at present be inconsistent, evidence-based guidelines within SCT units will need to be established. Whatever the practice is on individual units, there is little doubt that oral hygiene should be initiated during the first few days of hospital admission for the transplant. This allows the child and family to become familiar with the unit's chosen methods and allows the child time to adapt to new ways of cleaning teeth. The use of play specialists to familiarise the child with toothbrushes, dental sponges and mouth inspections should be assessed on an individual basis. The child's developmental stage will be crucial to the success of this process.

Chlorhexedine mouthwashes can be painful, as stomatitis and ulceration progress, but the nurse should encourage adherence and positive reinforcement of oral hygiene with the use of sticker charts, etc. Although a role that parents often undertake, there may be times when parents should be encouraged to opt out of doing mouth care as it becomes more difficult for the child so as to reduce stress for them. Toothbrushes remove plaque and food debris from the gum line. Soft-headed baby toothbrushes are best used by children whose platelet and white cell counts are suppressed. The care of lips and the products used to prevent drying and cracking, again, varies from unit to unit, though petroleum jelly is still the most common lubricant (Ezzone *et al.*, 1993).

Nausea and vomiting

Nausea and vomiting in the transplant child are often the result of the chemotherapy and radiotherapy used in the conditioning of the child. This is often expected and prophylactic antiemetics should be given in accordance with the unit's policy. Following the expected nausea and vomiting associated with the use of radiotherapy or chemotherapy, these symptoms frequently persist in the SCT child and can be multi-factorial including infection, pain due to mucositis, GVHD (particularly gut GVHD), veno-occlusive disease, TPN and swallowing of oral secretions. Multiple-drug therapy used in transplant including morphine, antibiotics and immunosuppressive agents such as ciclosporin are also thought to contribute to the refractory nausea and vomiting suffered by children undergoing SCT. It is clear that the causes of such prolonged nausea and vomiting remain elusive in the transplant setting and require further investigation. Moreover, it is important that the approach to antiemetic therapy is both structured and systematic to avoid an erratic polypharmacy approach where every possible antiemetic is thrown at the problem without proper evaluation of their efficacy (Gibson & Hopkins, 2005). It should be remembered that relief from nausea and vomiting might also be gained from non-pharmacological interventions such as guided imagery or sea bands, although these are sadly often given a fairly low priority by clinical staff.

Nausea is a subjective feeling which is difficult for the child to describe and thus difficult to relieve. Therefore, avoid exposing the child to the smell of known causes of nausea (e.g. food, perfume). Intravenous antibiotics are a common cause of nausea due to the heightened sense of smell following chemotherapy and the powerful odour that these drugs exude. Inform the child of when such drugs are to be given and allow time for distraction to take place; some children find smelling soap or comforters help. Sucking sweets or infusing rather than injecting antibiotics can prevent the taste distortion that some children experience.

Vomiting during the conditioning period may be well controlled with 5HT antagonists such as ondansetron. Persistent vomiting requires other antiemetic agents and both metoclopramide (both oral and IV) and cyclizine have been beneficial.

Hyoscine patches and IV lorazepam have also proved to be effective, particularly in older children. Support for the child and family is vital. Vomiting is distressing for both the child and family. It can cause further damage to already fragile oral mucosa and, if the platelet count is low, bleeding can occur from the membranes and petechial bleeds may occur especially around the eyes. The parents and child should be informed that this might occur. Input/output and fluid balance must be monitored accurately, as well as electrolyte balance.

Research into specific nausea and vomiting in the post-transplant child continues. The antiemetic flow guidelines are currently under review (see Figure 11.1 on p. 146). Table 11.1 presents the drugs used to combat nausea and vomiting.

Diarrhoea

Diarrhoea is a common early symptom of mucosal ulceration of the lower gastrointestinal tract. This can be particularly distressing particularly for the older child who may become incontinent if it is severe. Careful IV fluid replacement to prevent fluid and electrolyte depletion is paramount. The greatest risk to the child is infection due to loss of mucosal integrity and damage to the peri-anal skin area as a result of frequent diarrhoea. Routine stool specimens will isolate pathogens and allow the early instigation of treatment. The collection of these stool specimens is often combined in the surveillance screening undertaken during the pancytopenic phase following SCT and reports of abdominal pain, fever and abdominal tenderness should be investigated rigorously. Common viruses that cause protracted diarrhoea are rotavirus, adenovirus, astrovirus and small round cell virus. Scrupulous hand washing is vital to prevent spreading these viruses to other children in the unit.

Alterations in nutritional status

The child and family need to be prepared and educated for the loss of appetite and slow recovery following SCT. As mucositis progresses and the child's oral intake diminishes, reduction in nutritional status leading to weight loss will occur, therefore weighing the child once a day will give guidance as to when to give additional dietary support. The recognition of weight loss has led some units to instigate prophylactic TPN at an early stage in the transplant (Graham *et al.*, 1993). However, as discussed earlier, appropriate enteral nutrition via a nasogastric or gastrostomy tube offers some advantages over TPN and should therefore be the first course of nutritional support. However, if the child is suffering from severe vomiting and/or diarrhoea, TPN may be the most sensible short-term solution. On recovery of the child's white cell count and the resolution of mucositis, poor nutritional intake may persist. This is commonly because of the refractory

nausea children undergoing transplant seem to suffer from. The involvement and support of a dietician will be vital to ensure adequate calorie intake following SCT. This may involve continuing supportive measures, such as nasogastric tube feeds or high-energy sip feeds, after discharge from the transplant unit.

Pain

The child experiences pain during SCT for a variety of reasons. Veno-occlusive disease, mucositis, procedures and GVHD can all be a cause of pain. Adequate evaluation is vital to ensure a successful

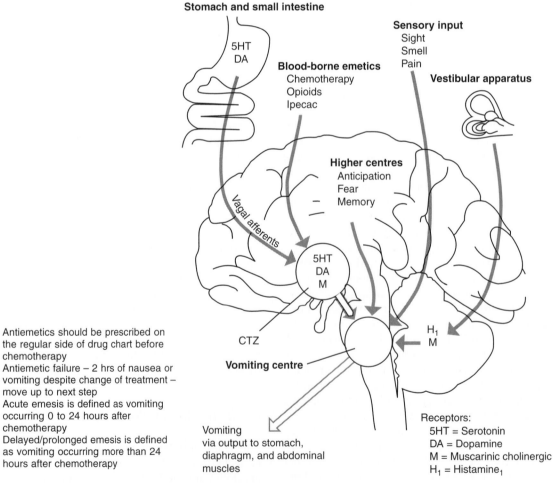

- Antiemetics should be prescribed on the regular side of drug chart before chemotherapy
- Antiemetic failure – 2 hrs of nausea or vomiting despite change of treatment – move up to next step
- Acute emesis is defined as vomiting occurring 0 to 24 hours after chemotherapy
- Delayed/prolonged emesis is defined as vomiting occurring more than 24 hours after chemotherapy

Figure 11.1   Guidelines for use of antiemetics with chemotherapy for bone marrow transplant patients.

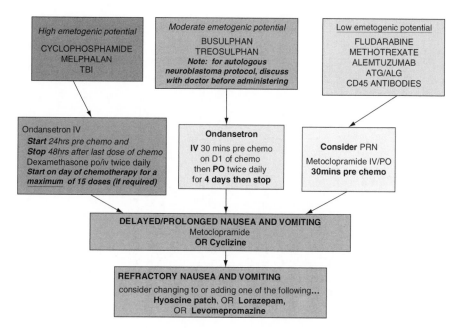

Figure 11.1   (Continued)

outcome with a child in pain; evaluation not only of the level of the child's pain but also of the interventions and assessment applied to treating the pain. A variety of assessment tools are available for measuring children's pain: CHEOPS (McGarth et al., 1985); the Faces Scale (Wong & Baker, 1988) and the Eland Color Scale (Eland, 1988). Whichever instrument is used it must be reliable, provide consistent information, be user-friendly and be appropriate for the child's cognitive level.

The choice of appropriate pain control often follows the World Health Organization (WHO) ladder approach to cancer pain (Patterson, 1992). However, individual unit guidelines vary and the initial use of analgesics such as paracetamol may be avoided, as their antipyretic effect may be perceived as masking the signs of infection. Often, as the cause of the child's pain progresses and the pain worsens, a step-up approach to analgesia is needed, leading to the use of opiates as effective control of the child's pain.

The use of opiates for pain control in SCT is often necessary, particularly for controlling the pain associated with mucositis. These drugs may be administered intravenously or subcutaneously according to unit policy. The use of patient-controlled analgesia pumps (PCA) in older children provides both adequate pain relief and some degree of patient control (Gureno & Reisinger, 1991), an important factor for older children during SCT when so much surrounding this procedure is beyond their control.

Pancytopenia

Following infusion of bone marrow or stem cells the child will be at considerable risk from both infectious and haemorrhagic complications. These two complications are as a result of the myeloablative therapy used in the conditioning regimes of either chemotherapy alone or chemo-radiotherapy with, in the allogeneic setting, the use of further immunosuppressive therapy such as ciclosporin. Furthermore, the occurrence of GVHD and its treatment will cause increased immunosuppression for the child.

Haematological complications

As discussed earlier, the most common haemorrhagic problem to occur during the initial pre-transplant phase is haemorrhagic cystitis caused

Table 11.1 Drugs to combat nausea and vomiting

DRUG	DOSE	ADVERSE EFFECTS* (*See BNF for more information)	COMMENTS	PREPARATIONS
CYCLIZINE	ORAL: < 1 year, 1 mg/kg — 3 times daily 1–6 years, 12.5 mg — 3 times daily 6–12 years, 25 mg — 3 times daily > 12 years, 50 mg — 3 times daily IV: 1mg/kg — 3 times daily Subcutaneous: 3mg/kg in 24 hours as continuous infusion	– drowsiness – blurred vision – dry mouth – urinary retention – restlessness – insomnia – tachycardia	Particularly for emesis of raised intracranial pressure Compatible with diamorphine for infusion Avoid using Hyoscine	Preparations: Tablets 50mg Injection 50 mg/ml
DEXAMETHASONE	IV bolus/Oral: 1–12 years: 0.1mg/kg two–three times daily for 5 days Maximum of 15 doses for each course	– adrenal suppression – gastric irritation – osteoporosis	Give first dose with Ondansetron, 15 mins before chemotherapy	Injection 8mg/2ml Tablets 500 microgram 2mg
HYOSCINE HYDROBROMIDE	Topically: <4 years: 1/2 of a patch every 72 hours, applied to a clean, dry, hairless area of skin behind the ear, avoiding any cuts or irritation >4 years; Apply one patch every 72 hours	– weight gain – drowsiness – dry mouth – dizziness – blurred vision – difficulty with micturition – somnolence	Wash hands after applying and the skin area after removal Scopaderm patches can be cut Transcop patches cannot be cut. If half a patch prescribed, occlude other half with Opsite or similar dressing (not IV 3000)	Transdermal Patches 1mg absorbed/72 hours
LEVOMEPROMAZINE	Oral/IV: 1–12 years: 0.25mg–1mg/kg three to four times daily (max 37.5mg per day) >12 years: 12.5mg–50mg three to four times daily (max 200mg per day)	– asthenia – dry mouth – hypotension – raised ESR	Particularly for emesis when all other options exhausted	Tablets 25mg Injection 25mg/ml

Drug	Dose	Side effects	Notes	Formulations
LORAZEPAM	Slow IV bolus: 0.02–0.04mg/kg every 8 hours Oral: 90 % of IV dose	- drowsiness - amnesia - confusion and ataxia - pain with intravenous injection	For anticipatory nausea and vomiting start 24 hrs before chemotherapy Maximum 48 hrs supply as TTO.	Injection 4mg/ml Tablets 1mg
METOCLOPRAMIDE	Oral/IV:	- extrapyramidal effects	Treat dystonic reactions with IV bolus of BENZTROPINE in children over 3 years; (contra-indicated in children <3 years)	Tablets 10mg
low dose	1–12 years: General antiemetic: 100–170 micrograms/kg three times daily This dose can be increased to 200 microgram/kg four times a day.	- hyperprolactinaemia - drowsiness - restlessness	100 micrograms/kg, (maximum dose = 2mg) In children <3 years use PROCYCLIDINE IV bolus 1 month–2 years 500microgram–2mg 2–12 years 2–5mg Reduce dose in renal and hepatic failure	Oral solution 5mg/5ml (sugar and colour free, contains sorbitol) Injection 5mg/ml
ONDANSETRON	Oral/IV: 5mg/m^2 twice daily increasing to three times a day if necessary	- constipation - headache - transient rise in liver enzymes - hypersensitivity reactions	Continue for 24 hours after last chemotherapy dose (48 hours if drug known to cause delayed emesis) Should only be used for chemotherapy-induced nausea and vomiting	Injection 4mg/2ml 8mg/4ml Tablets 4mg, 8mg Melt tablets 4mg, 8mg Syrup (sugar free) 4mg/5ml

by the use of high-dose IV cyclophosphamide. While this is usually an early transplant complication, late-onset haemorrhagic cystitis has also been reported. For this reason, a daily urinalysis to observe for microscopic blood should be carried out. The aetiology of this later haemorrhagic cystitis may be the cyclophosphamide but a viral cause should not be ruled out. Adenovirus, CMV and BK viruses, as well as GVHD, have all been implicated in these cases. Treatment includes hyperhydration and bladder irrigation as well as maintaining adequate platelet and haemoglobin levels. Some success has been noted with the use of short-term oestrogen, although the exact mechanism for this is unclear (Veys & Rao, 2004).

Epistaxis (nosebleeds) is also a common haemorrhagic transplant complication. Triggered primarily by a low platelet count, some children seem to be more susceptible to this and in severe cases may need an appropriate ENT (ear, nose and throat) referral. Some relief may be gained from the use of tranexamic acid and topical application of ice can also help.

Rectal bleeding can occur, particularly in conjunction with gut GVHD, and stools should be observed for evidence of both old and fresh blood. It should be noted that bleeding could cause a great deal of distress and panic in both children and parents, as it can be very frightening to witness. Reassuring families that this is an expected and common occurrence as well as prompt assessment of the child's cardiovascular status should therefore be a priority.

Transfusions of both blood and platelets will be necessary until the donor marrow becomes fully engrafted and functional. The level at which the child will need transfusing will depend on both the transplant unit's policy and the child's condition. For example, haemoglobin of 8 g/dl or a platelet count of 20×10^9/l or less should be transfused. However, a child with an infection, fever or an existing clotting problem may need to have a platelet count maintained at 50×10^9/l or higher. Whatever the unit's policy regarding the level at which the child must be transfused, it is essential that both blood and platelets are irradiated and of the appropriate CMV status. By irradiating these two products the lymphocytes within them will be destroyed and therefore unable to cause an immune response in the child, thus preventing the child developing transfusional GVHD.

Cytomegalovirus (CMV), which can be transmitted in blood products, is the main cause of morbidity and death in patients treated with allogeneic stem cells. In the UK approximately 40–50 % of the adult population is CMV positive. For the CMV negative child who receives marrow from a CMV negative donor, it is essential that CMV negative products be given. For a child who is CMV positive or whose donor is CMV positive, the ideal situation would also be to transfuse CMV negative products although no additional benefit has been shown in this situation as in the UK all blood products are leucodepleted, greatly reducing the rate of CMV complications. If there is a shortage of CMV negative products the use of a leukocyte filter for blood or platelet transfusions (the virus is transmitted through leukocytes) will greatly reduce the risk of transmitting CMV.

Infection

The risk from the wide range of infections occurs at three distinct phases and coincides with the child's haematological and immunological recovery post-transplant (Wujcik et al., 1994; Veys & Hann, 1997). The three phases for infection are:

- neutropenic phase;
- post-engraftment phase;
- late phase.

The neutropenic phase lasts approximately 0–21 days post-SCT and occurs during the period of the gastrointestinal mucositis. The post-engraftment phase lasts from approximately days 30 to 100 post-SCT. Late-phase infections occur from day 100 and may last until immune recovery occurs at 1–2 years post-SCT. However, if the child is treated for chronic GVHD, recovery of T cell function will be further delayed so the risk of infection may become a long-term problem. During the neutropenic phase the child is at risk from a wide spectrum of infections (Table 11.2). Prophylactic treatment varies between units, however, the treatment for febrile neutropenia or proven infection appears to be universally very similar. Once the child's axillary temperature reaches the level for antibiotic commencement (as decided upon by the

Table 11.2 Infectious complications post stem cell transplant

Phase	Infection	Organism
Neutropenic (days 0–21)	Gram-positive bacteria	Staphylococcus epidermidis Staphylococcus aureus
	Gram-negative bacteria	Pseudomonas aeruginosa Escherichia coli
	Fungal	Candida albicans Aspergillus
	Viral	Herpes simplex (HSV) Rota virus Respiratory Syncytial Virus (RSV)
Post-engraftment (days 30–100)	Viral	Cytomegalovirus (CMV) Adenovirus, Epstein-Barr virus (EBV) Pneumoncystis carinii
Late (days 100+)	Viral Encapsulated bacterial organisms	Varicella Zoster (VZV) Streptococcus pneumoniae Haemophilus influenzae

Sources: Barnes (1992a, b), Wujcik *et al.* (1994), Veys & Hann (1997).

unit but generally 38–38.5°C) a first-line broad-spectrum antibiotic regimen is commenced which will cover both Gram-negative and Gram-positive bacteria. Additional antibiotic, antiviral or antifungal therapy will be commenced according to:

- the child's clinical condition;
- the child's response to first-line antibiotics;
- the results of various cultures and X-rays;
- the results of the C-reactive protein level (CRP).

(Barnes, 1992a, b)

Recombinant G-CSF, which is a naturally occurring hormone, has been included in the drug regime post-SCT (Singer, 1992), although clear benefit to the use of growth factors following allogeneic SCT has yet to be demonstrated. G-CSF is given intravenously once a day (commencing between day 1 and day 8 post-transplant, depending upon the unit) to boost early bone marrow engraftment. An early marrow engraftment reduces the length of time the child is neutropenic, therefore reducing the risk of neutropenic fever and infections. There is a direct correlation between the length of time the child is neutropenic and the acquisition of a fungal infection such as aspergillus (Barnes, 1992a, b). However, children receiving stem cells from a haplo-identical donor do not routinely receive G-CSF. This is largely because G-CSF promotes neutrophil recovery at the expense of T cell recovery. Children receiving haplo-identical transplants are already more likely to have prolonged T cell depletion and the risk of viruses becomes too great to delay recovery of T cells any longer than necessary.

During the post-engraftment phase (days 29–100 post-transplant) the child's new bone marrow will start functioning and producing neutrophils, thus decreasing the risk of bacterial and fungal infections. However, both cell-mediated and humoral functions take several months to recover and full immunity may take at least one year to recover post-SCT. Furthermore, if the child is receiving steroids as part of treatment for GVHD, their immunity will be further compromised, resulting in an increased risk of developing a viral illness. The most common viral infection at this stage is CMV, causing an interstitial pneumonia, which carries a greater than 50% mortality rate.

Cytomegalovirus

This may occur as a result of:

- primary infection;
- reactivation of infection if the child was CMV positive prior to SCT;

- reactivation, if the child was CMV negative and received CMV positive donor stem cells or blood product.

The following may all lead to an increased chance of developing CMV:

- increased intensity of conditioning regimens;
- the child being CMV positive prior to SCT;
- the donor being CMV positive;
- the child being treated for GVHD.

In children, the incidence of CMV is lower than in adults. This may be due in part to children and their sibling donors being younger and therefore more likely to be CMV negative. Second, the incidence of acute GVHD in children, which increases the risk of CMV infection, is far less than in adults. The most likely risk of reactivation of CMV is from a seropositive donor or recipient (Wingard, 1990).

The signs and symptoms of CMV pneumonitis include:

- low-grade fever;
- dyspnoea;
- dry cough;
- respiratory failure.

Weekly monitoring of blood by using the Polymerase Chain Reaction (PCR) that has the benefits of being highly sensitive (Cathgomas *et al.*, 1993) from admission to up to six months post transplant will allow for early treatments to be put in place. The diagnosis of CMV pneumonitis needs to be confirmed to rule out other chest problems such as pneumocystis carinii pneumonia (PCP). It is confirmed by the child undergoing a bronchoalveolar lavage (BAL) and/or lung biopsy to confirm the diagnosis. A diagnosis of CMV in the child's nasal pharyngeal aspirate (NPA) and/or urine can be detected on cultures. In addition to CMV pneumonitis (although much less common), the child may also develop a CMV enterocolitis, hepatitis, chorioretinitis, encephalitis and pancytopenia.

Prophylactic treatment for high-risk children, who are CMV negative, and received CMV positive cells or who are themselves CMV positive is with high-dose IV aciclovir eight-hourly with IV immunoglobulin to prevent reactivation of the virus (Schmidt, 1992; Prentice *et al.*, 1997). The treatment of choice for children who are excreting CMV in their urine, have positive blood cultures or who develop CMV pneumonitis is IV ganciclovir and IV immunoglobulin (Wingard, 1990). If this combination is not successful in reducing the viral load or the myelosuppression of the drug is too severe, then the ganciclovir can be altered to IV foscarnet or indeed to a combination of half-doses of both ganciclovir and foscarnet. The long-term treatment of CMV with increasing high doses of antiviral therapy can lead to both antiviral resistance and toxicity. The toxicity often primarily affects myelopoiesis, resulting in prolonged neutropenia and further infections.

At present, research is being undertaken into developing the safety and efficacy of giving children CMV-specific cytotoxic T cells (CTLs). The aim of infusing CMV-specific CTLs is to allow earlier reconstitution of the child's viral immunity, with the hope that the more toxic antiviral drugs (ganciclovir, foscarnet and cidofovir) can be avoided (Einsele *et al.*, 2002). For children who are considered at high risk of becoming CMV positive, CMV-specific CTLs will have been made, pre-transplant, by using 200 mls of fresh peripheral blood from the stem cell donor. These cells have, on the whole, been given to children who continue to have rising CMV levels despite optimum therapy (Veys & Rao, 2004). The incidence of CMV infections has been dramatically reduced due to the use of both CMV negative and filtered leukodepleted blood products, along with the improvement of antiviral therapies.

Adenovirus

In children, adenovirus is the most common cause of either respiratory or gastrointestinal illness. This may occur as a result of:

- primary infection
- reactivation of the virus.

This may occur at any time during the transplant period especially during the first 100 days. Children are most at risk of developing adenovirus because of:

- the donor being a mismatched donor;
- the donor being a haplo-identical donor.

In both these settings there is significant depletion of the donor T cells from the infused stem cells, furthermore there is a continued need for ongoing immunosuppression that may include steroids. The signs and symptoms of adenovirus are:

- diarrhoea (often severe);
- fever;
- abnormal liver function (in extreme cases of fatal hepatitis).

The diagnosis of adenovirus needs to be confirmed and not mistaken for gastrointestinal GVHD as the use of steroids to treat GVHD exacerbates the spread/load of the adenovirus infection. A diagnosis of adenovirus in the child's NPA or stool can be detected on routine monitoring. Weekly monitoring of blood for adenovirus using the PCR method should be set in place from admission up to six months post transplant. As yet there is no prophylactic drug therapy to prevent adenovirus. Treatment using one or a combination of the two IV antiviral drugs ribavirin and cidofovir has shown very positive results. However, should the adenovirus become disseminated, these drugs may provide little benefit, and therefore the treatment in this case would be to reduce or stop the immunosuppression. Research is being undertaken to give children with adenovirus, which is unresponsive to drug therapy, a series of 'T cell add back' using cells taken from the donor at the time of the initial stem cell donation. The aim of the T cell add back is to prevent a disseminated adenoviraemia by boosting the child's T cell recovery.

Epstein-Barr Virus (EBV)

EBV is one of the herpes viruses (Human Herpes Virus 4). EBV typically targets mature B-lymphocytes and squamous epithelial cells of the oral cavity, pharynx and genital tract. The virus inserts itself into the DNA of B lymphocytes and induces them to proliferate. EBV is a worldwide human virus and once infected (usually via close saliva contact), the virus will lie dormant and the infected individual will be a lifelong carrier in whom the virus always has the potential to reactivate. In a healthy individual, EBV may simply cause a fever or swollen glands, or indeed no symptoms at all. This is primarily because cytotoxic and natural killer cells control B cell proliferation. However, in immunosuppressed individuals, symptomatic disease, which is often severe, will occur. Moreover, T cell depletion with alemtuzumab, ciclosporin and steroid therapy further exposes the transplant patient to a high risk of EBV. Signs and symptoms of EBV include fever, sore throat, enlarged lymph nodes, splenomegaly, hepatomegaly, nausea and fatigue. Diagnosis of EBV is usually through blood tests, although nasal pharyngeal swabs and biopsy of lymph nodes can be used. Treatment may include the monoclonal antibody, rituximab. Other antiviral drugs including cidofovir, foscarnet and/or ganciclovir have little or no effect. Infusing cytotoxic T cells (CTLs) that specifically target EBV has also been used with some success.

Lymphoproliferative disorder (LPD), which causes the development of lymphomas which may be rapid or slow growing, is a serious complication triggered by a combination of EBV and immune suppression. Treatment with antiviral therapy, chemotherapy, immunoglobulin, rituximab and CTLs may be required.

To continue to protect the child from these common infections, there are a number of prophylactic medications now used both pre-, during and post-SCT, many of which the child will be required to take orally (Table 11.3).

The effectiveness of prophylactic therapies depends upon the concordance of the child. Often, pre-transplant the child is able to comply, but unfortunately, as nausea and vomiting followed by mucositis occurs, adherence weakens. Not only is the child feeling miserable and ill but adherence may be the only form of control they have. To help the child continue with as many oral drugs as possible in a stress-free manner, the use of a sticker chart is often recommended. It is also helpful to award a sticker for each painful procedure, such as mouth care, peripheral blood sampling, or taking oral medications. Once an agreed number of stickers has been achieved, the child has a 'dip' in a treasure chest, which is filled with amusing novelty toys and games.

Older children will require a different approach and there is nothing to be achieved by using the seriousness of their condition to frighten them into adherence (Blotcky et al., 1985). If treated in a mature way, and if explanations are provided with patience and clarity at the commencement of

Table 11.3 Drug therapy related to infection prophylaxis

Drug therapy	Prophylaxis against
Antimicrobials	
cotrimoxazole (oral)	Pneumocystis carinii pneumonitis
ciprofloxacin (oral)	Gram-negative bacterial infections
Antiviral	
aciclovir (i.v. /oral)	Cytomegalovirus (CMV)
	Varicella Zoster virus (VZV)
Palivizumab (IM)	Respiratory Syncytial Virus (RSV) given monthly to 'high risk' children (e.g. SCIDS)
Antifungals	
itraconazole (oral)	Aspergillus
fluconazole (oral)	Candida
amphotericin (oral/ inhalation)	Candida, Aspergillus
nystatin (oral)	Candida
Others	
immunoglobulin (i.v.)	To improve post-transplant immunity reduces the length of the neutropenic phase
granulocyte colony stimulating factor (G-CSF) (i.v.)	

treatment and maintained throughout treatment, adherence should be more realistically achieved. Hopefully, if the child's pain and/or nausea and vomiting are well controlled and he feels well supported by both parents and staff, the days when oral medications are missed will be minimal.

Veno-occlusive disease

Hepatic veno-occlusive disease (VOD) is a major complication, which can occur in up to 20% of children undergoing BMT (McDonald *et al.*, 1984). VOD is generally associated with the use of alkylating agents, particularly busulphan, in the conditioning regimens pre-transplant (Ringden *et al.*, 1994, cited in Bearman, 1995; Wadleigh *et al.*, 2003). It is believed that their metabolites damage the endothelial lining of both the sinusoids and terminal hepatic venoules, leading to necrosis of the hepatocytes (Bearman, 1995; Wadleigh *et al.*, 2003). The hepatic veins become increasingly occluded by cellular debris causing the blood flow from the liver to back up and the protein-rich fluid content

of the blood to leak out into the peritoneal cavity, resulting in ascites (Grandt, 1989; Baglin, 1994). As with GVHD there are some recognised factors to predict which children may develop VOD, such as having:

- a mismatch or unrelated donor marrow;
- high doses of busulphan (>16mg/kg);
- a second transplant following on from a failed first transplant;
- a pre-existing infection during conditioning therapy;
- a pre-existing chemical or viral hepatitis.

There is little doubt that there is a fine balance between risking rejection due to low busulphan levels and risking VOD if the levels are too high. Recent developments have included the introduction of IV treosulphan in an attempt to minimise toxicity. The effect of oral busulphan seems to vary greatly between patients and IV busulphan is also becoming more commonplace (Veys & Rao, 2004). A diagnosis of VOD is usually based on clinical signs and symptoms and includes:

- unexplained weight gain;
- ascites;
- hepatomegaly;
- increase in bilirubin;
- refractory thrombocytopenia;
- increase in almine amino-transferase (ALT);
- hypoalbuminaemia;
- clotting abnormalities.

Although a Doppler ultrasound may confirm occlusion of blood vessels and reversal of blood flow, the findings are often inconsistent and unhelpful and clinical judgement carries more weight (Veys & Rao, 2004). The diagnosis of VOD can range from mild to moderate or severe. Early onset VOD tends to carry greater morbidity and mortality risk. The child may not develop all the symptoms but the more severe the symptoms are, the more severe the form of VOD. It usually occurs within the first three weeks post-transplant and lasts for approximately 10–14 days from the onset of the liver dysfunction (McDonald *et al.*, 1985). Jaundice and encephalopathy are both late signs and symptoms. The diagnosis of VOD is usually made on clinical grounds and the differential diagnosis includes infectious or chemical hepatitis or GVHD of the liver. However, it is only in VOD that there is unexplained weight gain and fluid retention (Bearman, 1995). There are two techniques available to confirm the diagnosis of VOD. The first is a non-invasive procedure using Doppler ultrasound, which shows reversal of hepatic portal venous flow. Alternatively, a liver biopsy can be performed. However, as these children are usually thrombocytopenic and may also have clotting abnormalities due to liver dysfunction, a liver biopsy is not recommended.

The management of the child with VOD is the joint responsibility of nursing and medical staff. Early detection and support measures by both teams may help to decrease the damage to the liver, the aim being to reverse liver disease rather than allowing it to prove fatal (Bearman, 1995). In children who are at high risk of developing VOD there may be an indication for prophylactic treatment with oral ursodeoxycholic acid or IV defibriotide. Recent studies suggest that prophylaxis with low-dose heparin has not prompted the desired reduction in the incidence of VOD and is a practice that has been abandoned in many transplant centres (Veys & Rao, 2004). Treatment used to be primarily supportive until the liver function recovered. While supportive care remains paramount, IV defibriotide has been used recently to successfully treat VOD (Richardson et al., 1998). Defibriotide is antithrombolytic, anti-ischaemic and anti-inflammatory in its action, but has no systemic anti-coagulant effect that means the risk of bleeding is minimised (Bearman, 2000).

As defibriotide does not have an immediate effect, supportive care remains a priority for the child with VOD. Both intravenous fluid volumes and sodium content must be restricted to minimise third spacing (i.e. fluids found outside of the intravascular space) and maximise renal perfusion. To reduce symptomatic ascites, diuretics such as IV furosemide and IV spironolactone can be given. However, to maintain intravascular volume, IV albumin may need to be given concurrently. In the event of gross ascites that is not responding to albumin, diuretics and fluid restriction, careful paracentesis with intravascular colloid replacement may need to be performed. This will remove the peritoneal fluid, thus improving the child's respiratory function and ensuring the child's comfort (Bearman, 1995). This may avert the need for mechanical ventilation and an intensive care admission. Antithrombin has been shown to be useful in some patients and it may also be wise to counterbalance clotting dysfunction by administering IV vitamin K over several consecutive days.

In the case of severe VOD in a child whose condition continues to deteriorate, studies have shown that the use of recombinant tissue plasminogen activator (rtPA) has been successful in a number of cases (Baglin et al., 1990). However, it is widely believed that the catastrophic bleeding this may induce is too hazardous (Veys & Rao, 2004). The outcome for the child with VOD can range from full recovery to fulminant hepatic failure and death. Markers for a better prognosis are later onset, peak bilirubin levels $<105\ \mu\text{mols}/1$ and ALT levels <286 U/l. Unfortunately, the presenting signs and symptoms that are a feature of VOD are also indicative of several possible causes. Raised liver enzymes are associated with certain drugs (particularly the imidazole group of drugs such as itraconazole), lipid toxicity if the child is on TPN, liver GVHD and cryptosporidium infections affecting the liver. It is therefore vital that clinicians continue to monitor for all possible causes of liver dysfunction so that appropriate interventions are instigated.

From a nursing perspective the following should be in place to address the effects of VOD:

- Ensure twice-daily weight recording and girth measurement.
- Make an accurate recording of the fluid balance chart.
- Restrict intravenous and oral fluids.
- Restrict IV sodium chloride.
- Give diuretics, e.g. IV furosemide and IV spironolactone.
- Administer pain relief, e.g. subcutaneous or IV morphine.
- Assess the child for petechiae and bleeding.
- Give platelets, albumin and fresh frozen plasma, as directed.
- Maintain adequate respiratory function for the child.
- Assist with paracentesis, if required.
- Provide support for the child and family.

Graft versus host disease (GVHD)

GVHD is a reaction of donor cells to histocompatible differences between the donor and the host (Witherspoon & Storb, 1993). GVHD was a major complication in the early days of BMT (Barrett, 1993) and today it continues to be a complication of allogeneic transplants. This situation is likely to continue with the increasing use of unrelated and mismatched donors.

Originally, GVHD was seen as a T cell-mediated disease, brought about by infiltration of effector cells into target tissues with their resultant destruction (Treleaven & Barrett, 1993). It has now been shown that the situation is far more complex with involvement of natural killer (NK) cells, macrophages and cytokines (Witherspoon & Storb, 1993). Cytokines are produced in response to the conditioning regime prior to stem cell reinfusion. The release of inflammatory cytokines such as tumour necrosis factor (TNF) and interleukin 1 (IL-1) increases the HLA expression and up-regulates the immune response. This enhances the recognition of donor histocompatibility by the donor T cells. The activated T cells proliferate and secrete cytokines, mainly interleukin 2 (IL-2), which in turn activates more donor T cells and mononuclear cells. This is the afferent pathway of GVHD. The mononuclear cells are induced to produce IL-2 and TNF, which again stimulates further T cell activity. In this way a positive feedback loop is initiated amplifying the immune response and increasing tissue damage. The individual contribution of lymphocytes, macrophages and cytokines in mediating tissue damage during the efferent phase of GVHD remains unknown (Veys & Hann, 1997). Furthermore rapidly expanding cells sensitive to GVHD may also express HLA antigens, which may be up-regulated by both bacterial and viral infections. This link might provide the answer to an exacerbation of GVHD in the face of active adenoviral and CMV infections (Meyers et al., 1986). The resulting damage is focused on the rapidly dividing cells of the epithelium, gastrointestinal tract and liver.

Two forms of GVHD are described: acute and chronic. Acute GVHD (aGVHD) occurs in the first 100 days following transplant and may range from a mild and self-limiting or a fatal disorder (Veys & Hann, 1997). In its mild form, treatment may be symptomatic, with control of itching and monitoring of the condition. If the child becomes systemically unwell or the GVHD progresses, oral steroids may be added and increased or reduced as necessary. With progressive GVHD, which has failed to respond to steroids, other treatment approaches, including the use of monoclonal antibodies, thalidomide and IL-2 receptor antagonists have been used. Chronic GVHD (cGVHD) occurs beyond day 100 of the transplant. It may occur earlier, in isolation or as a progression of aGVHD. Chronic GVHD affects more organ systems than aGVHD and the effects on the child appear to be similar to autoimmune diseases such as scleroderma. The nursing implications for both forms will be described separately below.

The diagnosis of GVHD is usually clinical, however, skin, gut or liver biopsy may be used to confirm diagnosis. Biopsy results, nevertheless, are not always definitive and need to be put into context with clinical findings. Biopsies, however, may rule out a differential diagnoses of drug toxicities, veno-occlusive disease and viral infection (including CMV colitis and cryptosporidium). Both individual organ grading and overall GVHD grading is used (Figure 11.1). Patients with grades III and IV GVHD have a reduced chance of survival and grade IV GVHD is generally fatal.

Acute GVHD

There are recognised risk factors used to predict the severity and occurrence of GVHD:

- mismatched or unrelated donor (increasing level of HLA mismatch, the greater the risk of GVHD;
- racial mismatch;
- intense conditioning regimens;
- donor–recipient sex mismatch (increased GVHD in female donor to male recipient);
- increasing age of donor and recipient;
- infections with DNA viruses (CMV and HSV);
- cytokine administration;
- sunlight (can exacerbate skin GVHD).

Prevention of GVHD is undertaken according to the perceived risk. At present, a variety of methods are used to achieve this, involving either T cell depletion of the donor stem cells prior to infusion or the use of ciclosporin plus or minus methotrexate in the patient post stem cell infusion. The chosen method of GVHD prevention is a matter of choice for individual units and the chosen methods applied in response to the specific requirements of that transplant.

Skin GVHD

Onset is 7–10 days following transplant. Acute skin GVHD varies in intensity from a mild to a severe form with desquamation of large areas of the body. Frequently, the first sign is a rash or increased redness of the face, neck, including ears, palms, soles and limbs. This can progress to a maculopapular rash on the upper and lower body causing itching and discomfort to the child. Severe GVHD of the skin can progress to generalised erythroderma and desquamation (taking on the manifestation of second-degree burns). From a nursing perspective the following nursing care should include:

- Educate the parents in the prevention and early detection of skin GVHD.
- Daily skin care with an emollient bath oil to maintain skin integrity.
- Encourage the use of skin moisturisers, at least once a day.
- Assess the skin daily for any rash.
- Symptom control of itching with antihistamines (small babies may need to wear cotton gloves to prevent secondary infection). Loose cotton clothing can help to reduce skin irritation.
- Ensure the child has adequate sun protection applied correctly; the education of parents on discharge is vital. During the summer high factor UVA 5-star sun cream and long-sleeved shirts and trousers should be worn when outside, even on cloudy days.

Gastrointestinal GVHD

Onset is 10–21 days following transplant. Gastrointestinal GVHD often, but not always, follows skin GVHD. Presenting signs include diarrhoea with abdominal cramps, nausea and loss of appetite. From a nursing perspective the following nursing care should include:

- Awareness of the gut signs of GVHD is needed to differentiate mucositis and GVHD (GVHD stools are green and watery with strands of gut lining present).
- Assess the amount, colour and consistency of the stools.
- Maintain an accurate intake/output and fluid balance.
- Observe the child for dehydration, blood loss and signs of infection.
- Monitor the electrolyte balance.
- Ensure the peri-anal area is cleaned following episodes of diarrhoea. Maintain skin integrity as per unit policy.
- Rest the gut; provide nutrition with TPN.

Further gastrointestinal involvement can lead to increasing amounts of diarrhoea (stools are often green with mucus to begin with, becoming increasingly watery with strands of epithelial lining). As the involvement of the gut progresses, severe fluid loss, blood loss and bowel perforation may occur, requiring intensive medical and nursing care. Severe gut GVHD carries a high incidence of morbidity and mortality.

Liver GVHD

Onset is 30+ days following transplant, liver GVHD rarely occurs as an isolated event but usually as a progression from resolving gut and or skin GVHD. Liver involvement in GVHD occurs as a result of the destruction of the hepatic bile ducts and mucosa (Wujcik et al., 1994). Elevated liver enzymes, enlarged liver, jaundice and right upper quadrant pain can be an early indication of liver GVHD but may be due to ciclosporin, other drug toxicity or liver infection. From a nursing perspective the following nursing care should include:

- Provide analgesia and monitor its effectiveness.
- Position the child on the left side to decrease liver pressure.
- Provide comfort measures for itching as a result of jaundice.
- Provide support and comfort to the parents and the child.

The prevention of aGVHD frequently involves the use of ciclosporin, possibly combined with other drugs, such as oral steroids, methotrexate or mycophenolate mofetil (MMF). Treatment of GVHD consists of, in the first instance, topical steroids for mild skin GVHD to systemic treatment if the child's skin lesions progress or there is evidence of gut or liver involvement. Initially oral steroids, i.e. prednisolone, are started increasing to high doses of IV methylprednisolone in severe cases. For steroid refractory GVHD there have been some good results with the use of monoclonal antibodies such as infliximab and dacluzimab (Veys & Rao, 2004). The side effects of drug therapies may compound those already apparent with aGVHD and these are:

- *Increased hirsutism* (especially facial hair). Ensure the child and parents are aware of this as it may be upsetting for them. The parents and child should be reassured that this excess hair will go once the drugs are stopped.
- *Hypertension.* Monitoring of the child's blood pressure should continue on discharge even if this has not been a problem as an inpatient. It should be ensured that the community team is aware of the need to monitor blood pressure. Antihypertensive drugs may be needed to control this symptom.
- *Cushingoid appearance.* The child and the family should be supported during this time. Reassurance should be given that this alteration in body image is temporary and the child's appearance will return to normal once the ciclosporin and steroids are discontinued.
- *Increased risk of infection* (particularly fungal and viral). The child and parents need to understand the need to be concordant with drug therapies and to continue observing protective precautions as recommended by the unit.

Hyper-acute graft v host disease

Hyper-acute GVHD is an amplified version of aGVHD and is most commonly seen in the first week; in particular, the first 72 hours post-infusion of stem cells. It is usually seen in children who have an HLA mismatched donor and manifests itself as an extreme version of aGVHD. The child will have sudden onset respiratory problems, including de-saturation, fever, skin rashes, diarrhoea and a raised bilirubin. Treatment is supportive with oxygen therapy and steroids.

Chronic GVHD

Chronic GVHD (cGVHD) is unusual in children, however, the risk of occurrence increases with age. For children under the age of 10 years receiving a sibling transplant and receiving GVHD prophylaxis of methotrexate and ciclosporin, the incidence is as low as 13 % rising to 28 % in adolescents (Sullivan *et al.*, 1991). The reason for the younger child being at less risk of cGVHD is not known (Mehta, 2004). Chronic GVHD is defined as GVHD occurring 100 days post-transplant. However, clinical and histological features may occur 30 days post-BMT (Barrett, 1993). It may occur alone or in conjunction with aGVHD (Atkinson, 1991). Risk factors include increased age of donor, degree of HLA mismatch and previous aGVHD (Veys & Hann, 1997). The primary feature of cGVHD is an increase in collagen deposits causing sclerosis and atrophy of the dermis. More organs are affected than in aGVHD and clinical signs reflect the organ affected. These may include joint and muscle contractures, skin colour changes, malabsorption and liver damage due to bile duct destruction (Frederick & Hanigan, 1993) (Table 11.4).

Risk factors for cGVHD

The main risk factor for developing cGVHD following SCT are:

- a preceding acute GVHD;
- HLA matching between patient and donor;
- age of the donor.

There is some debate as to whether GCSF mobilised peripheral blood stem cells increase the incidence of cGVHD (Mehta, 2004). Treatment is both specific and symptomatic. Alternating oral steroids and ciclosporin is an effective regimen and aims to minimise drug-related side effects (Sullivan *et al.*, 1991). For those with a poor response to this regime, thalidomide, MMF (mycophenolate mofetil), FK506 (tacrolimus), infliximab and PUVA (Psoralen ultra violet A radiation) have been used (Vogelsang & Hess, 1994; Vogelsang *et al.*, 1996; Greinix *et al.*, 1998; Zecca & Locatelli, 2000). Symptom control is necessary to maintain the child's comfort and quality of life. This includes

Table 11.4 Signs and presenting symptoms of cGVHD

Signs	Presenting symptoms
Skin	
scleroderma	Red discoloration of the skin, stiffness of connective tissue,
lichen planus	joint contractures.
skin colour	Dry white patches on the skin.
alopecia	Can be increased or decreased
	Sparse, uneven hair – both head and body.
	Dry eyes and mouth.
Sicca syndrome	White dry patches on oral mucosa, often mistaken for oral candida.
lichenoid lesions	Painful friable mucous membranes (this may also affect the vagina, oesophagus, external auditory canal).
premature dental decay	Dry mouth, difficulty in swallowing, and reduction in saliva
mucositis	
xerostomia	Gastrointestinal tract
Malabsorption	
anorexia	Weight loss, diarrhoea
dysphagia	Difficulty in swallowing may be due to narrowing of oesophagus
Musculoskeletal	
muscular atrophy	Weakness and wasting painful joints, knees and hips
Lungs	
obliterative pulmonary bronchitis	Decreased activity tolerance
Liver	
bile duct abnormalities	Cirrhosis liver failure
Immune system	Recurrent encapsulated infections

Sources: Frederick & Hanigan (1993); Barrett (1993).

a multidisciplinary team approach from occupational therapists and physiotherapists in order to maintain mobility and prevent contractures.

Due to the low levels of circulating antibodies that are a feature of cGVHD and the immunosuppressive nature of the treatment, the risk of viral, bacterial and fungal infections is increased. Prophylaxis against pneumocystis and encapsulated organisms is also needed, alongside continued immunoglobulin replacement therapy (Barrett, 1993). Response to treatment and the long-term outlook depend upon the number of organs involved and the platelet count; thrombocytopenia less than $50 \times 10^9/l$ is also an indication of poor prognosis (Veys & Hann, 1997).

The occurrence of cGVHD can have emotional as well as physical effects. The child never becomes well after transplant, leading to depression and low self-esteem. This can affect all family members, as the affected child remains dependent on the parents for both physical and psychological support. For the sibling donor, extended feelings of guilt may be shown at having a part to play in the debilitation of their sibling through donation. Nursing intervention includes recognising the family at risk of stress due to caring for a child with cGVHD and the implementation of support mechanisms.

GVHD, both acute and chronic, still remains despite many new approaches, one of the major obstacles to survival post SCT. However the absence of GVHD can also pose a problem for the child with leukaemia, as it is thought that GVH enhances the graft v leukaemia (GVL) effect (Munker et al., 2002).

Graft versus leukaemia (GVL)

One of the specific advantages of SCT concerns the phenomenon of the graft versus leukaemia (GvL) effect. Following SCT there is a high rise in cytokines, including interleukin-2 (IL-2), natural killer (NK) interferons and tumour necrosis factor (TNF). This 'cytokine storm' is thought to be responsible for unrestricted cytotoxicity towards leukaemia cells. On activation, T cells demonstrate a wide range of cytotoxicity towards tumour cells. GvL is thought to be the result of minor donor T cell recognition and elimination of host leukaemic cells' histocompatibility antigen differences on the surface of cells. This phenomenon is most readily seen in adults with chronic myeloid leukaemia (CML) both from donor T cells infused at the time of transplant and with donor T cell infusions following relapse of CML post-transplant. It may have a role to play in BMT for childhood leukaemia but the full implications and appropriate use in the clinical setting will be the subject of further medical research (Caudell & Adams, 1990; Magarth, 1994; Veys et al., 1994).

Relapse and the role of a second stem cell transplant

Relapse following SCT or failure of the stem cells to engraft is a devastating event for the child and the family, it is, however, a common cause of transplant failure (Sandler & Joyce, 2004; Veys & Rao, 2004). Multiple transplants are not uncommon in the USA (Magarth, 1994), but are rare in the UK. Parents will often seek more treatment in the hope of a cure, however toxicity is considerable. The decision to undertake a second transplant must consider many aspects, and no one answer or solution will be suitable for all children. For children who relapse within six months of a first transplant, long-term survival following a second procedure is less than 10% and with a treatment mortality of >60% (Veys & Rao, 2004). However, for children who relapse more than six months after their first transplant, a second procedure is a possibility with generally a 20–30% disease-free survival (Sandler & Joyce, 2004).

Factors influencing the decision to proceed to a second transplant are assessed on an individual basis but may include:

- the availability and potential risks (both psychological and physical) to the donor;

- the risk of toxicity to the patient in proceeding with the second transplant;
- the probability of the second transplant being successful (Prentice et al., 1996).

Therefore the use of reduced intensity conditioning, once the child is in remission may offer a better chance of cure and with minimal organ toxicity. The aim of the procedure would be to manipulate the graft and increase the GvL effect by reducing the GVHD prophylaxis and using T replete stem cells. Donor registries do allow adult donors to donate bone marrow or peripheral stem cells twice and to donate T cells to the patient in light of a relapse, however, the use of GCSF in unrelated adult donors is an area of continued debate. The use of sibling donors in these circumstances is a more difficult decision, on both moral and practical grounds. The use of central lines for small children unable to cope with leukopheresis from a peripheral cannula may expose these children to another general anaesthetic. The psychological stress involved for this tiny group of sibling donors is an area where future research needs to be focused.

Donor lymphocyte infusions (DLI)

For children with chronic myeloid leukaemia who relapse following SCT the infusion of donor T lymphocytes may achieve a remission without having to use further chemotherapy. If there is neither GVHD nor response, the infusions can be given at 12-weekly intervals with a larger increment of cells given at each infusion. One problem that may arise is the chance of the child developing marrow aplasia or severe GVHD. To date there has been little success in using DLI in children with acute lymphoblastic leukaemia, however, there may be some hope for children with Philadelphia-positive or infant ALL. Within the acute leukaemias, for DLI to work the child must be in remission, therefore some prior chemotherapy to achieve this state is vital (Kolb et al., 1995; Veys & Rao, 2004).

References

Atkinson P (1991) 'Chronic graft versus host disease – review' Bone Marrow Transplantation 5: 69–82

Baglin T (1994) 'Veno-occlusive disease of the liver complicating bone marrow transplantation (Review)' *Bone Marrow Transplantation* 13(1): 1–4

Baglin T, Harper P & Marcus R (1990) 'Veno-occlusive disease of the liver complicating ABMT successfully treated with recombinant tissue plasminogen activator (rt-PA)' *Bone Marrow Transplantations* 5(3): 439–441

Barnes R (1992a) 'Infections following bone marrow transplantation' *in*; Treleaven J & Barrett J (eds) *Bone Marrow Transplantation in Practice*. London: Churchill Livingstone, pp. 281–287

Barnes R (1992b) 'Treatment of bacterial, fungal and viral infections in hospital' *in*: Treleaven J & Barrett J (eds) *Bone Marrow Transplantation in Practice*. London: Churchill Livingstone, pp. 299–306

Barrett J (1993) 'Graft versus host disease' *in*: Treleaven J & Barrett J (eds) *Bone Marrow Transplant in Practice*. London: Churchill Livingstone, pp. 257–272

Bearman S (1995) 'The syndrome of hepatic veno-occlusive disease after marrow transplantation (Review article "Blood")' *Journal of the American Society of Hematology* 85(11): 3005–3020

Bearman S (2000) 'Veno-occlusive disease of the liver' *Current Opinion in Oncology* 12(2): 101–109

Beck, S (1979) 'Impact of systematic oral care protocol on stomatitis after chemotherapy' *Cancer Nursing* 2(10): 185–199

Blotcky AD, Cohen DG & Conatser C (1985) 'Psychosocial characterisation of patients who refuse cancer treatment' *Journal of Consulting Clinical Psychology* 53(5): 729–731

Cathgomas G, Morris P, Pekle K *et al.* (1993) 'Rapid diagnosis of cytomegalovirus pulmonary pneumonia in marrow transplant recipients by bronchoalveolar lavage using the polymerise chain reaction, virus culture, and the direct immunostaining of alveolar cells' *Blood* 81: 1909–1914

Caudell K & Adams J (1990) 'Cyclosporine administration practices on bone marrow transplant units: a national survey' *Oncology Nurses Forum* 17(4): 563–568

Eilers J, Berger A & Peterson M (1988) 'Development, testing and application of the oral assessment guide' *Oncology Nurses Forum* 15(3): 325–330

Einsele H, Ehinger G & Hebart H (1995) 'Polymerase chain reaction monitoring reduces the incidence of cytomegalovirus diseasd and the duration and side effect of antiviral therapy after bone marrow transplantation' *Blood* 86: 2815–2820

Eland J (1988) 'Pain in children' *Nursing Clinics of North America* 25(4): 871–884

Ezzone S, Jolly D, Repogle K, Kapoor N & Tutschka P (1993) 'Survey of oral hygiene regimes among bone marrow transplant centers' *Oncology Nurses Forum* 20(9): 1375–1381

Frederick B & Hanigan MJ (1993) 'Bone marrow transplantation' *in*: Foley GV, Fochtman D & Mooney KH (eds) *Nursing Care of a Child with Cancer*. Philadelphia: WB Saunders, pp. 130–178

Gibson F (1989) 'Parental involvement in bone marrow transplant' *Paediatric Nursing* 1(7): 21–22

Gibson F, Cargill J, Allison J, Cole S, Stone, J, Begent J & Lucas V (2006) 'Establishing content validity of the oral assessment guide in children and young people' *European Journal of Cancer* 42: 1817–1825

Gibson F & Hopkins S (2005) 'Feeling sick is horrible, and being sick is very frightening . . . say Jasper and Polly (Pearman, 1998)' *European Journal of Oncology Nursing* 9: 6–7

Graham H, Pecoraro D, Ventura M & Meyer C (1993) 'Reducing the incidence of stomatitis using a quality assessment and improvement approach' *Cancer Nursing* 16(2): 117–122

Grandt N (1989) 'Hepatic veno-occlusive diseases following bone marrow transplantation' *Oncology Nursing Forum* 16(6): 813–817

Greinix HT, Volc-Platzer B, Watkins P, *et al.* (1998) 'Successful use of extracorporeal photophoresis (ECP) in the treatment of chronic graft versus host disease. *Blood* 92: 3098–4104

Gureno M & Reisinger C (1991) 'Patient controlled analgesia for the young pediatric patient' *Pediatric Nursing* 17(3): 251–254

Kanfer E (1993) 'The diagnosis and management of early complications' *in*: Trealeven J & Barrett J (eds) *Bone Marrow Transplantation in Practice*. London: Churchill Livingstone, pp. 247–256

Kolb HJ, Schattenburg A, Goldman J, Hertenstein B, Jacobsen N, Arcese W, Ljungman P, Ferrant A, Verdouk L, Niederweiser D, Rhee F, Mittermuellur J, de Whitte T, Holler E & Ansari, H (1995) 'Graft versus leukaemia effect of donor lymphocyte transfusions in marrow engrafted patients' *Blood* 86(5): 2041–2050

Magarth I (1994) 'Bone marrow transplantation for leukaemia: a lame horse for use of high technology medical care' *The Lancet* 345(8950): 601–602

McDonald GB, Sharma P, Mathews DE, Shulman HM & Thomas ED (1984) 'Veno-occlusive disease of the liver after bone marrow transplantation: diagnosis, incidence, and predisposing factors' *Hepatology* 4(1): 116–122

McGarth P, Johnson G, Goodman J, Schillinger P, Dunn J & Chapman J (1985) 'CHEOPS: a behavioral scale for rating postoperative pain in children' *in*; Fields HL, Dubner R & Cervero F (eds) *Advances in Pain Research and Therapy*. New York: Raven Press, pp. 395–401

Mehta P (2004) 'Graft versus host disease after stem cell transplantation in children' *in*: Mehta P (ed.) *Paediatric*

Stem Cell Transplantation. Boston: Jones & Bartlett, pp. 401–410

Meyers JD, Flournay N & Thomas ED (1986) 'Risk factors for cytomegalovirus infection after human marrow transplantation' *Journal of Infectious Diseases* 153(3): 478–488

Munker R, Gunther W & Kolb J (2002) 'New concepts about graft-versus-host and graft-versus-leukaemia reactions; a summary of the 5th international symposium held in Munich March 2002' *Bone Marrow Transplant 30*: 549–556

Patterson K (1992) 'Pain in paediatric oncology patients' *Journal of Pediatric Oncology Nursing 9*(3): 119–130

Prentice G, Gluckman E, Powles RL *et al.* (1997) 'Long-term survival in allogeneic bone marrow transplant recipients following aciclovir prophylaxis for CMV infection' *Bone Marrow Transplant 19*: 129–133

Prentice HG, Atra A, Cornish JM, Gibson B, Kinset S, Pinkerton R, Potter MN, Will A & Veys P (1996) 'Donor leukocyte infusion as immunotherapy of acute leukemia relapsed after allogeneic bone marrow transplant' Protocol of the UKCCSG paediatric bone marrow transplant group-pilot/dose finding study (2nd Draft)

Richardson PG, Elias AD, Krishnan A, Wheeler C, Nath R, Hoppensteadt D, Kinchla NM, Neuberg D, Waqller EK, Antin JH, Soiffer R, Vredenburgh J, Lill M, Woolfrey AE, Bearman SI, Iacobelli M, Fareed J & Guinan EC (1998) 'Treatment of severe veno-occlusive disease with defibriotide: compassionate use results without significant organ toxicity in a high-risk population' *Blood 92*(3): 737–7441

Sandler E & Joyce M (2004) 'Acute lymphoblastic leukaemia' *in*: Mehta P (ed.) *Pediatric Stem Cell Transplantation.* Boston: Jones & Bartlett, pp. 187–207

Schmidt G (1992) 'Prophylaxis of cytomegalovirus infection after bone marrow transplantation' *Seminars in Oncology Nursing 19*: 20–26

Singer J (1992) 'Role of colony stimulating factors in bone marrow transplantation' *Seminars in Oncology Nursing 8*(1): 27–31

Sullivan KM, Agura E & Anasetti CM (1991) 'Chronic graft versus host disease: late complications of bone marrow transplantation' *Seminars in Hematology 28*(2): 250–259

Treleaven J & Barrett J (1993) 'Introduction to bone marrow transplantation' *in*: Treleaven J & Barrett J (eds) *Bone Marrow Transplantation in Practice.* London: Churchill Livingstone, pp. 3–10

Veys P & Hann IM (1997) 'Bone marrow transplantation for leukaemia' *in*: Plowman PN & Pinkerton R (eds) *Paediatric Oncology: Clinical Practice and Controversies* (2nd edn). London: Chapman & Hall Medical, pp. 617–627

Veys P & Rao K (2004) 'Advances in therapy: megatherapy allogeneic stem cell transplantation' *in*: Pinkerton R, Plowman PN & Pieters R (eds) *Paediatric Oncology* (3rd edn). London: Arnold, part 3A, pp. 513–517

Veys P, Sanders, F & Calderwood S (1994) 'The role of graft versus leukaemia in bone marrow transplantation for juvenile chronic myeloid leukaemia' *Blood 84*: (suppl.) 337A

Vogelsgang G & Hess A (1994) 'Graft versus host disease: new directions for a persistent problem' *Blood 84*(7): 2061–2067

Vogelsgang GB, Wolff D, Altomonte V, *et al.* (1996) 'Treatment of chronic graft versus host disease with PUVA' *Bone Marrow Transplant 17*: 1061–1067

Wadleigh M, Ho V, Momtaz P & Richardson P (2003) 'Hepatic veno-occlusive disease: pathogenesis, diagnosis and treatment' *Current Opinion in Haematology 10*(6): 451–462

Wingard J (1990) 'Advances in the management of infectious complications after bone marrow transplantation' *Bone Marrow Transplantation 6*: 371–383

Witherspoon R & Storb R (1983) 'Bone marrow transplantation' *in*: Lachman P, Peters K & Rosen Walport M (eds) *Clinical Aspects of Immunology* (5th edn). Boston: Blackwell Scientific

Wong P & Baker CM (1988) 'Pain in children: comparison of assessment scales' *Pediatric Nurse 14*(1): 9–17

Wujcik D, Ballard B & Camp-Sorrell D (1994) 'Selected complications of allogeneic bone marrow transplantation' *Seminars in Oncology Nursing 10*(1): 28–41

Zecca M & Locatelli F (2000) 'Management of graft versus host disease in paediatric bone marrow transplant recipients' *Paediatric Drugs 2*: 29–55

Zerbe M, Parkerson S, Ortleib M & Spitzer T (1992) 'Relationships between oral mucositis and treatment variables in bone marrow transplants' *Cancer Nursing 15*(3): 196–205

12 Discharge Planning and Psychosocial Issues for the Family

Nikki Bennett-Rees and Sian Hopkins

Discharge planning

The experience of a SCT, for both the child and the family, takes place over a long period. The experience begins with the search for a donor and this may take many months and be emotionally exhausting for the child and family. Hopes and expectations are raised and dashed in the search for and identification of a suitable donor. With the success of finding a donor, the transplant follows. This often takes place at a regional transplant centre, which may be some distance from the home and away from the support of family and friends. The extensive medical and nursing support needed following transfusion of the marrow or stem cells and in the wait for engraftment requires weeks, possibly months, of hospitalisation. At last the child and the family reach the physical criteria required by the unit to be allowed to go home. This is the day everyone has been waiting for. However, the complexities of discharge following SCT should begin pre-admission. It is crucial to ensure that the family have a suitable home to return to, for both them and their child post SCT. For example, is the home free from damp/animal infestation and is any building work required or indeed planned? Has home tuition been set up

so that when the child returns home there are no delays in continuing with home schooling? If the family have pets, are they healthy, with vaccinations up to date?

On discharge from a transplant unit parents may face a myriad of concerns and anxieties related to treatment, prognosis and changes in their lives resulting from the transplant experience. Once home the practicalities of family life need to be resumed. The financial cost of the transplant often becomes apparent on discharge, even in countries with free medical care the cost implications for families undergoing stem cell transplant are vast. Usually one parent (often the mother) gives up a wage or takes a career break during the transplant period. This loss of income can have major implications for the family; the financial costs of a home and family carry on and although put on hold during the hospitalisation of the child, they reappear once the family is home. This may lead to a change to the previous lifestyle of the family, affecting all its members, particularly healthy siblings who may lose out on previously granted treats or pastimes. On discharge there is a transition from an acute to a chronic phase of care, requiring an alteration in the coping mechanisms demanded of the family and the child. White

Cancer in Children and Young People   Edited by Faith Gibson and Louise Soanes
© 2008 John Wiley & Sons, Ltd

(1994) has identified six major themes of concern to parents on discharge from the unit:

- the return home;
- working with this;
- changing relationships;
- learning the rules;
- the new norms;
- the uncertain future.

Returning home

The return home is often seen by families as a mixed blessing. Reporting 'it's good to be home, to be a family again in familiar surroundings and in charge of our lives again' but also expressing concerns about leaving the safety and security of the unit with the 'experts on tap'.

Changing relationships

If the transplant has occurred far from home, the follow-up care may be coordinated at a local paediatric unit. In some cases this might be the original referring hospital in which the child has been cared for in the past. If this is the case, relationships with staff will have been formed and the routines and environment of the hospital will be familiar to the child and family. However, for those children with little or no previous experience of hospital, for example, children with metabolic disease or children for whom the follow-up hospital is not their referring hospital, the involvement of another hospital can be an added stress. New relationships will need to be formed with staff of this hospital and a new philosophy of care learned. Parents can be helped in this with the support of paediatric community nurses from the shared care or tertiary hospital. In such cases the family becomes a teacher, explaining the past experiences of the child and the practicalities of SCT to new staff. The potential inexperience of staff in the follow-up hospital in relation to the field of SCT can lead to further stress and anxiety for the family.

Learning the rules

Learning the rules of discharge can be a major component of the discharge experience for parents.

The vulnerability of parents leaving the safety of the hospital, often perceived as clean and germ-free, to enter the outside world again can be a time of fear. Physical care of the child is now their sole responsibility; monitoring vital signs and the symptoms of GVHD and choosing when to act on them is now their responsibility.

New norms

The skills parents have previously learned and once undertaken in order to care for their child while sick may need to be relearned prior to discharge, for instance, the timing and safe administration of the many oral drugs required after a transplant and caring for central venous lines. Skills such as these may have once been second nature, but now physically and emotionally exhausted following the transplant, parents may have forgotten how to carry them out; or tasks may have been performed by staff on the transplant unit, so leading to loss of confidence. Staff should not make the assumption that because parents have successfully carried out such tasks before, they are capable, willing or confident about resuming them on discharge. New skills need to be learned, such as giving naso-gastric feeds. The monitoring of adequate calorie intake and other supportive care also needs to be learned by parents prior to discharge.

The uncertain future

The sense of responsibility for the physical well-being of the child can lead to unrealistic expectations by parents as to how safe they can make their home in order to prevent complications and infections occurring. The extended use of hospital-based infection precautions, such as methods of washing clothes, and the adoption of hospital-type cleaning routines have been reported and in one case a child's bedroom was rebuilt as the old wood was seen by the parents as a potential infection risk. Reluctance to return the child to school and the prolonged use of restrictions on the child's activities may prevent the child's reintegration into 'normal life'. To help these families make sense of the transplant experience and to help in the child's reintegration to normal life careful discharge planning is required.

Although a significant event, SCT is a temporary period in a family's life. Helping a family to make sense of this period and return to society post-transplant begins before the transplant and requires a multidisciplinary approach, which is often coordinated by a nurse. Hare *et al.* (1989) suggest that the period and quality of preparation can have a significant effect on the family's attitude towards treatment and recovery. Discharge interviews are recommended by some authors (Heiney *et al.*, 1994; Sormati *et al.*, 1994); these interviews can act as debriefing sessions for the family and help them to begin to make sense of the transplant experience. The staff leading the discharge planning need to acknowledge that the transition from the acute to the chronic phase of the SCT and the return to the new norm may not be smooth. The nurse leading these sessions needs to be someone the family already knows and with whom they have a working relationship. This may be their primary nurse, key worker, social worker or transplant coordinator. This person will need to be confident in their ability to coordinate the care of the child and the family's reintegration to home life. Skilled communication is called for, as is understanding of the role of the resources and functions of the multidisciplinary team. Each family will require careful assessment, planning and implementation of a care plan as discharge approaches. The family's involvement is paramount to the success of discharge planning. For those families for whom English is not the first language, the use of interpreters for both oral and written information should be considered in advance and cultural advocates may be necessary to provide coordinated discharge from hospital.

The child whose post-transplant care is to be shared with other hospitals and agencies may require multidisciplinary discharge planning meetings, in which the anticipated transition can be discussed openly and supportive measures implemented. Prior to discharge, professionals within the multidisciplinary team for whom SCT is not the norm may be apprehensive about receiving the child into their care. This should be recognised as a cause of stress to staff and support mechanisms should be identified for them. Staff in such areas will need input from the discharging unit about the precautions and possible complications of SCT. Such information should include practical advice, for example, restrictions on diet, immunisation and sun protection, as well as general advice on physical and psychological responses to SCT.

At the discharge meetings acceptance of each other's areas of responsibility and limitations should be recognised and respected. In both areas a named link person/key worker would be beneficial, and effective communication systems should be established before discharge of the family from the unit. As early discharge from units may be a feature of the future, due to pressure on resources and the expansion of transplants in paediatrics, this situation may become more frequent. The link person/key worker coordinating the discharge should be easily contactable by parents and staff and have a named associate to cover in their absence. Effective communication within the unit will help in the continuity of care and reduce confusion and stress for all those involved.

The first year after transplant has been shown to be the most stressful in emotional, physical and psychological terms (Pot Mees, 1989); support during this period is likely to be the most intense. As the family adjusts to the new norms, the intensity of involvement by the supportive agencies can be reduced; naturally there will be some families for whom longer-term intervention is needed due to the physical results of treatment, such as the side effects of TBI and GVHD, or the psychological trauma of a difficult or complicated transplant. Long-term support groups for parents have been used in some centres with beneficial results (Andrykowski *et al.*, 1995).

For parents, the need is for concrete information to help them cope with the physical and psychological care of their child and the knowledge that their fears and concerns will be acknowledged and acted upon (White, 1994). As discharge approaches and the child's physical health improves, care by parents can be increased and nursing intervention slowly withdrawn. 'Step down' units or transfer to a quieter, more distant area of the unit can aid in the transition to home with less nursing intervention. Responsibility for drug administration by parents can be implemented with help and support from staff and the learning (or relearning) of skills, such as caring for central venous lines and nasogastric feeds, undertaken.

Confidence is needed by both sides that the recognition of complications post transplant, such as GVHD, and the required action, are understood and that other carers the child may have, for example, grandparents, are aware of the need for precautions such as adequate sun protection and skin care. Support and reinforcement are once again vital if parents are to be confident in their child's care after discharge. Written information is needed to support the verbal information given, with a named person to contact if necessary. This may be included in a parent information folder or booklet. Again, consideration for families for whom English is not the first language needs to be taken into account. The use of multidisciplinary outpatient clinics can be of benefit to both families and staff alike in providing a cohesive transition to home and the opportunity for parents to talk over their fears and concerns with the 'experts'. For successful transition from hospital to home, awareness is needed by both the family and the staff. The family will require information that the transition from hospital to home may not be as smooth as they expect. Information about what to expect, both from their own and the child's reaction to returning home, will need to be discussed with them. Speaking to a family recently discharged from the unit may help to highlight areas only apparent to those who have experienced transplant at first hand. Coping mechanisms and strategies for coping with setbacks (both physical and psychological) will need to be identified. The transition from hospital to home can be managed well, allowing the family to reintegrate with support and education from the multidisciplinary team with the minimum of trauma.

Finally, as the day for discharge approaches and the isolation precautions have been reduced, parents must be given sound discharge advice, balancing the continued need for the child's protection against infection with the need to resume a 'normal' life.

Psychosocial effects of stem cell transplant on the family

Few studies have looked specifically at the experience that families live through when their child has had a SCT (Dermatis & Lesko, 1990); most literature revolves around families whose child has cancer. However, increasing numbers of children who do not have cancer are undergoing SCT. Clearly this is an area where research is needed in order to ensure that the transplant episode is as manageable as possible. Stem cell transplantation presents many challenges to both children and their families; it can affect many areas surrounding quality of life issues from the acute stage through to long-term recovery. It is on discharge from the transplant unit that families often realise the full impact that the transplant has had on their lives. A change in perspective occurs. The trivia of life that once seemed important, such as cars breaking down and delayed trains, no longer seem as crucial; one mother described it thus, 'the small things don't matter any more, after this [the transplant] the rest is just not important.'

This change in philosophy can be accompanied by an alteration in spirituality. This may not take the form of religion but may be expressed as a growth in inner strength, conviction and life goals (Ferrell et al., 1992a, b). If faith was important to the family before, it may be reinforced by the experience of transplant. In some cases belief in a greater being and prayer may have been used during the transplant and their use be afforded some responsibility for its success; these coping mechanisms may or may not be continued after discharge (Brack et al., 1988). The spiritual issues of SCT can also lead to the question of 'Why did our child survive and others die?', so-called 'survivor guilt' (Whendon & Ferrell, 1994). Being aware that other families on the unit are not as lucky to be discharged with a well child may lead parents and children to ask why they were chosen to survive instead of others. Survivor guilt has been reported to lead to feelings of despair in some survivors of SCT (Ferrell et al., 1992b). The discussion of survivor guilt is included in the following section looking at a potentially negative response to SCT, post-traumatic stress disorder (PTSD).

The perception (by both nurses and the family) that the transition from hospital to home will always be smooth is unrealistic and in some cases may be so difficult as to result in post-traumatic stress disorder (PTSD) (Heiney et al., 1994). PTSD is defined as a 'psychological traumatic event that is outside the normal range of usual human experience'. Often used to describe reactions to man-made or natural disasters, it can also be used to describe any overwhelming life-threatening event. The presentation of PTSD is the development of a set of characteristic symptoms which include re-experiencing the event, avoidance, detachment, physiological arousal and feelings such as anger, guilt, depression and grief. Factors contributing to PTSD include decreased social support, the extent to which the sufferer played a part in the event and the origin of the stressor. Heiney *et al.* (1994) examined PTSD in the aftermath of SCT in paediatric patients and their families. In this work she found that seven factors in the transplant period affected the development of PTSD:

- degree of life threat;
- duration of trauma;
- degree of bereavement and loss;
- displacement from home and family;
- potential for recurrence;
- role of the parent in the trauma;
- exposure to death and destruction.

These issues are discussed briefly below. The transplant, an attempt to prevent death or improve quality of life, carries a risk of mortality and morbidity that continues throughout life with the occurrence of complications, rejection and the fear of relapse (Sherman *et al.*, 2004). Parents report lying awake at night worrying what to do if a relapse occurs, if the graft is lost due to infection, or the uncertain response to transplant. Parents are involved in their child's care during transplant and give consent to the procedure. This involvement and the witnessing of complications and trauma for the child can lead to stress and feelings of helplessness by parents. The displacement from home and support networks can lead to feelings of isolation and detachment. In the place of usual support networks friendships are formed with other families on the unit. Some of the children in these families may die during their transplant. This, in turn, leads parents to face not only the possibility that their own child may die but also the death of children whom they know well, an experience rarely faced by families in twenty-first-century Western society. The relationships formed with other families on the unit are especially significant during the transplant period. On discharge, relationships with old friends and neighbours are

resumed and this is taken to be a sign of returning to normal by others. Families report that the loss of contact with people with whom they have shared a common experience is difficult to adjust to, 'People who are in the same boat as you are lost', is how one mother described this loss of support.

Relationships within the family may also have altered during the child's admission. The parent who stayed in hospital and the sick child may have almost become a single family. A relationship can be formed in which each party knows the other more intensely than before or than other members of the family know them. The readjustment to their previous roles within the family can take both time and energy. In their parent's absence, older siblings may have taken on the role of parent to younger siblings, and fathers may have taken on roles previously carried out by the mother. In effect, the parent and child may return to a household in which the roles they once occupied have been filled. One mother, after a prolonged transplant admission, commented that on her return 'it was almost as if they didn't need me any more'.

The transplant period of separation has also been described as having a negative effect on marital relationships and the personality of the parents (Freund & Seigel, 1986). The transplanted child has to readjust to being one of the family again, and no longer the centre of attention. Relationships with and between siblings will also require adjustment. Siblings who have been sent to stay with relatives will need to adjust to the family rules again and a period of conflict may occur as old roles and domains are regained or adjustments made to permanent changes to family dynamics. In addition, for the mother, adjustment to the changed home environment may be compounded with her return to work. This can be additionally stressful, as leaving the child previously in her care can give rise to feelings of fear and guilt (Pot Mees, 1989).

Once home, many families do adjust to the new norm and rapidly gain confidence in their child's care, instigating changes and moving on from the hospital. The reintegration to school/college is one area that may be a significant event for the family. The point at which the child is allowed to return to school/college will vary from unit to unit. Often, once immunosuppressive drugs have stopped and the immune system is re-established, the school/college can be restarted. However, the fear of infection is one of the main reasons cited for the delay in restarting school/college and outbreaks of infections such as chickenpox may cause the child to be withdrawn from school again. For the child, adaptation to their peer group can be stressful. Old friendships will have moved on, the rules and culture of school/college, as with the family, will once again have to be relearned and academic work interrupted by the transplant will need to be regained. The provision of home tuition while the child is well but still immunosuppressed can help to reintroduce academic work. Once this hurdle has been overcome, confidence in reintroducing other activities usually grows, 'Once he started school, it seemed silly not to allow him to do the other things, we just slowly started them up again things like football and Cubs, so far there's been no problem.'

Following SCT, it can often take a year for the family to readjust to the experience (Pot Mees, 1989). This experience, which has not been shared by the family as a whole, will mean that each member child, the parent who stayed in hospital, the parent who stayed at home, the sibling donor, and the sibling who was not a donor, will all have their own private feelings about the transplant. The year following the transplant will be a time of upheaval and resettlement for the family as they re-form. This year can be likened to the 'golden hour' in emergency medicine, in that what happens during that time is vital for the long-term implications for the family's health, both as individuals and as a whole. Planning for the family's discharge is a key area of responsibility for the transplant nurse.

References

Andrykowski M, Brady M, Greiner C, Altmaier E, Burish T, Antin J, Gingrich R, McGarighe C & Henslee Downley P (1995) ' "Returning to normal" following bone marrow transplantation: outcomes, expectations and informed consent' *Bone Marrow Transplantation* 15(4): 573–581

Brack G, LaClave L & Blix S (1988) 'The psychological aspects of bone marrow transplant' *Cancer Nursing* 11(4): 221–229

Dermatis H & Lesko LM (1990) 'Psychological distress in parents consenting to child's bone marrow transplantation' *Bone Marrow Transplant* 6: 411–417

Ferrell, B, Grant M, Schmidt G, Rheiner M, Whitehead C, Fonbuenu P & Foreman S (1992b) 'The meaning of quality of life for bone marrow transplant survivors part 2: improving quality of life for bone marrow transplant survivors' *Cancer Nursing* 15(4): 247–253

Ferrell, B, Grant M, Schmidt G, Rheiner M, Whitehead C, Fonbuenu P & Foreman S (1992b) 'The meaning of quality of life for bone marrow transplant survivors part 2: improving quality of life for bone marrow transplant survivors' *Cancer Nursing* 15(4): 247–253

Freund B & Siegel K (1986) 'Problems in transition following bone marrow transplantation: psychosocial aspects' *American Journal of Orthopsychiatry* 56(2): 244–252

Hare J, Skinner D & Kliewer D (1989) 'Family systems approach to paediatric bone marrow transplantation' *Children's Health Care* 18(1): 30–36

Heiney S, Neuberg R, Myers D & Bergman L (1994) 'The aftermath of bone marrow transplantation for parents of pediatric patients: a post traumatic stress disorder' *Oncology Nurses Forum* 21(5): 843–847

Pot Mees C (1989) *The Psychosocial Effects of Bone Marrow Transplantation in Children.* Delft: Eburon

Sherman A, Simonton S & Latif U (2004) 'Psychological adjustment after stem cell transplantation' *in*: Mehta P (ed.) *Paediatric Stem Cell Transplantation.* Boston: Jones & Bartlett, pp. 99–115

Sormati M, Dungan S & Ricker P (1994) 'Pediatric bone marrow transplantation: psychological issues for parents after a child's hospitalisation' *Journal of Psychological Oncology* 12(4): 23–41

Whendon M & Ferrell B (1994) 'Quality of life in adult bone marrow transplant patients: beyond the first year' *Seminars in Oncology Nursing* 10(1): 42–57

White A (1994) 'Parental concerns following a child's discharge from a bone marrow transplant unit' *Journal of Paediatric Oncology Nursing* 11(3): 93–101

13 Staff Support in Stem Cell Transplant Units

Sian Hopkins

Caring for children and their families facing haematopoetic stem cell transplant, as with other areas of high-dependency nursing, is stressful. Some sources of stress are common to nursing as a profession and others are unique to the speciality. Common stressors identified within the nursing profession on a general level include workload, low morale and dealing with death and dying as well as the global issues of economic and corporate restraints which seem to have become the hallmarks of working within the National Health Service (NHS) today (Tyler & Ellison, 1994).

Within the paediatric SCT speciality, these general stressors are compounded by those specific to this speciality and include working with children who may be both acutely and chronically sick and coping with rapid advances in technology and treatments available (Molassiotis & Van der Akker, 1995). Nurses must also deal with children who may face death not simply as a result of their condition, but paradoxically may die due to the very treatment given in an attempt to save their life (Kelly *et al.*, 2000). Patenaude *et al.* (1979) summarise the stressors faced by SCT nurses as:

- uncertainty regarding the benefits and outcomes of the treatment;
- intensity of the emotional involvement with families and patients;
- ethical dilemmas surrounding SCT;
- interpersonal relationships and communication between staff and, in some cases, families.

Furthermore, children undergoing SCT often spend long periods of time on a unit which may be very distant from home. This, coupled with stringent isolation and visting restrictions, can result in families being separated for months at a time. Consequently, the usual support networks offered by extended families are often temporarily replaced by members of nursing staff. While this may be both positive and therapeutic for both parties, it can be particularly stressful to the nurse as families form intense relationships in which the professional boundaries become blurred and this may contribute to the risk of burnout in staff (Kelly *et al.*, 2000).

Formation of such intense relationships may lead to the loss of professional boundaries, in which each party is unsure of their role (Ruston *et al.*, 1996; Ford & Turner, 2001). Over-involvement by the nurse may lead to advocacy giving way to paternalism. The nurse may lose sight of the need to involve the parents in the decision-making process, and in an attempt to protect the family, make decisions or offer opinions on their behalf. In some situations, this may occur without the family's consent or knowledge. Such situations are

Cancer in Children and Young People   Edited by Faith Gibson and Louise Soanes
© 2008 John Wiley & Sons, Ltd

dangerous for all involved. The parents become disempowered in the care of their own child and the nurse takes on a role that cannot be maintained (Hawes, 2005). Over-involvement occurs slowly and is often a two-way process between the parents and nurse. Indications for such involvement include the refusal of parents to allow nurses other than the 'favoured' nurse to undertake care of the child, exceptions to ground rules being demanded from or granted to parents, nurses coming in when off duty to care for the child and the formation of an exaggerated sense of responsibility towards the child's care (Ruston et al., 1996).

Strategies to avoid such situations include a unit culture that is open and honest with both the family and the staff involved. This includes advocating the belief encompassed in the partnership model (Casey & Mobbs, 1988; Coyne, 1995) that families are autonomous and the child's prime advocate. In situations of stress, such as SCT, the parents need to be supported by nurses who recognise their responsibilities and can fulfil their role within a partnership, demonstrated in the nurse's readiness to negotiate care and their ability to involve the parents in the decision-making process (McKinnon & Schlucter, 2004). The ability of nurses to reflect upon their actions and to identify situations where their professional role may be under threat by over-involvement is also an essential aspect of therapeutic boundary setting in SCT.

Patient care issues related to such complexities as the decision to withdraw from active treatment are one of the most stressful areas of HSCT nursing. End-of-life decisions are not uncommon and issues such as quality of life and benefit versus risk often provoke a degree of conflict between individuals and between professional groups (Forte, 1997; Bowman, 2000). Personal values of individual practitioners are complicated by an ever-changing workforce creating an atmosphere where moral conflict is high (Bowman, 2000). Yet, in an era characterised by a multidisciplinary approach, it becomes vital that difficult decisions should be appropriately negotiated and rigorously inter-professional. Only then can conflict become transformed into meaningful discussion and collaboration to provide morally justifiable and sensitive care (Woolridge and Burrows, 1999; Masri et al., 2000).

Ethical decision-making in particular seems to lie primarily within the medical rather than nursing domain (McAlpine et al., 1997; Ferrand et al, 2003). A nurse's lack of involvement in ethical decisions or conflict with medical judgements regarding aggressive or experimental interventions translates into high levels of emotional and moral distress causing both occupational and personal stress (Molassiotis & Van der Aker, 1995; Vogel Smith, 1996). This is because nurses are forced to act upon decisions they find morally unacceptable (Oberle & Hughes, 2000; Goodman, 2003) or they feel powerless to translate moral choices into actions, therby incurring high levels of guilt. Within the SCT field this guilt can become particularly potent as nursing staff administering drugs can often feel culpable for the numerous physical side effects caused by transplant treatments.

Interpersonal staff conflicts on transplant units have been identified as one of the main sources of occupational stress within SCT (Molassiotis & van der Akker, 1995). As with the partnership between parent and nurse, similar partnerships are needed between members of the multidisciplinary team with each group of health-care professionals recognising that they are an expert not the expert, and respecting their boundaries of professional responsibility. More collaboration between the professions requires better awareness and understanding of the ethical diffficulties faced by the other. This becomes even more important in the modern-day health-care system where roles and responsibilities between nurses and doctors are becoming increasingly blurred (Melia, 2004). While the benefits of increased collaboration and communication between the professions would clearly improve levels of job satisfaction and decrease emotional distress, there is clearly an overriding benefit to be gained for the child and family when difficult moral decisions need to be made.

Educational needs of nurses in blood and bone marrow transplant units

Lack of knowledge may initiate feelings of insecurity and incompetence, and is compounded by the few textbooks available on the subject of paediatric SCT. Nurses caring for the child and family are required to be effective in their care and for this to happen, specialist education is required. Though education alone cannot create expert SCT practitioners, Benner (1983) notes that skilled nursing requires a sound educational base. The outcome of offering such a foundation means quicker skill acquisition and safer practice.

Specialist paediatric SCT courses are offered by some nurse education institutions throughout the UK. Such courses allow nurses 'time out' from the busy ward environment giving them a valuable opportunity for reflection. The work of Benner (1983) and Schön (1991) identifies the use of structured reflection as a vehicle for nurses to rediscover and explore their practice and enable them to identify what makes the nurse effective (Benner & Wrubel, 1989). Such courses also give nurses time to network with other national centres. Networking allows practitioners to examine and benchmark best practices within the field, leading to care that is consistent and cohesive between different units. Finally, the application of nursing theories and examination of relevant research involved in these courses can enhance the nursing knowledge of both inexperienced and experienced practitioners. Stem cell transplant units need nurses capable of offering multifaceted and holistic care required by children and their families. This level of care is only achievable through rigorous evidence-based practice that is relevant to the needs of the child and family.

While theoretical knowledge is evidently of paramount importance to become an effective practitioner within the SCT setting, the practical knowledge required is also vital. This ranges from the small everyday issues of routines and practices within individual units to the larger issues of advances in science and technology.

Newly appointed staff to a SCT unit are confronted by an overwhelming sea of new practices and terminology, and even staff experienced within the speciality may have to deal with rapid changes in practice. The nurse may consequently find they change from proficient practitioner or even expert to novice overnight. The period of novice may be short-lived as previously learnt coping mechanisms come into play, but even the temporary loss of role can give rise to stress (Benner, 1984) and access to appropriate support and education becomes paramount.

It is well established that new members of staff benefit from a period of preceptorship for a negotiated period of time in order to adapt to a new clinical area (United Kingdom Central Council for Nursing, Midwifery and Health Visiting [UKCC, now referred to as the Nursing and Midwifery Council], 1994). This may then be extended to formal clinical supervision benefiting staff in both their professional and personal development (Butterworth & Faugier, 1992). However, it is clear that although a preceptorship period is vital to support a new nurse in SCT, both newly qualified nurses and more experienced staff also benefit from some sort of clinical support role such as a practice educator or clinical facilitator (Wilkins & Ellis, 2004; Lambert & Glacken, 2005). The presence of an experienced member of staff who is supernumerary can support the team through direct bedside education of skills such as IV therapy. Furthermore, she/he can take over patient care for a member of staff for a period of time allowing them some valuable time out to pursue areas of interest such as shadowing clinical nurse specialists or visiting relevant clinics. This not only enhances their basic knowledge, but also gives staff a degree of respite from a busy and stressful ward environment. Clearly, clinical support must also extend to student nurses who often require high levels of supervision within any high-dependency area. Once again, the presence of a designated clinical support nurse can enhance the student's experience, thereby promoting a positive recruitment and retention message.

References

Benner P (1983) 'Uncovering the knowledge embedded in clinical practice' *The Journal of Nursing Scholarship* 15(2): 36–41

Benner P & Wrubel J (1989) *The Primacy of Caring, Stress and Coping in Health and Illness.* Reading, MA: Addison-Wesley

Bowman K (2000) 'Palliative care in the intensive care unit' *Journal of Palliative Care* 16: 17–23

Butterworth T & Faugier J (1992) *Clinical Supervision and Mentorship in Nursing.* London: Chapman & Hall

Casey A & Mobbs S (1988) 'Partnership in practice' *Nursing Times* 84(44): 67–68

Coyne I (1995) 'Parental participation in care' *Journal of Advanced Nursing* 21(4): 716–722

Ferrand E, Lemaire F, Regnier B, Kuteifan K, Badet M, Asfar P, Jamer S, Chagnon J, Renault A, Robert R, Pochard F, Herve C, Brun-Buisson C & Dulvaldestin F (2003) 'Discrepancies between perceptions by physicians and nursing staff of intensive care end-of-life decisions' *American Journal of Respiratory and Critical Care Medicine* 167: 1310–1315

Ford K & Turner D (2001) 'Stories seldom told: paediatric nurses' experiences of caring for hospitalised children with special needs and their families' *Journal of Advanced Nursing* 33(3): 288–295

Forte P (1997) 'The high cost of conflict' *Nursing Economics* 15(3): 119–123

Goodman B (2003) 'Mrs B and legal competence: examining the role of nurses in difficult ethico-legal decision-making' *Nursing and Critical Care* 8(2): 78–83

Hawes R (2005) 'Therapeutic relationships with children and their families' *Paediatric Nursing* 17(6): 15–18

Kelly D, Ross S, Gray B & Smith P (2000) 'Death, dying and emotional labour: problematic dimensions of the bone marrow transplant nursing role?' *Journal of Advanced Nursing* 32(4): 952–960

Lambert V & Glacken M (2005) 'Clinical education facilitators: a literature review' *Journal of Clinical Nursing* 14(6): 664–673

Masri C, Farrell C, Lacroix J, Rocker G & Shemie S (2000) 'Decision-making and end-of-life care in critically ill children' *Journal of Palliative Care* 16: 45–54

McAlpine H, Kristjanson L & Poroch D (1997) 'Developing and testing of the ethical reasoning tool (ERT): an instrument to measure the ethical reasoning of nurses' *Journal of Advanced Nursing* 25(6): 1151–1161

McKinnon DD & Schlucter J (2004) 'Parent and nurse partnership model for teaching therapeutic relationships' *Pediatric Nursing* 30(5): 418–420

Molassiotis A & Van der Akker T (1995) 'Psychological stress in nursing and medical staff on bone marrow transplant units' *Bone Marrow Transplant* 15 (3): 449–454

Oberle K & Hughes D (2000) 'Doctors' and nurses' perceptions of ethical problems in end-of-life decisions' *Journal of Advanced Nursing* 33(6): 707–715

Patenaude A, Szymanski S & Rappeport J (1979) 'Psychological costs of bone marrow transplantation in children' *American Journal of Orthopsychiatry* 49(3): 409–422

Ruston C, McEnhill M & Armstrong L (1996) 'Establishing therapeutic boundaries as patient advocates' *Pediatric Nursing* 22(3): 185–189

Schön DA (1983) *The Reflective Practitioner*. Aldershot: Avebury

Tyler PA & Ellison RN (1994) 'Sources of stress and psychological well being in high dependency nursing' *Journal of Advanced Nursing* 19(3): 469–476

United Kingdom Central Council for Nursing, Midwifery and Health Visiting (1994) *The Future of Professional Practice: The Council's Standards for Education and Practice Following Registration*. London: UKCC

Vogel Smith K (1996) 'Ethical decision-making by staff nurses' *Nursing Ethics* 3(1): 17–24

Wilkins AM & Ellis G (2004) 'Enhancing learning environments by maximising support to mentors' *Nursing Times* 100(26): 36–38

Woolridge M & Burrows D (1999) 'Withdrawing treatment in the ITU: staff opinions of the decision-making process' *Nursing in Critical Care* 4(6): 286–293

14 Further Developments in Stem Cell Transplantation

Nikki Bennett-Rees, Sian Hopkins,
Lesley Henderson and Jinhua Xu-Bayford

Gene therapy

Gene therapy is a new treatment option currently undergoing clinical trials at designated centres worldwide. Initially conceived as treatment for hereditary single gene defects, the first human gene therapy studies were conducted on patients with ADA deficient severe combined immuno-deficiency (ADA-SCID) in the early 1990s (Blaese et al., 1995; Bordignon et al., 1995; Kohn et al., 1995; Fischer et al., 1997). Most recent studies in X-linked severe combined immunodeficiency (SCID-X1), ADA-SCID and X-linked chronic granulomatous disease (CGD) have shown that haematopoietic stem cell gene therapy can offer an excellent immune system and clinical recovery (Cavazzana-Calvo et al., 2000; Gaspar et al., 2004; Pott et al., 2006). In some children, the use of low intensity preconditioning, coupled with gene therapy as used for ADA-SCID and X-CGD, offers considerable hope for many other haematological and immunological disorders.

What is gene therapy?

Gene therapy involves replacing a defective gene with a functional, normal gene using recombinant DNA technology. This functional gene then provides the correct enzyme or protein, consequently eliminating the underlying cause of the disease. Or sometimes gene therapy can be used to add a new property to a cell, for example, to make it sensitive to a drug. There are several approaches to gene therapy:

- a normal gene is inserted into a non-specific location of genome;
- an abnormal gene is replaced with a normal gene through homologous recombination;
- an abnormal gene is repaired through selective reverse mutation which returns the gene to its normal function;
- the regulation of a gene can be altered by turning it on/off.

Cancer in Children and Young People   Edited by Faith Gibson and Louise Soanes
© 2008 John Wiley & Sons, Ltd

Gene therapy prospects for primary immunodeficiencies

Primary immunodeficiencies (PID) are a group of disorders in which inherited genetic defects compromise the child's immunity (Fischer 2004). PID disorders have the potential to be corrected by gene therapy because of their defined molecular defects. The development of gene therapy has been driven by established complications, long-term side effects and mortality following conventional allogeneic stem cell transplantation, particularly in the HLA-mismatched setting. Recently, several studies have shown that gene therapy can have major beneficial therapeutic effects. However, as with any new treatment the potential for toxicity needs to be anticipated. In recent years the genetic basis of almost three-quarters of all PID has been established. The most severe forms of PID are known as severe combined immunodeficiency (SCID), in which T lymphocyte development is compromised. Affected infants often become seriously unwell in the first few months of life with opportunistic infections, chronic diarrhoea and failure to thrive. Without treatment, most of these babies will die in the first year of life. X-linked or SCID-X1 accounts for 50 % of all SCID cases and occurs in approximately 1 in 50–100,000 live births. Haematopoeitic stem cell (HSC) transplantation offers a high survival rate if a well-matched donor is available (Buckley *et al.*, 1999; Antoine *et al.*, 2003). However, for the majority of children, this is not the case, and survival from mismatched family transplants is significantly lower and associated with more complications. This is due to the toxicity arising from the administration of chemotherapy to achieve adequate engraftment.

What does the gene therapy process involve for the child?

In general, gene therapy is an option when a suitable well-matched donor is not available, but there are differences between the various conditions.

The current entry criteria into the gene therapy trial for patients with SCID are:

- confirmed diagnosis of SCID-X1/ADA-SCID;
- genetic defect identified;
- no matched sibling, matched family or fully matched unrelated donor;
- ethical approval from GTAC (the Gene Therapy Advisory Committee).

The basic principle of gene therapy is to introduce a working gene into bone marrow cells by using viruses. These viruses have been specially engineered to remove the diseased parts in the laboratory, so that they are unable to grow and infect other people. They simply carry the new gene into cells, and are often called 'vectors' for this reason.

For the child, gene therapy is a relatively straightforward procedure which involves taking bone marrow from the affected child, and then, under GMP laboratory conditions, manipulating and correcting these cells in cell cultures. The treated cells (sometimes called transduced cells) are returned a few days later by transfusion into the child via a central venous catheter. As in SCT these new stem cells find their way to the bone marrow spaces where they start to produce healthy immune cells. This is known as somatic gene therapy (Figure 14.1) as altered genetic material is only present in the child's own immune system and cannot be passed on to offspring.

Nursing care for the child and family undergoing gene therapy

Gene therapy remains a largely experimental and innovative treatment. It is currently undergoing clinical trials in children with primary immunodeficiencies. At present, only one hospital within the UK is treating children using this form of therapy. However, because it is such a rapidly expanding field, the expertise in caring for these children will develop, to allow more individualised care pathways (i.e to nurse in full or semi-isolation) to be developed. Children with ADA-SCID or CGD are nursed in hospital (in the same way as a child post-allogeneic SCT) for approximately four to six weeks. But the infant with X-linked SCID will only be in hospital for four days, however, on discharge home he will continue to be cared for in semi-isolation.

Gene Therapy

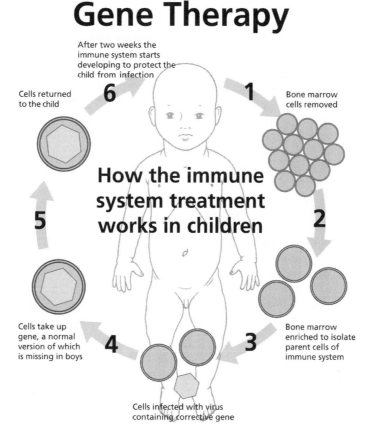

After two weeks the immune system starts developing to protect the child from infection

6

1

Bone marrow cells removed

Cells returned to the child

How the immune system treatment works in children

5

2

Cells take up gene, a normal version of which is missing in boys

4

3

Bone marrow enriched to isolate parent cells of immune system

Cells infected with virus containing corrective gene

Figure 14.1   Gene therapy.

Physical preparation of the child

The physical preparation of the child undergoing gene therapy is the same as for the child undergoing allogeneic HSCT. This includes all the initial tissue typing to eliminate any potential sibling donor. Psychological preparation may be limited due to the child's young age. However, the child might well benefit from an assessment with either the unit occupational therapist or physiotherapist, which will help determine if the child is reaching his milestones, or if he needs some extra input to achieve normal development. In addition, an assessment with the play therapist will enable suitable toys or activities to be used in order to enable the child to progress with his expected developmental skills.

Preparation of the family

Preparation of the family begins once a diagnosis of ADA or X-linked SCID has been established. The child, any full siblings and parents will be tissue-typed. If there are no fully matched siblings, an unrelated donor search will be put in place. During the time it takes to establish any potential unrelated donor, the medical team will approach GTAC (the Gene Therapy Advisory Committee, which is the regulatory authority for gene therapy clinical trials) to seek approval for gene therapy. If the child is accepted onto the trial programme, the parents will have a joint meeting with both a consultant in immunology who is involved with gene therapy, and a consultant in paediatric SCT. During this meeting both aspects of treatment, i.e.

gene therapy and conventional SCT, are discussed with the parents and this information is followed up with relevant written information. In addition, the internet can provide a wealth of information about gene therapy. This information helps parents to have a greater understanding of both gene therapy, and conventional SCT, and enables them to formulate questions to bring to hospital consultations. If the parents' choice is for their child to proceed to gene therapy, they will have an appointment with an independent counsellor to ensure they fully understand the process of gene therapy. The counsellors are medical professionals who are neither involved in the clinical trials, nor work in the centre undertaking gene therapy. Anecdotal discussion with some parents whose child has undergone gene therapy highlighted some of the areas which helped them to decide which treatment option was right for them as:

- percentage of survival following gene therapy is higher than following a matched unrelated SCT;
- fear of chemotherapy;
- fertility issues for the child;
- shorter hospitalisation with gene therapy;
- safer treatment option, at least in the short term.

As this is such a new treatment option there is no available data on fertility or endocrine function for children undergoing gene therapy. Clearly it may take many years for such information to be collated, that may also feature in parents' decision-making.

Once the decision to proceed to gene therapy has been confirmed, and the child is clinically stable and free of infections, the admission to the unit will be determined by the following:

- availability of the vector to attach the gene;
- laboratory resources to prepare the cells;
- theatre space for the child to have a bone marrow harvest;
- availability of a bed on the appropriate unit.

While waiting for admission, the child will continue with his physical work-up, along with the parents meeting staff who will help them prepare for their admission and on-going care of their child (Table 14.1). It is vital that the parents know and understand about the care their child will need

Table 14.1 General preparation of families for gene therapy

For non-conditioned gene therapy
Hickman® line insertion
Hickman® line dressing
Hospitalisation and isolation

For conditioned gene therapy
Hickman® line insertion
Hickman® line dressing
Back-up bone marrow harvest
Hospitalisation and isolation
Nausea and vomiting
Naso-gastric tube
Mouth care
Hair loss
Finger pricks

to enable them to participate in as much of their child's care as they feel able to do.

Care of the child undergoing gene therapy for X-linked SCID

The child with SCID-X1 undergoing gene therapy is usually between 6–12 months old, thriving and free of infection. The inpatient stay is minimal and much of the care is at home ensuring the child is kept infection-free and able to continue achieving his milestones within a recognised timeframe. A typical hospital care pathway is:

- Sunday – Admit to the ward in a specialist centre.
- Monday – To theatre for insertion of a Hickman® line and bone marrow harvest.
- Monday/Tuesday – Discharge home if well.
- Friday – Readmit for infusion of transduced cells.
- Saturday – Discharge home.

The cell volume to be infused is generally between 60–100 mls and can be infused over 30–45 minutes using a blood-giving set. There should be no need to give any 'pre-medication' prior to infusing the cells, but it would be wise to have prescribed oral paracetamol, IV chlorphenanine and IV hydrocortisone in the event that the child has a reaction. The ongoing care for this child, once discharged, is shared between the hospital undertaking the gene therapy and the shared care hospital and community nursing team. Initially the child will be seen weekly by the gene therapy unit progressing to every two, then three, weeks as his immunity begins to improve. Regardless of whether the child is in hospital or at home they will need to be cared for in semi-isolation until they have adequate immune reconstitution (Table 14.2). Once the child's CD4 count is greater than 300, all prophylactic medication, apart from oral penicillin and IV immunoglobulin, can stop. Similar to children having SCT, the penicillin will probably be a lifelong medication.

Table 14.2   Immune reconstitution post gene therapy

4–6 weeks, natural killer (NK) cells start recovering
12 weeks, T-cells start recovering
6 months, CD4 count should be greater than 300

Care of the child undergoing gene therapy for ADA-SCID or CGD

For children diagnosed with either ADA-SCID or CGD, the process is different due to the fact that they receive Chemotherapy conditioning (for example, IV melphalan) to help engraftment of the transduced cells. Prior to gene therapy the children with ADA-SCID have a weekly IM injection of PEG ADA, often for many months. The PEG ADA improves the child's immune function, and it is this immunity that needs to be removed by giving IV melphalan. In the case of the child with CGD, it is the diseased neutrophils which need to be removed with the IV melphalan. As part of the child's physical work-up a back-up bone marrow harvest will be taken approximately six weeks pre-gene therapy. In the future it is hoped that there will be no need to store the child's marrow, but as gene therapy remains an experimental treatment, for those children who have melphalan conditioning, it is a precaution in the event that the child fails to recover his own cells.

From admission to the unit for gene therapy, until discharge, the child will be an inpatient for aproximately six weeks, and nursed in an isolation room in the same way as the child post SCT.

A typical care pathway for a child having melphalan conditioning is:

- Sunday – Admit to the ward in a specialist centre
- Monday – Bone marrow harvest
- Tuesday – Rest day
- Wednesday – IV melphalan
- Friday – Reinfuse transduced cells.

As so few children have had this therapy, the nursing care of the child until count recovery has been based on the care given to children having autologous PBSCs. Clearly the melphalan will cause a degree of side effects similar to, but generally less severe than, those seen in children following high dose therapy and autologous rescue for solid tumours (Table 14.3).

Table 14.3   Side effects seen post-melphalan conditioned gene therapy

Nausea and vomiting, resulting in weight loss
Mucositis, affecting mouth and gut
Neutropenia, with the potential for life-threatening infections
Potential pancytopenia, requiring red cell and platelet
   transfusions
Hair loss

Given these side effects, the nursing/medical care will revolve around keeping the child infection-free, pain-free and well nourished. Should the child require any blood product support, cells will need to be irradiated and of the appropriate CMV status. Generally blood counts are low for up to eight days post-infusion of cells and recovery occurs between 2-4 weeks post melphalan.

For the child with ADA-SCID, prophylactic medication stops when the CD4 count is greater than 300, which in some cases may take up to two years. In CGD, the appearance of gene-corrected cells may occur within three to four weeks. For the child with CGD, prophylactic medication will continue until it is judged that immune reconstitution is adequate. Children with CGD often have aspergillus, and it is unknown how long post immune reconstitution that the child needs to continue anti-fungal therapy.

Parental support

As numbers of children within the UK undergoing gene therapy remain small, much of the support parents receive has been from other parents who have been through the same treatment. While the unit multidisciplinary team offers information and support, parents often feel that a greater understanding and family-based support comes from other parents living through the same treatments and experiencing isolation. In the years to come as treatment with gene therapy expands, maybe to include other diseases, support networks will no doubt grow. As medical and nursing staff learn what the future holds for these children, our ability to support parents and help them face any potential late effects will be to the same level of expertise as the support and care given to those families and children undergoing HSCT.

Risks and side effects of gene therapy

Of a total of 38 children (21 SCID-X1 patients, 11 ADA-SCID patients and 6 X-CGD patients) treated to date in Europe, three SCID-X1 patients developed T cell lymphoproliferative disease about three years after the gene therapy. Two of these children have been treated and are in remission, and one child died from a leukaemic relapse.

The development of leukaemia as a result of gene therapy associated insertional mutagenesis has raised concerns regarding the toxicity of retroviral vector-based gene delivery. These side effects are now being studied in detail and measures to prevent such events through alternative vectors are being developed. Even so, somatic gene therapy has produced remarkable therapeutic effects. This, in turn, offers considerable hope for the treatment of many inherited immunological and haematological disorders. It is therefore likely to encourage rapid progress in terms of technological development and clinical efficacy. The use of any new therapy, including gene therapy, ultimately depends on the balance of risks against those of alternative treatments. New strategies to overcome toxicity issues are likely to establish gene therapy as an effective treatment regimen for many forms of PID. The balancing of clinical risk and benefit is illustrated in Figure 14.2.

As in all types of treatments, especially experimental therapy, long-term follow-up of patients is vital. The information gained will provide a more accurate assessment of the benefits of gene therapy over alternative approaches such as allogeneic stem cell transplantation.

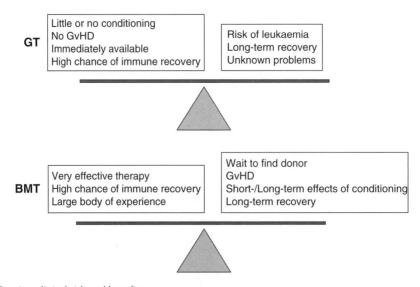

Figure 14.2   Balancing clinical risk and benefits.

The future

Stem cell transplantation is characterised by rapid developments in treatment and drug therapies so it is difficult to predict what new innovations will appear in the next few years. However, while gene therapy has exposed the speciality to a completely new technology, it is unlikely to fully replace the 'traditional' transplant techniques. Clinicians have an obligation to reduce the toxicity endured during the transplant experience and this includes several unresolved issues such as:

- What is the optimal conditioning regimen?
- What is the optimal cell dose to be infused?
- What is the optimal GVHD prophylaxis? (Kletzel, 2004)
- What other diseases may gene therapy be successful in treating?

Some of these issues remain largely within the medical domain. However, nursing research is beginning to address the 'lived experience' of stem cell transplantation for both the child and the family in an attempt to minimise the negative impact that transplant often carries. For example:

- treatment of latent and refractory emesis;
- establishing optimal diet restrictions and nutritional support;
- establishing optimal protective isolation and hygiene techniques;
- examining the issue of post-traumatic stress disorder in transplant families;
- examining what families experience and the effect this has on family dynamics.

There is no doubt that rigorous research is required to address these and other nursing issues. Furthermore, it is imperative that better collaboration is established between national and international transplant centres to establish care that is both consistent and of the highest standard.

References

Antoine C, Muller S, Cant A *et al.* (2003) 'Long-term survival and transplantation of haemopoietic stem cells for immunodeficiencies: report of the European experience 1968–99' *Lancet 361*(9357): 553–560

Blaese RM, Culver KW & Miller AD *et al.* (1995) 'T lymphocyte-directed gene therapy for ADA-SCID: initial trial results after 4 years' *Science 270*(5235): 475–480

Bordignon C, Notarangelo LD, Noble N *et al.* (1995) 'Gene therapy in peripheral blood lymphocytes and bone marrow for ADA-immunodeficient patients' *Science 270*(5235): 470–475

Buckley RH, Schiff SE, Schiff RI *et al.* (1999) 'Hematopoietic stem-cell transplantation for the treatment of severe combined immunodeficiency' *New England Journal of Medicine 340*(7): 508–516

Cavazzana-Calvo M, Hacein-Bey S & de Saint BG (2000) 'Gene therapy of human severe combined immunodeficiency (SCID)-X1 disease' *Science 288*(5466): 669–672

Fischer A, Cavazzana-Calvo M, de Saint BG *et al.* (1997) 'Naturally occurring primary deficiencies of the immune system' *Annual Review of Immunology 15*: 93–124

Gaspar HB, Parsley KL, Howe S *et al.* (2004) 'Gene therapy of X-linked severe combined immunodeficiency by use of a pseudotyped gamma retroviral vector' *The Lancet 364*(9452): 2181–2187

Kletzel M (2004) 'Immune ablative (mini) transplants in pediatrics' *in*: Mehta P (ed.) *Pediatric Stem Cell Transplantation.* Boston: Jones & Bartlett, pp. 319–335

Kohn DB, Weinberg KI, Nolta JA *et al.* (1995) 'Engraftment of gene-modified umbilical cord blood cells in neonates with adenosine deaminase deficiency' *Nature Medicine* (10): 1017–1023

Pott MG, Schmidt M, Schwarzwaelder K, Stein S, Siler U, *et al.* (2006) 'Correction of X-linked chronic granulomatous disease by gene therapy, augmented by insertional activation of MDS1-EVI1, PRDM16 or SETBP1' *Nature Medicine 12*(4): 401–409

Part 3

Surgery

Commentary

General Surgery

Charlie Rogers

Introduction

The role of surgery within the field of paediatric oncology has changed from being the only treatment available for children with solid tumours to being an integral part of the child's total treatment plan. Chapter 15 gives a very thorough description of how this has occurred and how surgery now fits alongside chemotherapy and radiotherapy as a treatment for childhood cancer.

This commentary identifies how the information presented may help the paediatric oncology nurse in his or her day-to-day practice under the following headings: diagnosis, continuity of care, pain and central venous access. It aims to highlight where practice may differ from that described by the author and to encourage readers to take up the challenge of changing and developing practice when necessary, in order to provide a high standard of care for their paediatric oncology patients undergoing surgery.

Diagnosis

The period of diagnosis is particularly stressful for the child and family. For the parents, there is uncertainty about what is wrong with their child and what the future might hold. The child who is

undergoing investigations and sometimes painful procedures may be distressed and frightened by what is happening to him. This chapter is very helpful in that it informs the nurse of the reasons for and the significance of the biopsy and investigations involved in making a cancer diagnosis. This information can help the nurse prepare the child and family prior to any procedures by explaining exactly what is going to happen. It is also useful as a reference for others involved in this process, such as the play specialist. Such specific information can help the nurse answer the child's/family's questions, thus helping to reduce any fear of the unknown. In practice, the doctor usually informs the parents about the investigations their child is to undergo, but does not always have the time to explain everything in detail.

The more the nurse can understand what the child and family are experiencing around the time of diagnosis, where often the prognosis is also addressed, the more they can support them through this stage.

Continuity of care

As outlined by the author, a further time when the child/family require specific psychological preparation is prior to the planned surgery for the

Cancer in Children and Young People   Edited by Faith Gibson and Louise Soanes
© 2008 John Wiley & Sons, Ltd

excision of the tumour. Very often, this occurs on a different ward, or even within a different hospital, where the environment will be unfamiliar to the child and family.

The author emphasises the importance of good communication between the oncology and surgical specialities in order to maintain continuity of care and, for the family, confidence in both caring teams. In practice, the doctors liaise with their surgical colleagues as it is one identified consultant talking to another. It is more of a challenge for nurses, however, due to the many different nurses from both specialities involved in caring for the child. To aid the communication between the nursing teams, it may be helpful to have an identified nurse from each team to meet and discuss any specific nursing or psychosocial issues prior to surgery. Making time to address an individual patient's concerns/issues can help to provide a smooth transition from the paediatric oncology unit to the surgical ward.

From a practical viewpoint, for the paediatric oncology nurse working on a very busy unit, it may prove difficult finding the time to link up with the named surgical nurse. It may be more appropriate for the key worker, as identified by national guidance in the UK (National Institute of Health and Clinical Excellence, 2005), to make this link. The key worker has the responsibility of liaising with the different care teams involved in the treatment of the child with cancer and this is likely to be undertaken by the Paediatric Oncology Outreach Nurse Specialist (POONS) although this will vary between paediatric oncology centres. The key worker could also accompany the child/family to any outpatient consultations with the surgeon, thus enabling them to know what information has been given and answer any questions as necessary.

When addressing the psychological care of the child/family prior to and during surgery, the author describes how interventions such as role play and relaxation techniques can help the child cope with this stage of treatment. It is also important to address any anxiety the child/family may experience as a result of being cared for in an unfamiliar environment. Some families may only have experience of the paediatric oncology unit and be anxious about such issues as having to adjust to unfamiliar nursing and medical staff, being looked after by nurses not experienced in paediatric oncol-

ogy or having to abide by different ward 'rules'. Ways of reducing this anxiety include showing the child and family around the surgical ward prior to admission, introducing them to different staff members and ensuring they understand the ward 'rules' and the reasons for them. Talking to surgical nursing colleagues about the child's diagnosis and experiences can help them to understand what the child and family are going through and identify their individual needs.

A further challenge for the paediatric oncology nurse is to help explain to the child/family what the surgery involves and what they are likely to experience. Chapter 15 provides detailed information about post-operative nursing care and potential complications resulting from the different types of surgery, which is a useful reference when seeking detailed information. The information about specialist surgery and related nursing care is also helpful for children's surgical nurses who are inexperienced in caring for children undergoing surgery for cancer.

Pain

The importance of accurately assessing a child's pain and providing effective pain relief can never be underestimated. The author provides a detailed account of what needs to be addressed when assessing a child's pain and emphasises the importance of discussing pain management options with the child and family prior to surgery in order to help allay any fears or misconceptions and identify individual patient needs. This section encourages the reader to think about their own practice and to look at how they could improve the way they assess and treat the pain experienced by each child they look after, who is undergoing surgery or a painful procedure.

In relation to pain assessment tools, there are several reliable and valid tools available to assist the nurse in identifying the child's pain experience (Twycross et al., 1998). It is not the type of tool which is crucial, however. What is crucial is that the tool chosen is used consistently and effectively by the nurses caring for the child, as part of the overall pain assessment, and that pain management strategies are then altered accordingly so that any pain experienced is relieved.

The role of parents in assessing the child's pain can be questioned. The author states that parents have a vital role in interpreting the child's experience as they know their child best. This is very often the case, but for some parents they may be too stressed to make an accurate assessment or may have little experience of seeing their child in pain (Eland, 1985). It is important therefore, for the nurse to be aware of this and work with the parents to ascertain how much they would like or feel able to be involved in their child's pain assessment. It is also important to discuss openly with parents what they feel about their child's pain and to give them the opportunity to discuss their concerns. Effective communication is vital in this situation.

The author emphasises the importance of having a children's pain management team to support the clinical areas in delivering safe and effective pain management. This can be seen as the gold standard, yet many hospitals do not have this service. The challenge, therefore, is for nurses to look at what resources are available in their area and to use these to deliver safe and effective pain management for all children undergoing surgery for cancer.

Central venous access

Chapter 15 gives an excellent description of the two different types of central line in common use, the external catheter and the implantable port, and the differences between them. This is helpful for nurses unfamiliar with central lines as, with this knowledge, they are in a position to explain about central lines to the child and family, thus helping them to make an informed choice.

The author highlights the importance of involving the child and family in deciding which type of central line the child will have. This is supported by McInally (2005) and Sanderson (2004). In practice, it can be questioned whether families are really given all the information and the time to make an informed choice. Once a diagnosis has been made, the medical consultant may be keen to get a central line in to start treatment and he or she may not be in a position to explore the different options available with the family. The challenge for nurses is to work with the medical staff to ensure that each family is given the time and the oppor-

tunity to discuss which type of line would be most appropriate for their child.

It is important to acknowledge that resource implications may also influence the type of central line a child receives. For example, a centre may only be allowed to use Hickman® lines because they are cheaper to purchase than Portacaths®. However, as described by the author, there is some clinical evidence that the risks of infection are greater in external catheters than in ports and so the additional cost of treating these infections in a Hickman® line may actually outweigh the extra cost of the port. Thus in the long run, a Portacath® may work out cheaper. The challenge for nurses is to have the evidence to support this and to take this evidence to their Trust/hospital in order to ensure that Portacaths®, as well as Hickman® lines, are available for their patients, thus allowing them a choice.

A further challenge for nurses is to provide continuity of care when caring for a central line. As the author points out, in the absence of national guidance, robust local policies must be developed to standardise all aspects of central line care, to avoid variations in practice that can be confusing to patients. It would be fairly straightforward to develop guidelines for one area, such as the paediatric oncology centre (POC), where everyone does the same and the child and family know what to expect. What is more challenging is when the child goes back to their Paediatric Oncology Shared Care Unit (POSCU) and their central line is treated in a different way. As long as the care is safe, lack of continuity may not be a problem. However, it may cause increased anxiety for the family to see their child's central line being cared for in different ways, especially if they care for the line themselves and have been shown different techniques. National guidance is needed to overcome these potential problems.

In relation to complications of central lines, the author focuses on infection and clot formation. In practice, for a minority of children the complications they develop as a result of having a central line outweigh the benefits of the line itself. For example, a child who persistently develops clots within their line may require anticoagulation therapy such as daily, subcutaneous, low molecular weight, Heparin injections which they may find very distressing. It is important for the nurse to be aware of this and realistic about potential complications. How often do we hear a doctor saying to the child 'once you have this line, there will be no more needles', and then the child ends up with daily subcutaneous injections? The challenge, when preparing a child and family for the insertion of a central line, is to inform them of the advantages of the line but also of the potential complications, thus giving them a realistic view.

Conclusion

This chapter gives us plenty of food for thought about the physical and psychological care needed by children with cancer undergoing surgery and how best to provide this care. It gives us a challenge for the future, which is to continue to improve collaboration between the surgical specialists, both medical and nursing, and the paediatric oncology multi-disciplinary team to ensure continuity of care for the patient and family throughout the whole cancer treatment trajectory.

References

Eland J (1985) 'The child who is hurting' *Seminars in Oncology Nursing* 1: 116–122

McInally W (2005) 'Whose line is it anyway? Management of central venous catheters in children' *Paediatric Nursing* 17(5): 14–18

National Institute for Health and Clinical Excellence (NICE) (2005) *Improving Outcomes in Children and Young People with Cancer.* London: NICE

Sanderson L (2004) 'The experience of children with a central venous catheter' in Gibson F, Soanes L & Sepion B (eds) *Perspectives in Paediatric Oncology Nursing.* London: Whurr Publishers Limited, pp. 283–310

Twycross A, Moriarty A & Betts T (1998) *Paediatric Pain Management: A Multi-disciplinary Approach.* Abingdon: Radcliffe Medical Press Limited, pp. 56–76

15 General Surgery

Rachel Hollis, Sharon Denton and Gill Chapman

Introduction

Up until the early years of the twentieth century, and before the advent, first, of radiotherapy and then of chemotherapy, surgery was the only treatment available to children with solid tumours. Complete, radical surgical excision of a malignant tumour held the only chance of cure. This was only possible in the early stages of localised disease, when a tumour could easily be detected and readily accessed by the surgeon. Mortality rates at surgery were high and cure rates very low, only around 5 % in Wilms' tumour, for example, today one of paediatric oncology's greatest success stories.

The history of the treatment of Wilms' tumour (or nephroblastoma) illustrates the changing and developing role of surgery in the treatment of the solid tumours of childhood. Tumours of the kidney were first described in medical literature in the early nineteenth century. There was a steadily growing recognition that a variety of differently described renal tumours was actually a single entity, nephroblastoma, and this was brought together in a definitive review by Max Wilms in 1899, of a tumour which continues to bear his name. The first nephrectomy carried out on a child with a renal tumour was performed by Mr Jessop at the General Infirmary at

Leeds in 1877. Excision, with a high surgical mortality, remained the only treatment available until 1915, when for the first time radiotherapy was given after surgical excision.

Radiotherapy developed alongside improved surgical techniques and in the 1940s survival rates reached around 20 %. Chemotherapy was first used in the 1950s, with single-agent dactinomycin (actinomycin-D), followed by the addition of vincristine. By the late 1960s a combination of surgery, post-operative radiotherapy and adjuvant chemotherapy had pushed survival rates to nearly 40 %. As successive clinical trials continued to refine treatment, and explore the use of different combination treatments, survival rates steadily improved, and five-year survival today is around 80 % (Thoms, 2004). The treatment of Wilms' tumour can be seen as a model for the development of multimodality therapy in childhood malignancy as surgery became seen as one arm of treatment, to be used in association with radiotherapy and chemotherapy.

As national and international clinical trials began to look at the treatment of childhood cancer in a more coordinated way, it became apparent that paediatric tumours generally demonstrated a better response to radiotherapy and chemotherapy than did adult malignancies. The role of

Cancer in Children and Young People Edited by Faith Gibson and Louise Soanes
© 2008 John Wiley & Sons, Ltd

surgery has changed in response to these developments. When used in isolation, the primary aim of surgery had always been complete resection of a solid tumour. Part of the cost of those cure rates has been, in some cases, major and mutilating surgery, resulting in either loss of function, or major cosmetic insult, sometimes both. As radiotherapy techniques have changed and as multi-agent chemotherapy protocols have proved effective across a range of diseases, the role of surgery has developed and become more defined. Advances in paediatric surgical techniques and the increasing expertise of the specialist surgeon, alongside developments in paediatric anaesthesia have played their part in improving cure rates and decreasing morbidity in many forms of childhood malignancy. In the field of general surgery there have been moves to minimise the late sequelae of surgical interventions without jeopardising the hope of further improving cure rates. The question in surgery has changed from 'Can it be removed?' to 'When should it be removed?' and even 'Should it be removed at all?' Resection of the primary tumour is often still required, but the timing of that resection is frequently delayed, for example, in hepatic tumours, neuroblastoma, Wilms' tumour and soft tissue sarcomas. The preservation of organ function has become an important principle, while maintaining the primary need for disease control (Weiner, 1999).

One of the most important developments in the treatment of childhood cancer has been the increased referral of children to specialist cancer centres (Stiller, 1994). The paediatric surgeons working in these centres have therefore been able to develop expertise in their surgical management which has contributed to decreased surgical morbidity. It has also meant the greater integration of the surgeon into the wider multidisciplinary team caring for children, young people and their families. One of the greatest lessons of the recent past is the importance of the multidisciplinary approach from the earliest days of diagnosis (Mott et al., 1997). The collaborative working practices of the surgeon, the oncologist, the radiologist, pathologist, and other scientific staff alongside the wider multidisciplinary team are fundamental to the delivery of optimal treatment programmes and paediatric surgery has developed several distinctive roles which will be further explored below.

The challenge of surgical care in paediatric oncology

The place of surgery in paediatric oncology has moved from an isolated, often heroic, intervention to an increasingly integrated part of the overall management of children with cancer. This can sometimes lead to difficulties for nurses and families when the paediatric oncology patient requires a specific surgical intervention. The increasing specialisation of children's nurses is leading them to develop skills, knowledge and clinical expertise in particular areas. Paediatric oncology and paediatric surgery are two specialities in their own right and it is rare to have nurses whose skills bridge the two. Children will often move, therefore, between the paediatric oncology ward and the surgical ward. There are particular challenges here for the nursing teams operating in these two distinct, frequently geographically distant, settings. Communication between teams and individuals caring for these children is of vital importance in maintaining continuity of care and, for the family, confidence in both caring teams (Callahan & De la Cruz, 2004).

Some children will initially be referred to the paediatric surgeon, either because there is no suspicion of cancer, or because the child presents with a number of differential diagnoses, resulting from a distended abdomen, for example. As the likelihood grows that the child has some form of malignancy, some families may find it difficult to be on a ward where many children will be undergoing relatively straightforward surgical procedures. They will begin to look for further information and support from the oncology team. It is at this stage that good liaison is critical to ensure that the child and the family receive appropriate and consistent information as the process of diagnosis and staging continues. At some point it will probably be appropriate for the child to be transferred to the oncology ward and this move should be negotiated with the family, who may react in a variety of ways. For some, it will give the opportunity to be in an environment with other families in the same position, where they perceive the expertise to be in treating their child. For others, however, it may be difficult to leave an area where they have made relationships with staff and found support. It may also mean confronting the reality of their child's diagnosis. Denial is a natural element of many people's reaction, and being on an 'ordinary' ward can reinforce that particular coping mechanism. Moving on to the oncology ward can be hard for some families and it may sometimes be appropriate to delay that move until the family is ready for it.

The move from an oncology unit to a surgical ward is likely to take place at a later stage in the child's illness, at the time of primary tumour surgery. The issues involved in this transfer of care will be further outlined below. However and whenever the change in clinical setting occurs, the most important factor for the child and the family will be good, consistent communication between them and the wider multidisciplinary team as surgical interventions play their part along the patient pathway.

Surgery as a diagnostic tool

In most paediatric solid tumours, tissue analysis is of critical importance, not just in confirming the pathological diagnosis but also in gaining further biological information which may indicate the potential behaviour of the disease. This information is increasingly used to modify or intensify treatment according to a particular child's prognosis. The role of the surgeon is vital in providing the pathologist with the best possible material in order to arrive at the most accurate diagnosis, so that the child may receive optimum treatment. Tissue diagnosis is a critical component of the preliminary 'work-up' of a child with a solid tumour, and should be integrated with other investigations. The child and family will be subjected to a range of procedures, the aim of which is to determine the nature of the disease (diagnosis) and evaluate its spread (staging). Careful planning of the investigations and appropriate preparation of the child and family require the cooperation and expertise of all members of the multidisciplinary team (Pinkerton et al., 1994). The importance of early referral of the child to a specialist centre cannot be overemphasised and at this stage can help to prevent unnecessary or repeated investigations.

On first presentation of a child with a suspected solid tumour, a considerable amount of information can be gained without invasive procedures, through accurate history-taking and careful clinical examination. Determining whether a mass is palpable, if it is painful, whether it is mobile, if it has grown quickly or been there for some time and whether there are enlarged lymph nodes, can give early indications of a differential diagnosis. Blood pressure may be raised in a child with an abdominal mass indicating either a Wilms' tumour or neuroblastoma. Phaeochromocytoma can also produce an elevated blood pressure, but this is rare in children. Pallor and bruising may indicate disease in the bone marrow and this would point towards a diagnosis of neuroblastoma, particularly where the characteristic periorbital bruising is evident.

Moving on from clinical examination, biological tumour markers may help to further the process of diagnosis. These markers are tumour-associated compounds found in either the serum or the urine of children with particular malignancies. Examples are the excretion of urinary catecholamines and their metabolites in neuroblastoma, Alpha-fetoprotein (AFP) in the blood of children with hepatoblastoma, and AFP or beta-human chorionic gonadotrophin hormone (β hCG) in germ cell tumours. Such markers are of clinical significance at the time of diagnosis and can also be used in the evaluation of response to therapy. They may assist in the detection of minimal residual disease following apparent complete resection. In follow-up, the presence of a raised tumour marker may indicate tumour recurrence before this can be detected clinically.

The information obtained from a child's history and clinical examination will be used to determine the need for further radiological investigation, and guide the most appropriate imaging techniques. The growth and development of medical imaging in the past 25 years have provided a range of methodologies on which to call. There is now a technique for most clinical problems and the challenge for the clinician, in consultation with the radiologist, is to identify the type of imaging suited to a particular tumour, both at diagnosis and for subsequent follow-up. Plain X-ray films retain their importance, especially in the detection of tumours of the chest and bone, but have been superseded in many respects by more sophisticated technologies. Ultrasound is of particular importance in the assessment of abdominal tumours, and high resolution scanning is required in order to obtain comprehensive information on which to base diagnosis. Computerised tomography (CT scanning) and magnetic resonance imaging (MRI) have both played an increasing role in the documentation of the extent of the primary tumour and the accurate assessment of tumour response (Pinkerton *et al.*, 1994). MRI scanning is particularly useful where there is soft tissue involvement, and also prevents additional unnecessary radiation. CT and MRI scans are used predominantly in the evaluation of primary tumours, although they are also used to detect metastases, most notably chest metastases by CT scanning. In tumours that metastasise to bone, technetium bone scans are widely used to detect bony lesions. The use of radioisotopes has increased the quality of the information available to the clinician looking at the extent of disease. Within paediatric oncology, the use of isotope scanning has been particularly important in neuroblastoma. Metaiodobenzylguanidine (mIBG) is a compound taken up by tumours of the central nervous system, and so is a useful imaging agent in neuroblastoma (and phaeochromocytoma) where, labelled with radioactive isotopes, it has been shown to be effective in assessing the extent of disease and sometimes in locating the primary tumour.

The new technique of Positron Emission Topography (PET scanning) has yet to be fully evaluated in children. In the UK it is now being used in the follow-up of chlidren with Hodgkin's disease and in some difficult to evaluate non-Hodgkin's lymphoma.

Scans and imaging provide a great deal of information about the nature and spread of a tumour and the interpretation of such information is both an art and a science in its own right. The radiologist is an important member of the multidisciplinary team in the planning and interpretation of these investigations. Some of the imaging procedures outlined above, in particular CT and MRI scanning, involve complex, frightening, sometimes noisy machinery, and require children to keep still for considerable lengths of time. For small children, this often means sedation and general anaesthetic. Input from play specialists in the form of preparation and distraction can help to reduce the requirement for such interventions. If scans are carried out under general anaesthetic other staging investigations, such as bone marrow aspiration and trephines, or lumbar puncture, should be

carried out at the same time. If appropriate facilities and personnel are available, tumour biopsy can sometimes be performed under that one anaesthetic.

In most types of solid tumour the definitive diagnosis is usually made on tissue biopsy from the primary tumour site. Even where diagnosis is almost certain on the basis of positive tumour markers and primary tumour imaging (as may sometimes be the case, for example, in neuroblastoma), biopsy will still be required. The accuracy of diagnosis in childhood cancer is of critical importance and can be difficult to make in some paediatric tumours, which may be poorly differentiated and require sophisticated analysis to arrive at a positive identification (Parkes *et al.*, 1997). It is recognised that the more information there is available on the identification of a disease and the nature of a paediatric tumour, the more specific and effective treatment can be. It is not just the broad diagnosis, for example, Wilms' tumour, which is required, but more specific information regarding the molecular and genetic make-up of the cells involved which can help the pathologist and the scientists to identify more clearly the nature of that particular tumour, in that particular child. Within Wilms' tumour, for example, it is necessary to distinguish between favourable histology and unfavourable histology (Mitchell *et al.*, 2000). In rhabdomyosarcoma, the embryonal variant has a far better prognosis than the alveolar type. In neuroblastoma, the amplification of the oncogene N-myc is particularly useful as an indicator of poor prognosis and other significant biological features are increasingly being recognised (Brown, 2001).

In order to obtain all the information required about a tumour, a range of tests will be needed. Histology and immunochemistry can generally be carried out on fixed samples, but there is an increasing requirement for fresh tissue for cytogenetic and other biological studies. Many of the specialist techniques needed for the diagnosis of tumours in children require specimens to be handled and prepared in a particular manner. Where fresh biopsy samples are required by the pathologist and scientist, it is self-evident that there must be close collaboration with the surgeon carrying out the biopsy to ensure they are collected. It is important to make sure that the quality of the biopsy and the material gained are adequate for all the tests required in any particular tumour type. It is equally important that the technique used to carry out the biopsy is as safe as possible and appropriate to the child's clinical condition. There has been some disagreement among surgeons and oncologists on the most appropriate type of biopsy in certain paediatric solid tumours. The Surgical Group of the United Kingdom Childhood Cancer Study Group (UKCCSG), parent organisation of today's Children's Cancer and Leukaemia Group (CCLG) attempted to define a consensus on the principles of tumour biopsy (UKCCSG, 1996). This paper makes the point that the primary role at biopsy is to make a diagnosis as a basis for individual patient treatment, but that biological research studies and the storage of tissue for future studies are also important in furthering the understanding of the tumours of childhood and adolescence, so contributing to developments in treatment. When taking additional samples for current and future research, parents and patients must always be informed of the purpose of all tissue which is to be taken, and give explicit consent for the storage of these samples (McIntosh *et al.*, 2000; Medical Research Council, 2001). The individual trial or study protocols for the treatment of particular tumours prescribe certain types of biopsy, which should be carried out following national or best practice national guidelines. The different options for biopsy are as follows:

- *No biopsy*: This may be appropriate for some germ cell tumours where a diagnosis can be made on tumour markers alone. In neuroblastoma, biopsy is preferred because of the importance of biological information, but occasionally the diagnosis will be clear from tumour markers, primary tumour imaging and bone marrow aspiration. If a child's clinical condition is such that a biopsy would carry undue risk, it is hard to justify this further intervention. In the case of some lymphomas, particularly where there is diffuse disease, examination of ascitic fluid or pleural effusion may produce sufficient cells for morphological analysis and immunophenotyping and so avoid the need for surgical procedures (Patte, 2004). The current European protocol for suspected localised Wilms' tumour allows initial chemotherapy to be given without histological confirmation, for fear of the biopsy rupturing

and spreading the tumour, although the recommendation for UK specialists is to carry out a needle-core biopsy. On rare occasions a mediastinal lymphoma may cause life-threatening obstruction and will require immediate therapy before a biopsy can be safely attempted.

- *Fine needle aspiration cytology (FNAC)*: In the UK. this is rarely used, as such biopsies are held to provide inadequate samples, and lead to difficulties in interpretation. In Europe, however, this technique is more widely employed as a less invasive intervention.

- *Wide needle core biopsy (e.g. Trucut, Temno)*: This is usually a multiple biopsy, ideally under radiological guidance using ultrasound or CT. It may be used in liver tumours, Wilms' tumours and other solid tumours. Increasingly a 'co-axial' technique is being used, where a single wide-bore needle is inserted into the tumour, through which a thinner needle-core biopsy needle can be repeatedly passed, to get multiple biopsies with only a single tumour capsular puncture.

- *Laporascopic/thoroscopic biopsy (needle or incisional)*: These specialised techniques require considerable clinical expertise, and may be used where an open, incisional surgical biopsy is thought to be too invasive. Often described as minimally invasive surgery (MIS), there is increasing evidence for the use of such techniques in children, particularly in the biopsy of intra-abdominal and thoracic lesions for tissue diagnosis (Spurbeck *et al.*, 2004).

- *Open incisional surgical biopsy ± needle cores*: This remains the biopsy of choice for most types of solid tumours in the UK as it is the least likely to lead to diagnostic problems caused by inadequate tissue samples. Certain considerations should, however, be borne in mind when planning such a biopsy. Skin incisions should be planned to allow the scar to be excised at the definitive resection. A deep narrow wedge is generally preferable to a wide, superficial biopsy and if the biopsy can include the interface of the tumour with adjacent normal tissue this is often helpful to the pathologist.

- *Complete resection*: This may be the only satisfactory biopsy in some germ cell tumours, certain cystic renal tumours, and ganglio-neuroblastoma.

All these biopsy techniques carry with them potential risk of complications: bleeding from the tumour, damage to adjacent organs, or the subsequent development of adhesions. Advocates of the techniques of minimally invasive surgery suggest that these risks are lessened by their use (Holcomb, 1999). Any form of biopsy is a form of rupture of the tumour and so brings the theoretical risk of local spread. The biopsy site should generally be placed where it can be excised at subsequent surgical resection. When identifying the type of biopsy to be carried out, the risks of the procedure should be taken into consideration and every attempt made to minimise distress to the child. It should also be remembered, however, that inadequate samples may lead to a delay in treatment and the need for repeat biopsies. The more accurate the information that can be gained on the nature of the tumour, the more closely treatment can be tailored to the need of the individual child. When preparing a child for biopsy, there are particular anaesthetic and surgical risks which should be identified and managed in order to minimise the risk of the complications of this procedure (Table 15.1).

Surgery as a treatment modality

For many of the solid tumours of childhood, surgery remains the definitive and in some cases still the only treatment in curing the disease. The timing and the nature of many surgical procedures have increasingly been refined with developments in chemotherapy and radiotherapy. In most solid tumours surgery is a part of a controlled clinical trial or study protocol which aims for the best chance of cure, while trying to minimise long-term effects of treatment, by preserving function and improving cosmetic effect. The primary objective in treating most solid tumours remains complete surgical resection and the completeness of removal of the primary tumour is held to be an important prognostic factor for many types of malignancy. The way in which this is attempted will vary widely, depending on the size, the location and the nature of the tumour. For some localised tumours, complete surgical excision remains the best and most satisfactory option. The greatest changes to surgical strategy have occurred in those tumours found to be sensitive to chemotherapy and, to

a lesser extent, radiotherapy. When these other treatment modalities were first introduced, surgery remained the first line of treatment. Tumours were removed where possible and first radiotherapy and then chemotherapy were used to try to prevent any recurrence of disease (adjuvant treatment). If a tumour could not be completely removed, as much as possible was resected (debulking). Radiotherapy and chemotherapy were then used to treat residual disease, with varying degrees of success. Current approaches to surgical management are generally more likely to involve pre-operative (neo-adjuvant) treatment with chemotherapy in order to shrink the tumour prior to resection.

Developments in chemotherapy have made it possible to reduce the size of many paediatric tumours, so facilitating complete tumour resection with decreased morbidity, and better likelihood of preserving organ function. Chemotherapy can also help to reduce local invasion by the tumour and so allow greater preservation of adjacent healthy tissue and less risk of damage to neighbouring organs. With a reduction in size, there is generally less risk of rupture of the tumour and because the blood flow to it is reduced, there is also less risk of haemorrhage. With the use of pre-operative chemotherapy, tumours that were unresectable at diagnosis will therefore frequently become so. In some cases, there will be such a good response to chemotherapy that the residual tumour becomes unable to be detected clinically or radiologically. In such cases surgery may still be necessary, as there may be residual macroscopic or microscopic disease apparent only through surgical exploration. It is important to define the extent of any remaining disease in order to plan subsequent treatment.

The timing of surgical intervention in the overall treatment of children with cancer remains the subject of much study, comparative work and some disagreement among oncologists and surgeons. The studies and clinical trials coordinated by the CCLG and on an international level by the International Society of Paediatric Oncology (SIOP), and other collaborative groups, include surgery as part of the overall management of children with particular diseases. In some of these studies one of the trial questions may be looking at the right time to attempt surgical excision of the primary tumour. The following is

Table 15.1 Risk factors prior to surgical tissue biopsy

Physiological parameters	Potential problems	Treatment options
Blood counts	Bone marrow suppression: • Anaemia • Thrombocytopenia • Neutropenia	Transfuse packed red cells if symptomatic, or at request of anaesthetist/surgeon Platelet transfusion if $< 50 \times 10^9$ Alert to risk of infection
Blood pressure	Hypertension due to • Neuroblastoma • Wilms' tumour Hypotension caused by hypovolaemia secondary to rupture of tumour	Antihypertensive agents Fluid resuscitation and packed cell transfusion
Renal function	Acute obstruction due to tumour Tumour lysis syndrome	Relieve pressure if possible (urinary catheter or nephrostomy) Manage tumour lysis according to unit protocols
Respiratory function	Compromised by large chest mass	Close monitoring of respiratory function Oxygen therapy as required Early review by intensive care team
Gastrointestinal function	Acute bowel obstruction caused by abdominal mass	Nil by mouth and nasogastric tube
Pain	Pressure from tumour	Analgesia as required

an outline of the role of surgery in the current management of the more common solid tumours of childhood and its relation to other treatment modalities. This will include a brief review of some ongoing studies and trials.

Wilms' tumour

Wilms' tumour, as outlined previously, has been one of the great success stories of paediatric oncology. It has been treated by the three major modalities of surgery, radiotherapy and chemotherapy, but the challenge remains; how to use them most effectively, how to continue to increase survival if possible, and how to reduce the effects of therapy on children with a good prognosis. Despite advances in chemotherapy, the surgical excision of Wilms' tumour is, and will almost certainly remain, the treatment of choice. However, there is considerable debate about the timing of surgery, particularly in relation to preoperative chemotherapy (Mitchell, 2004). Historically, the surgical treatment of Wilms' tumour has always been immediate nephrectomy unless the tumour

was either metastatic at presentation, spreading into the inferior vena cava and thus inoperable, or bilateral; this remains the approach in North America. European groups (through SIOP) have suggested benefits from pre-operative chemotherapy in reducing the size of the tumour, so that it becomes more resectable. As well as facilitating the surgical procedure, this approach may actually 'downstage' a child with Wilms' tumour, thus reducing the need for subsequent chemotherapy. The disadvantages of this approach are that during the pre-operative chemotherapy there is obviously less information about the tumour itself. The diagnosis may prove to be inaccurate, the histological features which predict tumour response may be unclear, and the local extent of spread is unknown.

In all situations, with or without pre-operative chemotherapy, a child with a Wilms' tumour will eventually come to surgical resection. This may be more complicated if there is intracaval tumour, where cardiac bypass procedures may be required, or by extensive bilateral tumour. There is a risk of renal failure following surgery for bilateral disease, and on rare occasions, a child may need dialysis, and subsequent kidney transplant. Because of the fact that occasionally Wilms' tumour can develop in the remaining kidney of a child who has already had one kidney removed for a Wilms' tumour, some European centres are evaluating conservative surgery. This entails removing all the tumour without removing all the kidney, even in unilateral tumours.

Soft tissue sarcomas

Soft tissue sarcomas are a heterogeneous group of tumours which arise from a number of different epithelial tissues (Carli *et al.*, 2004). The most common form of soft tissue sarcoma in childhood and adolescence is the rhabdomyosarcoma. Treatment strategies have been derived from multi-institutional clinical trials, on a national or international basis. These trials have resulted in more sophisticated use of radiotherapy, more effective chemotherapy, and have looked at ways of combining these modalities with surgery to maximise survival and reduce treatment-related side effects. The optimal timing and intensity of each phase of treatment must be planned to take into account the site of the primary tumour, its histology, and the potential late effects of treatment (Carli *et al.*, 2004).

Initial surgical excision should only be attempted if the tumour can be removed completely, safely and without mutilation. This is rarely possible, the main exception being in paratesticular tumours, which may be completely excised. In most cases, the initial surgical intervention will be a biopsy, with delayed surgical excision following shrinkage of the tumour by chemotherapy, and possibly radiotherapy. Chemotherapy is used both as treatment for possible systemic disease and to optimise local therapy, particularly with regard to organ conservation where possible, for example, in tumours of the bladder. The timing of delayed surgery is determined by response to treatment, and by the study design of particular treatment protocols and is obviously dependent on the location, the size and the extent of the tumour. Where resection is incomplete, or is not possible due to the site of the tumour, the child may go on to have further adjuvant treatment. Occasionally, the response to chemotherapy and radiotherapy may be inadequate to the extent that the child will require a mutilating procedure, such as amputation or pelvic exenteration, but such an outcome is increasingly unusual. Soft tissue sarcomas in different sites require variable methods of local control which can be summarised according to general principles (Table 15.2).

Table 15.2 Local control in soft tissue sarcomas

Site	Usual strategies of local disease control
Orbit	Primary chemotherapy
	Radiotherapy if incomplete response
	Surgery rare
Parameningeal – Head and neck	Primary chemotherapy
	Radiotherapy commonly used
	Surgery if considered resectable, complex techniques often required
Non- parameningeal – Head and neck	Primary chemotherapy
	Surgery if considered resectable, complex techniques often required
	Radiotherapy as 2nd line treatment
Bladder and prostate	Primary chemotherapy
	Surgery if considered resectable, may be mutilating
	Radiotherapy if unresectable or residual disease
Paratesticular	Immediate surgery
	Adjuvant chemotherapy
Limbs	Primary chemotherapy
	Occasionally immediate surgery, otherwise surgery for local control
	Radiotherapy if unresectable or residual disease

Advances in the pathological diagnosis of soft tissue sarcomas have identified a range of different sarcomas, such as the peripheral primitive neuroectodermal tumours, which respond in a similar way to rhabdomyosarcoma and are treated using the same strategies. Other types of rare soft tissue sarcoma are paediatric variants of adult tumours, for example, synovial sarcoma and fibrosarcoma. They are frequently less sensitive to chemotherapy and surgical management plays a more important role, with radiotherapy where resection is incomplete.

Neuroblastoma

Neuroblastoma is a malignant tumour derived from the sympathetic nervous system. It is the most common extracranial solid tumour in children, with a median age at presentation of 2 years old (Pearson & Pinkerton, 2004). Surgery is extremely important in the management of neuroblastoma, but the timing and strategy for resection are dependent on a number of factors, including the stage of the disease at presentation. There is now an internationally accepted International Neuroblastoma Staging System (INSS) which has been critical in allowing collaborative research and the comparison of studies and treatment trials in this particularly complex disease (Brodeur *et al.*, 1993):

1. Stage 1: Localised tumour with complete gross excision
2. Stage 2a: Localised tumour with incomplete gross excision
3. Stage 2b: Localised tumour with incomplete gross excision and ipsilateral nodal involvement (*on same side as tumour only*)
4. Stage 3: Localised unilateral tumour which is unresectable, or crosses the midline with or without regional lymph node involvement; or localised unilateral tumour with contralateral regional lymph node involvement (*other side from tumour*); or midline tumour with bilateral extension by infiltration or by lymph node involvement
5. Stage 4: Any primary tumour with dissemination to distant lymph nodes, bone, bone marrow, liver, skin and/or other organs

6. Stage 4S: (Infants under 1 year old only) Localised primary tumour with dissemination limited to skin, liver and/or bone marrow.

Classification and staging are further complicated in neuroblastoma by the increased understanding of the molecular pathology of this particular disease, which has led to a recognition of features which have an impact on the clinical outcome of treatment. In particular, amplification of the oncogene MYCN is recognised as being associated with a particularly poor outlook (Brown, 2001). There is growing international recognition of the need to develop a classification system that would employ molecular pathology in the further stratification of patients into more clearly defined risk groups (Pearson & Pinkerton, 2004). In neuroblastoma, above all there is a need to improve survival in the poor risk groups, and a recognition that there are patients who are over-treated, and perhaps some patients who do not actually require treatment at all.

Surgery remains the initial, and often the only, treatment for non-metastatic, resectable tumours (Stages 1 and 2). It is now generally accepted that this includes patients staged as 2b after surgery if the histology is good. The current large collaborative European Neuroblastoma Study uses surgery alone with most Stage 1 and 2 tumours. If Stage 2 patients have MYCN amplification, then they are treated on high-risk neuroblastoma protocols, which includes intensive chemotherapy (Pearson & Pinkerton, 2004).

The standard treatment for patients with Stage 3 disease is to have pre-operative chemotherapy to shrink the tumour enough to proceed to complete surgical excision. Recent studies suggest that complete surgical resection is in itself a good prognostic factor. It is suggested that in the future, patients with good prognosis Stage 3 disease in whom complete surgical resection is possible may have no other treatment. On the other hand, if patients in this group are found to have MYCN amplification, their treatment will be intensified by the use of high-risk protocols.

The outlook for children with Stage 4 disease, over the age of 1 year, remains poor. There is a common treatment strategy across a number of collaborative groups; initial chemotherapy is followed by attempted surgical excision of the primary tumour. Maximal surgical resction is the aim, as it appears that this might have prognostic significance. Surgery is followed by high dose chemotherapy with peripheral blood stem cell (PBSC) rescue. This is then usually followed by local irradiation, and in some cases a course of cis-retinoic acid to promote differentiation of the tumour (Pearson & Pinkerton, 2004).

Infants have a much better prognosis than older children, although the outcome in any individual child is hard to predict. In Stage 4S disease, some tumours will regress spontaneously, in others it will progress, and may require active treatment. The role for surgery is unproven, as localised tumours may require less aggressive treatment in infants than in children over the age of 1. One of the aims of current infant studies is to ensure that they do not receive unnessary treatment, including surgery, that is more dangerous to them than the tumour itself.

Liver tumours

Most primary liver tumours in children are malignant, the most common being hepatoblastoma, followed by hepatocellular carcinoma. The aim of surgical treatment is complete tumour resection, but this can be a high-risk procedure and less than 50 % of tumours are resectable at diagnosis (Shafford & Pritchard, 2004). The increased use of aggressive pre-operative chemotherapy regimens, usually containing cisplatin and doxorubicin, means that in over 70 % of children there is enough shrinkage or necrosis of the tumour to allow for complete resection (Reynolds, 1999). It should be noted that alongside developments in chemotherapy there have been technical advances in liver surgery which have helped to make resection an attainable goal in more cases (Vos, 1995). Resectability depends on the location of the tumour, and its vascular supply. The usual types of resection are right or left full or partial lobectomy. In children, the liver has a great capacity for regeneration, and in some cases a trisegmentectomy may be carried out, which takes out the left medial lobe, as well as all of the right lobe. Where is not a possibility, either because all four segments of the liver are affected, or if the tumour involves the hilum of the liver, complete tumour removal is only possible if liver transplantation is carried out. As results of liver transplant for malignancy have improved, this is increasingly considered as an option, carried out only in a quaternary treatment centre (Otte et al., 2004). Survival rates for children with hepatoblastoma treated by liver transplant have improved, and are now between 60 and 80 % (Shafford & Pritchard, 2004). In some centres, living related donors are used. The advantage of this procedure is that transplant can be scheduled to fit in with the chemotherapy regimen.

Germ cell tumours

Germ cell tumours originate in embryonic cell division and arise from the pluripotent germ cell population which in foetal life migrate from the yolk sac endoderm to the genital ridge where they populate the developing testis or ovary. The tumour may occur in the ovary or the testis, but may also be found in distant sites due to the aberrant migration of cells along the gonadal ridge, which, in the developing embryo, lies adjacent to the vertebral column. This explains why, in children, about two-thirds of tumours occur outside gonadal sites, most commonly in the sacrococcygeal area, in the retroperineum, the mediastinum, the neck and the pineal region of the brain (Mann, 2004). Germ cell tumours are classified according to the degree of differentiation of the cells that make up the tumour, and there is considerable difference in the treatment of the different types of tumour, which range from the well-differentiated teratoma, to the completely undifferentiated embryonal carcinoma (Mann, 2004). Malignant germ cell tumours in children develop in cells that show differentiation towards either the yolk sac, and these cells produce alpha-fetoprotein (AFP) or the placenta; these cells produce beta-human chorionic gonadotrophin (βhCG). These tumour markers are extremely useful in the initial diagnosis, and subsequent monitoring of disease.

Surgery has a clear role in the management of most of germ cell tumours (GCT), but only extracranial tumours will be considered here. When a GCT is suggested by initial investigation and imaging, a complete surgical excision is performed wherever that is possible; this should always preserve major organs in the first instance. If imaging suggests that complete excision is not possible, a biopsy should be carried out. Further treatment then depends on the histology, the site, and the stage. The broad principles of management are surgical resection for localised disease, chemotherapy for metastatic or residual disease and neoadjuvant chemotherapy with delayed surgical excision where tumours are initially unresectable (Rescorla, 1999). Within these broad principles are different considerations to take into account in the different types of tumour.

Testicular tumours are resected by inguinal orchidectomy, with high ligation of the spermatic cord. In most cases, surgical excision alone is likely to be curative, although the majority of tumours are malignant, mostly yolk sac tumours which produce AFP. Boys with malignant disease are therefore followed up closely after surgery, with monitoring of AFP. Those patients who develop raised AFP, or clinical evidence of residual disease, or relapse, are treated by chemotherapy, with excellent results.

Ovarian tumours make up about a third of GCTs in children, with a peak in early adolescence. Yolk sac tumours are more common and AFP is again a useful marker. In localised disease, unilateral salpingo-oophorectomy may be curative without the need for radiotherapy or chemotherapy. However, this is a tumour which responds well to chemotherapy, and where there is extensive disease, chemotherapy can be used to avoid the need for extensive surgery such as bilateral oophorectomy or hysterectomy.

Sacrococcygeal tumours make up 40% of all GCTs, and around half of these are present at birth, the majority of them benign mature or immature teratomas (Mann, 2004). High AFP levels in normal neonates means that this is a poor indicator of malignancy in this age group. Complete surgical resection is curative in most cases, although this may be difficult, as it must include removal of the coccyx, while avoiding damage to the lumbar sacral plexus. Complete excision of malignant teratomas is more difficult, and as these tumours are very responsive to chemotherapy, delayed surgical excision is preferred. Mediastinal germ cell tumours can be very bulky at presentation, possibly with significant respiratory compromise, in which case treatment is a matter of urgency. Measurement of serum markers, showing raised AFP or βhCG, may be enough evidence on which to make a diagnosis where an attempt at surgical excision, or even a biopsy, would carry too high a risk. Effective chemotherapy can shrink most of these tumours to a size where later surgical resection is possible.

Non-Hodgkin's lymphoma

The primary role for surgery in non-Hodgkin's lymphoma (NHL) is restricted to biopsy for tissue diagnosis, although this may be provided by bone marrow, ascitic fluid or pleural effusion cytology. NHL responds well to chemotherapy and there is therefore no role for initial debulking of abdominal disease, or attempted resection of the tumour, as happened in the past. Such intervention can cause unnecessary morbidity with no therapeutic effect (Patte, 2004).

Occasionally, T cell NHL can present with rapidly progressing upper airway obstruction, which may require an emergency tracheostomy. In general, however, this disease will respond so quickly to the initiation of treatment that such an invasive procedure will be unnecessary. Intestinal NHL may present with bowel obstruction either because of the mass itself, or because the mass has become the basis for an intussusception. Limited resection to relieve the obstruction may be appropriate, but radical surgery is not indicated, and biopsy alone followed by chemotherapy may suffice.

Following chemotherapy for B-cell NHL a residual mass may require excision, or at least a generous biopsy, in order to make a final determination of whether complete or partial remission has been achieved (Patte, 2004).

Retinoblastoma

Retinoblastoma is the most common eye tumour in children. It is a tumour of neuro-ectodermal origin which arises in retinal tissue. Its treatment depends on the extent of the tumour and is as conservative as possible, using increasingly sophisticated radiotherapy techniques and adjuvant chemotherapy.

The spread of disease at diagnosis is frequently so extensive that enucleation may be the only option (Doz *et al.*, 2004). Enucleation is a complex specialist intervention and requires careful subsequent management. The specialised techniques required in both radiotherapy and surgery require that retinoblastoma is managed in quarternary treatment centres with the required expertise and resources. By this centralisation children receive the expert care they require, and families receive appropriate support in dealing with surgery and its effects. When children require chemotherapy, however, this may be delivered more locally.

Surgical treatment of metastases

The most common site of metastases in paediatric solid tumours, both at presentation and at relapse, is the lung. If control of the primary tumour can be achieved, then surgical treatment of metastases may be attempted, and has produced good results. This is one of the areas where minimally invasive surgery, using thorascopic techniques, has been used successfully. It is suggested, however, that this technique should not be used in patients with metastatic osteosarcoma, as radiological imaging can underestimate the number of lesions present (Spurbeck *et al.*, 2004). In these patients open thoractomy should be the procedure of choice, and is still frequently used for other metastatic lesions. Bilateral metastases can either be removed in a single procedure, through a median sternotomy approach, or by staged lateral thoracotomies a few weeks apart. The risks of two procedures must be balanced against the risks of surgical trauma to both lungs occurring at the same time.

Preparing the child and the family for surgery

The child undergoing planned surgery for excision of a tumour requires both psychological and physical preparation. The change of clinical setting, to a surgical ward, which happens for many children and families requires careful management. The issue of pain assessment and control should also be addressed prior to surgery.

Psychological care of the child and the family

In the early stages after the child's diagnosis the parents may experience a sense of numbness and shock precipitated by the sight of their child appearing acutely ill. Information and advice given at this time may need to be repeated and emphasised regularly. When surgical intervention is required, discussions should be held with the family with both surgeon and the oncologist present where this is possible. A nurse should also be present to ensure continuity of information.

The importance of holistic care is now well recognised (Barnes, 2005). Throughout the child's stay, it is important to remember that they are part of a family unit and that care should include close family members. Parents should be encouraged to continue their role in care. Siblings should not be forgotten as their lives, too, will change dramatically. Everyday routines will be disrupted while their brother or sister may endure lengthy hospital stays, intensive treatment and the follow-up required. Siblings may feel insecure, and left out. They need particular care and attention from the time of diagnosis onwards.

Help from the play specialist should be sought early for the child, brothers and sisters (Dolan, 1993). They may be seen by the child as a non-threatening member of staff and the playroom thought of as a 'safe area' where only pleasant things happen. Age-appropriate play can be invaluable in preparation for surgery. Role play can help to prepare the child for surgery and the dressing-up box can include uniforms, oxygen masks, theatre hats, stethoscopes and much of the paraphernalia of surgery. Coping mechanisms can be introduced in the form of play, for example, using play dough to squeeze, or visual imagery during painful procedures. Relaxation techniques can be valuable for both the child and the family and there are many tapes, videos and CDs available for this purpose.

Despite recent research showing their value, very few hospitals have a dedicated unit for teenagers and young people, who may therefore be nursed on paediatric surgical wards (Smith, 2004). If possible, teenagers wanting privacy should be nursed in a single room, preferably with their own bathroom facilities.

Pain assessment and control

Pain assessment is pivotal to effective pain management. It facilitates diagnosis, directs the choice of which method(s) to employ and enables monitoring of the effectiveness of particular interventions (Finley & McGrath, 1998; World Health Organisation, 1998).

Wherever possible, pain assessment and management should be discussed during admission procedures. A pain history allows the nurse to gain insight into any previous experience of pain that the child may have encountered, including strategies that have or have not been previously effective. The history can also provide a behavioural baseline to assist in subsequent pain assessments and will identify words that the child and family may use for pain, e.g. poorly, ouch, hurt (Royal College of Nursing, 1999). This is an opportunity to discuss the various pain management options and should be supported by written information in the form of parent- or child-friendly leaflets. This may allay fears and misconceptions that the child and family may have regarding pain management and provide information to support the child's and family's ability to give informed consent.

Pain is a subjective phenomenon; assessment tools can interpret the subjective experience of pain into objective, meaningful measures. An appropriate assessment tool should be chosen by the child, family and nurse by taking into account the child's developmental stage and ability to use it. The child's pain experience can be communicated using this tool to allow for assessment of pain and evaluation of management strategies. Where the child is unable to verbalise their pain, behavioural observational tools can be used. Recent studies have produced tools suitable for use with children with special needs (Twycross et al., 1999). Parents have a vital role in interpreting the child's pain experience as they know their child best and alongside the nurse's experience this can help to translate the child's self-report into a meaningful assessment. The Royal College of Nursing (1999) has developed clinical guidelines on the recognition and assessment of acute pain in children; these guidelines provide recommendations of evidence-based strategies to support assessment. *The National Service Framework for Children, Young People and Maternity Services: Standard for Hospital Services published by the Department of Health* (DoH, 2003) describes the minimum standard that providers of hospital-based care for children in the UK should employ when addressing chidren's pain management.

Alongside the expected surgery, there may be times where the child is subjected to painful events, e.g. venepuncture or drain removal, therefore planning is important to minimise pain occurring around these events. The pain of venepuncture can be managed by use of surface anaesthetics, e.g. EMLA® (eutectic mixture of local anaesthetics: prilocaine and lignocaine) or tetracaine 4% gel.

Entonox® (50% nitrous oxide and 50% oxygen) is an inhaled gas that can provide immediate and effective analgesia, which may be useful for short planned procedures such as drain or catheter removal (Finley, 2001; Duff & Bliss, 2005). Entonox® is usually self-adminstered via a demand valve, allowing the child to individually regulate their own analgesia. Entonox® can promote the child's sense of control, which can have a positive effect on their coping abilities (Hodgkins & Lander, 1997). The effects of Entonox® are short-lasting, therefore it is important to also administer appropriate analgesia prior to commencing the procedure, in order to manage any post-procedural pain or discomfort. In the surgical setting pain management techniques are often dictated by the surgery that the child is to undergo, so that oral analgesia may be appropriate for a minor procedure such as insertion of an indwelling central venous device, whereas major surgery, such as tumour resection, requires more complex management techniques which may include epidural infusion or intravenous morphine infusion.

Epidural analgesia is achieved by the placement of a fine catheter in the epidural space, into which local anaesthetic, with or without opioids, is infused. The resultant band of analgesia over the wound provides excellent pain relief. Only specialist centres can support an epidural service, and not all patients will be offered post-operative epidural analgesia, due to specific contraindications.

Infusions of morphine are also effective in managing severe pain. The manner in which the infusion is delivered is dependent on the child and their developmental stage. If a child is receiving a continuous morphine infusion, regular assessment of the child's pain and condition should be made and the hourly rate adjusted accordingly, to provide adequate analgesia. Patient-controlled analgesia (PCA) means that the child can obtain a bolus dose from the syringe driver as they need it. Children as young as 5 years have been able to effectively use PCA; the child must be able to understand the concept and be physically able to use the demand button (Royal College of Paediatrics and Child Health [RCPCH], 1997). Patients who are unable to use PCA may be suitable for nurse-controlled analgesia (NCA); this is where the nurse provides bolus doses according to the child's need. With NCA the time between the availability of the bolus dose is extended, to address the subjectivity of the pain experience and reduce unwanted side effects such as over-sedation.

The child with cancer who is undergoing surgery may present with particularly complex needs. An individual pain management plan should be devised for each child taking into account any previous pain interventions and current pain medication, their current physiological status including the haematological picture and the type and site of surgery.

The aim of post-operative pain management is to provide 'child friendly, multimodal pre-emptive pain and symptom management for all' (Morton, 2001, p. 13). The analgesic ladder (WHO, 1998) provides a framework on which to base drug choice on pain severity, e.g. in mild pain paracetamol is appropriate as a drug of choice whereas in severe pain a strong opioid, plus paracetamol, and a non-steroidal anti-inflammatory drug such as ibuprofen would be a regimen of choice. Advances in local anaesthetic techniques such as infiltrations and nerve blocks, provide peri- and post-operative fields of analgesia, which can reduce the amount of systemic analgesia that a child may require (Wilson & Doyle, 1998). The analgesic ladder allows for a step-up and step-down approach to pharmaceutical pain management as directed by the child's pain, and their overall post-operative recovery. Some drugs such as paracetamol and certain non-steroidal anti-inflammatory drugs are commonly used in the surgical setting, whereas they may not be appropriate at other stages in the child's treatment. This needs to be carefully explained to the child and family with the rationale behind each situation, to prevent subsequent confusion and inappropriate medication.

Pain management is best provided by using a holistic approach, where a combination of pharmacological and non-pharmacological strategies are employed to improve the child's pain experience. Non-pharmacological interventions can be useful adjuvants in managing surgical pain and may include play, distraction, positioning and comfort measures, heat or cold therapy. Regular assessment of the child will enable the nurse to judge whether the interventions implemented to promote pain management are effective.

Every hospital providing children's surgical services should have in place a children's pain management team, whose role is to support the clinical areas in delivering safe and effective pain management and act as a resource to monitor and improve current approaches, through guideline development, standard setting, audit and research (RCPCH, 1997; Royal College of Anaesthetists, 2001).

Physical preparation of the child for a general anaesthetic

Surgical interventions in children with cancer pose a significant challenge to both the anaesthetist and the surgeon. The aim of pre-operative assessment, preparation and care is to ensure that the child is in the best possible physical condition to undergo both the anaesthetic and the surgical procedure.

The type of tumour and the consequences of therapy may both indicate particular requirements in anaesthetic care. For example, in the case of neuroblastoma, the tumour may secrete catecholamines which can cause a rise in blood pressure. Careful monitoring of blood pressure and the administration of antihypertensive agents may be necessary. In the case of phaeochromocytoma, sudden gross hypertension may cause cardiovascular collapse at the time of surgery. Tumours involving the airway, for example, nasopharyngeal rhabdomyosarcoma, have the potential to compromise the airway.

Bone marrow suppression, caused either by the disease or by cytotoxic drugs, can also cause problems for both the anaesthetist and the surgeon. For example, children may be thrombocytopenic, and so more prone to bleeding, or neutropenic, and more prone to post-operative infections. Some children may require blood or platelet transfusions prior to surgery. The medication required by the child with cancer can also alter anaesthetic management. Steroid therapy can lead to adrenosuppression and intravenous hydrocortisone may be necessary in the peri-operative and immediate post-operative period. Bleomycin, in the presence of oxygen therapy, can cause pulmonary fibrosis and may lead to respiratory failure. In such cases, minimum oxygen concentration must be administered to maintain oxygenation. Treatment with anthracyclines can cause cardiomyopathy and thus compromise cardiac function; this may require investigation prior to surgery. Other chemotherapy agents may cause renal toxicity, and urine and blood tests may be needed to establish the child's renal function, and identify any electrolyte abnormalities prior to undergoing the procedure, and consequent anaesthesia.

On admission to the surgical unit, the child will require similar preparation to that for any child requiring routine general surgery. Baseline observations of vital signs and pulse oximetry should be taken and an accurate height and weight recorded. Blood tests and other investigations as indicated above will be carried out and any required correction made.

In the pre-operative period, details will need to be given regarding fasting. Traditionally, patients used to fast from diet and fluids for a minimum of six hours. Research indicates that although food, including milk, should be avoided for six hours, clear fluids may be taken up to two hours pre-operatively (Bates, 1994; Ham, 2005). During the fasting period the continuation of mouth care should be encouraged. This maintains the child's comfort by keeping the mucosa moist and also serves to reduce the feeling of thirst.

The theatre team may provide an opportunity for the child and the family to visit the anaesthetic room and parts of the theatre suite. Information and reassurance given to the family pre-operatively can be of benefit in the post-operative period (Edwards, 1998). If it is likely that the child will require a period of time in the intensive care unit, then arrangements should be made for the family to visit this area, to meet the nursing staff and to familiarise themselves with this potentially frightening environment.

Parents or carers should be allowed to accompany their child to theatre and, if they wish, provision should be made for at least one of them to stay with the child in the anaesthetic room until they are asleep. Repeated general anaesthetics can lead to psychological problems due to fear and anxiety for the child. Pre-operative preparation is of paramount importance, as is a calm, efficient but welcoming environment in the anaesthetic room (Kain et al., 1998). Pre-medication is not routinely used in children, although it may be beneficial to administer oral midazolam to the extremely anxious child (Mitchell et al., 1997). If a tumour is enlarging, it may begin to occupy vital organ space and this may lead to a mediastinal shift, with chest tumours or splinting of the diaphragm with abdominal tumours. This may cause respiratory or cardiac compromise and in such cases the surgeon and anaesthetist may not have the luxury of time to ensure that the child is in optimum health prior to surgery, due to a developing emergency situation.

At the time of surgery, there are a number of complications that may arise and may lead to a need to modify a planned procedure. This may include rupture of major blood vessels requiring grafting or rupture of the tumour which may later lead to modification of the treatment regime. Parents should be kept informed of progress as far as possible, and thus it is important that they can be easily located if necessary. A prolonged anaesthetic may result in a longer stay in the recovery area, thus increasing the time the child is away from the ward. When the condition of the child allows, the parents should be allowed to stay in the recovery room with them until transfer is appropriate (Edwards, 1998; Melody, 1999). As the recovery room can be a frightening place for parents unfamiliar with this environment, it is helpful if they are given information about what they are likely to see when they visit their child post-operatively. Once the surgery is complete, it is important that the surgeon visits and provides a comprehensive description of the findings and the procedure.

Post-operative nursing care

Recent advances in surgery mean that children will often require high dependency care from nurses with advanced skills following surgical interventions. Specialised nursing care allows for a safe and full recovery from the anaesthetic and surgical procedure. During this post-operative period the care of the child progresses from a high level of nurse dependency to a greater emphasis on family-centred care which requires nursing support rather than management. Care should be tailored to meet the individual needs of the child and the family. There are general considerations which must be acknowledged to promote recovery (Table 15.3) and specific care is required following surgery to particular sites and tumour types.

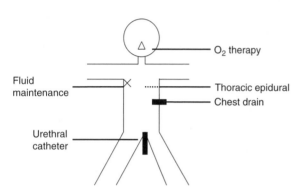

Figure 15.1 Chest surgery.

Surgery to the chest

Surgery to the chest (Figure 15.1) includes the resection of soft tissue sarcomas such as primitive neuroectodermal tumours (PNET) and chest metastases where thoracotomy is indicated. The main post-operative consideration with all chest surgery is to maximise effective respiration and oxygenation. In the immediate post-operative period, this may entail ventilatory support in the intensive care setting. Within 24 hours the child is usually transferred to the surgical ward.

Observations of respiration should include rate, depth, effort and pattern of chest expansion. Humidified oxygen therapy is administered as prescribed to maintain acceptable oxygen saturation levels. Any deterioration in condition can be measured by blood gas analysis. Chest drains are placed to empty the pleural space of air or fluid, the presence of which will prohibit full lung expansion (Brandt *et al.*, 1994). These should be managed according to local guidelines. Drainage of air, blood or fluid from the pleural space requires an air-tight system with gravity or application of low-flow suction. Chest drains should be observed for oscillation and/or swinging with respiration. Blockage of the system may occur due to kinking of the drainage tube or presence of blood clots. Any excessive blood loss should be replaced intra-

Table 15.3 Post-operative care considerations

Problem	Aim of care	Nursing care	Family involvement
Potential respiratory difficulty following general anaesthetic	Maintain adequate oxygenation	Maintain airway with appropriate positioning until fully conscious	Observation of conscious level
		Suction as necessary	
		Care of humidified oxygen therapy as prescribed	
		Monitor oxygen saturation	
		Observe colour, respiratory rate and effort	May be more aware of change in child's colour
		Report unequal chest expansion	
		Encourage early mobilisation and liaise with physiotherapist	Assist with mobilisation
		Administer intravenous antibiotics if prescribed	
Potential bleeding and hypovolaemic shock	Early detection and treatment to ensure haemodynamic stability	Record vital signs and report if not within acceptable parameters for age	Give reassurance regarding wounds, drains, etc

		Check peripheries for coolness and mottling. Aim for capillary refill in less than two seconds	
		Record wound drainage; report if excessive and/or fresh blood	Distract child from pulling drains
		Give colloids/blood/platelets as prescribed as per protocol. Note need for filters or pre-medication	
Pain due to surgery	Manage pain to enable comfort and rest	Care of chosen system according to local protocols, e.g. epidural, PCA, continuous morphine infusion	Help with assessment tools
		Assess pain score and act accordingly, noting effectiveness	Give comfort and support
		Ensure child is nursed in a comfortable position with drainage tubes, catheters, etc. placed safely	Provide personal things from home e.g. toys, blankets
		Promote a restful environment	Help with distraction and play
		Liaise with play specialists to provide distraction and relaxation	
		Consider complementary therapies	
Reduced oral intake due to GI disturbance and GA	Maintain hydration	Maintain nil orally until bowel sounds return as instructed by surgeon	Provide mouth care
		Care of IV infusion as prescribed	Encourage drinks, ice lollies when allowed
		Monitor fluid balance chart and report any significant imbalance	Do not drink in front of child when nil orally
		Aspirate naso-gastric tube one-four hourly, depending on drainage, and replace ml for ml with IV fluids as prescribed	
		Administer anti-emetic as prescribed	
		Monitor hypovolaemia/oedema	
		Monitor blood sugars if required	
Potential deterioration of renal function	Maintain adequate urine output	Record urine output, aiming for 0.5 ml/kg/hour	Encourage child to sit on potty/toilet
		Care of indwelling catheter. Ensure taped securely, not kinked, and observe for haematuria and clots	Help in changing nappies
		Assist with blood sampling for U&Es as requested	Can be taught catheter care
		Report if child has not passed urine 12 hours post-op	Give teenager privacy
		Observe for palpable bladder	
		Assist with standing/using commode	
Reduced oral intake	Provide adequate nutrition	Liaise with dietician regarding establishing NG feeds or need for TPN	Continue care of NG feed if familiar
		Maintain accurate weight	Give suggestions for favourite foods
		Encourage oral intake as appropriate	
		Daily urinalysis and bloods if on TPN	
Potential wound infection	Promote infection-free healing	Remove dressing after 24 hours if wound not visible	Provide comfort and support during dressing changes
		Complete wound assessment chart	Distract child from playing with dressings and touching wounds

Table 15.3 (Continued)

Problem	Aim of care	Nursing care	Family involvement
		Daily dressing to wound drains using aseptic technique	
		Observe wound for any inflammation and record temperature four-hourly	
		Obtain swab for culture if discharging	
		Administer prescribed antibiotics	
		Remove wound drains as instructed	
Reduced mobility	Maintain skin integrity	Perform pressure area care and change of position two-four hourly whilst in bed	Assist with washing, cleaning teeth, etc
		If epidural present, pay particular attention to heels and bottom	Provide cool, comfortable nightwear
		Ensure optimum pain relief to enable early mobility	Take child for walks using pushchair/wheelchair
		Use appropriate pressure-relieving aids and moving/handling equipment e.g. rope ladder, banana board, etc	
		Provide assistance with hygiene needs	
		Liaise with physiotherapist	
Boredom and anxiety	Provide reassurance and stimulation appropriate to age	Explain all procedures and provide as much choice as possible with certain aspects of care	Presence at bedside and involvement as desired
		Provide toys, games, books, music, etc	Arrange for close friends to visit
		Enlist help of play specialist, school teacher, and psychologist	Have access to telephone
		Maintain privacy for teenagers	Encourage periods of respite away from ward
		Consider relaxation techniques	

venously with colloid. The presence of a chest drain should not hinder early mobility. With careful handling and positioning of the underwater seal drain, i.e. below chest level to prevent backflow of fluid into the pleural space, the child should be encouraged to sit out of bed for short periods the day following surgery.

Thoracotomies are painful incisions, therefore effective pain management is essential. Thoracic epidurals with an opioid-local anaesthetic mixture offer very good pain relief (De Cosmo *et al.*, 2005) and should be maintained until drain removal (Ochroch & Gottschalk, 2005). Alternative analgesia methods may be employed such as a Patient Controlled Analgesia System (PCAS) or continuous opioid infusion in combination with regular oral analgesia. Chest physiotherapy is essential to prevent the development of respiratory tract infections. Physiotherapy will help the lungs to re-inflate effectively but should be planned to coincide with optimum pain relief. Any concerns over the chest should be addressed promptly with full chest examination, chest X-ray and administration of antibiotics as indicated. Removal of chest drains are performed as soon as the surgeon is satisfied the air leak has resolved, usually 2–3 days post-operatively if no complications have arisen. An occlusive dressing should be applied and observed for leakage. Repeat chest X-ray post-removal is indicated and observation of respiratory rate and effort documented until medical staff are satisfied that effective respiratory function has been re-established.

Surgery to the abdomen

This includes biopsy or resection of Wilms' tumour (Figure 15.2), neuroblastoma and hepatoblastoma (Figure 15.3). Providing the surgery is relatively complication-free, the post-operative recovery from a nephrectomy for Wilms' tumour can be surprisingly rapid. On return to the ward, hydration is maintained intravenously until the child's oral intake is sufficient. Oral fluids are usually allowed on the first post-operative day, followed by a light diet as tolerated. Accurate documentation of fluid balance is aided by the presence of a temporary urethral catheter which will be inserted during surgery. Kidney function should be monitored by daily blood urea and electrolyte analysis, noting any significant increase in urea and creatinine levels. Careful monitoring of blood pressure and the administration of any anti-hypertensive medication required should be continued.

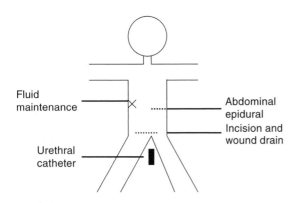

Figure 15.2   Wilms' tumour.

Epidural pain relief combined with oral analgesia is very effective for abdominal surgery. As with any surgery, regular observation of the wound should prevent, or at least, diagnose any infection quickly. Wound drains require daily aseptic dressings until removal. Every effort should be made to prevent the child from touching and removing the clean dressing. Dressings should be performed when pain relief is at an optimum level, the play specialist can be enlisted to provide distraction while this is performed.

Where bilateral nephrectomy is indicated, input from the nephrology team is sought early. Place-

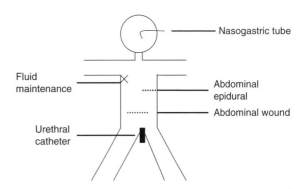

Figure 15.3   Neuroblastoma and hepatoblastoma.

ment of a peritoneal dialysis catheter can be performed at the end of surgery. It may be necessary for a permocath to be inserted if haemodialysis is required. The current recommendation for a child who has had bilateral nephrectomy for Wilms' tumour is to wait at least one to two years after completion of chemotherapy before renal transplantation (Kist-van Hothe *et al.*, 2005).

Resection of abdominal tumours can lead to a prolonged paralytic ileus. This may be exacerbated by chemotherapeutic agents such as vincristine and opiates such as morphine. The child will therefore return from theatre with a nasogastric tube to drain gastric contents until peristalsis returns. If drainage is excessive the surgeon may instruct that the amount is replaced accordingly by intravenous infusion. If the child was fed nasogastrically pre-operatively, this should be re-established as soon as possible. Liaison with the dietician will ensure that optimum nutrition is provided. If the paralytic ileus is prolonged and the child is unable to tolerate nutrition orally or via nasogastric feeds, this may indicate a need for total parenteral nutrition (TPN).

The site of the tumour may indicate the need for a stoma (either temporary or permanent). Appropriate advice from the stoma nurse should be sought pre-operatively. Correct placement of the stoma is essential if it is to be accepted by the child (Borkowski, 1998). A choice of appliances can be shown and basic care discussed at an early stage.

Depending on the extent of tumour involvement of the vascular system, there may be a need to graft major blood vessels during surgery. Post-operative monitoring should therefore include circulatory observations of the lower limbs. Colour and temperature of the feet and presence of pedal pulses should be recorded.

Where surgery has involved the liver, careful monitoring of clotting factors is required, with the possible need of parenteral replacement. Hypogly-caemia may also occur and so blood sugars should be closely monitored.

Surgery to the pelvis

Surgery to the pelvis (Figure 15.4) includes biopsy or resection of soft tissue sarcomas such as rhab-domyosarcoma and PNET, and germ cell tumours. It may involve the urinary tract and or the repro-ductive system. Urological nursing often involves caring for indwelling catheters (urethral or supra-pubic) and ureteric stents with external drainage. Bleeding is common and clots may lead to block-age of the drainage system. To maintain patency, stents and catheters may need to be flushed with 10–20mls of normal saline. Securing drainage tubes with tape helps to prevent dislodgement. Additional security is provided if the catheter has been sutured in place at the time of surgery. Frequently the catheter tip may irritate the blad-der mucosa, causing bladder spasm. This is very distressing for the child as it is difficult for them to localise the site of the discomfort. It can usually be controlled by the administration of an anti-cholinergic agent, most commonly oral oxybutynin (Thompson & Lauvetz, 1976). Other interventions such as the administration of intra-vesical local

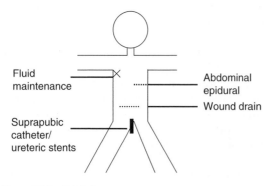

Figure 15.4 Pelvic tumours.

anaesthetics, and the use of muscle relaxants have been also been shown to be effective (Chiang *et al.*, 2005).

Removal of the drainage system is performed on the ward after appropriate analgesia has been given. Following catheter removal the child should be monitored until they are passing urine regu-larly and fluid balance is maintained. Extensive urinary surgery may necessitate the formation of a urinary stoma as will be discussed below.

Discharge planning

Discharge from hospital is planned in advance to enable a smooth transition from the surgical ward to the community or home. It may warrant a further change in the clinical setting by, for exam-ple, transfer back to the medical oncology ward. Close liaison between all parties should be encour-aged to ensure that timing for discharge is appro-priate and occurs when the child is deemed fit for discharge by parents, nursing staff, surgeons, oncologists, and the child concerned. The child and parents are given verbal advice on wound care, medication and return to activities such as contact sports and school. A contact number for advice and queries should also be given. An outpatient appointment will be made at a combined surgi-cal/medical oncology clinic, for follow-up assess-ment of the child. Paediatric oncology outreach nurse specialists have a vital role in ensuring a smooth transition from ward to home and a strong link between the two. They liaise with the surgical team before the child's discharge and coordinate community services. They may visit the family at home shortly after discharge, or offer telephone support.

Late effects of surgical treatment

Stoma formation

On rare occasions the surgical treatment for blad-der tumours is total cystectomy; this will mean that a urostomy or an ileal conduit will need to be formed. The psychological preparation of the child requiring stoma formation should begin as soon as the surgeon is aware that a cystectomy is the treatment of choice. Preparation includes clear and concise explanations about the care of the urostomy; it is helpful if the stoma specialist nurse is introduced at the earliest possible time (O'Connor, 2005). Extensive bowel resection may also result in stoma formation with similar principles of overall management and the need for good, early preparation where this is possible.

For a very young child or baby, explanation and teaching should be directed at the family members who will be performing the care. The older child, who has more awareness of body image, will require more direct involvement and counselling and may benefit from meeting another child with a stoma (Willis, 1998). After surgery, the programme of education about the care of the stoma continues, and dolls or teddies are often useful in demonstrating procedures. The stoma specialist nurse can offer support to the child and the family in grieving, and in coming to terms with the child's altered body image. Children should be encouraged to help with their stoma care as soon as is possible, as familiarity may help lead to a sense of normality.

Bladder neuropathy

Due to the effects of the tumour, surgery or treatment with chemotherapy or radiotherapy, the child may have a resultant bladder neuropathy. In the past, the treatment of choice was continuous urethral catheterisation. However, this has associated complications of urethral erosion, urinary infections and fears of leakage or disconnection and the embarrassment of wearing a catheter bag. In most case, intermittent self-catheterisation (ISC) is preferred over continuous catheterisation. ISC is performed throughout the day at regular intervals. The child (or carer) empties the bladder by the insertion of a catheter which is then immediately removed; they are taught to do so by nurses who have themselves undertaken specialised training. Videos and leaflets are available to reinforce the advice given by the nurse. The child is taught the anatomy of the urinary system and the nurse explains the procedure of ISC, including the care and supply of catheters and observes the child/carer perform ISC. A mirror is often helpful when identifying the urethral opening in girls (Winder, 1994). This programme of education

continues until the child/carer is able and confident to perform ISC on their own, thus leading to a greater sense of control over the process. ISC leads to a more normal pattern of bladder emptying and, as a result, can improve the child's body image and lifestyle (Edwards et al., 2004).

Fertility

Surgery to the reproductive system necessitating organ removal may involve a threat to fertility, which can be compounded by other treatment modalities. In the very young child this may be a difficult concept for the parents to cope with and may be seen as a low priority. In future life, however, it may be of paramount importance to the survivor of childhood malignancy who can barely remember the original illness. Sensitivity in broaching this subject is important and referral to a specialist team, which may include a counsellor, psychologist and gynaecologist, may be appropriate. Nursing staff should be aware that for teenagers, infertility may be viewed as a high priority but embarrassment may prevent them from discussing it. Opportunities should be provided for the subject to be discussed and then at the appropriate time the various options available can be considered.

Malabsorption

Resection of large amounts of intestine may lead to malabsorption resulting in nutritional deficiency. The child may require long-term nutritional support at home, either through enteral feeding using modular products or by TPN. Care should be aimed at providing the required feed at home, with involvement of the dietician, the general practitioner and local children's community nursing teams.

Adhesions

Formation of bowel adhesions due to scar tissue is a common complication of all abdominal surgery. The child may present with acute abdominal pain and severe dehydration due to persistent vomiting, indicating intestinal obstruction. Intravenous fluid replacement therapy should be commenced immediately to prevent hypovolaemic shock and to correct any fluid and electrolyte imbalance. The pain experienced may vary in nature from being described as mild and cramp-like, to severe, continuous and localised. This will depend on the type of obstruction. If the obstruction does not resolve with conservative management, by keeping the child 'nil by mouth' and inserting a nasogastric tube, kept on free drainage, then surgery will be indicated to divide the adhesions.

Body image

When the surgeon is considering the type of surgical procedure to be used, attention should be given to the placement of the incision to minimise the effect on body image. Scarring cannot be avoided, but careful planning can reduce the cosmetic insult, perhaps with a scar placed where it can be covered by clothing, for example, a 'bikini-line' incision, or an incision in a natural skin crease. Occasionally future plastic surgery may be needed to reduce surgical scarring.

Surgery in supportive care

The supportive care aspects of surgery in paediatric oncology are important across all treatment modalities. Surgeons play a key role in the management of the central venous access which is essential to the management of children and young people with cancer. As surgeons have become more integrated members of the oncology team, they have taken an important role in helping to manage some of the short-term effects of intensive treatment regimes, for example, the management of gut toxicity and colitis following chemotherapy, and the treatment of abscesses and other lesions caused by infection.

Central venous access

The introduction and continuing development of indwelling central venous access devices (CVADs)

have been essential to the advances in treatment seen in paediatric oncology in the past three decades. The administration of aggressive multidrug chemotherapy protocols, and the complex supportive care they necessitate, would be impossible without the availability of robust, permanent venous access (Dillon, 1999).

There are two types of central line in common use. The external catheter (Hickman® or Broviac type) is composed of cuffed silastic tubing, tunnelled under the skin from the anterior chest wall into the cephalic subclavian or internal jugular vein, with the tip lying near the right atrium. The line is held in position by a dacron cuff, which encourages the formation of fibrous tissue ingrowth into the cuff, and has an external segment. It may have one or more lumens. The alternative is a wholly implantable subcutaneous port, attached internally to a silastic catheter, accessed by insertion of a needle; this can be either a single lumen or a double lumen (which has two separate ports). In recent years there have been developments in both types of line arising from the increased sophistication of both medical technology and surgical techniques of line placement. These developments have given rise to a number of clinical features which should be considered when choosing the most appropriate line for a particular child (Table 15.4).

The choice of line will be influenced by a number of factors, taking into account these different clinical features (McInally, 2005). A child undergoing a particularly complex or aggressive treatment regimen, who is likely to require continuous access over weeks or even months, would be better with a dual lumen, external catheter. A child with a solid tumour, or acute lymphoblastic leukaemia (ALL), receiving 'standard' intermittent chemotherapy may find an implanted port less restrictive. Older children and young people, for whom body image is of particular importance, may also find a port less intrusive. For some children, particularly those with a developed needle-phobia, the accessing of the port with a needle would be a major disadvantage. The use of local anaesthetic applications on ports is, however, very effective and children should be assured of this. For some younger children the process of simply changing dressings on an external catheter can be distressing, whereas when the implanted port is not in use, no inter-

Table 15.4 Comparison of the clinical features of central venous access devices

External catheters (Hickman® or Broviac® type)	Implantable ports (Portacath® type)
Designed for continuous use	Designed for intermittant use
Regular dressing required	Dressing required only when 'port' in use
Weekly flushing recommended	Flushing once a month recomended
Some restriction on activity (e.g. swimming) and lifestyle	Less restriction on activity and more 'normal' lifestyle
Dislodgement of catheter possible	Dislodgement of port rare but separation of catheter reported
No needle required to access	Needle required to access; possible risk of dislodgement
Extravasation rare	Extravasation following needle dislodgement reported
Significant impact on body image	Less impact on body image
Suggested higher infection rate (especially multi-lumen line)	Suggested lower infection rate

vention is needed. There is some clinical evidence that the risks of infection are greater in external catheters than in ports (Dillon, 1999; Squire *et al.*, 2005). This is probably related to the fact that with the external device the exit site is a portal of entry for skin flora, and that the hub by which it is accessed is inevitably exposed (Shapiro, 1995).

All these factors need to be taken into account when considering the insertion of a central venous access device. Children and families should be involved in the decision-making process, and so need to be fully informed of the advantages and disadvantages of each type of device. When clinical condition and treatment plan permit, the child and the family should be given a choice of what sort of line they will have.

Historically, external catheters have been more widely used in paediatric oncology patients, and this probably remains the case in most centres within the UK although the audit of cental line use reported in this chapter dates from 1996 (Tweddle *et al.*, 1997). Anecdotal and local evidence would suggest that ports are becoming more widely used, following a number of studies which demonstrated that they can be used successfully in children with leukaemia as well as solid tumours and may offer certain advantages (Shapiro, 1995). In a number of centres in the UK as well as in North America, the implanted port has become the preferred device in children with ALL, as studies suggest a lower incidence of complications, as well as improvements in the patient experience (McInally, 2005; Squire

et al., 2005). The lower infection rates reported in implanted ports appear to be significant. Quality of life may also be improved, with fewer restrictions on activity and less maintenance of the catheter. They appear to offer a more attractive option to some with a more 'normal' lifestyle and minimal alteration to body image.

The information-giving process is an important first step in the process of preparing the child and the family for the insertion of a central line. They need first to understand what a central line is and why it is necessary. For children, play can be very important in this process. Dolls or teddies with central lines in place can demonstrate the difference between the types of line (also helpful to parents!) and help children to become familiar with them. So, too, can seeing other children with lines in place and the family will often find it useful to discuss lines with another family and hear 'first hand' about their use and the care needed at home. Information given must clearly be tailored to the age of the child or young person and the understanding of the family (McInally, 2005). For teenagers and young people, offering a choice of line where this is possible can be helpful in restoring a measure of control in their treatment and it is therefore of critical importance that they receive the information they need to help them make the right choice. Pictures, diagrams, models and the 'real thing' may all be helpful in this process.

Before surgery, consideration should be given to the siting of the catheter, as the impact on physical appearance and body image can be minimised by careful surgical placement (Daniels, 1995). This also affects ease of access, particularly with internal ports. Central lines should be inserted by an experienced surgeon who carries out this procedure on a regular basis, in order to minimise potential complications (Tweddle *et al.*, 1997). Where it is possible, line insertion should be carried out when the child is neither neutropenic nor thrombocytopenic, in order to reduce the risks associated with bleeding, bruising and infection. This is clearly not always possible, as the child's clinical condition and the need for treatment will often dictate the need for a line. When the child has a low platelet count, the administration of pre- and post-operative platelet transfusions will be required to try to avoid these problems. The issue of pain control should be discussed before surgery, in order that it may be effective post-operatively.

Surgical techniques for the insertion and fixation of central lines have developed alongside the growing expertise of those carrying out these procedures. Increased collaboration between surgeons working in the regional centres treating children has led to moves towards standardising these techniques, and formulating national guidelines.

There remain at present wide local variations in the type of line used, the way it is inserted, the way it is secured, and the different aspects of subsequent management. While it is hoped that national guidelines will be established in the future to address these issues, there are certain basic principles essential to good practice in the handling of central venous access devices. Aseptic technique is of paramount importance from the time of insertion onwards. The frequency with which lines are cleaned and dressed subsequent to insertion is a local variable, as is the type of dressing used. Studies which have looked at the frequency of early dislodgement of external lines indicate the importance of a robust method of securing lines in the early days after insertion, allowing time for the exit site to heal and the cuff to become established *in situ* (Tweddle *et al.*, 1997). The use of a cuff stitch has been recommended (Weiner *et al.*, 1992). There is a suggestion that a stitch at the exit site might also be beneficial, although it has proved to be difficult to test such aspects of surgical technique in a controlled, randomised trial.

A variety of dressings are available to cover the exit site of an external catheter, or a port when it is accessed. There is no conclusive clinical evidence as to whether gauze and tape or occlusive film dressings, are superior when it comes to the securing of lines, or the prevention of infection (Gillies *et al.*, 2003). Indeed, there is a suggestion that no dressing at all may be necessary (Bravery & Hannan, 1997). There is clinical evidence that chlorhexidine is the most effective antiseptic when cleaning exit sites (Chaiyakunapruk *et al.*, 2002).

Catheter hub contamination is recognised as an important contributory factor to catheter-related infection; central lines are capped by a variety of different obdurators and connectors, many of which aim to provide a closed, needle-free system for both blood sampling and the administration of drugs and fluids. These devices were originally developed with the primary aim of preventing needle-stick injury, and there has been no convincing study to show the benefit of such devices in preventing infection (Flynn, 2000). It should be remembered that such devices are guaranteed for only a limited number of punctures, records need to be kept of this and obdurators changed on a regular basis. Minimising the number of times the catheter is accessed, and improving staff compliance with a sound, aseptic, non-touch technique can help to reduce the incidence of infection (Puntis *et al.*, 1991).

There remains considerable discrepancy over the flushing of central lines when not in use. There is some evidence that a Hickman® type line only needs to be flushed once a week with a heparinised saline solution and indeed there are centres which do not routinely flush these catheters at all (Tweddle *et al.*, 1997). Any instructions for flushing from the manufacturers of individual devices should be followed. An implanted port should be flushed with a heparinised solution once a month, in accordance with manufacturer's instructions.

Research is still needed to develop evidence-based practice in all aspects of the management of central lines to provide evidence on which to base clinical practice. In the absence of national guidance, robust local policies must be developed to standardise all aspects of central line care, to avoid variations in practice that can be confusing to patients and practitioners alike. The risk of potential complications associated with central venous lines can be minimised with the development of a sound policy for handling and training whether it is aimed at health-care professionals, parents, or children themselves (Dougherty, 1996).

Once a central line has been inserted, the family and the child need to be taught how to care for it, in accordance with such local policy. This teaching needs to be carried out in a standard way, but at the pace of the individual child or family, well supported by the nurse caring for them (Pike, 1989). By encouraging them to become involved with treatment in this way and take on this aspect of care, the family or the child themselves can regain some sense of control over the process. This may be one of the first steps in transferring some of the child's care from the hospital setting back to home. Lines must always be well secured and many families and the staff caring for them have devised a range of 'pockets' and pouches in which to keep the line out of the way.

Complications of central venous access

The types of central venous access devices now common in clinical practice have brought great benefits to children, but are not themselves without risk. They bring with them a number of potential complications which can be divided into two main categories: infectious and mechanical.

Infectious complications are the most commonly reported problem with venous access devices (Dillon, 1999). There are several distinct types of infection related to central venous catheters. Superficial infections at both the tunnel and the exit site are often an early complication, although they can occur at any time during the lifetime of a line. Infection can also occur at the pocket of an internal port and is particularly difficult to treat. Catheter-related infections are frequently signalled by fever and rigours associated with use of the line and may be identified by positive blood cultures which can indicate colonisation. As stated previously, a number of studies have shown overall lower rates of infection with internal ports in comparison to external catheters (Shapiro, 1995). As this author points out, however, this may be partly related to the population of patients in each group. As external catheters tend to be used in patients

with leukaemia and those undergoing intensive chemotherapy regimens, they tend to be generally more at risk of infection associated with prolonged and profound neutropenia. Other risk factors for the development of line infections include the child's age, and the length of time for which lines are in use. Gram-positive organisms, particularly the *Staphylococcus* species, are the most common pathogens, followed by Gram-negative organisms (Das *et al.*, 1997).

There continues to be much debate between clinicians and microbiologists about the treatment of catheter-related infections and the indications for the removal of an infected catheter. It is frequently possible to treat catheter-related bacteraemias with antibiotics, administered through the device; when a dual lumen device is in place, antibiotics should be given through alternate lumens, as this ensures maximal exposure of the pathogens. The persistence of positive blood cultures or the reappearance of a particular organism on more than one occasion would be reasons to remove the line. Ongoing studies in the UK and elsewhere are investigating the best way of using antibiotics where a line is thought to be infected, evaluating the use of antibiotic 'locks' as an alternative to systemic treatment. Certain organisms, notably *Staphylococcus aureus* and species of *Candida* are almost impossible to eradicate with antibiotics alone and removal of the catheter will then normally be required. When lines are removed because of infection, an interval should be left before a new line is inserted, as otherwise it too is likely to become infected. Any serious infection of the tunnel of an external line, or the pocket of an internal port, is likely to lead to its removal.

A number of studies have reported an association between infection and the presence of thrombus formation. This is thought to result from the development of a fibrin 'sheath' on the catheter surface, to which organisms such as *Staphylococcus aureus* and *Candida albicans* can adhere (Bagnall-Reeb & Perry, 2002). This has prompted a number of studies into the use of thrombolytic agents such as urokinase to help in clearing infection in central lines (Ascher *et al.*, 1993). This is now an accepted intervention in some North American institutions, but further studies are needed to establish the efficacy of this approach, and it is not widely practised in the UK.

Sampling or blood withdrawal problems can occur in both types of central venous access device, and may be caused by the formation of a fibrin sheath, or a clot which acts as a sort of one-way valve at the catheter tip, or because the tip is up against the wall of the blood vessel. Repeated flushing and aspiration of the catheter, change of position of the child, or the instillation of 5000 units of urokinase into the catheter may solve this problem. Thrombolytic therapy, principally the instillation of urokinase, may help to clear a line that has become occluded as a result of thrombus formation. Lines may also become blocked through other causes, such as lipid clots caused by prolonged parenteral nutrition; there is some evidence that they can be cleared with the use of alcohol instilled in the line. Where precipitation is thought to have occurred in the line, hydrochloric acid or sodium bicarbonate may also be used to free a blocked line. Such interventions should always take place according to a properly formulated protocol.

Clot formation is now recognised as a more widespread problem than had previously been thought with an increasing recognition of the risk of venous thrombosis formation at the catheter tip, and the possibility of subsequent thromboembolic events. Imaging and an echocardiogram should therefore be considered to establish the cause of the occlusion in a blocked catheter, particularly in the presence of infection. Thrombosis may develop in the upper extremities and local thrombosis of the subclavian vein may present with the development of collateral circulation with prominent superficial veins over the chest wall and clavicle. Risk factors for thrombus formation include the type of line used (larger lumen catheters carry a greater risk), and the use of medication known to affect coagulation, principally asparaginase.

Nutritional support

Central venous access is required for the administration of parenteral feeding, but surgeons may be involved in methods of enteral feeding as well. Enteral feeding is preferred wherever possible, as it helps to maintain the integrity and function of the gastrointestinal tract. When children require enteral nutritional support, nasogastric feeding is usually the first option, but when there is likely to be a long-term feeding requirement, or where vomiting is a particular problem, gastrostomy tubes are increasingly considered. Gastrostomy feeding tubes can be placed either endoscopically, or surgically, and the percutaneous endoscopic gastrostomy (PEG) tube is becoming more widely used in the oncology setting (Skolin et al., 2002). PEG tubes can be more appropriate for young people where body image is a priority; the visible presence of a nasogastric tube can significantly lower self-esteem. Particular care should be taken of the gastrostomy site as this is a potential source of infection. The exit site should be cleaned daily with boiled and cooled water and an antiseptic ointment should be applied for the first one to two weeks. It should be observed for early signs of inflammation and discharge. Carers and the child should be taught how to care for the PEG as recommended by the manufacturer. The dietician will calculate nutritional requirements and give advice on the appropriate feeding regimen. Following insertion, when peristalsis has returned, small bolus feeds given during the day are gradually increased as tolerated. Additional continuous overnight feeds may then be introduced if appropriate.

Management of infection

The surgeon should be clearly identified as an important member of the multidisciplinary treatment team in the management of a number of infectious complications in children with cancer.

Neutropoenic enterocolitis

When children become neutropenic, they are at risk of infection affecting the whole of the mucosa of the intestine. Neutropoenic enterocolitis, also known as typhlitis, is an infectious, and potentially life-threatening process which is characterised by a distended abdomen, abdominal pain, and large loops of inflamed distended bowel. It varies greatly in severity, and at its worst can lead to a necrotising process which can lead to infarction and perforation of the wall of the bowel. In the face of profound neutropenia and thrombocytopenia, management of this condition will be, where possible, by the conservative measure of resting the bowel, to allow healing to take place. On occasion, however, urgent surgical intervention will be required. An experienced surgeon should, therefore, be involved in the child's management from the onset of such symptoms and decisions about treatment taken in close cooperation and consultation with the oncologist. It has been suggested that the neutropenic patient with abdominal pain can present the greatest diagnostic challenge a surgeon can meet, and that although imaging can be helpful, the most important monitoring of these patients is by physical examination and constant re-evaluation (Dillon, 1999). Surgical intervention is indicated in patients with clear evidence of intestinal perforation, or in severe cases showing clinical deterioration despite active medical management, or where there is persistent gastrointestinal haemorrhage despite correction of thrombocytopaenia or other clotting abnormalities (Shamberger *et al.*, 1986). It should be remembered that children undergoing chemotherapy can develop other 'surgical' conditions such as appendicitis, or adhesions with small bowel obstruction, and this may be very hard to distinguish from enterocolitis.

Nursing care of these children requires well-developed clinical assessment skills, alongside an understanding of the underlying disease process, so that significant changes are recognised and reported to other members of the multidisciplinary team in a timely manner (King, 2002).

Perianal abscess

Local infection in the perianal region is a relatively common problem during episodes of neutropenia. Symptoms can include intense pain and discomfort, although physical signs may be minimal, partly because of the lack of neutrophils (Dillon, 1999). There may, however, be induration and erythema, and in severe cases ulceration may occur, with the risk of tissue necrosis. Most infections are caused by a mixture of organisms, with *Pseudomonas aeruginosa* frequently involved. In the majority of cases, treatment is conservative, but regular observation for tissue necrosis or abscess

formation must be undertaken. In these circumstances, surgical intervention may be required.

Pulmonary infections

Pulmonary infections are often seen in children undergoing particularly intensive protocols, notably those undergoing myelo-ablative chemotherapy with stem cell rescue. Fungal infections such as *Aspergillus* or *Candida* can cause particular complications, and carry a high morbidity and mortality. The surgeon will on occasion be asked to help in the diagnosis of such infections. Bronchoscopy and bronchoalveolar lavage is an effective way of obtaining culture results in many patients, and this procedure may be carried out by either a respiratory physician, or a surgeon. If bronchoscopy findings are negative, then either a thorascopic or an open lung biopsy may be considered, and these patients will require appropriate preparation and subsequent care as discussed above.

Surgery to avoid the complications of radiotherapy

In the planning of external beam radiotherapy, consideration is always given to normal tissue structures and the radiation dose they will receive. In certain situations there is a role for surgery in moving certain critical organs to ensure that they do not receive high doses of radiation with attendant damage, and repositioning them for the duration of treatment. Several mechanisms have been devised, using tissue expanders, for moving normal bowel out of a radiation field. This has a particular application in pelvic Ewing's sarcoma, where it is necessary to target the tumour with a high dose of radiation. The technique of ovarian plication has also been developed to 'hitch' the ovaries out of the area of pelvic irradiation (Tait, 1992).

In some children, radiation doses will be delivered using brachytherapy, where a radio-isotope is placed within the tumour, or in close proximity to it, in order to give a continuous, concentrated dose of radiotherapy. Here the surgeon may be required to carry out physical placement under the guidance of the radiologist.

Future trends in surgery

The continued development of treatment for children with cancer in the developed world has focused on two major aims: to improve cure rates for the 25 % of children who do not survive, and to reduce long-term effects of treatment and improve the quality of life for those who do. Future trends in surgery, alongside the other primary treatment modalities, will address these aims in each of the different areas outlined in this chapter.

As scientific progress continues to be made in the process of tissue analysis, and the understanding of tumour biology, so the requirements of tissue biopsy have become more clear and more precise. Increased sub-specialisation within the surgical profession is designed to ensure that children and young people are referred to centres with appropriate expertise in undertaking these procedures, as has been emphasised by recent national guidance in the UK (National Institute of Health and Clinical Excellence, 2005).

Minimally invasive surgical techniques are becoming more widely used in tissue diagnosis, and increased experience with such techniques in the hands of identifed surgeons should lead to reduced risk of complications for children (Holcomb, 1999). The increased role of surgeons in the setting up and conduct of clinical trials in the treatment of paediatric solid tumours has led to a more defined understanding of the place of surgery in the overall clinical management of children. Treatment will increasingly be tailored to the nature of the particular tumour in the particular child. In some cases this may mean a greater role for surgery in the complete resection of tumours. In other cases it may mean identifying groups of children who should not be operated on, as happened with non-Hodgkin's lymphoma, and is now under review in infants with neuroblastoma.

As surgeons develop further expertise in particular fields, there will be continued improvements in surgical techniques, with the hope of increased collaboration and communication leading to more standardised procedures based on best clinical practice.

Technological advances in medicine offer a number of exciting possibilities in the further development of surgical techniques. Developments in the clinical application of new techniques and technology in both robotics and telemedicine are being explored in the hope of increasing their role in particularly complex and demanding surgery (Bagnall-Reeb & Perry, 2002).

In many types of tumour there have been moves away from mutilating surgical treatment to more conservative options, for good reason and with positive effects. As the late effects of radiotherapy and chemotherapy and their associated toxicities become more apparent, it may be that the role of surgery will be re-evaluated, with surgeons working much more closely as part of the multidisciplinary treatment team. The role of surgery in supportive care will continue to evolve as many aspects of treatment become more complex, requiring the close involvement of all members of the multidisciplinary team (Dillon, 1999).

Surgery in many cases can be one of the most emotionally critical points of treatment for the child and family. It is a defined and concrete intervention with a clear aim, and often immediate results. It thus presents an enormous challenge to nurses working in both the oncology and the surgical setting to ensure that the child and family are prepared for and supported through this critical episode of care.

References

Ascher D, Shoupe B, Maybee D & Fischer G (1993) 'Persistent catheter related bacteremia: clearance with antibiotics and urokinase' *Journal of Pediatric Surgery* 28: 627–628

Bagnall-Reeb H & Perry S (2002) 'Surgery' *in*: Baggot C, Kelly K, Fochtman D & Foley G (eds) *Nursing Care of Children and Adolescents with Cancer*. Philadelphia, PA: WB Saunders, pp. 90–115

Barnes E (2005) 'Caring and curing: pediatric cancer services since 1960' *European Journal of Cancer Care* 14: 373–380

Bates A (1994) 'Reducing fast times in paediatric day surgery' *Nursing Times* 90(48): 38–40

Borkowski S (1998) 'Pediatric stomas tubes and appliances' *Pediatric Clinics of North America* 45(6): 1419–1435

Brandt M, Luks F, Lacroix J *et al.* (1994) 'The paediatric chest tube' *Clinical Intensive Care* 5(3): 123–129

Bravery K & Hannan J (1997) 'The use of long-term central venous access devices in children' *Paediatric Nursing* 9(10): 29–35

Brodeur G, Pritchard J, Berthold F *et al.* (1993) 'Revision of the international criteria for neuroblastoma diagnosis, staging and response to treatment' *Journal of Clinical Oncology* 11: 1874–1881

Brown N (2001) 'Neuroblastoma tumour genetics: clinical and biological aspects' *Journal of Clinical Pathology* 54: 897–910

Callahan C & De la Cruz L (2004) 'Central line placement for the paediatric oncology patient: a model of advanced practice nurse collaboration' *Journal of Pediatric Oncology Nursing* 21(1): 16–21

Carli M, Cecchetto G, Sotti G *et al.* (2004) 'Soft tissue sarcomas' *in*: Pinkerton R, Plowman P & Pieters R (eds) *Paediatric Oncology* (3rd edn). London: Arnold, pp. 339, 347–348

Chaiyakunapruk N, Veenstra D, Lipsky D & Saint S (2002) 'Chlorhexadine compared with povidone-iodine solution for vascular catheter-site care: a meta-analysis' *Annals of Internal Medicine* 136(11): 792–801

Chiang D, Ben Meir D, Pout K & Dewan P (2005) 'Management of post-operative bladder spasm' *Journal of Paediatrics and Child Health* 41(1–2): 56–58

Daniels L (1995) 'The psychosocial implications of central venous devices in cancer patients' *Journal of Cancer Care* 4: 141–145

Das I, Philpott C & George R (1997) 'Central venous catheter related septicaemia in paediatric cancer patients' *Journal of Hospital Infection* 36: 67–76

De Cosmo G, Mascia A, Clemente A, *et al.* (2005) 'Use of levobupivicaine for the treatment of postoperative pain after thoracotomies' *Minerva Anaesthesiology* 71(6): 347–351

Department of Health (2003) *The National Service Framework for Children, Young People and Maternity Services: Standard for Hospital Services*. London: Department of Health, pp. 27–28

Dillon P (1999) 'Challenge of supportive surgical care in pediatric oncology' *Seminars in Surgical Oncology* 16(2): 193–199

Dolan A (1993) 'A day in the life of a hospital play specialist' *British Journal of Theatre Nursing* 3(3): 31–32

Dougherty L (1996) 'The benefits of an IV team in hospital practice' *Professional Nurse* 11(11): 761–763

Doz F, Brisse D & Stoppa-Lyonet X (2004) 'Retinoblastoma' *in*: Pinkerton R, Plowman P & Pieters R (eds) *Paediatric Oncology* (3rd edn). London: Arnold, pp. 326–330

Duff A & Bliss A (2005) 'Reducing distress during venepuncture' *in*: Davis T (ed.) *Recent Advances in Paediatrics 22*. London: Royal Society of Medicine Press

Edwards J (1998) 'Parents in recovery: a paediatric recovery nurse's view' *British Journal of Theatre Nursing* 8(6): 5–6

Edwards M, Borzyskowski M, Cox A & Badcock J (2004) 'Neuropathic bladder and intermittent catheterisation: social and psychological impact on children and adolescents' *Developmental Medicine and Child Neurology* 46(3): 168–177

Finley G (2001) 'Pharmacological management of procedure pain' *in*: Finley G & McGrath P (eds) *Acute and Procedural Pain in Infants and Children*. Seattle: ISAPP Press

Finley G & McGrath P (eds) (1998) *Measurement of Pain in Infants and Children*. Seattle: IASP Press, p. 1

Flynn P (2000) 'Diagnosis, management and prevention of catheter-related infections' *Seminars in Pediatric Infectious Diseases* 11: 113–121

Gillies D, O'Riorden E, Carr D *et al* (2003) 'Central venous catheter dressings: a systematic review' *Journal of Advanced Nursing* 44(6): 623–632

Ham B (2005) 'Children do well with shorter fast before surgery' *Child Health News* 27 April

Hodgkins M & Lander J (1997) 'Children's coping with venepuncture' *Journal of Pain and Symptom Management* 13(5): 274–285

Holcomb G (1999) 'Minimally invasive surgery for solid tumours' *Seminars in Surgical Oncology* 16(2): 184–192

Johnson H (1992) 'Stoma care for infants, children and young people' *Paediatric Nursing* 4: 8–11

Kain ZN, Caramico LA, Mayer LC, Genevro JL, Bornstein MH & Hofstadler MB (1998) 'Preoperative preparation programs in children: a comparative examination' *Anaesthesia and Analgesia* 87(6): 1249–1255

King N (2002) 'Nursing care of the child with neutropenic colitis' *Journal of Pediatric Oncology Nursing* 19(6): 198–204

Kist-van Hothe J, Ho P, Stablein D *et al.* (2005) 'Outcome of renal transplantation for Wilms' Tumour and Denys-Drash syndrome: a report of the North American Pediatric Renal Transplant Cooperative Study' *Paediatric Transplantation* 9(3): 305–310

Mann J (2004) 'Germ cell tumours' *in*: Pinkerton R, Plowman P & Pieters R (eds) *Paediatric Oncology* (3rd edn). London: Arnold

McInally W (2005) 'Whose line is it anyway? Management of central venous catheters in children' *Paediatric Nursing* 17(5): 14–18

McIntosh N, Bate B, Brykczynska G *et al.* (2000) 'Guidelines for the ethical conduct of medical research involving children: Royal College of Paediatrics and Child Health: Ethics Advisory Committee' *Archives of Disease in Childhood* 82: 177–182

Medical Research Council (2001) *Human Tissue and Biological Samples for Use in Research: Operational and Ethical Guidelines*. London: MRC

Melody A (1999) 'Parents in recovery areas: a review of the literature' *British Journal of Theatre Nursing* 9(8): 351–358

Mitchell C (2004) 'Wilms' tumour' *in*: Pinkerton R, Plowman P & Pieters R (eds) *Paediatric Oncology* (3rd edn). London: Arnold, pp. 420–422

Mitchell C, Jones P, Kelsey A *et al.* (2000) 'The treatment of Wilms' tumour: results of the United Kingdom Children's Cancer Study Group (UKCCSG) second Wilms' tumour study' *British Journal of Cancer* 83: 602–608

Mitchell V, Grange C & Black A (1997) 'A comparison of midazolam with trimeprazine as an oral premedicant for children' *Anaesthesia* 52: 11–23

Morton N (2001) 'Simple and systematic management of postoperative pain' *in*: Finley G & McGrath P (eds) *Acute and Procedural Pain in Infants and Children.* Seattle: ISAPP Press

Mott M, Mann J & Stiller C (1997) 'The United Kingdom Children's Cancer Study Group – the first twenty years of growth and development' *European Journal of Cancer* 33: 1448–1452

National Institute for Health and Clinical Excellence (NICE) (2005) *Improving Outcomes in Children and Young People with Cancer.* London: NICE

Ochroch E & Gottschalk A (2005) 'Impact of acute pain and its management for thoracic surgical patients' *Thoracic Surgery Clinics* 15(1): 105–121

O'Connor G (2005) 'Teaching stoma-management skills – the importance of self-care' *British Journal of Nursing* 14(6): 320–324

Otte J, Pritchard J & Aronson D (2004) 'Liver transplantation for hepatoblastoma: results from the International Society of Paediatric Oncology (SIOP) study (SIOPEL-1) and review of the world experience' *Pediatric Blood Cancer* 42: 74–83

Parkes S, Muir K, Cameron A *et al.* (1997) 'The need for specialist review of pathology in paediatric cancer' *British Journal of Cancer* 75: 1156–1159

Patte C (2004) 'Non-Hodgkin's lymphoma' in Pinkerton R, Plowman P & Pieters R (eds) *Paediatric Oncology* (3rd edn). London: Arnold, pp. 256–259

Pearson A & Pinkerton CR (2004) 'Neuroblastoma' *in*: Pinkerton R, Plowman P & Pieters R (eds) *Paediatric Oncology* (3rd edn). London: Arnold

Pike S (1989) 'Family participation in the care of central venous lines' *Nursing* 3(38): 22–24

Pinkerton C, Cushing P & Sepion B (1994) *Childhood Cancer Management.* London: Chapman & Hall

Puntis J, Holden C, Smallman S *et al.* (1991) 'Staff training: a key factor in reducing intravascular catheter sepsis' *Archives of Disease in Childhood* 66: 335–337

Rescorla F (1999) 'Pediatric germ cell tumours' *Seminars in Surgical Oncology* 16(2): 144–158

Reynolds M (1999) 'Pediatric liver tumours' *Seminars in Surgical Oncology* 16(2): 159–172

Royal College of Anaesthetists (2001) *Guidance on the Provision of Paediatric Anaesthetic Services.* Bulletin, 8 July. London: RCA

Royal College of Nursing (1999) *Clinical Practice Guidelines: The Recognition and Assessment of Acute Pain in Children.* London: RCN

Royal College of Paediatrics and Child Health (1997) *Prevention and Control of Pain in Children.* London: BMJ Publishing

Shafford E & Pritchard J (2004) 'Liver tumours' *in*: Pinkerton R, Plowman P & Pieters R (eds) *Paediatric Oncology* (3rd edn). London: Arnold, pp. 453–457, 460–461

Shamberger R, Weinstein H, Delorey M & Levey R (1986) 'The medical and surgical management of typhlitis in children with acute nonlymphocytic (myelogenous) leukemia' *Cancer* 57: 603–609

Shapiro C (1995) 'Central venous access catheters' *Surgical Oncology Clinics of North America* 4(3): 493–451

Skolin I, Hernell O, Larsson M, Wahlgren C & Wahlin Y (2002) 'Percutaneous endoscopic gastrostomy in children with malignant disease' *Journal of Pediatric Oncology Nursing* 19(5): 154–163

Smith S (2004) 'Adolescent units – an evidence-based approach to quality nursing in adolescent care' *European Journal of Oncology Nursing* 8(1): 20–29

Spurbeck W, Davidoff A, Lobe T *et al.* (2004) 'Minimally invasive surgery in paediatric cancer patients' *Annals of Surgical Oncology* 11(3): 340–343

Squire R, Aki U & Teong P (2005) 'Implantable ports versus cuffed external catheters in the management of children and adolescents with acute lymphoblastic leukaemia' *Pediatric Blood and Cancer* 45: 39–45

Stiller C (1994) 'Centralised treatment, entry to trials and survival' *British Journal of Cancer* 70: 352–363

Tait D (1992) 'Minimization and management of morbidity from radiotherapy' *in*: Plowman P & Pinkerton CR (eds) *Paediatric Oncology: Clinical Practice and Controversies.* London: Chapman & Hall, p. 592

Thompson I & Lauvetz R (1976) 'Oxybutinin in bladder spasm, neurogenic bladder and enuresis' *Urology* 8(5): 452–454

Thoms JR (ed.) (2004) *CancerStats Monograph.* London: Cancer Research UK

Tweddle D, Windebank K, Barrett A *et al.* (1997) 'Central venous catheter use in UKCCSG oncology centres' *Archives of Disease in Childhood* 77: 58–59

Twycross A, Mayfield C & Savory J (1999) 'Pain management for children with special needs: a neglected area?' *Paediatric Nursing* 11(6): 43–45

United Kingdom Childhood Cancer Study Group (1996) 'Biopsy of paediatric solid tumours' (unpublished)

Vos A (1995) 'Primary liver tumours in children' *European Journal of Surgical Oncology* 21: 101–105

Weiner E (1999) 'Editorial to Special Issue: Pediatric Surgical Oncology' *Seminars in Surgical Oncology* 16(2): 71–72

Weiner E, McGuire P, Stolar C *et al.* (1992) 'The CCSG prospective study of venous access devices: an analysis for insertion and causes for removal' *Journal of Pediatric Surgery* 27: 155–164

Willis J (1998) 'Growing up with a stoma' *Nursing Times* 94(27): 61–63

Wilson G & Doyle E (1998) 'Local and regional anaesthetic technique' *in*: Morton N (ed.) *Acute Paediatric Pain Management: A Practical Guide*. London: Baillière Tindall

Winder A (1994) 'Achieving independence' *Nursing Times* 90(22): 50–52

World Health Organisation (1998) *Cancer Pain Relief and Palliative Care in Children*. Geneva: WHO, p. 15

Commentary

Neuro-oncology

Jennie Sacree

Brain and spinal tumours account for about 20% of all childhood cancers. They are the most common solid tumour and the second most common malignancy. The incidence of central nervous system (CNS) tumours appears to be rising in Western industrial countries (McKinney et al., 1998; Keene et al., 1999), although the reasons for this remain unclear at present. Improved diagnostic imaging may contribute to this, but other environmental factors – such as exposure to ill-defined causal agents – may also be responsible.

A second group of children should also be included here and that is those who have a secondary CNS tumour following radiotherapy for a different childhood malignancy – usually Acute Lymphoblastic Leukaemia (ALL) (Bhatia et al., 2002).

The diagnosis of a brain tumour in a child is a devastating blow to any family, one that precedes a usually long and traumatic journey through many departments, beginning with scanning/diagnosis though surgery and then further treatments; chemotherapy or radiotherapy or both, before a long-term outcome may be more obvious. That hospital staff need to understand the processes and treatments these children and their families may go through on this journey is as important as understanding the underlying patho-physiology of the particular tumour in question.

In summary, Chapter 16 discusses brain tumours, and is a well-presented, logical account that guides the reader through the journey a family, and the staff they come into contact with, are likely to experience. It starts with incidence, presentation, location, type, signs and symptoms, and proceeds through investigations, the role of the multidisciplinary team, pre-, intra- and post-operative care and complications. It then takes the reader through a real-life experience of a family and the cancer journey they undertook. The chapter continues with further therapies and neurological and late-effect sequelae, and finishes with a positive outlook for neuro-oncology in the future.

The initial section covers location, presentation and acute management of resultant hydrocephalus and increased intracranial pressure. This is followed by good description of types of tumour which is comprehensive and clearly set out. The chapter walks the reader nicely through the investigations that a child and his family may be exposed to during their initial admission, radiological, blood work, etc. However, there could possibly have been a little more discussion of blood tumour markers and the significance and levels likely to be seen in certain tumours.

Cancer in Children and Young People   Edited by Faith Gibson and Louise Soanes
© 2008 John Wiley & Sons, Ltd

MRI and CT scanning are described in some detail. Maybe the newer forms of MRI could have been explored a little more here, with three Tesler scanners and scans becoming more widely available. These are most likely to be the way forward, giving a much more focused and expressive picture, especially with the detail they give in the posterior fossa region and also with small tumours in eloquent areas. With this newer technology becoming available, it is hoped this will give the detailed MRI information in a much quicker form. At present, a CT scan of the head is possible in 20 seconds but an MRI takes around 30 minutes. In the next five years the technology to do MRI scans in a few minutes should be possible. This will have an important effect on the way we scan children, and the way we use MRI in place of CT.

An excellent and concise section on neurological observations, which forms an integral part of the care of a child with a tumour and later post-operatively, follows.

The section on play could have included a little more about what the play specialist is able to do specifically with different age groups and specific brain tumours, and perhaps the particular aids they use when the child is being prepared for radiotherapy and the mask making. Also a mention could have been made of the importance of inclusion of the whole family and siblings in play with the specialist, thus allowing the whole family to use play to work through their emotions and worries. Working with the play therapist will also enable them to be more aware of the specific worries of their child who is undergoing the surgery and subsequent therapy.

Pain post-operatively is addressed, although perhaps wound pain could have been mentioned, as pain post-operatively is often more from the wound than a headache. Oral and non-opiate medications have a place in post-operative management and also simple relaxation techniques. The use of alternative therapies probably has a role within this setting although there is very little specific research on alternative and complementary therapies with children and brain tumours; however, plenty of work in this area has been carried out with children in oncology (Courtney Wolfe Christensen *et al.*, 2006).

Post-operative nursing care and complications cover all aspects of the post-operative journey and include:

- Electrolyte imbalance which is most likely to occur following midline tumour surgery, where there may be interference of the pituitary gland by the surgeon.
- Mention of this and of diabetes insipidus following such surgery is made.
- Post-fossa mutism is a part of 'Posterior Fossa Syndrome' and is briefly mentioned. It can occur in up to 10% of post-fossa surgery in some form or another. It is extensively researched and explored but only briefly mentioned in the chapter. It is more common in medulloblastoma, but is thought to be exacerbated in any post-fossa tumour surgery where the vermis is split and manipulated.

The next section describes Jack's journey. This is an excellent commentary on what happens in real time from admission, through surgery and the post-operative phase, up to the point at which diagnosis is made histologically and adjuvant treatment is being discussed. This will help everyone understand how rapidly a child and his family start the 'brain tumour journey' and move through the first phase. It would have been helpful to conclude the story with an outline of the time frame of the rest of his therapy, particularly as this contrasts so sharply with the velocity of the beginning of his journey.

Follow-on therapy is then discussed in some detail, with excellent sections on chemotherapy and radiotherapy. Chemotherapy for CNS tumours is not as well established as in other solid tumours, such as Wilms' tumours, and the reasons for this are discussed within the chapter. This is an area of marked interest within the discipline as scientists now understand better how to break down the blood–brain barrier and allow access of chemo-agents to the tumour cells (Estlin & Veale, 2003). There is much new work being undertaken in this area and phase 2 and phase 3 international trials are now taking place which will take forward this type of knowledge.

Radiotherapy has been around for much longer and for a time was the only treatment available for certain types of tumour, although this is now changing with the greater knowledge and understanding of chemotherapy routes and methods of working. The specific complications of CNS radiotherapy are clearly covered.

Some of the final few paragraphs of the chapter relate to the subject of late effects. This is perhaps one of the most valid aspects of brain tumour surgery and adjuvant therapy – how we leave the child in order for them to continue the rest of their lives. As more and better therapies become available and understood, we are treating more patients and they will have a higher survival rate. This can only be a good thing if the late effects of the treatment do not outweigh survival. All aspects are dealt with in detail here.

The closing paragraph of Chapter 16 deals in an optimistic way with the future of neuro-oncology. Overall, this chapter presents a timely, informative and at times thought-provoking overview of brain tumours, their aetiology, progression, initial treatment and follow-on therapies.

References

Bhatia S, Harland NS & Pabustan OB (2002) 'Low incidence of second neoplasm among children diagnosed with acute lymphoblastic leukaemia' *Blood* 99: 4257–4264.

Courtney Wolfe Christensen BS, Mullins LL, Scott JG & McNall-Knapp RY (2006) 'Persistent psychosocial problems in children who develop posterior fossa syndrome after medulloblastoma resection' *Pediatric Blood and Cancer* 49: 723–726

Estlin EJ & Veal GJ (2003) 'Clinical and cellular pharmacology in relation to solid tumours of childhood' *Cancer Treat Rev* 29: 253–273

Keene DL, Hsu E & Ventureyra E. (1999) 'Brain tumours in childhood and adolescence' *Paediatric Neurology* 20: 198–203

McKinney PA, Parslow RC, Lane SA, Bailey CC, Lewis I *et al.* (1998) 'Epidemiology of childhood brain tumours in Yorkshire, UK 1974–1995: geographical distribution and changing patterns of occurrence' *British Journal of Cancer* 78: 974–979

16 Neuro-oncology

Lindy May and Beth Ward

Introduction

Rickman Godley undertook the first successful craniotomy for removal of a brain tumour in 1884; however, the patient died of meningitis 10 days later (Ainsworth, 1989). The procedure of craniotomy was initiated by primitive man, who used this method in an attempt to rid ill tribal members of demons. Today, craniotomy/craniectomy still constitutes the primary therapy for tumour eradication (National Institute for Health and Clinical Excellence [NICE], 2006) but is often just the starting point of treatment, which consists of radiotherapy and/or chemotherapy in addition to surgical resection.

This chapter will describe some of the main central nervous system (CNS) tumours found in children, along with associated presenting signs and symptoms; treatment options will be discussed and pre-operative and post-operative issues outlined. Discharge planning, adjuvant therapy and a mention of late effects will close the chapter. A case study which highlights the complex pathway a child may take from diagnosis to treatment has been included.

Overview of brain tumours

Paediatric brain tumours are the most common solid tumour found in children under 15 years of age and the second most common group of neoplasms. In most populations they represent 20–25% of childhood cancers (Rutka & Kuo, 2004). Historically, these tumours have been treated with surgery and/or radiotherapy, but chemotherapy is now routinely used either on its own or more usually in conjunction with the above treatment. The use of chemotherapy for CNS tumours was initially limited by the belief that drugs needed to cross the blood–brain barrier to be effective. Many strategies have been developed in an attempt to circumvent the blood–brain barrier or to disrupt it in order to enhance drug delivery to the target tumour site within the central nervous system. These include the use of mannitol and vaso-active compounds, and administration of very high doses of chemotherapy. However, more recent work has suggested that tissue transport is increased in brain tumours and consequently water-soluble chemotherapy agents may have a greater role than was previously supposed (Walker, 2004).

Cancer in Children and Young People   Edited by Faith Gibson and Louise Soanes
© 2008 John Wiley & Sons, Ltd

The effect of chemotherapy on intellectual loss and neural impairments to children treated with brain tumours is still under investigation, although a positive developmental outcome has been reported in very young children treated with chemotherapy alone (Copeland *et al.*, 1999). Influencing factors in the treatment protocols today include the child's age, the degree of surgical resection and the histological characteristics of the tumour. While multi-modality therapy has increased the outcome for many children with brain tumours, some remain refractory to current therapeutic modalities. A high rate of disease control has been achieved for low grade gliomas, ependymomas, germ cell tumours and medulloblastomas, but considerable therapeutic challenges remain when treating the remaining groups (Rutka & Kuo, 2004). Neuro-radiology and in particular MRI scanning, have been essential aids in advancing treatment, and surveillance MRI scanning is now a routine procedure.

Compared with other types of childhood cancer, improvements in survival of children with CNS tumours have been modest. However, in the United Kingdom, for those children who survived five years following treatment between 1971 and 1995, the probability of them surviving a further ten years was 89 % (Robertson *et al.*, 1994). Today, research-based clinical practice aims to improve these statistics, while caring comprehensively for the child, with an attempted cure being the objective. However, along with increased survival for the child with a brain tumour comes the recognition of significant long-term consequences of the treatment, and these include physical, psychosocial, neuropsychological and neuro-cognitive effects.

Aetiology of brain tumours

Tumours of the brain comprise about one-fifth of all cancers during childhood, however, there has been an increase in their incidence in the past 15 years, of 15 %. This finding may be due to improved diagnostic services rather than any real biological changes, for example, small benign tumours are now being isolated on MRI scanning. The only known factors that predispose to the development of brain tumours are certain genetic factors, such as neurofibromatosis type 1 and 2, tuberous sclerosis and Li-Fraumeni syndrome (Byrne, 1996). Ionising radiation, including exposure in utero, is known to increase the risk of tumours; further exposures and characteristics include pesticides, and polyomaviruses (Bunin, 2003).

Presentation of brain tumours and acute management

The variations in presentation exhibited by the child with a brain tumour are dependent on the following three factors:

- compression or infiltration of specific areas of cerebral tissue;
- related cerebral oedema;
- development of raised intracranial pressure.

Depending on the type and location of the tumour, one or all of the above symptoms may occur. The diagnosis of a brain tumour is often difficult to establish in a child, since many of the signs and symptoms may mimic those of the more common childhood illnesses. This delay in diagnosis will frequently lead to anger and/or guilt on behalf of the parents, and much reassurance is required to allay the fears that an earlier diagnosis might have changed the outlook (May, 2001).

Signs and symptoms may further vary depending on the age and development of the child, and the size and location of the tumour, although most children will suffer headaches.

Focal neurological signs

Some 50–60 % of childhood brain tumours originate in the posterior fossa; these include astrocytomas, medulloblastomas and ependymomas. The remaining 40–50 % are supratentorial and include optic pathway tumours, hypothalamic tumours, cranio-pharyngiomas and astrocytomas. Primitive neuroectodermal tumours (PNETs) can occur at any site.

Posterior fossa tumours

The main tumours in the posterior fossa include PNET (Primitive Neuroectodermal Tumour) including medulloblastoma, ependymoma and astrocytomas. Due to the position of these lesions, children will present with ataxia, headache, and early morning vomiting and visual disturbance. Hydrocephalus is common.

Brain stem tumours

These include astrocytomas of varying malignancy and in addition to the above symptoms, will cause cranial nerve deficits, in particular, difficulties with speech and swallowing. Long tract signs can also occur (Farmer *et al.*, 2001), with disturbance to motor and sensory neurones connecting the brain and spine.

Supratentorial cortical tumours

These include astrocytomas, ependymomas, PNET and many more. They are commonly associated with hemiparesis, visual disturbances, seizures and intellectual difficulties.

Supratentorial/mid-line tumours

These include astrocytomas and are commonly associated with pituitary disturbance, visual changes and raised intracranial pressure due to hydrocephalus.

Increased intracranial pressure and hydrocephalus

If any of the three components in the skull (blood, brain and cerebrospinal fluid) vary in volume due to oedema, haemorrhage or hydrocephalus, the intracranial pressure varies. This results in an increase in head circumference in the baby whose skull sutures are not yet fused. In the child with fused sutures this results in symptoms such as headaches, vomiting, papilloedema

and an altered level of consciousness. Tumour growth can cause a direct volume increase, resulting in cerebral oedema and raised intracranial pressure. This is the rationale for the use of corticosteroids such as dexamethasone has a valuable short-term role in the management of these children but long-term administration is often associated with high levels of morbidity (Glaser & Buxton, 1997).

Hydrocephalus refers to the progressive dilatation of the ventricles due to production of the cerebro-spinal fluid (CSF) exceeding its rate of absorption. A blockage due, for example, to a tumour, prevents the normal flow of cerebrospinal fluid and results in hydrocephalus. This is a frequent symptom of brain tumours in children and will often be the trigger that prompts admission to hospital, due to a sudden deterioration in conscious level. Solid or cystic tumours can attain considerable size, the effects of which may be exaggerated by hydrocephalus or cerebral oedema. In infancy, non-specific features are common, including irritability and vomiting, with slowly progressing raised intracranial pressure; babies may display a tense anterior fontanelle, downward diversion of the eyes (called 'sunsetting') failure to thrive and increasing head circumference.

Removal of the tumour may resolve the hydrocephalus, but an emergency insertion of an external drainage system for CSF drainage may be required initially. Alternatively, a third ventriculoscopy may be an option and is sometimes performed at the same time as tumour resection, thus eliminating the need for a shunt. Ventriculostomy involves passing an endoscope into the third ventricle and making a hole in the floor, allowing CSF to flow out into the prepontine cisterns. The success rate for third ventriculostomy in patients with tumoural obstructive hydrocephalus is 70% (Chumas et al., 2001).

For those children requiring a permanent shunt, complications of blocking (40% within the first year of insertion) and infection (1–10% risk and far higher in the neonatal period; Drake et al., 2000) cause increased morbidity and potential mortality. Consequently the neuro-oncology nurse must have an understanding of the mechanics of shunts and their possible complications. These complications include infection, blockage, disconnection, fracturing or migration of the shunt and very occasionally, tumour dissemination via the shunt (Back *et al.*, 2005). Shunt malfunction may mimic the signs of the brain tumour (such as vomiting, headache and drowsiness) and diagnosis may well be impossible without a scan. This may necessitate either sedation or general anaesthesia in the uncooperative child, followed by surgical replacement of the shunt if required. Children presenting with pyrexia and neutropenia with a shunt placed must have the possibility of a shunt infection assessed. CSF is taken for culture only if such an infection is strongly indicated, as introducing infection by sampling is a risk.

The child with a brain tumour presents additional concerns when receiving chemotherapy. The risk of increased intracranial pressure from hyper-hydration must be balanced against the risk of chemotherapy side effects due to inadequate hydration. The presence of a ventricular-peritoneal shunt for the treatment of hydrocephalus might be an asset in the presence of hyper-hydration, assisting in reducing raised intracranial pressure. Antiemetics with a sedative side effect are often used with chemotherapy but their benefits must be balanced against the possibility of 'missing' the drowsiness caused by shunt malfunction. Both parents and nurses must be encouraged to report subtle changes in a child's behaviour promptly, so that appropriate investigations can be instigated as required.

Tumour types

Astrocytomas

Astrocytomas account for approximately 50% of childhood brain tumours and are sub-classified by grade (1–4, with 1 being the lowest grade) or histological description such as pilocytic, diffuse, anaplastic and glioblastoma. The outcome for the child in terms of morbidity and mortality depends on both the tumour type and location (Rilliet & Vernot, 2000). Astrocytomas occur throughout the central nervous system with presenting symptoms related to the tumour location. Hydrocephalus is common due to obstruction of the ventricular system by the tumour.

Pilocytic astrocytomas can occur in the optic chiasm and the posterior fossa, the latter when totally resected, resulting in long-term survival and probable cure for the child. Low-grade astrocytomas, which are not totally resected due to their anatomical position, may require further treatment with low-dose chemotherapy and/or radiotherapy in the expectation that tumour growth will be halted or reduced.

Glioblastomas (high-grade gliomas) are highly malignant and consequently difficult to cure and the outlook is bleak for the majority of these children.

Medulloblastoma (primitive neuroectodermal tumours of the posterior fossa)

This is a common malignant brain tumour in children and accounts for 20% of childhood brain tumours. The peak incidence is between the ages of 5 and 8 years with a second peak in adolescence and young adults with a male predominance. These tumours are highly malignant, arising from the anterior aspect of the inferior right vermis and inferior medullary velum. They may extend through the fourth ventricle to invade the brain stem and obstructive hydrocephalus is common. Symptoms of any tumour in the posterior fossa, including medulloblastoma, are early morning vomiting, ataxia, headaches and often visual disturbances.

Medulloblastomas are radiosensitive and chemosensitive. Initial surgical treatment is undertaken, including the management of hydrocephalus. Chemotherapy for children under 3 years old and radiotherapy and/or chemotherapy for those children over 3 years old are resulting in improved outcomes for these children.

Prognosis: medulloblastomas respond well to treatment and treatment regimes are continuing to improve the prognosis for this tumour group. These tumours are known to recur, however, and the presence of spinal metastases at diagnosis increases this risk and lowers the overall chance of survival (Koeller & Rushing, 2003).

Ependymomas

Ependymomas can occur throughout the central nervous system, but most commonly occur in the posterior fossa. They are tumours predominantly of the younger patient with 50% being under the age of 5 (Nazer *et al.*, 1990). They arise from ependymal cells lining the ventricles and are characteristically found in the fourth ventricle. Hydrocephalus is common and spinal metastases often occur. Total surgical resection is often difficult due to the anatomical position and frequent local recurrence occurs. The grade of ependymomas has not been proven to be of prognostic significance and a 'watch and wait' policy will very occasionally be implemented in a non-metastatic, totally resected tumour. Following surgical resection all other children would receive radiotherapy (if over 3 years old) and chemotherapy (if under 3).

Prognosis: this is dependent on the degree of surgical resection and the presence or absence of metastases.

Brain stem tumours

Symptoms include multiple cranial nerve involvement and occasionally hydrocephalus. The development of MRI scanning has allowed better visualisation of the brain stem, and although the majority of brain stem tumours are malignant with a poor outlook, there are a small number which are cystic, focal and operable. Clinical controversy continues over the risks and benefits of biopsy within the brain stem for purely diagnostic purposes. Many tumours are difficult to treat and surgery is limited to the relief of raised intracranial pressure in some children and tumour resection in a small and specific minority.

Prognosis: Surgery should be undertaken for exophytic, low-grade midbrain and medullary tumours, but not for pontine gliomas due to their anatomical position. Radiation is curative in the minority of children with brain stem tumours and therefore is only palliative in the remainder. Chemotherapy is given within clinical trials but the outlook remains poor for most children with brain stem tumours.

Mid-line tumours

The anatomical site of these tumours, plus their histological diagnosis, makes the signs and symptoms they exhibit very variable, and the treatment given is based on their histology. Included are deep-seated tumours, such as craniopharyngiomas, germ cell tumours, optic pathway, hypothalamic and pineal tumours. Their symptoms include endocrine abnormalities, visual disturbances, cognitive impairment, personality and memory changes. Although most of these tumours are benign, their position makes surgical resection difficult or impossible and radiotherapy and/or chemotherapy may be the only treatment possible. Craniopharyngiomas are the most common of these tumours, accounting for 6–8% of all childhood brain tumours. They are difficult to resect and there is usually significant long-term endocrine disturbance. Radiotherapy is sometimes used, as are intracystic radioactive implants and chemotherapy (such as bleomycin).

Prognosis: a complete surgical resection of these complex tumours offers the highest chance of cure, but often results in significant physical and cognitive changes. These tumours are persistent and an incomplete resection reduces the chances of long-term survival. The exception is the group of germ cell tumours, where surgical resection/biopsy is not warranted for secreting germ cell tumours.

Investigations into brain tumours

CT scan

Computed Tomography (CT) has been the cornerstone of neurological diagnostic procedures and continues to be of huge importance (Jaspan, 2004). The head is scanned in successive layers by narrow X-ray beams that pass through the skull and are transmitted or absorbed depending on the tissue density. The X-rays are converted into light photons by an array of scintillation crystals (the 'scanner'). The photons are, in turn, converted to electrical signals that are stored on a computer. The information is digitised and manipulated by the computer and the resulting display image photographed on Polaroid or standard film or communicated as images on PACS systems. A CT scan will illustrate changes in the location of structures, abnormalities and displacement of these structures and changes in tissue density. However, the definition of structures in the posterior fossa and spine is limited and the child is subjected to ionising radiation.

MRI scan

Magnetic Resonance Imaging (MRI) is perhaps a safer technique than the CT scan since no radiation is used, and it is becoming more widely available. MRI provides greater definition than the CT scan, particularly of the posterior fossa and spine. The patient is placed in a strong magnetic field and is then subjected to precise bursts of computer-programmed radio frequency waves. It is effective in detecting tumours, tumour necrosis and central nervous system degeneration. The images received are extremely accurate in their detail of anatomical information and the physiology and biochemistry of living tissue.

The child requiring either a CT scan or MRI may require sedation if they are unable to lie still for the required time. This may pose problems for the child who has raised intracranial pressure and a general anaesthetic may be safer in these situations. Involvement of a play specialist if available, appropriate explanation, the use of photographs of the scanners, relaxation techniques and diversion therapy can often result in a successful CT scan without sedation (Pressdee et al., 1997; de Amorim e Silva, 2006); but the noise of the equipment and the length of time required to keep still for MRI means that most toddlers and young children will require sedation or anaesthesia. Of note, MRI can be performed when metal clips are in situ; however, it is advisable to discuss this with the radiologist as the image may be distorted.

Neurological assessment

The aim of a neurological assessment is to determine the following:

- to identify the presence of any central nervous system dysfunction and hence anticipate further dysfunction that may be aggravated by surgery;

- to compare existing data to determine any changes (this may be particularly appropriate in a child with a brain stem tumour, where deterioration may be sudden and consequent treatment should be prompt);
- to detect any life-threatening situations (children with secondary hydrocephalus may quite suddenly reach a level of raised intracranial pressure which is no longer acceptable and respiratory arrest will occur if intervention is not undertaken);
- to provide a baseline profile on which further care will be based.

Neurological assessment should comprise a recognised coma scale, such as the Glasgow Coma Scale, or associated coma scales such as the Great Ormond Street Hospital for Children NHS Trust Coma Chart (Figure 16.1). The latter was research-based and utilises one concise chart for all age groups; it is based on cognitive rather than chronological age. Coma scales standardise observations for the assessment of level of consciousness and the National Paediatric Neuroscience Benchmarking Group devised a commonly agreed coma chart for children.

Pupillary signs and motor function of the upper and lower extremities are based on assessment of eye opening, best verbal response and motor response. Observations of vital signs must also be recorded in conjunction with neurological observations and these may alert the nurse to problems caused by or in association with a change in intracranial pressure. Although there is a recognised association of raised intracranial pressure with bradycardia and hypertension, this is often a late sign in children. A drowsy or irritable child with slow pupil reaction should alert the nurse to a rise in intracranial pressure. Infants and small babies with tachycardia and a low blood pressure may be displaying signs of systemic hypovolaemia following surgery, or their symptoms may be due to a sudden loss of cerebrospinal fluid resulting in a reduction in intracranial pressure; neurological observations in conjunction with recordings of vital signs will help ascertain the cause and necessary treatment to be given. A GCS of 14–15 is normal, but a score of less than 14 should raise concerns. A GCS of 8 or less indicates resuscitation is required, including the possibility of

Name				
Hosp. No				
DOB		**Coma Scale**	Great Ormond Street **NHS**	
Ward	(Affix patient label)		Hospital for Children	
			NHS Trust	
Consultant		Referring Hospital		Weight		Kg

The coma scale is scored on a total of 15 points. A score of less than 12 should give rise for concern. This is a universally accepted tool for measuring coma. A decrease in coma scale will be associated with a decreased level of consciousness. This needs to be considered along with the child's vital signs. Further information about the coma scale can be found in the related clinical procedure guideline

A.   Eyes Open
If the eyes are closed by swelling, please write 'C' in the relevant column, thus indicating the reason for a lower score.

B.   Best Verbal Response
In the left hand margin are two separate scales: on the far left is the scale for babies and infants and on the right is the scale for older children.
The following section gives an explanation of the best verbal response of infants.

   a. Smiles
      This can be used to describe an alert, contented infant as not all will smile at a stranger. The interaction between parents/carers and the infant should therefore be taken into account.

   b. Appropriate Cries
      The infant may be unable to settle.

   c. Inappropriate Cries
      The infant may have periods of being drowsy, but at times is heard to cry out. This is not always associated with being disturbed. The cry may be high pitched.

   d. Occasional Whimper
      Less frequent than above and may be associated with deep painful stimuli, required to gain a motor response.

   e. None
      No verbal response.

C.   Best Motor response to Stimuli
The age and cognitive abilities of the child must be taken into account.

D.   Pupils
When recording pupil size it is important to remember the effects of drugs, e.g. morphine will cause pinpoint pupils and atropine drops will dilate pupils for up to 6 hours.

E.   Limb Movements

   a. If a child has a permanent hemiparesis please indicate this in the relevant column, e.g. weakness, even though it is normal for the child.
   b. A child with a severe developmental delay may score lower on the coma scale, as his motor response may be poor.

| Version No: 0.2 | Version date: 5th April 2004 | Document development lead: | Jacqueline Robinson, Practice Educator, Neurosciences |

Figure 16.1   Coma chart, coma scale and comments chart
Source: From the Great Ormond Street Hospital for Children NHS Trust.

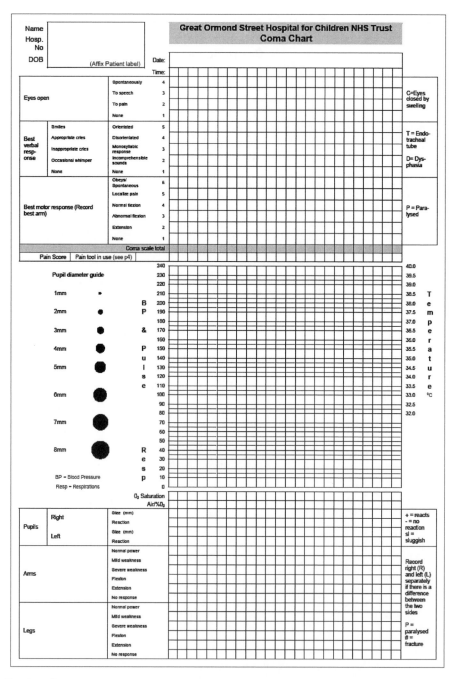

Figure 16.1   (Continued)

Record of Significant Events

Developmental Age:

Coma Scale Prior to Illness:

Date	Time	Description of Significant Event (E.g. post seizure, pain, headache, vomiting etc.)	Signature

Figure 16.1   (Continued)

intubation and ventilation to protect the airway as a child with reduced conscious level is unable to protect their airway.

Altered respiratory patterns occur with both raised and lowered intracranial pressure and mechanical ventilation may be required for the patient with reduced respiratory drive, or the unconscious patient. Hyperpyrexia is not uncommon, due to damage to the hypothalamus (following surgery or trauma). The presence of blood in the CSF is also known to result in pyrexia, the aetiology of which is unknown. Whatever the cause, pyrexia must be treated promptly, as the resulting rise in metabolic rate increases the oxygen and metabolic requirements of an already compromised brain.

Play therapy

Anthony Oakhill (1988) looked at play specifically related to children undergoing neurosurgical procedures and found that:

> Research has shown significant stress reduction in play preparation programmes that provide giving information, demonstrating procedures and having the child play with equipment for the neurosurgical procedure he is about to undergo. This cognitive, psychological approach helps the child acknowledge and play through his fantasies and misconceptions.

A play specialist is often the best person to discuss anxieties with a child and discover any preconceptions that may already be present. Play is an excellent medium through which the child can display their fears (Lawlor, 2003). The provision of play therapy is one of the top priorities in providing for a sick child's recovery and wellbeing (Dix, 2004). Preparation for surgery is essential and should be performed whenever possible as it may reduce some of the child's fears, and prepare the child for the post-operative period; children cope better with the anticipated, however brief the explanation may have been. They have huge fears of the unknown and many of these fears are based on fantasy which can be alleviated once discovered. Play also provides an emotional outlet

for the child and enhances their coping mechanisms, particularly utilising humour (Greenburg, 2005). Play is seen by the multidisciplinary team as a vital contribution to the child's recovery since it promotes normal development in both sickness and health and provides a comforting sense of normality which helps the child adjust to a strange environment (Woon, 2004). Reduction of stress in patients, parents, doctors and nurses is evident when a play therapy programme has been established (Dugdale, 2002).

The multidisciplinary team

Diagnosis of a brain tumour is often difficult to establish as many of the presenting symptoms mimic childhood illnesses, such as malaise and vomiting. The mean time from onset of clinical history to diagnosis varies but has been up to 20 weeks, with the involvement of various specialities before this (Edgeworth et al., 1996). Parental anxiety and distrust of professionals can consequently occur, and engagement with the family at the beginning of the information-giving process can sometimes help diffuse the situation. Parents also need to express their grief at the loss of their healthy child and the possible loss to death.

Input from the multidisciplinary team commences at the time of the child's admission. Once the diagnosis of a brain tumour has been confirmed radiologically, various medical and nursing teams will need to assess the child. Whichever medical team the child has been originally referred to, they will probably require input from multiple sources over the course of treatment.

The clinical nurse specialist (CNS) may not be involved until a definite histological diagnosis has been reached (see below). The anxiety and uncertainty at this early stage of the disease will cause enormous distress and exhaustion to the family and the ward nurse can assist by listening to their worries, answering their questions where possible and supporting them at this traumatic time. Anxious parents will result in an anxious child and appropriate information needs to be given, including details of procedures and surgery. Hospitalised sick children will often behave in a manner younger than their years, and the location and effect of the tumour may add to this;

information, therefore, needs to be appropriate for the child's developmental and emotional state and may need to be repeated to both child and parents.

Pre-operative care

In addition to radiological studies, blood profile and cross-match will be undertaken, as well as serum markers for germ cell tumours. Endocrine advice will be sought if appropriate, as electrolyte imbalance can occur; ophthalmology may be requested as a baseline for future assessment, and other members of the multidisciplinary team may be involved such as physiotherapists and speech and language therapists.

The child with a newly diagnosed brain tumour and their family (including siblings) will have been overwhelmed with information and explanations. They will also have met many new people at an exhausting, confusing and very frightening time. It is, therefore, understandable that explanations need to be repeated and consistent as the full implications of diagnosis and prognosis are impossible to take in at once. The family needs to be encouraged to take one step at a time and to involve the child as and when appropriate (Coyne, 2006).

Consent to surgery is often a traumatic undertaking and the presence of a nurse alongside the surgeon can allow reiteration of accurate information to the family later. Neurosurgery carries with it small but real risks of haemorrhage, cerebral damage and death. Balanced against this is the likelihood of death without surgery. Signing the actual consent form can be highly emotional, with much discussion as to which parent wishes to sign it. In addition, the management of pre-operative stress in parents will have a direct effect on the child's stress (McCann & Kain, 2001). A relatively calm parent will be of optimum support to the child.

Intra-operative care

An increased understanding of the pathophysiology of raised intracranial pressure, and how best to control this, has been aided by new anaesthetic agents and various monitoring techniques. The anaesthetist's task is often made more difficult by the position of the child on the operating table (sitting upright, for example, with the associated risk of air embolus).

During anaesthesia, controlled ventilation provides optimum operating conditions for performing craniotomy/craniectomy, by reducing intracranial pressure. Considerations include the effect drugs have on cerebral metabolism, cerebral blood flow, intracranial pressure and vasomotor tone. Other intra-operative concerns include the introduction of controlled hypothermia (thus decreasing cellular metabolism and the need for oxygen), hyper-ventilation (thus reducing brain bulk intracranial pressure) and venous air embolus (a potential problem associated with the sitting position frequently used for posterior fossa surgery). Surgery may take several hours and it is the responsibility of the theatre nurse, in addition to the anaesthetist, to ensure correct positioning of the child, both to allow access for surgery and to ensure the patient's protection and avoidance of pressure area sores; this includes positioning of the limbs, protection of the eyes by closing and covering them, and the usual attention to theatre protocol, such as the use of diathermy. The theatre nurse needs to be familiar with the constantly new and updated neurosurgical equipment such as navigation equipment and endoscopes. Correct assembly, cleaning and maintenance of this equipment are essential and involve appropriate training.

The anaesthetist and the neurosurgeon work closely during surgery. Any sudden haemorrhaging must be supported by the anaesthetist by prompt and appropriate replacement of blood/blood derivatives. An increase in intracranial pressure must be treated by hyperventilation or the administration of appropriate drugs such as mannitol. Any interference with the vital areas of the brain stem will produce an immediate irregularity or abnormality in the child's pulse and blood pressure; the anaesthetist will report this reaction immediately to the surgeon, who can then stop or proceed as appropriate. Should the child's condition deteriorate, the anaesthetist will advise the neurosurgeon while attempting to stabilise the child's condition. The theatre nurse can alert the ward nurse to any difficulties which might have arisen during surgery, although a detailed description should also be given by the anaesthetist and surgeon. Analgesia should be given at the end of surgery and before anaesthesia is withdrawn.

Post-operative management

The child will be nursed in the recovery room, the intensive care unit or the high dependency paediatric neurosurgical ward, depending on their condition, the individual hospital's organisation, and medical and nursing expertise available.

The objectives of immediate post-operative nursing management are:

- regular neurological assessment and early recognition and treatment of raised intracranial pressure;
- recognition and control of factors which could result in a rise of intracranial pressure;
- appropriate fluid management;
- recognition of potential complications and administration of the required intervention;
- safety of the child;
- administration of regular analgesia;
- comfort and support to both the child and family.

The child is observed closely for the first 24–48 hours following surgery as deterioration can be rapid and intervention must be prompt. The nurse works in conjunction with doctors and parents to provide the best care for the child, recognising that numerous problems can occur following surgery for a brain tumour, including the following:

1. *Airway, breathing and circulation*: Respiratory difficulties may arise due to airway obstruction or brain stem and cranial nerve involvement. This is a potential complication particularly following surgery to the posterior fossa or brain stem. Early identification of complications and appropriate treatment must be given and this may include intubation and ventilation if required. Hypovolaemia and anaemia may occur following surgery and fluid/blood products should be given as required. Cardiac arrhythmias are rare and are due to brain stem irritation or electrolyte imbalance, the former for which

there is no treatment and the latter which requires fluid/electrolyte management.

2. *Level of consciousness*: Any decrease in level of consciousness following surgery must be reported promptly as this may indicate a rise in intracranial pressure due to cerebral oedema (requiring an increase in steroids), haemorrhage (which may require emergency surgery) or hydrocephalus (which may require emergency surgery). The nurse must be efficient in assessing the child using the GCS and initiating emergency referral to the medical team as required. Neurological deficits (may be an early and late sign) or any acute changes in motor or sensory functions or communication should be reported and documented.

3. *Pain*: Headache will occur following craniotomy and a pain assessment must be undertaken. Analgesia is given in line with local hospital policy for children undergoing neurosurgery. However, some centres remain reticent in prescribing opiates to neurosurgical children as it has been thought in the past to reduce the level of consciousness and respiratory status. Studies and reviews continue to debate this issue.

4. *Electrolyte imbalance*: Electrolyte imbalance is common following craniotomy, due to haemodynamic instability, loss of cerebrospinal fluid, inappropriate antidiuretic hormone (ADH) or cerebral salt wasting. Hyponatraemia and hypo-osmolarity are a potent recipe for cerebral oedema with associated morbidity and mortality and careful fluid management is essential in reducing the likelihood of this occurring. Hydration is initially maintained via intravenous fluids; serum electrolytes and urine output must be measured and fluid management altered accordingly. Diabetes insipidus must be managed promptly with advice from an endocrine specialist.

5. *Nausea and vomiting*: This may have been one of the child's presenting symptoms and can persist following surgery, particularly if the floor of the fourth ventricle has been involved. Regular antiemetics should be administered intravenously and the child's fluid management supported intravenously as required.

Parenteral nutrition may be required in the malnourished child who is to commence high-dose chemotherapy.

6. *Seizures*: Seizures may occur due to the underlying cerebral abnormality, surgery, or because of electrolyte imbalance; hospital policy for seizure control should be implemented and the underlying cause managed. Seizures can be distressing and frightening to both child and family and reassurance and calm management will be helpful.

7. *CSF (Cerebro-Spinal Fluid) leak*: Should CSF leak through the wound, the doctor should be informed and the wound re-sutured if necessary to reduce the chance of infection. A pressure dressing will assist in the 'sealing' process.

8. *Cranial nerve deficits*: Any of the cranial nerves may be damaged during surgery but the commonest include irritation/damage to cranial nerves 9, 10 and 12 following surgery to the posterior fossa; this will result in difficulties relating to swallowing (including secretions), tongue movement and speech; this may be transient and the child should be supported during this phase. The speech and language therapist should be involved in assessing and managing the child, but in severe cases, a tracheostomy and gastrostomy/peg will be required. Vision may be affected, with the child complaining of altered/double vision (cranial nerves 2, 3, 4, 6) and this may be transient; alternate eye patching in the early post-operative days can be helpful and a referral to ophthalmology is recommended if the problem persists.

9. *Periocular oedema*: This will occur to varying degrees following frontal craniotomy and the child's comfort may be helped by applying cool packs over the eyes and maintaining the child in an upright position. Anxiety and fear are common if both eyes are oedematous and vision is occluded; family and child support is paramount.

10. *Nutrition and elimination*: Attention must be given to nutrition, but this is not a priority immediately post surgery. The administration of opiates and the fact that the child is immobile will result in constipation, and laxatives should be given as early as possible.

The use of steroids will increase the child's appetite and intake but further compound constipation.

11. *Comfort and safety*: The child may be confused and disoriented following surgery and cot sides should be used at all times. Parents should be encouraged to assist and comfort their child as early as possible to minimise distress and fear. They must of course be aware of their own exhaustion and coping abilities and encouraged to take regular food and rest breaks.

Specific supratentorial complications

Following surgery, the child is nursed at a 30% head-up tilt to allow for good venous return from the brain. Correct positioning of the Redivac drains is necessary to allow for free drainage without the siphoning effect caused by placing the drain too low beneath the patient's head. Occasionally suction may be applied to the drains to promote drainage.

Potential cranial nerve dysfunction may result in defects with eye movements which may be transient or permanent. Children adapt rapidly to such changes and should be encouraged and supported. Diabetes insipidus may occur if the pituitary has been involved. Seizures and hemiparesis are the other major areas of concerns; they may be temporary or permanent.

Specific infratentorial complications

Many children undergoing posterior fossa surgery are placed in the 'sitting position' for surgery, thus allowing the brain to sit in an anatomically normal position during surgery; an attempt is made to nurse these children head up post-operatively, although this is difficult to achieve in the agitated toddler. Potential cranial involvement may be multiple as described above and cerebellar ataxia is common and can be a long-term difficulty.

Cerebellar mutism/posterior fossa syndrome occasionally occurs and consists of aphasia with subsequent dysarthria, emotional lability, intense irritability, limb weakness and nystagmas (Steinbok *et al.*, 2003). Although some of the symptoms resolve spontaneously over time, ataxic dysarthia persists in many cases and has implications for counselling and support of family and patients.

Long-term concerns: morbidity and mortality

These include the following and are discussed in greater detail in the subsequent sections:

* neurological;
* personality changes;
* endocrinological changes;
* change of body image;
* change of family dynamics;
* quality of life;
* long-term prognosis.

The implications of these complications can be profound and the multidisciplinary team, both in hospital and in the community, will be closely involved with the family, working alongside the liaison nurse/CNS.

Jack's journey through CNS tumour treatment

The following patient journey is included to assist the reader in understanding the complex treatment for a child with a CNS tumour.

15 May 2005

Six-year-old Jack presented to his local casualty with a six-week history of progressive ataxia, early morning headache and vomiting. A CT scan undertaken revealed a posterior fossa tumour and hydrocephalus. He was referred urgently to a neurosurgical centre.

On arrival, Jack's GCS was 11, he was slow to rouse and confused. His parents were seen by the consultant neurosurgeon who explained Jack would need surgery for his tumour, but more immediately required surgery to relieve his hydrocephalus. Dexamethasone was commenced to reduce cerebral oedema. At 2 a.m. an external ventricular drain was inserted for CSF drainage.

Jack's condition was stable on return from theatre with a GCS of 13.

16 May 2005

Jack continued to improve during the day – his headaches were less and he commenced diet and fluids. His parents met again with the neurosurgeon who again discussed the plans for surgery. It was explained that tumour diagnosis (histology) would not be known for several days after surgery. The play specialist and nurses explained the drain to Jack and his parents.

16 May 2005

An MRI scan of brain and spine was undertaken, which Jack managed without sedation after a session with the play specialist. Surgery for tumour de-bulking was planned for the following day. Both parents and Jack were spoken to again in detail by the neurosurgeon and nurses and mortality and morbidity of the surgery were discussed with them. The play specialist prepared Jack for the days ahead, discussing his fears and learning about his existing coping strategies.

17 May 2005

Jack underwent a posterior fossa craniotomy for incomplete removal of tumour. Post-operatively he was nursed in the high dependency unit of the neurosurgical ward. His GCS remained stable at 12 although he was extremely irritable; pain was controlled with opiates. Intravenous fluids were administered and Jack was allowed nothing by mouth due to the possibility of cranial nerve damage altering his gag reflex. His external ventricular drainage continued. His parents were encouraged to assist with his nursing care such as mouth care and turning. Both were resident on the ward and were spoken to by the neurosurgeon who explained that tumour resection had been incomplete and that further treatment would be required.

18 May 2005

An MRI was performed as an indicator of tumour resection. Jack continued to be irritable and difficult to console. His parents were encouraged to care for themselves too, by taking regular breaks from the ward and resting as needed. Jack's gag was tested and he commenced oral fluids with intravenous fluids titrated accordingly. Analgesia was continued and Jack's nursing care organised around his resting periods as appropriate.

18–23 May 2005

Jack's condition continued to improve and he mobilised slowly with assistance from the physiotherapist. Neck pain is common following posterior fossa craniotomy and analgesia is required before mobilisation in the early post-operative days. He tolerated diet and fluids and his intravenous fluids were stopped. His external ventricular drain was raised daily to challenge his ability to cope without it and thus negate the requirement of a permanent shunt: many tumours in this location cause hydrocephalus but normal CSF flow can sometimes be restored once the tumour 'blockage' has been removed. Jack remained well and his external ventricular drain was removed on 23 May with no adverse effects.

24 May 2005

Histology confirmed a medulloblastoma and Jack's treatment was discussed at the multidisciplinary neuro-oncology meeting. His parents were then spoken to by the neurosurgeon in the presence of the neuro-oncology CNS. It was explained that a medulloblastoma was a malignant tumour and Jack would require radiotherapy and possibly chemotherapy for the best chance of survival; although tumour resection was incomplete, the tumour had not metastasised into his spine which was a positive sign. His parents were understandably devastated by the news. The ward sister and CNS spoke to his parents later in the day, listening to their fears and sadness and explaining the next steps, which would involve multifaceted care over a period of time.

Ongoing needs of a child with a brain tumour

Clinical Nurse Specialist (CNS) role

The care of children with brain tumours is complicated and extremely challenging, requiring a flexible and responsive approach to the individual needs of children and their families. The speciality bridges many disciplines, including neurosurgery, oncology, clinical oncology (radiotherapy), endocrinology, neuropsychology, physiotherapy, occupational therapy, play therapy, speech therapy and dietetics. The pivotal role of the clinical nurse specialist (CNS) facilitates the care of these children and their families throughout multiple treatments and long-term follow-up by providing constancy and continuity (NICE, 2005).

Information

It is recognised that timely, appropriate information is key to families being able to deal more effectively with the diagnosis of childhood cancer and that the delivery of this information should be viewed as a dynamic process, requiring active participation of both health-care professionals and families (Greenberg *et al.*, 2004). Having a large team of professionals involved in the delivery of information may prove overwhelming and it is therefore important to identify key professionals such as the neurosurgeon, oncologist and CNC to achieve continuity (Fisher, 1999). It has been suggested that parents should be the first targets for information, even when children are deemed competent in adolescence (Greenberg *et al.*, 2004). Children will often look to their parents for information.

Setting the scene

Guidelines support the value of setting the scene for disclosure of bad news (Baile *et al.*, 2000). A key step in the delivery of bad news is determining the family's perception, comprehension and current state of mind regarding the medical situation to date (Baile *et al.*, 2000). Research acknowledges that nurses are key to this information-gathering and the bedside nurse or the CNS is ideally placed to support this process (Arber & Gallagher, 2003). At the outset, it is important to clarify information that has already been given, bearing in mind that parents can only assimilate a small amount of information when in a state of stress and shock (Freeman *et al.*, 2003).

The family's viewpoint

It is acknowledged that the diagnosis of a brain tumour is often difficult to establish, as many of the symptoms may be non-specific and mimic other childhood illnesses. The mean time from onset of clinical history to diagnosis may be up to 20 weeks, with the involvement of various specialities before this occurs (Edgeworth *et al.*, 1996). This delay in diagnosis may cause parents to feel angry, leading to a mistrust of professionals. It is therefore essential to engage in the family's narrative at the beginning of the information-giving process. At this time, parents also need to express their grief at their loss of a healthy child and the possible loss to death.

Clearly, information relating to central nervous system tumours is complex and the format should therefore reflect the individual needs of the family. Important determinants such as parental education, primary language of communication, culture and social background influence the delivery and format of this information (Greenberg *et al.*, 2004). Interpreting services should be employed at the earliest opportunity as required. As well as being honest, accurate and open in the imparting of information, professionals also need to be sensitive to how much information the family want to know, this may be culturally determined.

The family's principal needs for information include:

- nature, biology and behaviour of the brain tumour;
- neuro-anatomy and implications;
- therapeutic interventions;
- radiotherapy;
- chemotherapy;
- clinical trials;
- family organisation;
- potential outcome.

(Greenberg *et al.*, 2004)

It is important that families have written material supporting the outline of their initial meeting, to assist their understanding and prompt further questions and discussion. It is helpful for them to have a basic understanding of the brain's functioning, which in turn will enable them to comprehend their child's symptoms.

Children's information needs

Brain tumours in children may cause speech and language disturbance that can range from difficulties with speech production, problems with word finding and difficulty understanding language. Information for the child therefore needs to be timely and the support of a speech and language therapist should be sought if the child's ability to communicate is affected by neurological impairment.

Information for the child needs to be simple, truthful and age-appropriate and delivered in stages, allowing the child to assimilate the 'next step' rather than a view of the overall treatment. Older children, however, are likely to understand the gravity of diagnosis and may ask direct questions about cure or the possibility of dying (Greenberg *et al.*, 2004). These questions should be answered honestly, instilling the reassurance of hope (i.e. 'without treatment there is a possibility that you would die, but we are hoping that treatment will offer cure').

Siblings

Concerns important to siblings can affect their ability to adapt to changes posed by the diagnosis of cancer (Freeman *et al.*, 2003). Siblings require information to understand what has happened, why it has happened and support in learning to cope with changes in their ill brother or sister (Freeman *et al.*, 2003). Children with a brain tumour may develop neuro-cognitive deficits and this may further impact on siblings.

Resources

With the rapid development of Internet accessibility, inevitably some health information has been distributed without regulation (Mazzini & Glode, 2001). Therefore one of the extended roles of the health professional team is to guide families to the most appropriate information. However, families still prefer hard copy of information to refer to (Greenberg *et al.*, 2004). There are a number of books available; some orientated to childhood cancer and some specifically to brain and spinal cord tumours.

Parental concerns and stressors

Problems associated with the on-going stress and insecurity of an unpredictable future can be a heavy burden on families. As parents struggle with feelings of despair and fear, followed by anger and sadness, health professionals must make allowances for subsequent episodes of unpredictable or irrational behaviour (De Sousa *et al.*, 2004).

With advancements in treatment for CNS tumours in the past 20 years, concern has been voiced that improvements in survival may not correspond with how well the family's needs are met (Freeman *et al.*, 2004). It is also acknowledged that symptoms from aggressive treatment, the sequelae of CNS tumours, as well as diagnosis can have a devastating effect on families (Walker *et al.*, 2004a). Quality of life studies have found that as many as 50% of children with brain tumours have a high risk of clinically significant emotional or behavioural problems (Kennedy & Leyland, 1999). A significant number of parents cite this as a major stressor in caring for their child (Freeman *et al.*, 2003). To help address these concerns, the role of the CNS should encompass an accurate assessment of psychological stressors and reactions of children and their family members to the diagnosis of CNS tumours (Hendricks-Ferguson, 2000).

Adjuvant treatment: specifics of treating a child with a CNS tumour

Developments in the management of children with central nervous system tumours are multidimensional. Definitive neurosurgical procedures, together with new radiotherapy techniques and improved chemotherapy protocols, have all contributed to an improvement in survival. Despite this, however, it is acknowledged that compared with other types of childhood malignancy, these improvements in survival in recent years have been modest, with most children surviving their tumour experiencing long-term neurological sequelae (Walker *et al.*, 2004a).

Corticosteroids

Corticosteroids have a valuable role in the management of children with CNS tumours, however, their administration is often associated with high levels of morbidity (Glaser & Buxton, 1997). The rationale for their use is to improve neurological function by reducing associated brain or spinal oedema, although the mechanism by which this occurs remains unknown. Approximately 25% of children presenting with CNS tumours will have clinical features of raised intracranial pressure (Edgeworth *et al.*, 1996). It is often appropriate to start corticosteroids while transfer to a neurosurgical centre is arranged.

The response to corticosteroids can be dramatic, with an improvement in signs and symptoms within as little as 24 hours. Treatment does not, however, increase survival time or cure rates. This dramatic improvement often fuels parental requests for the use of corticosteroids at a later stage in the child's care, especially at recurrence. This, however, requires careful discussion, weighing up the short-term benefits with adverse side effects. Severe mood and behavioural changes associated with corticosteroids can have a major impact on the child and family and are associated with a reduction in health-related quality of life. Insatiable appetite and weight gain can also be disturbing. Long-term sequelae, such as proximal myopathy (muscle weakness and wasting) and osteoporosis may compound difficulties during neurological rehabilitation and greatly affect mobility.

Chemotherapy

The role of radiotherapy to the developing brain has long been associated with long-term neurological sequelae; the younger the child, the greater the risk of damage. In response to these findings,

American oncologists in the late 1990s embarked on protocols, treating children younger than 2 years old with chemotherapy in an attempt to avoid or delay radiotherapy, therefore sparing the developing brain (Walker *et al.*, 2004b). However, administering chemotherapy effectively in the treatment of CNS tumours poses a number of problems.

To be effective, chemotherapy must reach its target. There are many challenges posed in successfully treating children with CNS tumours with chemotherapy, mainly compounded by the limited drug access to the brain through the protective mechanism of the CSF and the blood–brain barrier (the endothelial lining of blood capillaries) (Blaney *et al.*, 2004). To address this, recent advances in the delivery of chemotherapy agents have been three-pronged (Blaney *et al.*, 2004) concentrating on:

- the disruption of the blood–brain barrier with agents such as mannitol;
- administration of very high-dose intravenous chemotherapy;
- regional chemotherapy given intrathecally, intra-arterially and intratumourally.

The side effects of chemotherapy are discussed elsewhere in this book. Particular side effects pertinent to the care of children with CNS tumours include the following.

Nausea and vomiting

The use of antiemetics that act as serotonin antagonists, such as ondansetron, has greatly improved the management of chemotherapy-related nausea and vomiting. It is important, however, to monitor the child with a CNS tumour as protracted vomiting could indicate early signs of raised intracranial pressure necessitating urgent neurosurgical review. It should also be noted that children with tumours close to the 4th ventricle or brain stem, may be especially vulnerable to intractable nausea and vomiting and gastric oesophageal reflux, and will require additional antiemetic therapy (De Sousa *et al.*, 2004). Particular care should be taken with children who have dysphagia (speech and/or swallowing difficulties)

as there will be a high risk of aspiration with vomiting.

Hydration

Children with hypothalamic or pineal tumours require careful fluid management, the aim being to maintain an isovolaemic state, thus avoiding fluid and electrolyte shifts that may result in cerebral oedema.

Alopecia

Hair loss may prove particularly distressing for children with CNS tumours. Initially, hair will be partially shaved in preparation for surgery and subsequent hair loss through chemotherapy or radiotherapy will expose these surgical scars. It is important that the child and family are reassured that hair is likely to re-grow in time, but sparse hair re-growth may be experienced in the area of the high-dose radiotherapy field, most commonly the posterior fossa.

Neurotoxicity

Any added neurotoxicity can be devastating to children with existing neurological impairment and may significantly affect their mobility. In the older child, vincristine can cause peripheral neuropathy, leading to a loss of tendon reflexes, paraesthesia (tingling) and numbness in the fingers and toes and a reduction in dorsiflexion (backwards flexion of the foot). This can impact greatly on the child's ability to mobilise and may result in them becoming wheelchair-dependent for a period of time. The younger child meanwhile may present with ptosis (drooping of the upper eyelid). Any signs of neurotoxicity is an indication to reduce drug dose and all these side effects, although debilitating, are recoverable.

Ototoxicity

Ototoxicity results in hearing loss that is high frequency, bilaterally symmetrical and irreversible. It has been noted that capsulation, especially when coupled with cranial radiotherapy, can cause significant ototoxicity (Packer *et al.*, 2003).

Radiotherapy

Radiotherapy has long been accepted as having a significant contribution in the treatment of CNS tumours since Cushings first reported the curative potential of radiotherapy in the management of medulloblastoma in 1919 (Kortmann *et al.*, 2004). Radiation plays an essential role in the management of other childhood CNS tumours, especially when tumours cannot be entirely removed with surgery or there is a risk of microscopic spread. The side effects of treatment are discussed elsewhere in this book, but meanwhile there are a number of important issues when considering treatment to the cranial axis and whole CNS.

Treatment planning

Advances in brain tumour imaging, together with improvements in technology in the planning and delivery of radiotherapy, have led to childhood CNS tumours being successfully treated with conformal radiotherapy (Kirsch & Tarbell, 2004). Conformal radiotherapy targets and delivers the radiation dose specifically to the tumour, minimising the dose to the normal brain tissues, therefore limiting the long-term side effects of treatment.

Conformal radiation can be delivered by varying techniques that use high-energy X-rays (photons), such as three-dimensional (3D) conformal radiation therapy with fixed fields, stereotactic radiation therapy (SRT) using arc therapy, and intensity-modulated radiation therapy (IMRT). By delivering radiation with accurate target identification in this way, a smaller radiation field is selected and therefore less normal brain tissue is treated. 3D conformal radiation therapy can also limit the dose of radiation to the cochlea, which is key in the management of medulloblastoma where significant hearing loss from chemotherapy may be compounded by radiotherapy (Packer *et al.*, 2003).

Acute reactions

Acute reactions manifest as an exacerbation of the child's initial presenting symptoms, i.e. headaches and seizures. The aetiology of this remains unclear but may be related to localised cerebral oedema, causing an elevation of intracranial pressure. These effects tend to be short-lived, but may cause child or parent concern that treatment is failing.

Good information and reassurance at the outset of treatment are therefore required (Guerrero, 2005). A short course of corticosteroids may be required to alleviate symptoms. For those children experiencing seizures, serum anti-convulsant levels should be checked.

Early delayed reactions

Early delayed reactions are described as side effects occurring either during or, a few months following radiotherapy (Guerrero, 2005). These may include a loss of smell (owing to irradiation to the olfactory centre in the frontal lobes), otitis externa or media (owing to temporal irradiation) or irregularities in menstrual cycle (as a result of pituitary/hypothalamic irradiation).

Nausea and sensitivity to taste and smell

Nausea and vomiting are not a common side effect of cranial irradiation and therefore a child presenting with severe symptoms should be investigated for signs of raised intracranial pressure. More commonly children may describe a hypersensitivity to smells or an altered sense of taste as nausea. Hypersensitivity to smell is possibly caused by radiation to the olfactory nerve endings (cranial nerve 1) in the frontal lobes. Children with altered taste sensation may describe a 'metallic' taste. In this setting, it is important that children are examined for early signs of oral candidiasis, especially when on steroids. Once the aetiology of nausea is identified, antiemetics should be prescribed and an early referral to a dietician implemented to restore nutritional balance and prevent significant weight loss.

Hair loss

As with chemotherapy, children undergoing cranial irradiation will experience hair loss, usually 2–3 weeks into treatment. Alopecia is dose-dependent and therefore some hair loss due to high-dose fields may be permanent. Children can wash their hair during treatment but, to minimise skin irritation, a mild or non-perfumed shampoo should be used and the hair and scalp should be patted dry with a soft towel, avoiding the use of hairdryers.

Erythema

Erythema is described as flushing of the skin due to dilatation of the blood capillaries. This is likely to be the first side effect of cranial irradiation and precedes alopecia. This may cause some discomfort, requiring the application of aqueous cream or topical hydrocortisone 1% (Guerrero, 2005).

Somnolence syndrome

Somnolence syndrome is best described as excessive sleep, drowsiness, lethargy and anorexia. The process by which this occurs is not fully understood, but is thought to be a consequence of damage to the oligodendrogial cells. One of the major roles of oligodendrogial cells is the production of myelin for neuronal conduction. It is speculated that radiotherapy leads to a transient demyelination affecting the neuronal pathway thus leading to transient fatigue and exhaustion.

Somnolence may be experienced during radiotherapy or may evolve several weeks after completion of treatment and is noted as being one of the worst side effects of cranial irradiation (Guerrero, 2005). The severity is dependent on the total cranial irradiation dose and will therefore vary from child to child. Somnolence can be very debilitating, resulting in severe fatigue and the re-emergence of initial symptoms, leading to parental fear and anxiety that the tumour has recurred. Children may also feel emotionally vulnerable and tearful at this time and good, supportive nursing care is essential (Guerrero, 2005). Should the child have a ventricular-peritoneal shunt in situ for the treatment of hydrocephalus, excessive drowsiness may indicate a shunt dysfunction as opposed to radiation somnolence, and so develop into a neurosurgical emergency requiring a shunt revision.

Late effects of CNS tumours and acute rehabilitation needs

One in 1000 young adults is a cancer survivor, 10–15% of whom originally had a brain tumour (Spoudeas & Kirkham, 2004), but it must be acknowledged that survival alone is not indicative of quality of life (Walker et al., 2004b). The adverse effects of surgical treatment are usually apparent soon after surgery; whereas the effects of chemotherapy and radiotherapy may take a number of years to evolve. As long-term survival improves, it is becoming increasingly clear that many children have permanent neurological, neurocognitive, endocrinological and neuropsychological deficits (Packer et al., 2003).

Neurological sequelae: seizures

Seizures are reasonably common in children with brain tumours and may represent the main symptom at diagnosis. The risk of seizures is greatest in children with supratentorial tumours, increasing in incidence with age, from 22% in the younger child to 68% in adolescents (De Sousa et al., 2004). The occurrence is greatest in children with multiple neurological deficits and those children whose tumours are superficial in the cerebral hemisphere. It should be noted that there is a potential for interaction between anti-epileptic drugs and other medications such as analgesics, anti-inflammatory drugs and cytotoxic agents which may reduce anticonvulsant effects (French & Gidal, 2000).

Dysphagia

Both the effects of CNS tumours and subsequent treatment can affect the child's ability to feed (De Sousa et al., 2004). This can include impairment in mouth closure (cerebral tumours), disturbance in appetite (diencephalon tumours), co-ordination with chewing and swallowing (cerebella tumours) and bulbar palsy (brain stem tumours). Speech and language therapists and dieticians are the key to effectively managing dysphagia. It should be noted that dysphagia may also involve emotional and behaviour components which need to be addressed (De Sousa et al., 2004).

Motor deficits

Depending on the site of the brain or spinal lesion, motor deficits are characterised as spasticity, ataxia, dystonia or other abnormalities of posture, tone and movement (De Sousa et al., 2004).

These may lead to marked impairments of function, affecting daily living and educational activities such as dressing, feeding, pencil skills and keyboard skills. Paediatric physiotherapists and occupational therapists will use a number of different approaches that will encourage reacquisition of lost or deficient skills by encouraging practice and repetition.

Cranial nerve palsies

Cranial nerve palsies may result from a tumour arising from the nerves, the dissemination of an intracranial tumour, raised intracranial pressure, or may be the result of treatment, i.e. surgery, chemotherapy or radiotherapy (De Sousa et al., 2004). Approximately 25% of children will present with cranial nerve palsies at diagnosis. Multiple cranial nerve palsies are common in children with diffuse brain stem gliomas, meanwhile surgery for brain stem or posterior fossa tumours can cause residual cranial nerve palsies. Radiotherapy may lead to damage to the cranial nerves, although this is a rare, late complication (De Sousa et al., 2004). Chemotherapy agents such as vincristine can cause cranial neuropathies, the facial nerve being most commonly involved.

Visual loss

Tumours affecting the optic nerve can lead to progressive visual loss, which is described with reference to the visual fields. Facial weakness may lead to variable weakness of eye closure which in turn can lead to the risk of corneal damage. Impaired eye closure merits diligent eye care; artificial tears and taping the eyelid closed may prevent corneal abrasion.

Endocrine side effects

With improvements in survival rates following therapy for childhood brain tumours, there is a growing cohort of children surviving their tumour at risk of late effects (Gleeson & Shalet, 2004). Long-term endocrine problems in children with brain tumours can be varied and complex (Spoudeas

& Kirkham, 2004). Many studies have found that cranial irradiation plays a central role in causing endocrine dysfunction, but it is impossible to avoid irradiating the hypothalamic–pituitary axis in the treatment of children with most brain tumours (Gleeson & Shalet, 2004). The mechanism of radiation damage to the endocrine system is not well known. It may be related to direct injury to the cells responsible for hormone secretion, injury to the stroma or to the vascular channels that transfer hypothalamic hormones to the pituitary. Meanwhile, endocrine complications are uncommon when CNS tumours are treated with surgery alone (Anderson, 2003).

The most common problems are short stature due to both growth hormone deficiency caused by the effect of cranial irradiation and the effect of spinal irradiation on vertebral growth. Hypothyroidism occurs due to the involvement of the thyroid gland during spinal irradiation.

Recognition and the prompt management of associated side effects are essential to prevent further morbidity and impairment to quality of life (Gleeson & Shalet, 2004). With both the availability of synthetic growth hormone and its demonstrated ability to minimise growth retardation, and access to other relevant replacement therapies, it is essential that children are seen at designated endocrinology centres from the time of diagnosis and at regular intervals thereafter. If replacement therapy is required, its administration can greatly enhance the child's general quality of life (Spoudeas & Kirkham, 2004). Depending on the effect of radiotherapy on hormone production, some children may need medical support throughout puberty and as adults they may require fertility counselling and treatment; again, highlighting the need for long-term follow-up facilities.

Effect on intellect and education

Damage to the brain from both the tumour and treatment can affect cognitive and behavioural functioning (Savage et al., 2004). Radiotherapy is the main cause of cognitive dysfunction, but intrathecal methotrexate and surgery are also acknowledged to be contributory factors (Anderson, 2003). Retrospective studies into the long-term educational performance of children treated for CNS tumours demonstrate that the majority of children experience a decline in their school performance over time. It is also noted that a child's school performance in the first two years post-treatment is a poor long-term predictor of their final school performance/attainment. It is acknowledged that children below the age of 36 months may have the most severe cognitive effects from brain irradiation, which may be due to incomplete myelination of the white matter at the time of radiation therapy (Kirsch & Tarbell, 2004).

Children who have received craniospinal radiotherapy often have problems associated with poor short-term memory and recall. If teachers and/or parents observe a decline in the ability to keep pace with peers, it would be necessary to have a statutory assessment for a 'Statement of Special Educational Needs'. An educational Statement is a legally binding obligation (Department of Education, 1993; Department of Education and the Welsh Office, 1994; Education (NI) Order, 1996; Scottish Office, 1996). Where possible, any special help required by a child (special educational provision) should be provided within a mainstream state school alongside children of the same age.

Rehabilitation needs

If the burden of morbidity for children with CNS tumours is to be addressed, consideration needs to be given to meeting not only physical aspects of rehabilitation, but also those of psychological well-being. Research has demonstrated that children experience feelings of isolation from peer groups and may lack confidence socially. If ignored in the rehabilitative phase, these psychological problems can translate into functional difficulties such as poor attendance at school, attention deficits and overt eating disorders (De Sousa et al., 2004). It is therefore argued that rehabilitation for children with CNS tumours is lifelong (Walker et al., 2004a).

Currently, there is little evidence on which to base rehabilitative interventions for children, however, it is acknowledged that the management of children with CNS tumours has two main goals: the return of the child to as normal function as

possible and the reintegration of the child into family life and society (De Sousa et al., 2004).

The success of rehabilitative interventions depends on good communication between the child and family, as well as with the team of professionals supporting them. Rehabilitation also relies on the expertise of a team of professionals, and a concerted approach is required of the multidisciplinary team (De Sousa et al., 2004). The timing of interventions is key, and the initiation of rehabilitative measures early in the trajectory of a child's treatment needs to be offset by the risk of overwhelming children and families at diagnosis, a time when they are particularly vulnerable. Ultimately, co-ordinated, holistic rehabilitative care, delivered by a committed multidisciplinary team will contribute to improving the child's and the family's quality of life (De Sousa et al., 2004).

Second malignancy

The main risk to brain tumour survivors is the development of meningiomas at the edge of the radiation field or thyroid tumours following spinal irradiation. As there is a known carcinogenic potential of megavoltage irradiation and prolonged TSH stimulation, annual thyroid palpation and thyroid function tests are routinely carried out (Spoudeas & Kirkham, 2004).

Discharge planning

Communication across disciplines and agencies provides continuity; and communication must exist within and between each multidisciplinary team (NICE, 2005). It is important that professionals are aware that the primary responsibility for the coordination of care may alter from one subspecialty to the next during the course of treatment. It is clearly essential that the child and the family know which team, or which individual, is responsible for co-ordinating care at each stage (NICE, 2005). At discharge, the relevant ward or unit will follow its individual discharge planning protocol and the role of the CNS will be to act as a link in a large multidisciplinary team involving both hospital and community. This role will also involve the provision of advice and support to individual members of the teams. From the time of diagnosis the CNS will make contact and remain in communication with the following people:

- general practitioner (GP);
- health visitor/school nurse;
- paediatric community team;
- local paediatrician/hospital personnel;
- school/Local Education Authority;
- social worker;
- other support agencies/voluntary organisations.

Relapse and chemotherapy clinical trials

For many types of CNS tumours, particularly malignant glioma, disease progression at the primary site is the most common mode of relapse. Relapse is described as being more devastating to families than the original diagnosis, often signifying the loss of optimism associated with initial treatments (Greenberg et al., 2004). At this time, the implication of relapse, the child's neurological and general health status needs to be assessed and discussed openly with parents, as this will ultimately influence decision-making (Greenberg et al., 2004). Available protocols are invariably phase I and II trials, which may offer prolongation of life, but sadly rarely cure and therefore the exact nature of relapse should be clearly defined to facilitate parental and child decision-making.

The nature of relapse leads many parents to request second opinions, or urgently seek alternative treatments via the Internet. It is essential that parents and children are supported during this process, at a time of extreme vulnerability. As well as working collaboratively with families, clinicians are ethically and legally responsible for ensuring that the decisions made are in the child's best interest and, as with all treatment decisions, relapse and palliative care decisions must be informed choices. During discussions with parents and children, it is essential that hope is not completely extinguished, as this remains essential when coping with devastating news and the possibility of death. Although the hope of cure is no longer going to be realised, the focus can be shifted to the hope of good symptom control.

Relapse: the child

It is widely acknowledged that the burden of relapse is felt as intensely by children as by parents (Greenberg et al., 2004). At this time, it may prove difficult to provide information to children, as many parents will endeavour to protect them from the reality of the situation. This has to be carefully managed, respecting parental wishes, while encouraging a degree of openness with the child.

There is clearly great variability in a child's or an adolescent's ability to make decisions and to participate in decision-making but many children, given the opportunity, will be able express feelings and preferences relating to their care. What is key to this process is good communication and respecting the child's individuality, which is essential in effective ethical decision-making.

Palliative care

The speciality of paediatric palliative care has rapidly developed within the last decade in the context of the hospice movement, with the first children's hospice, Helen House, being opened in the UK in 1982. A steady growth of children's hospices has in turn led to the development of community hospice teams, enabling children to be cared for at home. The Association for Children with Life-limiting or Terminal Conditions and Their Families and the Royal College of Paediatrics and Child Health offer the following definition:

> Paediatric palliative care for children and young people with life-limiting conditions is an active and total approach to care, embracing physical, emotional, social and spiritual elements. It focuses on enhancement of quality of life for the child and support for the family and includes the management of distressing symptoms, provision of respite and care through death and bereavement.
>
> (ACT/RCPCH, 2003: 9)

When curative treatment is no longer possible, families require support from trusted professionals, enabling them to make informed choices about their child's palliative care. The majority of children and families opt to be at home during the palliative phase of care and to achieve this, the following are essential requirements for care:

- partnership in care;
- 24-hour access to expertise in paediatric and family care;
- 24-hour access to expertise in paediatric palliative care;
- a trusted professional as a key worker to co-ordinate care;
- immediate access to hospital.

Symptom management

CNS tumours are the commonest cause of death in the paediatric oncology population, and studies have demonstrated that a high incidence of neurological symptoms can be very distressing to the child, family and carers. Managing evolving symptoms can be challenging but these can be anticipated during the palliative phase of a child's care. Symptom guidelines are drawn up reflecting the site of the tumour, likely signs and symptoms and a step-wise approach to medication. These symptoms may include: headache, nausea and vomiting, progressive disability, visual deterioration, behavioural changes, seizures and dysphagia.

Considerable responsibility falls to parents when their child dies at home and strong professional support is essential. With careful planning and good team working, symptoms can be predicted and managed effectively, ensuring that children die peacefully in an environment where they feel most secure.

Psychological care

Although some parents may want to 'protect' children from the knowledge that they are going to die, it has long been recognised that children who are terminally ill invariably know. Silence can result in unnecessary suffering and many fears. With support, children of a very young age are able to work through their fears and anxieties, and obtain a sense of peace. Some children even have the ability to make their wishes for their death or funeral known to their family.

Siblings

It is widely acknowledged that siblings benefit in the long term from being involved in end-of-life care. At a time when parents are understandably overwhelmed with grief and preoccupied with their dying child, siblings are often left to stay with extended family or friends as measures to protect them from the reality of death. It is common for parents to presume that their healthy children are too young to understand, yet research has demonstrated that even young children have a concept of death and some of the protective measures taken by parents can actually hinder siblings' bereavement process. If they do not deal with their grief in childhood, it may interfere with the bereavement process, resulting in complex problems later in life.

Bereavement follow-up

After bereavement, the CNS service often supports the family with visits and telephone calls for a minimum of one year in order to cover all their personal anniversaries. This support is occasionally required into the second year. A point of contact is always made available, but it is essential for the professionals to withdraw, and not hinder the family's endeavours to make progress. Where necessary, families may be referred to professional bereavement support agencies or professional counselling services.

The future of neuro-oncology

It is predicted that the management of childhood brain tumours will change dramatically within the next few years (Packer & Reddy, 2004). While current treatments have improved outcomes in some brain tumours, progress in the management of CNS tumours generally has been modest when compared to advances in other childhood malignancies (Stiller & Bleyer, 2004). Advances in surgery, radiotherapy and chemotherapy are likely to marginally improve survival, and possibly improve quality of life for long-term survivors (Packer & Reddy, 2004) but a greater biological understanding of CNS tumours is key to the identification of new targets of treatment

(Walker *et al.*, 2004). As molecular factors underlying CNS tumours are better understood, it is envisaged that molecular-targeted therapy will become a major modality of treatment (Packer & Reddy, 2004).

Research to establish means by which to measure health-related quality of life (HRQL) is also essential in the future of neuro-oncology. It is recommended that this information is discussed prospectively, with parent and child questionnaires being one way of achieving this. Meanwhile, the question of how the collection and interpretation of data can impact on the lives of children and families urgently needs to be addressed.

The residual disability for children with CNS tumours is life-long, which clearly impacts greatly on the child's and family's psychological and social functioning. Coping with disability is not static or permanent and therefore providing on-going support is the key to the child and family's future. Despite a substantial growth in HRQL studies in children with cancer, further effort is needed to investigate how data can inform practitioners of the lived experience of children and therefore facilitate optimal on-going support from childhood and beyond.

References

Ainsworth H (1989) 'The nursing care of children undergoing craniotomy' *Nursing* 3(33): 5–7

Anderson NE (2003) 'Late complications in childhood central nervous system tumour survivors' *Current Opinion in Neurology* 16(6): 677–683

Arber A & Gallaher A (2003) 'Breaking bad news revisited: the push for negotiated disclosure and changing practice implications' *International Journal of Palliative Nursing* 9(4): 166–172

Association for Children with Life-limiting or Terminal Conditions and Their Families (ACT) & the Royal College of Paediatrics and Child Health (RCPCH) (2003) *A Guide to Development of Children's Palliative Care Services* (2nd edn). Bristol: ACT

Back MR, Hu B, Rutgers J *et al.* (2005) 'Metastasis of an intracranial germinoma through a ventriculoperitoneal shunt: recurrence as a yolk cell tumor' *Pediatric Surgery International* 12(1): 24–27

Baile WF, Buckman R, Lenzi R, Glober G, Beale EA & Delka AP (2000) 'SIKES – A six-step protocol for delivering bad news: application to the patient with cancer' *Oncologist* 5(4): 302–311

Blaney SM, Berg SL & Boddy AV (2004) 'Drug delivery' *in*: Walker D, Perilongo G, Punt J & Taylor R (eds) *Brain and Spinal Tumours of Childhood*. London: Arnold, pp. 228–245

Bunin G (2003) 'What causes childhood brain tumours? Limited knowledge, many clues' *Pediatric Neurosurgery* 32(6): 321–326

Byrne J (1996) 'The epidemiology of brain tumours in children' paper presented in the 7th International Paediatric Symposium for Pediatric Neuro Oncology, Washington, DC, Children's National Medical Center

Chumas P, Tyagi A & Livingstone J (2001) 'Hydrocephalus – what's new?' *Archives of Disease Child Fetal Neonatal Ed* 85: F149–154

Cooley C, Adeodus S, Aldred H, Besley S, Leung A & Thacker. L (2000) 'Paediatric palliative care: a lack of research-based evidence' *International Journal of Palliative Nursing* 6(7): 346–351

Copeland DR, Dowell RE & Fletcher JM (1999) 'Improved neuropsychological outcome in children with brain tumour, diagnosed during infancy and treated without intracranial radiation' *Journal of Child Neurology* 3(1): 53–62

Coyne I (2006) 'Consultation with children in hospital: children's, parents' and nurses' perspectives' *Journal of Clinical Nursing* 15(1): 61–71

De Amorim e Silva CJT, MacKenzie A *et al.* (2006) 'Practice MRI: Reducing the need for sedation and general anaesthesia in children undergoing MRI' *Australian Radiology* 50(4): 319–323

De Sousa C, May L & McGivern V (2004) 'Physical care, rehabilitation and complementary therapies' *in*: Walker D, Perilongo G, Punt J & Taylor R (eds) *Brain and Spinal Tumours of Childhood*. London: Arnold, pp. 463–480

Dix A (2004) 'Clinical management: where medicine meets play: let us play' *Health Service Journal* 114(5200): 26–27

Drake JM, Kestle JLW & Tuli S (2000) 'CSF shunts 50 years on – past, present and future' *Child's Nervous System* 16: 10–11

Drake JM & Sainte-Rose C (1995) *The Shunt Book*. New York: Blackwell Scientific

Dugdale A (2002) 'Child's play' *Emergency Nurse* 10(8): 19–20

Edgeworth J, Bullock P, Bailey P, Gallagher A & Crouchman M (1996) 'Why are brain tumours still being missed?' *Archives of Childhood Diseases* 74: 148–151

Farmer JP, Montes JL, Freeman CR, Meagher-Villemure K, Bond MC & O'Gorman AM (2001) 'Brainstem glioma: a 10 year institutional review' *Pediatric Neurosurgery* 34(4): 206–214

Fisher S (1999) 'Multidisciplinary teamwork' *in*: Guerrero D (ed.) *Neuro-Oncology for Nurses.* London: Whurr Publishers, pp. 36–37

Freeman PH, O'Dell C & Meola C (2003) 'Childhood brain tumours: parental concerns and stressors by phase of illness' *Journal of Pediatric Oncology Nursing* 21: 87–97

French JA & Gidal BE (2000) 'Antiepileptic drug interactions' *Epilepsia* 41(8): 530–536

Giovanola J (2005) 'Sibling involvement at the end of life' *Journal of Pediatric Oncology Nursing* 22(4): 222–226

Glaser A & Buxton N (1997) 'Corticosteroids in the management of central nervous system tumours' *Archives of Diseases in Childhood* 76(1): 320–324

Gleeson HK & Shalet SM (2004) 'The impact of cancer therapy on the endocrine system in survivors of childhood brain tumour' *Endocrine-Related Cancer* 11: 589–602

Grabb PA, Albright AL & Pang D (1992) 'Dissemination of supratentorial malignant gliomas via cerebrospinal fluid in children' *Neurosurgery* 30(1): 64–71

Greenberg ML, Hargrave D & Bond J (2004) 'Information needs for children and families' *in*: Walker D, Perilongo G, Punt J & Taylor R (eds) *Brain and Spinal Tumours of Childhood.* London: Arnold, pp. 501–521

Greenburg A (2005) 'Therapeutic play: developing humor in the nurse–patient relationship' *Journal of the New York State Nurses Association* 34(1): 25–31

Guerrero D (2005) 'Understanding the side effects of cranial irradiation and informing patients and carers' *British Journal of Neuroscience Nursing* 1 (3): 118–121

Hendricks-Ferguson VL (2000) 'Crisis intervention strategies when caring for families of children with cancer' *Journal of Pediatric Oncology Nursing* 17: 3–11

Jaspan T (2004) 'Diagnostic imaging' *in*: Walker D, Perilongo G, Punt J & Taylor R (eds) *Brain and Spinal Tumours of Childhood.* London: Arnold, pp. 108–162

Kennedy CR & Leyland K (1999) 'Comparison of screening instruments for disability and emotional/behavioural disorders with generic measure of health-related quality of life in survivors of childhood brain tumours' *International Journal of Cancer* 12:106–111

Kirsch DG & Tarbell NJ (2004) 'Conformal radiation therapy for childhood CNS tumours' *The Oncologist* 9(4): 442–450

Koeller K & Rushing E (2003) 'Medulloblastoma: a comprehensive review' *Radiographics* 23: 1613–1637

Kortmann RD, Freeman CR & Taylor RE (2004) 'Radiotherapy techniques' *in*: Walker D, Perilongo G,

Punt J & Taylor R (eds) *Brain and Spinal Tumours of Childhood.* London: Arnold, pp. 188–213

Lawlor P (2003) 'The importance of play in the A and E setting' *Irish Nurse* 15(10): 22–23

May L (2001) *Paediatric Neurosurgery: A Handbook for the Multidisciplinary Team.* London: Whurr Publishers, pp. 79–80

Mazzini MJ & Glode LM (2001) 'Internet oncology: increased benefit and risk for patients and oncologists' *Haematological Oncology Clinics of North America* 15(3): 583–592

McCann M & Kain Z (2001) 'The management of preoperative anxiety in children: an update' *Anesthesiology Analgesia* 93: 98–105

National Institute for Health and Clinical Excellence (NICE) (2005) *NICE Guidelines Set to Improve Services for Children and Young People with Cancer.* London: National Institute for Health and Clinical Excellence, No. 1

National Institute for Health and Clinical Excellence (NICE) (2006) 'Improving outcomes for people with brain tumours and other CNS tumours' *in*: NICE (ed.) *The Manual: NICE 2006/032.* Issued 28 June

Nazar G, Hoffman J & Becker E (1990) 'Infratentorial ependymomas in childhood: prognostic factors and treatment' *Journal of Neurosurgery* 72(3): 408–417

Oakhill A (ed.) (1988) *The Supportive Care of the Child with Cancer.* Bristol: IOP Publishing

Packer RJ, Gurney JG, Punko JA & Inskip PDl (2003) 'Long-term neurologic and neurosensory sequelae in adult survivors of a childhood brain tumour: Childhood Cancer Survivor Study' *Journal for Clinical Oncology* 21(17): 716–721

Packer RJ & Reddy A (2004) 'New treatments in paediatric brain tumours: current treatment options' *Neurology* 6(5): 337–389

Pressdee D, May L, Eastman E & Grier D (1997) 'The use of play therapy in the preparation of children undergoing MR imaging' *Clinical Radiology* 52(12): 945–957

Price J, McNeilly P & McFarlane M (2005) 'Paediatric palliative care in the UK: past, present and future' *International Journal of Palliative Nursing* 11(3): 124–126

Rilliet B & Vernot O (2000) 'Gliomas in children: a review' *Child's Nervous System* 16: 735–741

Robertson CM, Hawkins MM & Kingston JE (1994) 'Late deaths and survival after childhood cancer: implications for cure' *BMJ* 309(6948): 162–167

Rutka J & Kuo J (2004) 'Pediatric surgical neuro-oncology: current best care practices and strategies' *Journal of Neuro-Oncology* 69: 139–150

Savage RC, Ross BJ, Walker S & Wicks B (2004) 'Cognitive developments and educational rehabilitation'.*in*: Walker D, Perilongo G, Punt J & Taylor R (eds) *Brain and Spinal Tumours of Childhood*. London: Arnold, pp. 482–493

Spoudeas H & Kirkham FJ (2004) 'Toxicity and late effects' *in*: Walker D, Perilongo G, Punt J & Taylor R (eds) *Brain and Spinal Tumours of Childhood*. London: Arnold, pp. 433–463

Steinbok P, Cochrane D, Perrin R & Price A (2003) 'Mutism after posterior fossa tumour resection in children: incomplete recovery on long term follow up' *Pediatric Neurosurgery 39*(4): 179–183

Stiller CA & Bleyer WA (2004) 'Epidemiology' *in*: Walker D, Perilongo G, Punt J & Taylor R (eds) *Brain and Spinal Tumours of Childhood*. London: Arnold, pp. 35–50

Walker D (2004) 'Introduction' *in*: Walker D, Perilonogo G, Punt J & Taylor R (eds) *Brain and Spinal Tumours of Childhood*. London: Arnold, pp. 1–2

Walker D, Perilongo G, Punt JAG & Taylor RE (2004a) 'Future challenges' *in*: Walker D, Perilongo G, Punt J & Taylor R (eds) *Brain and Spinal Tumours of Childhood*. London: Arnold, pp. 515–521

Walker D, Punt J & Sokal M (2004b) 'Brainstem tumours' *in*: Walker D, Perilongo G, Punt J & Taylor R (eds) *Brain and Spinal Tumours of Childhood*. London: Arnold, pp. 291–314

Woon R (2004) 'Hospital play therapy; helping children cope with hospitalisation through therapeutic play' *Singapore Nursing Journal 31*(1): 16–19

Commentary

Primary Bone Cancer in Young People

Lin Russell

Only in 2006 were four cancers identified as 'true' teenage cancers (O'Dowd, 2006): osteosarcoma, Ewing's sarcoma, Hodgkin's lymphoma and germ cell tumours. Chapter 17 gives an excellent introduction to the two commonest primary bone malignancies.

Both these bone sarcomas most commonly affect young children and adolescents, whose needs are complex and hence provide a challenge to those who care for them. The author gives the reader an overview of the aetiology, investigative scans, blood tests and a comprehensive account of varied tumour protocols. These tumours are mostly treated with both chemotherapy and surgery, treatments which have many side effects and complications. These are discussed alongside the particular psychosocial needs of this client group. A diagnosis of cancer is a devastating one, even more so for a child or adolescent. Any member of a multidisciplinary team caring for these young cancer patients will find this a useful reference guide. It gives background information on care and informs the reader of the current health-care policy document and strategies which are at the forefront of contemporary health care. Due to the long treatment protocols these patients undergo and the need for regular blood tests in between chemotherapy cycles, many of these will be undertaken in the primary care setting, so this chapter will also be of interest to nurses and allied health-care professionals working within this setting.

Bone sarcomas are rare and often the initial phase of the cancer journey for both the child and their family is a long and complex one. This necessitates joint working both within and across cancer networks and shared between primary and secondary care. For at least two decades there has been a small number of supra-regional units across the country to treat these rare tumours. These preceded recommendations from the Chief Medical Officer (CMO) of Wales aimed at addressing deficiencies in the delivery of cancer services and improving patient outcomes (Calman & Hine, 1995). These recommendations have been implemented across England with the introduction of cancer centres and cancer units.

Patients with suspected sarcomas should be referred to a recognised bone cancer centre for diagnosis and management. These include patients whose symptoms are increasing, unexplained and persistent bone pain or tenderness, particularly at rest (and especially if not in the joint) or an unexplained limp. These should urgently be investigated by the primary health professional (DoH, 2000c). This approach is also supported by the guidance for children and young people

Cancer in Children and Young People   Edited by Faith Gibson and Louise Soanes
© 2008 John Wiley & Sons, Ltd

with cancer. They advise that persistent symptoms reported by the child or the parent (as they are usually the best observer of symptoms), or persistent parental anxiety, is a sufficient reason for referral, even if the health professional thinks it is most likely benign (NICE, 2005).

2006 saw the publication of the NICE *Guidelines for Sarcoma* (NICE, 2006) which complements recommendations made in 2005 to improve outcomes in children and young people with cancer (NICE, 2005). The development of the 'key worker' to support and be pivotal in the care pathway has been one of the most important recommendations from both publications supplementing the vision for cancer care as outlined in *The NHS Cancer Plan* (DoH, 2000b). The author describes the ways in which informed consent and patient education are essential and the role of the key worker is complex and diverse. This role is often undertaken by the specialist nurse or allied health professionals who have a wide and diverse range of skills. It is described how the key worker will:

- have in-depth specialist knowledge about sarcoma;
- act as an advocate;
- co-ordinate the diagnostic pathway;
- provide continuity;
- ensure the patient can access information and advice;
- be a core member of the multidisciplinary team;
- liaise with primary care.

The author emphasises the nurse's role as a key worker in providing an individual approach to disseminating information, supporting, listening and advising.

The cancer trajectory for young people diagnosed with a bone tumour is described in this chapter, and begins at the point of a clinical diagnosis. The reported delay in diagnosis may be accounted for by the low index of suspicion in both the primary and secondary care setting. Many patients make repeated visits to their general practitioner (GP) and due to the rarity of these tumours may be treated with simple analgesia and rest prior to being referred to a specialist team. Many young people may present themselves at their local accident and emergency department where they may often see the most junior doctor and have X-rays interpreted by a non-

specialist radiologist. This, alongside numerous differential diagnoses including, osteomyelitis and stress fractures, may account for significant delays in diagnosis. In 2000, the Department of Health issued suspected cancer referral guidelines including sarcoma. These guidelines were written by experts in the relative fields and circulated to all general practitioners to raise awareness and to encourage early referral (DOH, 2000c).

Once diagnosis has been established, the wide range of surgical options needs to be carefully considered. These we learn in the chapter will be dependent on the size and site of the tumour, the long-term prognosis and the child's interests and hobbies. As alluded to, endoprosthesis is not conducive to contact sports, football and rugby for example, but amputation, although a radical treatment, may in such cases be the treatment of choice. It is often seen as a failed option. However, as the author discusses, successful chemotherapy regimens have resulted in a decrease in the need for amputation and wider use of limb salvage.

All surgical treatments have differing problems and complications, for example, the child with a good prognosis may achieve a better long-term functional outcome with few complications and less need for future operations with an allograft as opposed to endoprosthesis. However, predicting long-term survival is not easy, those with a poor prognosis may benefit from a more 'quick-fix' option that is achieved by implanting an endoprosthesis. Many patients cannot believe they will survive and this again may influence the type of surgery they have. The same principle can be applied to the need to bank sperm. For example, a 14-year-old might not be focused on long-term relationships and wanting children at the time of diagnosis. We begin to understand the supportive and informative role the key worker will take.

The chapter discussed the length of time some patients undergo treatment, for some up to one year. This poses numerous ongoing problems for young people, schooling, peer pressure, physical body changes and misconceptions, often including 'can you catch cancer?' which may lead to loss of friends and isolation (NICE, 2005).

The government published *The NHS Cancer Plan* in 2000 (DoH, 2000b) outlining the vision for cancer care for the future. Included in this vision were the targets to reduce waiting times for patients accessing cancer services, specifically urgent referral by the general practitioner to a first appointment with a cancer specialist within 14 days and a target of 31 days to the commencement of treatment for children: this was to be mandatory for all cancers by 2005. These targets have therefore concentrated the efforts of health-care professionals and management alike on improving care for our client group. The average GP will normally not see a bone tumour in his working career. However, it must also be acknowledged that the patient themselves may delay before seeking medical assistance. Llewellyn *et al.* (2004) found that younger patients who considered themselves to be at low risk of cancer often mislabelled symptoms as insignificant. Goyal *et al.* (2004) also found that age influenced delay; in this study they compared children under and over the age of 12, and it was shown that the older age group demonstrated longer delay than the younger group. It was acknowledged, however, that this may be due to parental reporting of symptoms in the younger age group, as opposed to self-reporting among the adolescents in the older group.

Communication skills are key features for those professionals caring for cancer patients and services are measured against set standards which include advanced communication skills. Breaking bad news is an aspect of patient care which, if managed badly, can have profound effects. Buckman (1996) gives a definition of bad news as 'any news that drastically alters or changes the person's view of his or her future'.

Woolley *et al.* (1989), although a relatively dated study now, discuss how to break bad news to parents of children with an illness, and identified that, even years later, the memory of the discussion with the doctor about the illness lived on. This was even the case when patients were satisfied with the way it was given. This therefore highlights further what a dramatic effect the process of breaking bad news can have. Baile *et al.* (2000) have developed a step-by-step technique for clinical staff to follow in supporting patients through this difficult process.

Training and continuing professional development are key factors in maintaining and improving standards of care. NICE (2006, p. 97) states,

'Training should be developed and provided for all members of the core and extended multidisciplinary team.' Supportive information must also continue to develop and should be provided in a variety of formats and supported by information access on line.

The author describes surgical advances made in the past two decades especially with metal replacements. Advances in technology have meant improvements in patients' function, and a reduction in complications. The introduction of the hydroxiapatite collar has significantly reduced aseptic loosening (Unwin *et al.*, 1996; Grimer, 2005). The new non-invasive grower now reduces the number of operations, general anaesthetics and hospital admissions for young people. It can be lengthened in the outpatient setting by specialist nurses or physiotherapists. In two specialist centres where these health-care professionals perform such lengthenings, there is continuity of care as these nurses will be well known to the patient, having seen them on numerous occasions throughout their cancer journey.

Future developments will also include further research into anti-neoplastic drugs, for example Imatinib, an agent currently licensed for the treatment of newly diagnosed chronic myeloid leukaemia. Imatinib is a protein-tyrosine kinase inhibitor which may also inhibit the proliferation of Ewing's tumour cells mediated by the stem cell factor/KIT receptor pathway, and sensitises cells to vincristine and doxorubicin-induced apoptosis (cell death) (Gonzalez *et al.*, 2005). More studies need to be carried out to see if the different chromosomal translocations seen in Ewing's sarcoma have any influence on prognosis.

Challenges for the future include better provision of cancer care for children and adolescents. At present there are seven teenage cancer units across the country, all funded by the Teenage Cancer Trust. Transitional care for those entering adulthood and moving to adult services is also at the forefront of current policy (RCN, 2004). The incidence of children's cancer is on the increase from 15.4 % per 100,000 of the population in 1979 to 19.8 % in 2000 (O'Dowd, 2006), therefore service provision must also increase.

There has been a rapid growth in cancer nursing initially as a result of the Calman–Hine Report (1995) and latterly the improving outcomes guidance. Specialist nursing roles have developed exponentially in both primary and secondary care. A specialist, as described by Casteldine and McGee (1998), is someone who focuses their knowledge and skill on the specific medical and nursing needs of a particular client group. Sarcoma patients cross the boundaries of a number of sub-specialties, orthopaedics, oncology and care of the adolescent, resulting in a dearth of literature giving the reader such a broad overview of the patho-physiology and treatment options.

This chapter provides an excellent reference guide to enhance the knowledge of both nurses and other health professionals who will be supporting this client group throughout their cancer journey and are fundamental to the delivery of high quality care.

References

Baile W, Buckman R, *et al.* (2000) 'SPIKES – A six step protocol for delivering bad news: application to the patient with cancer' *The Oncologist* 5(4): 302–311

Buckman R (1996) 'Talking to patients about cancer' *British Medical Journal* 313: 699–700

Calman K & Hine D (1995) *A Policy Framework for Commissioning Cancer Services: A Report by the Expert Advisory Group on Cancer to the Chief Medical Officers of England and Wales*. London: Department of Health

Casteldine G & McGee P (eds) (1998) *Advanced and Specialist Nursing Practice*. Oxford: Blackwell Science

Department of Health (2000a) *The NHS Plan*. London: Department of Health

Department of Health (2000b) *The NHS Cancer Plan*. London: Department of Health

Department of Health (2000c) *Referral Guidelines for Suspected Cancer*. London: Department of Health

Gonzalez I, Andreu E, Panzio A, Inoges S, Fontalba A, Fernandez-Luna J, Gaboli M, Sierrasesumaga L, Martin-Algarra S, Pardo J, Prosper F & De Alava E (2005) 'Imatinib inhibits proliferation of Ewing tumor cells mediated by the stem cell factor/KIT receptor pathway, and sensitizes cells to vincristine and doxorubicin-induced apoptosis' *Clinical Cancer Research* 10: 751–761

Goyal S, Roscoe J, Ryder WDJ, Gattamaneni HR & Eden TOB (2004) 'Symptom interval in people with bone cancer' *European Journal of Cancer* 40: 2280–2286

Grimer R (2005) 'Osteosarcoma and surgery' *in*: Eden T, Barr R, Bleyer A & Whiteson M (eds) *Cancer and the Adolescent*. Oxford: Blackwell, pp. 121–129

Llewellyn CD, Johnson NW & Warnakulasuriya S (2004) 'Factors associated with delay in presentation among younger patients with oral cancer' *Oral Medicine, Oral Surgery, Oral Pathology* 97(6): 707–713

National Institute for Health and Clinical Excellence (2005) *Improving Outcomes in Children and Young People with Cancer*. London: NICE Cancer Service Guidance

National Institute of Clinical Excellence (2006) *Improving Outcomes for People with Sarcoma*. London: NICE Cancer Service Guidance

O'Dowd A. (2006) 'Clinical: true teen cancers identified' *Nursing Times*. 102(14): 8

RCN (2004) *Adolescent Transitional Care: Guidance for Nursing Staff*. London: RCN

Unwin P, Cannon S, Grimer R, Kemp H, Sneath R & Walker P (1996) 'Aseptic loosening in cemented custom-made prosthestic replacements for bone tumours of the lower limb' *Journal of Bone and Joint Surgery* 78-B(1): 5–13

Woolley H, Stein A, Forrest GC & Baum JD (1989) 'Imparting the diagnosis of life threatening illness in children' *BMJ* 298: 1623–1626

17 Primary Bone Cancer in Young People

Chris Henry

Introduction

Primary malignant bone sarcomas are rare but account for the second most common cause of death in young people after brain tumours, and are the fourth commonest malignancy (Whelan, 2005). They only occasionally occur under the age of 5 with a peak incidence aged 13–19 years. The male to female ratio is lower in the younger age group and higher in young adults, which may be linked to adolescent growth spurts (Birch, 2005). The two main types that occur in young people are osteosarcoma and Ewing's sarcoma, which are treated with adjuvant chemotherapy combined with surgery and/or radiotherapy. The five-year survival rate of 58% for young people with osteosarcoma in Europe has not improved since the 1980s, in spite of advances in molecular biology (Whelan, 2005). However, progress has been made in Ewing's sarcoma with an increase in five-year survival from less than 50% in the 1980s to more than 50% in the 1990s (Gatta et al., 2005).

Little is known about the cause of primary bone cancer and therefore few risk factors have been identified. High doses of irradiation have been linked to bone cancer but there was no increased incidence in the survivors of the atomic bomb in Japan (Piasecki, 1987). Radiation-induced bone sarcoma is more likely to occur in children as a complication of cancer treatment. Osteosarcoma of the jaw was reported to be more common in workers in the luminous watch dial trade who frequently pointed the tips of their brushes contaminated with radioactive material in their mouths (Souhami & Tobias, 1986). More recently, the possibility of a viral connection with osteosarcoma has been considered (Birch, 2005).

The incidence of bone cancer in young people is low and peaks during adolescence, representing 10–14% of cancers in the 13–19 age group. There has been a significant increase in Ewing's sarcoma in the past decade (Birch, 2005). It has been suggested that there could be a link with the rapid rate of growth in limb bones at this age and research has shown that a significant number of young people with osteosarcoma are taller than their average peers (Jurgens et al.1992; Craft, 2005). The site of the tumour in the skeleton may have a bearing on the prognosis. Patients with distal tumours appear to have a better outlook than those with more proximal tumours (Schwartz et al., 1993; Grimer, 2005). Tumours arising in the pelvic bones often present at a later stage, as the signs and symptoms may be less pronounced initially. As a

Cancer in Children and Young People   Edited by Faith Gibson and Louise Soanes
© 2008 John Wiley & Sons, Ltd

result, there may be a larger volume of tumour, with an increased risk of metastatic spread, making surgical management more challenging (Hosalkar & Dormans, 2005).

The highest incidence of osteosarcoma has been seen in Brazil. There is also a high rate in Italy, Finland and among Black Americans in the United States, whereas low incidence occurs in Japan, India, Hungary and Cuba (Mertens & Bramwell, 1994). Ewing's sarcoma is rare in Africans, Black Americans and the Chinese population (Schwartz et al., 1993; Birch, 2005).

Genetic factors may be significant in both osteosarcoma and Ewing's sarcoma. Current research into the molecular origins of cancer shows that young people with a history of hereditary retinoblastoma have an increased risk of developing osteosarcoma as a second primary tumour, as both tumours have the same genetic deletion in the same DNA sequence (Piasecki, 1992; Raymond et al., 2002). It has also been shown that osteosarcoma is one of the tumours that can occur in Li-Fraumeni cancer families. The main features of these families are soft tissue sarcomas in young people with the early onset of breast cancer in their mothers and close relatives, and are due to a TP53 gene germ-line mutation (Porter et al., 1992). The variation of the incidence of Ewing's sarcoma with ethnic origin may also be linked to genetic factors.

A variety of chemotherapy drugs, including high-dose methotrexate, cisplatin, doxorubicin, ifosfamide and etoposide, have been shown to be effective against both osteosarcoma and Ewing's sarcoma. Previous studies from the European Osteosarcoma Intergroup (EOI) have indicated that dose intensity, that is, the amount of drug given in a period of time, may be an important factor in disease-free survival (Ornadel et al., 1994). It has been possible to increase the dose intensity of certain drugs, by the availability of haemopoetic growth factors, such as granulocyte colony-stimulating factor (G-CSF), which can reduce the duration of myelosuppression (Craft, 2005). However, dose intensification has also shown serious side effects with no significant improvement in disease-free survival (Craft, 2005). Preliminary results from a randomised trial for osteosarcoma completed in 2003 showed no advantage in survival with an increased dose intensity of 25% (Whelan, 2005). Neutropenia may cause

delay or reduced doses of chemotherapy and put young people at risk of severe infections. The use of G-CSF to enable planned doses of chemotherapy to be given on time may be associated with better clinical outcomes (White et al., 2005). Clinical trials are important to elucidate the most effective combination of drugs and the optimal length of treatment.

Primary chemotherapy following diagnosis was established to allow time for an endoprosthesis to be made, and it has enabled the study of the efficacy of the drugs on the tumour at the time of its resection. It is accepted that 90% necrosis with 10% or less of viable tumour present indicates a good response to pre-operative chemotherapy while more than 10% of viable tumour left is considered a poor response (Jurgens et al., 1992; Hosalkar & Dormans, 2005; Whelan, 2005).

The increasing success of achieving tumour necrosis through the use of chemotherapy has resulted in a decrease in the need for amputation, the wider use of limb conservation surgery and its subsequent development. Studies show that limb conservation surgery, using autografts, allografts or endoprostheses, offers the same chance of survival as amputation, although there is a small risk of local recurrence. Although this is a significant risk factor for survival, it is less important than the response to chemotherapy (Grimer, 2005). The use of allografts, however, has been associated with more complications, especially in relation to infection, fractures and non-union (Roberts et al., 1991; Grimer, 2005).

Advances in surgical techniques have had an important effect on the treatment of young people with pelvic tumours. Wide local excision with bone grafting or the insertion of a hemi-pelvic endoprosthesis is now possible, and this has had a positive effect on both the function and prognosis of these patients. Previous treatment by chemotherapy and local radiotherapy, without surgery, has shown a greater risk of recurrence.

The treatment of lung metastases in young people with bone tumours has been improved by surgery. A metastatectomy via single or bilateral thoracotomies may be combined with further chemotherapy. Patients free of primary osteosarcoma with resectable lung metastases have shown event-free survival of 24% (Bacci et al., 2002).

Jurgens *et al.* (1992) suggest that this is of little value in patients with Ewing's sarcoma, as the presence of metastases is a reflection of resistance to chemotherapy at other sites.

Types of tumours and their presentation

Osteosarcoma

Osteosarcoma is the commonest primary bone tumour in young people, arising in the medullary cavity, with 91% in the metaphysis or ends of long bones, although this pattern changes with age (Raymond *et al.*, 2002). The commonest sites affected are the distal femur, proximal tibia and proximal humerus (Salisbury and Byers, 1994). The tumour mainly consists of malignant bone-producing cells called osteoblasts, which are subject to wide variations. These cells invade and destroy the cortex of the bone, and then find resistance to the outer covering of the bone called the periosteum. As the tumour continues to grow within a restricted area, a sun-ray pattern of new bone is formed. The periosteum responds by laying down a wedge of bone at the angle where it is pushed away from the bone. This angle of elevation is called the Codman's triangle (Figure 17.1). Both these phenomena can be seen on plain X-ray films with the tumour bone sometimes giving the appearance of cloud-like densities (Wittig *et al.*, 2002). Occasionally, a non-contiguous lesion may occur in the same bone as the primary site or in an adjacent bone. This is called a skip metastasis (Raymond *et al.*, 2002). A pathological fracture may occur in 5–10% of cases. Response to pre-operative chemotherapy is the most sensitive indicator of survival.

Ewing's sarcoma

Ewing's sarcoma is the fourth commonest primary bone tumour but the second most common in young people with 80% occurring under the age of 20 years (Ushigome *et al.*, 2002). The tumour usually arises in the diaphysis or shaft of a long bone but can also occur in other bones such as the scapula, pelvis and spine. It consists of round

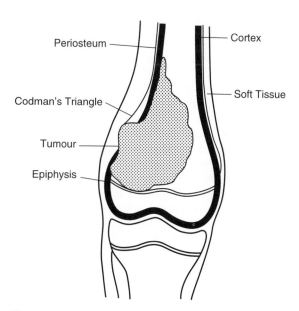

Figure 17.1   Osteosarcoma in the distal femur.

cells of unknown aetiology, and has a moth-eaten appearance on X-ray (Salisbury and Byers, 1994). Sometimes the periosteum resists the tumour and demonstrates an 'onion skin' layered appearance. It may also show a Codman's triangle, although this is more commonly seen in osteosarcoma. Ewing's sarcoma usually spreads into the soft tissues quicker than in osteosarcoma, and may be extensive. Unlike osteosarcoma, this tumour is sensitive to radiotherapy as well as chemotherapy and, although no longer used as first-line treatment, radiotherapy may be needed following a marginal excision of the tumour if there is less than a wide margin or if there is <90% necrosis.

Young patients may present with a history of fever and night sweats, especially in disseminated disease and blood tests may show leucocytosis and a raised ESR (Ushigome *et al.*, 2002). This, together with a low level of suspicion and inadequate biopsies, has led to a number of misdiagnoses of osteomyelitis (Tow & Tan, 2005).

Bone marrow aspirates are taken to screen for bone marrow infiltration. If these are present, high-risk patients may be considered for very high-dose chemotherapy with autologous bone marrow or peripheral blood stem cell support. Although high response rates have been recorded with the use of these melphalan-containing regimens, the role of very high-dose chemotherapy with bone marrow rescue is still uncertain and is being evaluated through clinical trials (Jurgens *et al.*, 1992; Craft, 2005).

Two important prognostic features have emerged from clinical trials for the treatment of Ewing's sarcoma. Metastatic disease at the time of diagnosis and poor response to initial chemotherapy show decreased disease-free survival. Other prognostic factors of less importance at diagnosis are tumour size of more than 8 cm, site of tumour, raised levels of lactose dehydrogenase (LDH), a high white blood cell count and a raised erythrocyte sedimentation rate (Schwartz *et al.*, 1993; Salisbury & Byers, 1994; Craft, 2005).

Patient history

Young people may first see their doctor after a minor trauma, which has drawn attention to a painful area. They may first notice an ache in the affected part, which increases in severity to become painful enough to wake them at night. Night pain should not be dismissed as 'growing pains' especially if it is only in one limb (Wittig *et al.*, 2002). The pain is usually localised to the tumour but may radiate elsewhere if it causes pressure on a nerve, especially in the sacral area of the spine. The sudden onset of pain may indicate a pathological fracture.

Because of the rarity of the tumours, a complaint of discomfort above or below the knee may not be immediately investigated and may be regarded as muscular strain from sporting activities. A study by Grimer and Sneath (1990) showed that, on average, a young person with osteosarcoma waited six weeks before consulting a doctor about the initial pain. It was then a further seven weeks before a diagnosis was made. With Ewing's sarcoma, they waited 21 weeks before deciding to consult a doctor, and 31 weeks for a diagnosis. The causes of delay in diagnosis were a low level of suspicion, inappropriate treatments and failure to detect the condition from X-rays. Currently, in spite of guidelines more recently being widely publicised and available for doctors regarding the key features for the early detection of bone tumours, there is no evidence that this has led to any reduction in the time delay (Grimer, 2005). Unfortunately delay

may lead to a greater bulk of tumour being present at diagnosis, which may indicate a poorer prognosis (Jurgens *et al.*, 1992).

Swelling is usually present at the tumour site, this will be firm, warm and tender to touch. If the tumour is near a joint, there may be limitation and guarding of movement. Other symptoms may include night sweats and recent weight loss. Due to the rarity of these tumours, it is recommended that at this stage, when plain X-ray films indicate a lesion, the young person should be transferred to a principal bone tumour treatment centre to ensure speedy and age-appropriate treatment (National Institute for Health and Clinical Excellence, 2005). The team involved in the surgical removal of the tumour should perform the biopsy (Grimer & Sneath, 1990; Wittig *et al.*, 2002).

Staging

Staging of the tumours may be carried out as an outpatient but if the young person is admitted to the ward for a few days, nursing staff and, if appropriate, play specialists will be able to prepare both patient and family for the various investigations. This ensures that correct information is given, that it is age-appropriate and adapted to the young person's pace and level of understanding and that they can be introduced to the support of the bone tumour team. Young people who receive open information at initial diagnosis have been shown to be less anxious and depressed and have a higher self-esteem than those who received it later (Ishibashi, 2001). Inpatient admission also facilitates a thorough assessment of pain and optimum relief. The use of a non-steroidal anti-inflammatory drug (NSAID) with paracetamol is effective in relieving mild to moderate tumour pain, but may need to be combined with an opiate for the relief of more severe bone and movement-related pain (Hanks, 2005).

Young people value an individual approach as it helps them to keep some control over a new and very frightening situation. The nurse may play a key role in disseminating information, while at the same time supporting, listening and understanding the wide range of emotions that the young person and family may express. They want to live and resent the interruption to normal life. They may show feelings of anger and feel that their normal life could be under threat, and may have difficulty expressing themselves and withdraw or hide behind anti-social or risk-taking behaviour. Adolescence is a critical time for young people to develop a positive sense of self, and this will be severely challenged by changes in body image, disruption of social and educational activities, loss of independence and autonomy and changes in relationships, especially with peers (Woodgate, 2005). If they do not have the opportunity to talk about secret fears and anxieties and off-load some of the emotional burden, they may become isolated (Peck, 1992).

Sharing information with young people poses problems of confidentiality, autonomy and truthfulness. Young people who have witnessed parents being taken to a separate room to be given information without them may express anger, and not believe that they have been told the whole truth. It can be underestimated how well young people are able to absorb and cope with difficult concepts, and this ability is reflected in the deep and searching questions they often ask. Younger children may misunderstand the cause of their illness and have difficulty keeping their friends because of the many myths and taboos about cancer (Ishibashi, 2001). Play can be a useful way to help them understand their illness and prepare them for their investigations and has been shown to reduce levels of distress and increase the young person's confidence and cooperation (Price & Spence, 2004). Trust can only be earned by the sharing of accurate and honest information. One of the most devastating effects of cancer on a young person is the loss of control over life and body; choices need to be made available for them to make decisions about treatments and future management (Peck, 1992; Hokkanen et al., 2004).

The diagnosis of cancer in a young person presents a crisis for all the members of the immediate and extended family. Parents expect to be able to look after and protect their children, and this is challenged by the uncertainty of a life-threatening disease and its associated treatment problems (Sloper, 1996). A full assessment of family and peer relationships, support systems, coping strategies, education, financial and leisure needs should be made before implementing the staging programme. This assessment should be transcultural in nature, with special attention paid to existing beliefs and attitudes to cancer. Theories about the cause of cancer can be significantly affected by culture, which in turn can influence the family's co-operation with the treatment plan (Sensky, 1996; Ishibashi, 2001). Child-rearing practices, family dynamics and the role of women will vary between societies and need consideration when giving information (Bird & Dearmun, 1995).

Families who have a young person with cancer are a high-risk group for family dysfunction, due to the severe stress involved. If family conflict existed prior to diagnosis, the illness increases the tension, making the risk of dysfunction more likely (Friedman, 1987). Illness can have both negative and positive effects on the strength and qualities of relationships, with equally high levels of distress for both fathers and mothers. Besides the effects of the illness and treatments, problems relating to employment, finance and social support place demands on family resources. Sloper (1996) found that these additional factors, rather than aspects of treatment, were more difficult for parents to deal with. Honest and open communication can help to prevent isolation and distancing of relationships within families, and help them to adapt to the inevitable changes in roles and responsibilities.

Language is another important consideration. Young people and their families from ethnic groups may not feel confident about communicating in English, and this may lead to additional stress and frustration (Bird & Dearmun, 1995). In this case, access to interpreters will need to be arranged. Sometimes another member of the family is suggested but this is not appropriate. Careful consideration should be given to who is chosen, as they are given a heavy burden of complicated, difficult and emotional information to impart. Inevitably, they will find this distressing at times and need support and guidance.

Investigations

Routine investigations can include plain X-rays, magnetic resonance imaging (MRI), computerised tomography (CT) of lesion and chest, radionuclide bone scan of the skeleton, blood tests and biopsy.

MRI scanning will show the extent of the tumour in the medulla of the bone and soft tissues, and must be taken before the biopsy and before any treatment is commenced as it can be used to assess cessation of tumour growth following initial doses of chemotherapy. The MRI scan is also important to show the relationship· of the tumour to major nerves and blood vessels, especially the neurovascular bundle behind the knee. If this is encased by tumour, then amputation may be the only surgical option (Wittig *et al.*, 2002). If limb conservation surgery is advised, these scans are used by the biomedical engineering unit, together with measurement films of both affected and unaffected limbs, in the manufacture of custom-made endoprostheses, allowing for the optimal resection of the tumour. Although the MRI scan is non-invasive, young people need to be prepared that they may feel claustrophobic in the tunnel, it can be noisy and because the scan can take up to 45 minutes to complete they may experience pain and stiffness around the tumour site. Consideration should be given to analgesia cover and pain levels should be assessed prior to the procedure.

The bone scan will show the site of the primary tumour and will detect or exclude sites of bone metastases. The presence of distant metastases in the bone, which is the second most common site, indicates late stage disease and is associated with the poorest prognosis (Wittig *et al.*, 2002). A radioactive marker is given intravenously, three hours before the scan, which will detect areas that are metabolically active. These are called 'hot spots' and may indicate the presence of a malignant tumour. Suspected sites should be further investigated with an MRI scan.

The need for a CT scan of the chest introduces the necessary discussion about the possibility of metastases and their first line involvement of the lungs. This may be difficult to approach before a proven diagnosis is established but young people will appreciate the explanation, and it can lead to a discussion about the meaning of malignancy and the reasons for the use of chemotherapy. Approximately 10–20 % of young people will have visible lung metastases on their first CT scan (Jurgens *et al.*, 1992). Unfortunately, the presence of lung metastases at the time of diagnosis indicates a poorer prognosis. This increases the need for support and information about the recent innovations in the successful management of lung metastases, in order to maintain a positive approach

to treatment. Routine blood tests are carried out including serum alkaline phosphatase (SAP) and serum lactic dehyrogenase (LDH). A raised SAP level at diagnosis in osteosarcoma may be one of the factors relating to poorer survival (Grimer, 2005), but a raised LDH level on its own is of less importance (Craft, 2005).

The most important investigation is the biopsy; improperly performed biopsies may cause misdiagnosis, amputation and local recurrence and have a negative impact on survival (Wittig *et al.*, 2002). The biopsy may be incorrectly sited so that conservative surgery cannot encompass it, or correctly positioned for surgical incision but in a site causing muscle contamination (Kemp, 1987). Grimer and Sneath (1990) found that problems relating to biopsy were ten times more common if they were carried out before referral to a tumour treatment centre. Cannon and Dyson (1987) found that local recurrence of tumour occurred in 38 % of cases in which the biopsy site could not be excised. Traditionally, an open biopsy was used to provide adequate material for histologic grading, but in more recent years a Tru-Cut needle core biopsy has been a popular option (Yang & Damron, 2004).

A review of 208 procedures by Stoker *et al.* (1991), showed that a needle biopsy performed by experienced practitioners was both safe and accurate, causing minimal disturbance to the tumour, reduction in morbidity and increased the potential for limb conservation surgery. A needle biopsy into a bony lesion is a painful procedure and a local anaesthetic is inadequate; young people require a general anaesthetic in spite of the associated risks. They should be warned that following the biopsy there may be some residual bleeding into the tumour, causing further swelling, and that this is not the tumour rapidly increasing. Tissue samples from the biopsy require complex, expert analysis and it may be up to two weeks before the results are available. This waiting period of uncertainty is very difficult for families who would benefit from the support of a key worker.

Treatment options

When all the investigations are complete, a decision has to be made promptly about treatment. With the rare exception of a low-grade tumour, all young people diagnosed with either osteosarcoma or Ewing's sarcoma will be referred immediately to a specialist oncology centre for neoadjuvant chemotherapy. Treatment will last for a period of up to nine months. The aim of chemotherapy is to cause tumour necrosis, reduce the volume of the tumour and have an immediate effect on any micrometastases, which might be present (Grimer & Carter, 1995). Combined with chemotherapy will be some form of surgical excision, if possible, generally after two to six cycles of chemotherapy, depending on the protocol, with radiotherapy being introduced, if appropriate, in the later phase of treatment.

This rapid referral for treatment underlines the importance of adequately preparing young people and their families before the diagnosis is established. Part of this preparation involves discussing the options for surgery. If the tumour is growing in close proximity to major blood vessels, then the possibility of amputation needs to be mentioned, even if limb conservation surgery is planned. Failure to mention this will result in anger and loss of confidence with treatment and practitioners if amputation becomes a reality, and does not allow adequate psychological preparation before surgery. The level of tumour response to chemotherapy will determine the options for surgery.

Initially, one of the most upsetting side effects of chemotherapy treatment for young people is the inevitable loss of hair, which is closely related to identity and may be viewed as loss of attractiveness. Loss of hair is a constant reminder of a cancer diagnosis and its visibility may draw negative reactions from society (Kuzbit, 2004). The fact that it is a temporary loss is of little consolation at this early stage and ideas about how other young people have adapted to this major change, such as cutting hair to a shorter style and the use of caps, hats, scarves, bandanas and wigs may help to lessen the impact (for further details, see Chapter 4).

A difficult topic, which needs discussion at this stage, is the possibility that the young person may become sub- or infertile following chemotherapy. This may be embarrassing for young people to talk about and hard to deal with at such a distressing time but issues of sexuality and fertility are of particular importance to the adolescent age group (Kim, 2003). Cisplatin and ifosfamide are two of the drugs that may cause gonadal damage but if a young person requires high-dose chemotherapy with melphalan and busulphan, then the risk of fertility being challenged is very high. Sperm banking facilities exist at most oncology centres but they are not generally adapted for use by young people. The opportunity to sperm bank is not always offered to young people on paediatric oncology wards which lack provision for teenagers (Wallace & Brougham, 2005). Edge et al. (2006) found that 67% of young people questioned had been able to sperm bank but those who were unsuccessful tended to be younger, with a higher level of anxiety at time of diagnosis, less understanding about the issue and had the greater difficulty talking about fertility.

Young female patients are less susceptible to the gonadotoxic effects of chemotherapy for bone cancer and the options if they are pre-pubertal are currently only experimental (Wallace & Brougham, 2005). Sexually mature young females may preserve their fertility by the collection of mature oocytes although this does not always lead to success in pregnancy as the cells are more damaged than if preserved as embryos. This process requires stimulation of the ovaries which takes several weeks and not only would cause an unacceptable delay in starting treatment, but is also only experimental in young people (Spears, 1994; Wallace & Brougham, 2005).

If young people require radiotherapy to pelvic sarcomas as part of their treatment, the temporary insertion of a 'spacer', a fluid-filled bag, to provide some protection to the gonads, may be used. This may be removed at the end of treatment. Careful and sensitive discussion about fertility issues will be needed and in young male patients assessment of sexual maturity, involving discussion with parents if appropriate, to determine which individuals should be counselled for sperm banking (for further details, see Chapter 2).

These are very difficult concepts for a young person to cope with when facing a life-threatening illness, with so much information having to be given in such a short time. However, a rapport built on honesty, sensitivity, empathy, availability and at times, humour, with the multi-disciplinary team, will remain a valuable source of continuing support throughout their long and protracted treatment.

Limb conservation surgery

Limb conservation surgery involves the wide excision of tumour bone and adjacent soft tissues. This bone may be replaced by the insertion of a metal implant called an endoprosthesis, which in young people with osteosarcoma often includes a joint to give adequate clearance from the tumour (Figure 17.2). An endoprosthesis has the option of an extendible telescopic section, which allows equality of growth and will require a minimally or non-invasive technique to lengthen it; however, debate exists as to the minimum age at which they should be used (Jurgens *et al.*, 1992; Piasecki, 1992).

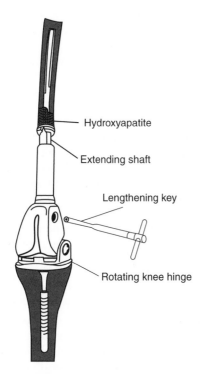

Hydroxyapatite

Extending shaft

Lengthening key

Rotating knee hinge

Figure 17.2   An extending femoral prosthesis.

Endoprostheses are most commonly used to replace tumours in the proximal and distal femur, proximal tibia and proximal humerus. In some instances it may be necessary to replace the whole femur or humerus. Part of the ileum, including acetabulum and proximal femur, may be replaced in pelvic tumours. Alternatively, if the tumour is above the acetabulum, excision of part of the ileum

and grafting with the patient's own fibula may be performed. If the tumour is in the pubic ramus, scapula or fibula, a local wide excision may be all that is required.

Tumours in the diaphysis of the bone where margins of excision do not involve a joint may be treated surgically without the use of endoprostheses. These tumours may be excised and bone transported from another area to be used as bone graft. For example, the patient's own fibula may be used for grafting following excision of a section of tibia. These autografts are much more successful than allografts, which have problems becoming incorporated into the host bone and re-achieving an adequate blood supply (Grimer & Carter, 1995).

Allografts offer a biological reconstruction after resection of the tumour. They are obtained from tissue donors; therefore the tissue is dead and they act as scaffolding (Grimer, 2005). The results are inconsistent and, although growth plates and joints may be preserved, there are problems relating to non-union, fractures, infection and arthritis (Grimer, 2005; Ramseier *et al.*, 2006).

Pre-operative issues

The timing of surgery between phases of chemotherapy requires close co-operation between oncologists and surgeons. Issues of infection and immunosuppression need to be resolved, so that the young person is as medically fit as possible to cope with the procedure and anaesthetic.

Young people may want to discuss fears relating to the anaesthetic and surgery. They commonly ask about waking up during surgery; not waking up at the end; post-operative pain; length of time in bed and restriction of activities. They are pleased to be having the tumour removed and a break from chemotherapy, but often concerned that it is no longer necessary as their pain has resolved with chemotherapy and they are more mobile. They may ask for a picture of the resected tumour for reassurance. It is important to establish their expectations of surgery and how they think it will impact on their lives. Options and choice for pain management, including the use of a continuous infusion epidural or morphine syringe driver, should be discussed pre-operatively, together with the advantages and disadvantages of each method. The possibility of urinary retention and how this may be resolved need to be included.

Concerns may be expressed about the position and size of the projected scar and a feeling of repulsion about having a large amount of metal inserted is not uncommon initially, especially if a knee joint is also being replaced. It may be helpful for young people to be able to handle a similar type of prosthesis and show it to friends and family. They need to be aware that it will set off the alarms at most airports. Photographs of previous patients, showing scars, appearance and involvement in normal activities such as riding bikes and swimming, are helpful in allaying fears and misconceptions.

Cytotoxic drugs may reduce serum calcium, magnesium and potassium levels and these may need to be supplemented. Cardiac arrhythmias are a possible complication of doxorubicin administration and results of recent echocardiograms should be available.

Lack of appetite and weight loss may cause concern, as poor nutritional status is less favourable to wound healing. Emesis, taste and smell aberrations, mouth ulcers from chemotherapy and the psychological effects of cancer, can all contribute to diminished food intake and consequent malnutrition in both Ewing's sarcoma and osteosarcoma (Tebbi & Erpenbeck, 1996). Cancer treatments can produce physiological changes, which can cause problems in wound healing. Lack of protein or vitamin C, reduced calcium and magnesium levels can all delay the healing process (Lotti et al., 1998).

Fear of surgery, the anaesthetic and post-operative pain may also decrease the desire to eat. It is therefore important to discuss and consider the use of dietary supplements and to try to provide a tempting menu suitable to the young person's needs. Young patients who have had problems maintaining weight and taking oral medications may be given alternative ways of supplementing nutrition by the insertion of a nasogastric tube or a gastrostomy peg. Poor intake of food may lead to conflict with parents, who may relate eating to a measure of health and feel rejected when food they have specially prepared is refused. However, with a welcome break from chemotherapy and a relief from some of the associated side effects, appetites usually improve and young people start

to enjoy food again, although taste alterations may persist.

Post-operative issues and possible complications

Pain management

The aim of post-operative pain relief is to give comfort to patients, allowing them to breathe, cough and move more easily. Multimodal pain therapy is the most important technique for the treatment of post-operative pain (Kehlet, 1994). This can be achieved by combining non-steroidal anti-inflammatory drugs and opiates.

An individual's reaction to pain is determined by past experiences, level of development and health status (McCready et al., 1991). Studies have shown that older children are able to think in more abstract terms and define pain as having both physical and psychological components (McGrath, 1990). This means that they may be more aware of feelings of helplessness, anxiety about how long the pain will last and its significance (Lansdown & Sokel, 1993). Young people facing surgical removal of their tumour frequently express fears of possible unrelieved pain after surgery, especially if they have experienced complete pain relief since starting chemotherapy.

Opiates may be effectively given via a patient-controlled analgesia device (PCA) or an epidural. Morphine is the drug of choice in a PCA, ideally combined with an antiemetic to prevent nausea. This form of analgesia has been well evaluated by young people undergoing orthopaedic surgery, as it gives them some choice and control over their relief from pain (Kaufmann Rauen & Ho, 1989). Studies have shown that young people use less analgesia post-operatively with a PCA than when drugs were administered by more conventional routes. The fact that they are active in controlling their pain may enhance the analgesic effect (McGrath, 1990).

Although effective, some young people dislike the 'spaced-out' feeling of opiates and this can make them reluctant to use the control. There may be some loss of pain control at night when they are asleep if the PCA does not have a background infusion. This can be helped by the use of a long-acting non-steroidal anti-inflammatory drug, providing there is not a history of asthma or gastritis from chemotherapy.

If surgery has involved the lower limb, young people may be offered a continuous infusion epidural as an alternative method of pain control using less opiate than a PCA. Research has shown this to be a superior method of relieving post-operative pain compared to a PCA for overall pain, pain at rest and for pain with activity (Wu *et al.*, 2005). This can be very effective and minimise systemic effects, although potential numbness of the legs may make neurological checks difficult. Special attention needs to be paid to areas that may become sore from pressure, such as the heel, as sensation may be temporarily impaired.

Culture and gender may have an influence on perceptions of pain. In Western cultures males are expected to feel less pain than females, whereas Jews and Italians may feel less inhibited (Gillies, 1992). Good pre-operative preparation, by giving information, answering questions, discussing fears and anxieties and giving the young people permission to complain of pain, should help to balance this and contribute to the overall effectiveness of pain relief.

Young people respond well to the use of a visual analogue scale as an assessment tool to discuss what an acceptable level of pain is for them and to evaluate how effective their analgesia is. Massage can provide not only psychological support through human contact, but can mediate the pain response. The quality of touch is important, and this can help in communicating with young people who find it difficult to express their feelings. When they are in pain, massage hand movements should be lengthened into long, slow strokes, which can soothe the sensory nerve endings and block the pain impulse (Day, 1995).

Nausea and vomiting

Nausea and vomiting may occur as a routine reaction to anaesthesia, anxiety and surgery but for the young person undergoing chemotherapy it holds more emotion, as a reminder of their ongoing treatment. Apart from antiemetic drugs, the use of acupressure wrist bands can be quite effective, and are usually welcomed by this age group as

an alternative (for further details, see Chapter 3). Consideration needs to be given to any residual gastritis from chemotherapy and an H2 antagonistic drug, such as ranitidine, may be indicated to reduce gastric hyperacidity, and prevent a stress ulcer occurring, especially if vomiting persists.

Urinary retention

Urinary retention may occur due to the use of an epidural infusion or intravenous opiates. A urinary catheter may be required and prophylactic antibiotics may be given pre-insertion and post removal. Gentamycin should not be used as it can affect the auditory nerve, which may already be compromised through the use of cisplatin. The potential risk of infection is always a concern in limb conservation surgery, where an endoprosthesis has been inserted.

Wound healing

Necrosis of the suture line is a potential problem post-operatively, following lower limb endoprosthetic replacement surgery. Theatre dressings may include layers of padding and stretch bandages, in the form of a pressure dressing, to provide support and prevent excessive swelling. If the bandages are too restrictive, however, allowing insufficient space for the knee to swell, the blood supply over the knee may be compromised, causing necrosis of the tissue which, if extensive, may require skin grafting. Regular neurovascular checks are essential, and complaints of excessive pain that is difficult to control may be an indication that dressings need to be released.

Wound healing may be delayed due to devascularisation of the skin following a wide skin incision and bony resection (Hockenberry & Lane, 1988; Lotti *et al.*, 1998). This may result in large blisters forming around the incision, which need careful management to aid healing and avoid infection. Wound healing should be complete before chemotherapy is resumed.

Neurological impairment and position of limb

Limb conservation surgery of more advanced tumours may involve resection close to the nerves, especially in the proximal tibia and fibula and sometimes the nerve will need to be sacrificed to gain adequate clearance. This may result in the inability to dorsiflex the foot, called 'foot drop', which requires the foot and ankle to be kept in a neutral position using a pillow or wedge, ensuring that the heel is kept free from pressure. A drop foot orthosis, inside a shoe, will be required for long-term support when walking. Careful assessment should be made post-operatively to establish any impairment in sensation and function, and measures taken to prevent the associated risks.

If surgery has replaced the proximal femur, there is a risk of dislocation of the hip. This can be prevented by keeping the leg in abduction, either by suspending it in slings and springs or using an abduction wedge. A post-operative hip orthosis may be needed when mobilising for approximately six weeks, until the muscles are strong enough to prevent such a dislocation.

Reduced mobility

A temporary reduction in mobility is inevitable following surgery but weight bearing with support is allowed in all but unstable procedures. A canvas splint will help to keep the knee straight until the quadriceps muscle is strong enough to control movements of the knee, and a hip orthosis may need to be worn for a while if muscle was removed during the hip replacement surgery. The physiotherapist has an important role in the multidisciplinary team, and will be crucial in the young person achieving optimal function. Exercise regimens are difficult to maintain when restarting chemotherapy, and structured goal planning can be of value to motivate young people and record their achievement. If an endoprosthetic knee has been inserted, it is essential to maintain full extension daily. If the knee becomes fixed in a flexed position, it will compromise mobility. Initially, a plaster of Paris back-slab may be required at night to maintain the position. If optimal function has not been achieved following completion of cancer treatment, a period of intense rehabilitation as an inpatient, with hydrotherapy, achieves good results. At this stage young people are physically well, feeling motivated and focused to regain maximum function.

Infection

Infection will always be the greatest threat to the successful outcome of endoprosthetic procedures, and routine intravenous antibiotic cover is given at the time of surgery. An infection around the prosthesis is difficult to eradicate, and may lead to chronic sinus formation and its ultimate removal. In extreme circumstances, a limb may need to be amputated (Grimer, 2005). Immunosuppression and an intravenous central line will add to this risk, although good practice and early recognition and treatment of infections will reduce this to a minimum. Young people need to be aware that their endoprosthesis will always be at risk from untreated infections such as tonsillitis, and that these should be treated promptly. Confusingly, a limb with an endoprosthesis in will always feel warmer to touch than the unaffected limb as the metal will conduct body heat.

A reactive hyperpyrexia may be present postoperatively as well as a tachycardia, neither of which are necessarily indicative of an infection; however, if clinically unwell, an infection in a central line must always be considered.

Amputation

A young person requiring an amputation of whole or part of a limb must be one of the most emotive experiences in orthopaedic surgery. Amputation at any age is distressing but, although the physical care is similar, the emotional needs differ significantly. Special concerns relate to physical appearance, acceptance by peers and achieving independence; greater adjustment appears to be needed by the younger age group (Felder-Puig et al., 1998).

During adolescence, young people are trying to cope with accepting normal physical changes to their bodies. The loss of all or most of body hair from chemotherapy together with weight loss is difficult but to lose part of their body is very traumatic and will initially lead to low self-esteem. Amputation holds fear of the unknown and some verbalise that they could not face life without their limb, although studies have shown how well they are able to adapt later (Grimer, 2005; Koopman et al., 2005). Concerns are expressed about peer relationships, swimming, activities, school, careers and how soon they will get an artificial limb. These feelings may lead to isolation, unpredictable behaviour and bouts of anger, which nurses need to be sensitive to and to be able to provide emotional support and understanding.

Pre-operative issues

Young people expecting to have an amputation of a part or whole limb need a great deal of preparation before surgery both with and separately from their families. The attitudes of nurses, peers, family and the whole multidisciplinary team will influence the way in which young people try to accept and adapt to their loss, and look positively to the future. They will need to know the exact level the limb is going to be removed, otherwise 'above the knee' may mean that literally to them, instead of possibly half the femur. This would not be obvious until all the dressings are removed for the first time and could cause great distress.

One of the first questions asked by young people and their families is how soon they can be fitted with an artificial limb. Some are upset that they will not be able to have it straight away. A plaster cast has to be taken from the stump, after the swelling has reduced, before the limb can be made. This will be about six weeks after surgery and will be arranged at their local limb-fitting centre. A short period of rehabilitation will then be necessary to learn to walk with it safely and correctly. This is always difficult to accommodate during an intensive chemotherapy regimen. It is important to discuss this with the young people, within an understanding of their cultural perceptions, of how they will be accepted within their peer group.

The opportunity to visit a limb-fitting department should be offered to see a prosthesis and discuss how the limb will function, and the range of activities they will be able to do. The staff in these centres are very understanding about the young person's need to look 'normal', and will work hard with them to achieve this, although while they are growing the prosthesis provided is fairly basic.

Young people may ask to meet another young person of a similar age who has previously had an amputation for cancer at the same level. This can be very helpful if they are willing to share their experiences. Ideally, the person should be the same gender, as there may be questions asked about sexuality; alternatively, they may ask for this meeting during the rehabilitation phase. Photographs showing the appearance of a stump, scars and an artificial limb are useful to have available and pictures of young amputees cycling, skiing, playing football and girls looking glamorous, or getting married, all help to promote a positive approach. All visual and educational material is useful, but extreme sensitivity is required to know if, when and how to introduce it. Positive information is that they can learn to drive earlier at 16 years, and this often becomes an important goal during rehabilitation, when it will provide greater independence.

Parents and siblings will find this pre-operative phase very difficult to manage, and may take longer than the young person to adjust. It is particularly important that the siblings are involved at every level, as research has shown that they have an improved level of adjustment if they have been given adequate information, allowed to be involved in the care and have been given special attention and emotional support (Von Essen & Enskar, 2003).

Post-operative issues

Pain management

A young person undergoing an amputation may experience three types of pain: stump pain, painful phantom limb sensations and emotional pain. If they are in agreement, the most effective form of pain control for stump pain is via an epidural infusion. It would appear that this has the added advantage of temporarily reducing the severity of phantom limb sensations. Debate exists as to the value of commencing analgesia prior to surgery, as pain in the limb before amputation has been correlated with the incidence and degree of phantom pain afterwards (Krane & Heller, 1995; Hazelgrove & Rogers, 2002, Middleton, 2003). Emotional pain and anxiety are inevitably strong factors influencing the experience of pain, and must be addressed when trying to achieve control.

Phantom limb pain

Phantom limb pain (PLP) is a form of neuropathic pain and is the sensory perception that the missing part of the limb is still there (Middleton, 2003). It is important that young people are able to distinguish between PLP and stump pain, as opiates are not effective against the former (Rounseville, 1992). Not all phantom limb sensations are painful and may be described as tingling, throbbing, burning, pins and needles, cramping and stabbing (Hazelgrove & Rogers, 2002). The more proximal the amputation, the stronger and more uncomfortable the sensations will be. Stress, anxiety and depression may intensify the sensations but do not cause them (Rounseville, 1992). Other factors that may exacerbate the condition are the weather and muscle spasm. Elevation of the stump, rest, heat and distraction may give some relief. Cramping pain may be caused by muscle tension in the stump, and can be helped by biofeedback treatment. Burning pain may be helped by drugs that increase the blood flow, such as vasodilators (Hazelgrove & Rogers, 2002).

Treatment for PLP may include drugs, transcutaneous nerve stimulation (TENS) and the use of deep relaxation and guided imagery. Traditionally, anticonvulsant drugs such as carbamazepine and clonazepam were used for the sharp, piercing type of pain, to prevent abnormal signals from reaching the brain and baclofen for the cramping or spasm-like sensations. Gabapentin is now the drug of choice. A tricyclic antidepressant such as amitryptyline may be used if the sensations cause insomnia and this may also help to counteract depression (Rounseville, 1992).

TENS, whereby electrodes are placed on the surface of the skin and a mild electric current is administered, has been shown to be of some help in giving relief from PLP although this has been of limited use (Hazelgrove & Rogers, 2002). Patients can alter the frequency, pulse widths and duration of the machine, and this may help them to feel more in control and offers an alternative to drugs.

Young people generally respond well to the idea of deep relaxation and guided imagery, as these are techniques they can learn to help themselves. They can be taught how to relax all the voluntary muscles and to try warm baths and massage. By distracting their thoughts away from the sensations, they may gain complete relief.

Others have found it helpful to pretend to massage the painful area where the limb should be, or the collateral limb.

Unfortunately, it may be necessary to try a variety of different ways to control LPP, but providing adequate time and support to explore all options, together with the knowledge that the sensations will lessen in time, will help young people to achieve long-term control without the use of medication.

Care of the stump

Swelling of the stump immediately post-operatively is controlled by the use of pressure bandaging and elevating the bed. A pillow should not be placed under the stump as this may cause hip or knee flexion contractures.

Painful sensations are usually felt in the stump when the theatre dressings are removed, and these are exacerbated by the intense feelings of anxiety at seeing the stump and wound for the first time; adequate analgesia cover will be required. Ideally the first dressing should be carried out where there will be minimal interruption and adequate time available to give support and information. The young person's need for sensitivity and privacy must be respected at all times.

Spontaneous wound healing and correct stump bandaging are essential for an artificial limb to be successfully fitted. The bandages help to mould the shape of the stump by applying even pressure to both sides and, when the stump is less sensitive, these are replaced by a firm elasticated sock called a 'Juzo'.

Exercises are required initially for balance if part of a lower limb has been removed and then to increase muscle tone and power in the remaining muscles in preparation for walking with the artificial limb. Practising this on the ward is the first stage in adjusting to being seen without a limb by peers. This can be a very positive experience as other young people are usually quick to encourage and praise their efforts.

The Van Nes rotationplasty

This surgical procedure was developed to convert an above-knee amputation into a more functional below-knee amputation, which gives considerable functional advantage (Lindner *et al.*, 1999; Grimer, 2005). It involves the removal of the tumour from the distal femur and the attachment of the proximal tibia after it has been rotated 180 degrees. The ankle joint functions as the knee joint in the artificial limb. The foot remains, pointing backwards and the toes may be electively removed for cosmetic purposes. The main advantages of this form of amputation, although uncommon in the United Kingdom, are a high level of function and lack of phantom limb sensations. The obvious disadvantage is the unusual appearance of the limb, which requires a particular form of prosthesis, which the young person would need immense support and guidance in accepting (Piasecki, 1992; Wicart *et al.*, 2005). It is becoming less popular in Europe as advances in endoprosthetic replacements become more widely known (Grimer, 2005).

Altered body image

Young people need to be able to socialise with friends and anything that prevents this happening will make them stand out from the rest and could affect their self-esteem (for further details, see Chapter 4). Physical attractiveness is an important factor for acceptance by peers. Race, religion and cultural background have an important influence on a young person's development, and the attitude of others will affect their own self-image and self-value (White, 1995).

When young people are diagnosed with a malignant bone tumour, their identity tends to lose importance as attention is focused on the disease process. They may feel as though they have lost control over their body. As they undergo chemotherapy and surgery, they try to adjust to considerable alterations in their appearance while at the same time trying to maintain a positive self-image (Woodgate, 2005). Young people have shown that it is extremely important to them to be kept fully informed about their illness, how it impacts on their future, and they should be given the opportunity to make decisions about their own future (Hokkanen *et al.*, 2004).

Regardless of the type of surgery, a young person's body will never be the same again. Scars and limb shape after surgery are important issues.

Spontaneous wound healing will contribute to a neat scar, which will be fairly extensive and need protection from the sun. In time this will be less noticeable and massaging cream into the scar tissue will help to keep it supple. Following conservation surgery the shape of the limb is usually good once the swelling has reduced but is not the same, and concern may be expressed over the wasting and reduction of muscle tissue. Any residual limp will be noticed and a regular physiotherapy programme is essential to achieve maximum function.

When an amputation is the only option, a young person's feelings of anger, fear, mutilation and grief will need to be dealt with, and the reactions of family, staff, friends and peers to their new image will be watched closely and will be important in helping them to regain their confidence and self-esteem. Mobilising as soon as possible and becoming independent will have a positive effect. Personal relationships will always be a worry for young people but their greatest concern is being accepted by peers when returning to school or college. Young people with an altered body image face a difficult challenge, and a lack of confidence may lead to regressive behaviour and a loss of academic performance. Support from teaching staff and, if possible, the school nurse, will be needed to prevent them from becoming isolated. Emphasis will need to be placed on their positive attributes rather than focusing on the illness, and a flexible approach may be needed to enable them to remain with peers, although they may not have reached the same level of achievement.

Discharge planning

Coordinated discharge planning is necessary for young people undergoing surgery for either limb preservation or an amputation. It is essential that oncologists be informed of the discharge date to enable them to plan post-operative chemotherapy. Ideally, a few days at home after discharge can be built into the plan, which will help them to prepare for the next phase of treatment.

Wound healing should be complete at this stage but central line care will need to be continued by the community care team. Communication, with them and the oncology unit following surgery, about ongoing surgical management issues and follow-up are important, together with any psychosocial issues that may have arisen during treatment.

Similar links should be made between other members of the multidisciplinary teams. Physiotherapists will arrange for continued therapy in both the community and oncology unit. Occupational therapists will liaise about any home alterations organised to aid mobility and independence. Social workers and counsellors will discuss work that needs to be continued, and the medical teams will exchange information relating to future management. Some oncology units have produced shared care folders for recording information such as treatment plans and blood test results. The hospital school may send a progress report to show what work has been covered. This is especially important with GCSE course work, and the teachers will liaise with the home tutor if appropriate.

Information about medication may need to be given, and precautions that need to be taken to prevent infection of the endoprosthesis. All young people want to be fully informed about restrictions on activities, in both the short and long term. Amputees should have been sent to a limb fitting centre and a resettlement officer, if appropriate, who can give advice about how, when and where to learn to drive and what modifications, if any, will need to be made to a car.

Follow-up surgical appointments are usually made to accommodate periods between chemotherapy and neutropenia. Good discharge planning will ensure safe continuity of care and help to minimise stress for young people and their families.

Late effects

Metastatic disease

Eighty per cent of young people show no apparent signs of lung metastases at the time of diagnosis but they may rapidly develop them within the first year, in spite of chemotherapy and surgery. This suggests that micrometastases are present at diagnosis and surgery (Schwartz et al., 1993). Lindner et al. (1999) evaluated 136 patients treated for osteosarcoma and found that the extent of pre-operative necrosis, surgical margins and tumour volume were the most important prognostic factors.

Adjuvant chemotherapy can contain or reduce lung metastases, allowing them to be resected. Young people who develop pulmonary metastases following chemotherapy have a poorer prognosis, although complete resection has been associated with long-term survival (Lewis, 1996). Other contributory factors to improved survival include a small number of metastases and a longer time from end of treatment to relapse. Additional chemotherapy using different drugs may be given prior to the metastasectomy. Young people presenting with bone metastases in both osteosarcoma and Ewing's sarcoma, either at diagnosis or relapse, have a fatal outcome in spite of therapies (Lewis, 1996).

Local recurrence

Studies have shown that limb conservation surgery and, in particular, endoprostheses, can be successfully used for local control, reducing the need for amputation (Mertens & Bramwell, 1994; Bacci et al., 2002). A review of 202 patients in the European Osteosarcoma Intergroup study showed no significant difference in survival rates between those treated surgically by limb conservation and those treated by primary amputation, although there were more marginal excisions and associated increases in local recurrence in those treated conservatively (Grimer et al., 2002). The significant findings in this study were that a raised alkaline phosphatase, tumours of the proximal femur and proximal humerus and a poor response to chemotherapy were the most significant prognostic factors for a poor outcome. Interestingly, no patient who had a good response to chemotherapy in the limb salvage group developed a local recurrence.

Roberts et al. (1991) found that the incidence of local recurrence in a review of 133 young patients treated with distal femoral prostheses was only slightly higher than that recorded for amputation. Although the patients with the recurrence subsequently had an amputation, the results still showed that following the insertion of the prosthesis, 88% of patients would not require an amputation at five years. In the same study, infection was shown to be the major complication, from surgery, a central line or wound breakdown while on chemotherapy. Two of these cases required amputation for persistent infection.

The presence of a pathological fracture in osteosarcoma has been regarded as a poor prognostic factor and an indication for ablative surgery (Scully *et al.*, 2002). Two reviews of young people with pathological fractures from osteosarcoma showed that although there was a correlation between local recurrence and the margins of resection in limb conservation surgery, this did not affect long-term survival when compared to patients treated by amputation who had no local recurrence, however, overall as a group they did have a decreased rate of survival (Abudu *et al.*, 1996; Scully *et al.*, 2002). Data from the second EOI study, which ran from 1986 to 1993, was unable to show that a pathological fracture was a risk factor for either survival or local recurrence (Grimer *et al.*, 2002).

Loosening of endoprostheses

A retrospective study of 1001 endoprostheses used as replacements for bone tumours showed that aseptic loosening was the main cause of failure of the implant requiring revision (Unwin *et al.*, 1996). The highest failure group due to aseptic loosening was after distal femoral replacements, and could be related to the amount of bone that was removed, the age of the patient and the site of resection. Younger patients with more than 60 % of bone resection in the distal femoral and proximal tibial groups were more at risk from loosening. Interestingly, there were no failures of proximal femoral replacements with more than 60 % of bone removed. This could be related to the natural curve of the femur and the quality of bone in the medullary canal, which allowed good fixation with cement.

Recent developments in endoprosthetic design have mainly focused on the extending mechanism to lengthen the shaft, with no surgical intervention, to achieve greater growth potential; the rotational element of the knee hinge, the coating of the prosthesis to prevent tissue reaction to the titanium alloy and the use of calcium hydroxyapatite ceramics (CHA). The risk of loosening of an endoprosthesis has decreased considerably with the use of calcium hydroxyapatite ceramics (CHA). These are non-toxic substances, which are biologically compatible with bone, produce little tissue reaction

and can be used in place of bone grafts (Uchida *et al.*, 1990). CHA is currently used to coat the end of the implant and X-rays have shown that the host bone is able to grow into the CHA and form a complete union. This significantly reduces the incidence of loosening by reducing forces on the cement bone interface (Unwin *et al.*, 1996; Grimer, 2005). However, this solid union is a disadvantage if the endoprosthesis needs to be replaced.

Leg length inequality

Limb length discrepancy will be inevitable when the tibial or femoral growth plate or physis is sacrificed. At the skeletal age of 8, it is estimated that potential growth from the proximal tibial physis is 4 cm and 9 cm from the distal femoral at maturity (Ramseier *et al.*, 2006). Research has shown that, when skeletally mature, these young people may be above average height for their age (Earl & Souhami, 1990). Since the 1970s endoprostheses with extendable telescopic shafts have been developed in the United Kingdom, to try to address this. Although successful, they require surgical lengthening, approximately 1.5 cm at each operation, with the potential risk of infection and the trauma for the young person of further hospitalisation.

The most recent and exciting development in the UK recently has been the successful use of a non-invasive endoprostheses with a telescopic shaft, which is lengthened non-surgically in the outpatient department. It is currently available for tumours in the femur and tibia and has been successfully implanted in young people from about the age of 8 years. This implant is designed with a magnetically driven gearbox. Length is achieved by placing the limb into a circular limb-extending machine, which generates a spinning magnetic field. The magnet in the endoprosthesis captures this motion; it passes through the gearbox, which turns the screw in the telescopic shaft. One millimetre of length is gained in 4 minutes. The average lengthening per session is 4 millimetres achieved in 16 minutes. This can take place in a nurse-led clinic at times to ensure minimal disruption to the young person's education. This method of lengthening prevents the risk of infection, is completely painless and allows a gentle, natural rate of growth.

If the younger patients continue to grow rapidly, they may require a replacement telescopic shaft or an adult size replacement at a later stage. It is possible to replace the telescopic shaft, when fully extended, to achieve additional growth in both types of extendible prosthesis. Leg length discrepancy can also be managed in young people who are tall for their age, by deliberately damaging a growth plate in the unaffected limb to slow down the rate of growth. Shortening of the unaffected limb in this group at maturity can be achieved by removing a wedge of femur.

Quality of life

One of the long-term disappointments for some young people with an endoprosthesis is the restriction placed on contact sports, especially if they were previously in school or county teams. In some schools great emphasis is placed on sporting ability, which in turn leads to popularity and peer acceptance. Fortunately, other sports such as swimming, cycling, golf and badminton are usually possible.

Realistic careers are another consideration for young people, depending on the type of surgery they have had. Education is usually compromised for a year, either as a deliberate decision or because of treatment difficulties; but some young people are able to continue studying and complete course work, taking exams between courses of chemotherapy and achieve satisfactory grades. Difficulties may arise in obtaining health, travel and life insurance, and this reinforces the uncertainty of their future prognosis. A survey looking at the quality of life of young people who had osteosarcoma, at least one year after treatment, showed that the overwhelming psychological problem was a fear of tumour recurrence and the possibility of more treatment (Nirenberg, 1985). However, the survey also showed that many patients had successfully completed their education, had careers and some had started families.

Felder-Puig et al. (1998) reviewed 60 patients who were diagnosed with bone cancer with their healthy peers, with varying ages below 30 years, from 1–20 years of treatment. The only illness-related variable that appeared to affect psychosocial adjustment was age at diagnosis.

Those patients diagnosed in adolescence had more problems relating to social well-being than patients diagnosed at an earlier age or as a young adult. This may be the result of the impact of the disease on the developmental tasks of adolescence, which establish personal identity, sexual and emotional maturity, independence and autonomy and future life opportunities (Woodgate, 2005). These patients appeared to live at home for longer and be less likely to marry and have children. This may reflect a strong attachment to and dependence on the parents. Their level of education was similar but many had difficulties finding a suitable occupation, and a number had to change jobs or preferred careers as a result of treatment. However, in spite of these changes, patients reported a high level of job satisfaction.

Koopman et al. (2005) investigated the health-related quality of life and coping strategies of young people at 3 and 8 years after the end of treatment for bone cancer. At 3 years they scored significantly lower than their healthy peers on motor functioning and autonomy, but at 8 years, although motor functioning remained lower, they scored higher on cognitive and social functioning and autonomy. Overall, they found that the young people adapted well after treatment for bone cancer, and were not at risk of developing long-term emotional or social problems.

Infertility

At some stage all young people will have concerns about their fertility. In general, male fertility is more likely to be affected, particularly with the use of high doses of alkylating agents which can cause dysfunction in spermatogenesis. These drugs are important in the treatment of bone sarcomas. This problem is also related to age at time of diagnosis. Pre-pubertal children are known to tolerate higher doses of these drugs and may therefore be more at risk (Jurgens et al., 1992); although girls treated before puberty appear less likely to have fertility problems than those treated after (Mosher & McCarthy, 1998). Young people have successfully become parents after completion of treatment even, in some cases, after a hemipelvectomy and the children have been healthy and normal, following uncomplicated pregnancies and deliveries (Nirenberg, 1985). The removal of ovarian tissue in young females and its re-implantation after cure are currently experimental, and may be available in the future (Wallace & Brougham, 2005), although there has been considerable concern about the possible risk of cancer cell transmission (Kim, 2003).

The outcome of pregnancies in survivors of osteosarcoma and Ewing's sarcoma are comparable to the general population and there has been no increased incidence of birth defects or cancer in the offspring (Mosher & McCarthy, 1998).

Osteoporosis

During normal health, bone mineral density (BMD) increases in childhood and adolescence until the peak bone mass is reached. Any serious disease, such as primary bone cancer, has the ability to interfere with this process. Holzer *et al.* (2003) reviewed 48 long-term survivors of osteosarcoma in whom 21% were found to be osteoporotic and 48% osteopenic. The significant factors were low body weight, early menarche and the type of endoprosthesis inserted. Patients with endoprosthetic replacements in the lower limb and proximal femur showed lower BMD values than those with a distal femoral replacement, and lower than other surgical procedures such as rotationplasty and amputation. The difference in body weight appears to relate to the load on weight-bearing bones, which will also be affected by periods of immobilisation known to reduce bone mass. Young people with osteosarcoma are treated with high-dose methotrexate which is known to suppress bone formation by inhibiting osteoblast production, and has been linked to osteoporosis in survivors of leukaemia. This was the first study to look at osteoporosis as a late effect in bone cancer and the regular measurement of BMD may be included in long-term follow-up in the future.

Other late effects from the chemotherapy may be cardiotoxicity from the anthracycline drug doxorubicin, renal tubular deficits from cisplatin and ifosfamide and auditory impairment from cisplatin (Mosher & McCarthy, 1998). For other specific late effects related to chemotherapy, see Chapter 5; and for those related to radiotherapy, see Chapter 3.

Future trends

Surgery

Seventy-five per cent of malignant bone tumours in young people occur near the growth plate. Joint-sparing surgery is evolving as it has been shown that, to a certain extent, the growth plate, or epiphysis can prevent the spread of the tumour but is not impenetrable. Joint-sparing endoprostheses are used, where appropriate, with a specially designed fixation close to the knee joint but preserving it (Canadell *et al.*, 1994).

External fixators may be used where the growth plate can be spared and, if the epiphysis has not been breached, the external fixator may be inserted above while the patient is having adjuvant chemotherapy, and distraction started to lengthen the metaphysis. Complete resection of the tumour, with clearance margins, is carried out when chemotherapy is finished and the area is grafted. Results so far have not shown any local recurrence (Canadell *et al.*, 1994). Problems may occur with infected pin sites, especially when the patient becomes immunosuppressed but the advantage of no endoprosthesis and preserved knee function is considerable.

Muscolo *et al.* (2005) reviewed 13 patients with high-grade osteosarcoma who had been treated with allografts preserving the epiphysis. They found recurrence in only one case but suggested that patients should be carefully selected with regard to a positive response to chemotherapy, and accurate pre-operative assessment of tumour extension to the epiphysis. Another advance in surgery is the excision of the tumour, and the subsequent irradiation of the tumour bone and its reinsertion, all in one procedure. Parents and young people need reassurance that the tumour cells have been completely killed. A review by Chen *et al.* (2005) of 29 patients of which 15 had received an irradiated autograft for a malignant bone tumour showed that only one patient had a local recurrence; the time to relapse was not stated. The non-union rate was significantly lower than an allograft, possibly because they were a perfect anatomical fit. Grimer (2005) suggests that this type of reconstruction will become more common, especially where other options are not readily available, such as the pelvis.

Research continues into the further development of the non-invasive extending prosthesis to reduce the size of the gearbox to enable it to be inserted into smaller prostheses, as well as its wider development for other orthopaedic conditions.

Chemotherapy

Future trends in chemotherapy for bone cancer will follow evaluation of the data from clinical trials. Survival rates for osteosarcoma have not significantly improved over the past 20 years. The European and American Osteosarcoma Study Group (EURAMOS), founded in 2001, was formed to try to improve survival rates by undertaking biological studies and conducting large randomised trials. A new randomised trial has started, called EURAMOS 1, which aims to optimise the treatment strategies for resectable osteosarcoma tumours based on histological response to pre-operative chemotherapy. This study hopes to show whether additional treatment with ifosfamide and etoposide to the current use of cisplatin, doxorubicin and methotrexate will improve event-free survival in patients who have had a poor response to pre-operative chemotherapy. It will investigate whether maintenance therapy, using interferon-alpha, will improve event-free survival in those patients who have responded well. In addition, the trial will record short- and long-term toxicities, time to disease recurrence, quality of life issues and measure molecular changes in the blood and tumour.

Impact of setting

Young people are an age group with their own unique set of needs. When they are diagnosed as having cancer, all their developmental tasks are threatened as they try to adjust to major changes in their lives (Evans, 1993). These young people deserve a special understanding, and need to be cared for by nurses who recognise how problems may affect their mood, behaviour and coping (Taylor & Muller, 1995). Young people with bone tumours should be nursed in age-appropriate units, with nurses specifically trained to care for this age group and speciality (Earl & Souhami,

1990). All teenagers interviewed by Burr (1993) on an adult and a children's ward stated that they would like to be cared for with their own age group. Mulhall *et al.* (2004) evaluated the first specialist teenage cancer unit in the country and found that it provided a supportive bond for adolescents and their families, that the facilities were focused on their needs and that the expertise and availability of an expert team of professionals, trained in this specialism, were central to creating an appropriate environment of care.

Gibson *et al.* (2005) found that young people wanted an environment that was more like home with more space and privacy, appetising food, age-appropriate toys and activities and to be away from younger children. They also wanted facilities that allowed them to keep in touch with their friends and have access to their level of education. The environment for young people is important for promoting peer support and interaction, although many young people have expressed a preference for single rooms when they have been available. The units should be relaxed and friendly, age-appropriate, supportive and flexible, with minimal ground rules. Nursing staff should be empathetic, adaptable and have a good sense of humour.

Body image and peer group identification are the developmental tasks that are most affected by having bone cancer (Nirenberg, 1985). Although many of the changes are temporary, it is the 'here and now' that is important to young people, and especially how their peers accept them. Young people have reported that having treatment for cancer has made them feel and act differently from their peers, not only because of the changes to their body but it has made them more mature (Nirenberg, 1985). Fedora (1985) found it very helpful to meet former patients who had completed treatment and adjusted to the physical changes. She also felt that staff should encourage and facilitate relationships with other peers, to move the focus away from being patients, onto supporting and encouraging others in their progress. This can be very successful on a mixed surgical unit where not all the young people have cancer but who have many other debilitating and distressing conditions. Woodgate (2005) found that the changing sense of self in young people was closely linked to their changing body, and that it was vital for friends and family to accept these changes, and respond to them as if they were the same person.

Good communication skills are needed by all the team involved in caring for a young person with cancer. Difficulties may arise if adults and young people do not identify with each other, and they will be unable to confide in someone they do not have a rapport with (Gillies, 1992). Young people usually welcome a frank and honest discussion about their condition, and it is important that the environment recognises and facilitates this, encouraging them to be involved in decision-making and planning their own care. Good communication is also required with the parents, who need to come to terms with the fact that although their children have a life-threatening illness, they still need control over their lives and to remain as independent as possible (Taylor & Muller, 1995).

Acute illness and the hospitalisation of a young person put a great strain on all family members, not least on the siblings. It is important that brothers and sisters share in the care of the sick sibling, especially if they are unlikely to survive, as it will help them to adjust to their loss (White, 1995). The diagnosis of cancer revolves around the sick patient; this means routines are changed and disruption to family life (von Essen & Enskar, 2003). Issues for siblings may include fear and uncertainty as to the outcome of the illness, fear of having the same cancer, jealousy, loneliness and resentment due to lack of attention and involvement (Craft, 1993). It is important that the holistic approach to the care of young people with bone cancer recognises these potential problems in the well sibling and is able to intervene, where appropriate, to help them to feel special and part of the process in an attempt to prevent or lessen the potential long-term adverse effects.

The environment should try to generate a sense of normality, particularly in relation to leisure and educational needs, offering a wide selection of activities. The role of education in hospital is as an important link with normal life (Wilson, 1993). It can provide stimulation, allow expression of emotions through writing and art and help to maintain or increase academic progress. Links are made with the patient's own school to ensure continuity of work and identify any weak areas that may be helped. The one-to-one tuition available in the larger hospital schools can be invaluable in helping young people with learning difficulties. Young people with bone cancer, who have opted out of school for a year, still may enjoy pottery, cookery, art and craft activities and access to computers.

Facilities to make drinks and light snacks and their own separate leisure area are evaluated well by young people, as well as a room where they can be quiet and reflect. They will also appreciate being able to e-mail peers and spend some private time with friends.

Nursing staff on special units for young people are in an ideal position to take an active lead in health promotion; however, to be effective they need to understand the social contexts in which young people function (Taylor & Muller, 1995). Displaying leaflets and booklets in a private area such as the toilet will ensure that issues relating to sexuality, smoking, nutrition, drug and alcohol abuse are addressed, and empower young people to seek out information and help them to understand it. A notice board is useful to display various helplines including the teenager cancer support groups and websites. Separate ward-based support groups for patients and parents can be helpful, dealing with a variety of issues of their choice.

Young people undergoing medical and surgical treatment for primary bone cancer can benefit greatly from being cared for in an age-appropriate environment by named nurses who understand and appreciate their role in facilitating young people to progress with their developmental tasks, especially in relation to psychosocial development. This role can help young people improve their self-image, achieve and maintain independence and will often develop into long-term support and interest in an attempt to make their hospitalisation a positive experience.

Young people have a right to open and honest communication, to informed choice and control, privacy, confidentiality and protection, which will lead to a trusting relationship providing physical and emotional support for them as they try to cope with the enormous stresses and uncertainties of their illness and treatments. It is crucial for young people to be able to maintain a sense of normality in their lives, and spend as little time as possible in hospital. Shared care, between disciplines in specialist units and the community, will benefit young people by providing a similar philosophy of care nearer home and friends enhancing quality of life. Effective communication between all key workers is vital to its success.

References

Abudu A, Sferopoulos N, Tillman R, Carter S & Grimer R (1996) 'The surgical treatment and outcome of pathological fractures in localised osteosarcoma' *Journal of Bone and Joint Surgery (Br)* 78-B: 694–698

Bacci G, Ferrari S, Lari S, Mercuri M, Donati D, Longhi A, Forni C, Bertoni F, Versari M & Pignotti E (2002) 'Osteosarcoma of the limb: amputation or limb salvage in patients treated by neoadjuvant chemotherapy' *Journal of Bone and Joint Surgery* 84-B: 82–92

Birch J (2005) 'Patterns of incidence of cancer in teenagers and young adults: implications for aetiology' *in*: Eden T, Barr R, Bleyer A & Whiteson M (eds) *Cancer and the Adolescent*. Oxford: Blackwell, pp. 13–31

Bird K & Dearmun A (1995) 'The impact of illness on the child and family' *in*: Carter B & Dearmun A (eds) *Child Health Care Nursing*. Oxford: Blackwell Science Ltd, pp. 101–115

Burr S (1993) 'Adolescents and the ward environment' *Paediatric Nursing* 5(1): 10–13

Canadell J, Forriol F & Cara J (1994) 'Removal of metaphyseal bone tumours with preservation of the epiphysis' *Journal of Bone and Joint Surgery (Br)* 76-B (1): 127–132

Cannon S & Dyson P (1987) 'Relationship of the site of open biopsy of malignant bone tumours to local recurrence following resection and prosthetic replacement' *Journal of Bone and Joint Surgery* 69-B: 49–52

Chen T, Chen W & Huang C (2005) 'Reconstruction after intercalary resection of malignant bone tumours: comparison between segmental allograft and extracorporeally-irradiated autograft' *Journal of Bone and Joint Surgery (Br)* 87-B: 704–709

Craft A (2005) 'Ewing's sarcoma' *in*: Eden T, Barr R, Bleyer A & Whiteson M (eds) *Cancer and the Adolescent*. Oxford: Blackwell, pp. 102–112

Craft M (1993) 'Siblings of hospitalized children: assessment and intervention' *Journal of Paediatric Nursing* 8(5): 289–296

Day S (1995) 'Complementary therapies' *in*: Carter B & Dearmun A (eds) *Child Health Care Nursing*. Oxford: Blackwell Science Ltd, pp. 237–246

Earl H & Souhami R (1990) 'Adolescent bone tumours' *The Practitioner* 234(1494): 816–818

Edge B, Holmes D & Makin G (2006) 'Sperm banking in adolescent cancer patients' *Archives of Disease in Child-hood* 91: 149–152

Evans M (1993) 'Teenagers and cancer' *Paediatric Nursing* 5(1): 14–15

Fedora N (1985) 'Fighting for my leg . . . . . . and my life' *Orthopaedic Nursing* 4(5): 39–42

Felder-Puig R, Formann A, Mildner A, Bretschneider W, Zoubek, Puig S & Topf R (1998) 'Quality of life and psychosocial adjustment of young patients after treatment of bone cancer' *Cancer* 83(1): 69–75

Friedman M (1987) 'Intervening with families of school-aged children with cancer' *in*: Leahey M & Wright L (eds) *Families and Life Threatening Illness*. Pennsylvania: Springhouse Corporation, pp. 219–235

Gatta G, Capocaccia R, Stiller C, Kaatsch P, Bervino F & Terenziani M (2005) 'Childhood cancer survival trends in Europe: a Eurocare Working Group Study' *Journal of Clinical Oncology* 23(16): 3742–3751

Gibson F, Richardson A, Hey S, Horstman M & O'Leary C (2005) *Listening to Children and Young People with Cancer*. London: Institute of Child Health, King's College London

Gillies M (1992) 'Teenage traumas' *Nursing Times* 88(27): 26–29

Grimer R (2005) 'Osteosarcoma and surgery' *in*: Eden T, Barr R, Bleyer A & Whiteson M (eds) *Cancer and the Adolescent*. Oxford: Blackwell, pp. 121–129

Grimer R & Carter S (1995) 'Paediatric surgical oncology 3: bone tumours' *European Journal of Surgical Oncology* 21(2): 217–222

Grimer R & Sneath R (1990) 'Editorial' *Journal of Bone and Joint Surgery (Br)* 72-B: 754–756

Grimer R, Taminiau A & Cannon S (2002) 'Surgical outcomes in osteosarcoma' *Journal of Bone and Joint Surgery* 84-B: 395–400

Hanks G (2005) 'Pain relief in cancer: recent developments' *Cancer Nursing Practice* March supplement: 12–15

Hazelgrove J & Rogers P (2002) 'Phantom limb pain: a complication of lower extremity wound management' *Lower Extremity Wounds* 1(2): 112–124

Hockenberry M & Lane B (1988) 'Limb salvage procedures in children with osteosarcoma' *Cancer Nursing* 11(1): 2–8

Hokkanen H, Eriksson E, Ahonen O & Salantera S (2004) 'Adolescents with cancer: experiences of life and how it could be made easier' *Cancer Nursing* 27(4): 325–335

Holzer G, Krepler P, Koschat M, Grampp S, Dominkus M & Kotz R (2003) 'Bone mineral density in long term survivors of highly malignant osteosarcoma' *Journal of Bone and Joint Surgery* 85-B: 231–237

Hosalkar H & Dormans J (2005) 'Surgical management of pelvic sarcomas in children' *Paediatric Blood Cancer* 44: 305–317

Ishibashi A (2001) 'The needs of children and adolescents with cancer for information and social support' *Cancer Nursing* 24(1): 61–67

Jurgens H, Winkler K & Gobel U (1992) 'Bone tumours' *in*: Plowman P & Pinkerton C (eds) *Paediatric Oncology*. London: Chapman & Hall Medical, pp. 325–350

Kaufmann Rauen K & Ho M (1989) 'Children's use of patient-controlled analgesia after spinal surgery' *Paediatric Nursing* 15(6): 589–637

Kehlet H (1994) 'Editorial: postoperative pain relief – what is the issue?' *British Journal of Anaesthesia* 72(4): 375–378

Kemp H (1987) 'Limb conservation surgery for osteosarcoma and other primary bone tumours' *in*: Souhami R (ed.) *Clinical Oncology*. London: Baillière Tindall, pp. 111–136

Kim S (2003) 'Ovarian tissue banking for cancer patients: to do or not to do?' *Human Reproduction* 18(9): 1759–1761

Koopman H, Koetsier J, Taminiau A, Hijnen K, Bresters D & Egeler M (2005) 'Health-related quality of life and coping strategies of children after treatment of a malignant bone tumor: a 5-year follow-up study' *Paediatric Blood Cancer* 45: 694–699

Krane E & Heller L (1995) 'The prevalence of phantom sensations and pain in paediatric amputees' *Journal of Pain and Symptom Management* 10(1): 21–29

Kuzbit P (2004) 'The importance of hair' *Cancer Nursing Practice* 3(8): 10–13

Lansdown R & Sokel B (1993) 'Commissioned review: approaches to pain management in children' *ACPP Review and Newsletter* 15(3): 105–111

Lewis I (1996) 'Medical management of bone tumours' *in*: Selby P & Bailey C (eds) *Cancer and the Adolescent*. London: BMJ Publishing Group, pp. 90–119

Lindner N, Ramm O, Hillman A, Roedl R, Gosheger G, Brinkschmidt C, Juergens H & Winkelmann W (1999) 'Limb salvage and outcome of osteosarcoma: the University of Muenster experience' *Clinical Orthopaedics Related Research* 358: 83–89

Lotti T, Rodofili C, Benci M & Menchin G (1998) 'Wound-healing problems associated with cancers' *Journal of Wound Care* 7(2): 81–84.

McCready M, MacDavitt K & O'Sullivan K (1991) 'Children and pain: easing the hurt' *Orthopaedic Nursing* 10(6): 33–42

McGrath P (1990) *Pain in Children: Nature, Assessment and Treatment*. New York: The Guilford Press

Mertens W & Bramwell V (1994) 'Osteosarcoma and other tumours of bone' *Current Opinion in Oncology* 6(4): 384–390

Middleton C (2003) 'The causes and treatments of phantom limb pain' *Nursing Times* 99(35): 30–33

Mosher R & McCarthy B (1998) 'Late effects in survivors of bone tumors' *Journal of Paediatric Oncology Nursing* 15(2): 72–84

Mulhall A, Kelly D & Pearce S (2004) 'A qualitative evaluation of an adolescent cancer unit' *European Journal of Cancer Care* 1(1): 16–22

Muscolo D, Ayerza M, Aponte-Tinao L & Ranalletta M (2005) 'Partial epiphyseal preservation and intercalary allograft reconstruction in high-grade metaphyseal osteosarcoma of the knee' *Journal of Bone and Joint Surgery (Am)* 87; Suppl. 1 (Pt 2): 226–236

National Institute for Health and Clinical Excellence (2005) *Improving Outcomes in Children and Young People with Cancer*. London: NICE.

Nirenberg A (1985) 'The adolescent with osteogenic sarcoma' *Orthopaedic Nursing* 4(5): 11–15

Ornadel D, Souhami R, Whelan J, Nooy M, Ruiz de Elvira C, Pringle J, Lewis I, Steward W, George R, Bridgewater J, Wierzbicki R & Craft A (1994) 'Doxorubicin and Cisplatin with granulocyte colony-stimulating factor as adjuvant chemotherapy for osteosarcoma: phase II trial of the European Osteosarcoma Intergroup' *Journal of Clinical Oncology* 12(9): 1842–1848

Peck H (1992) 'Please don't tell him the truth' *Paediatric Nursing* 4(2): 12–14.

Piasecki P (1987) 'Bone malignancies' *in*: Groenwald S (ed.) *Cancer Nursing: Principles and Practice*. Boston: Jones & Bartlett Inc., pp. 417–441 .

Piasecki P (1992) 'Update in orthopaedic oncology' *Orthopaedic Nursing* 11(6): 36–43

Porter D, Holden S, Steel C, Cohen B, Wallace M & Reid R (1992) 'A significant proportion of patients with osteosarcoma may belong to Li-Fraumeni cancer families' *Journal of Bone and Joint Surgery (Br)* 74-B: 883–886

Price J & Spence N (2004) 'Play in the community – quality care for the child with cancer' *Cancer Nursing Practice* 3(8): 31–34

Ramseier L, Malinin T, Temple H, Mnaymneh W & Exner G (2006) 'Allograft reconstruction for bone sarcoma of the tibia in the growing child' *Journal of Bone and Joint Surgery (Br)* 88-B: 95–99

Raymond A, Ayala A & Knuutila S (2002) 'Conventional osteosarcoma' *in*: Fletcher C, Unni K & Mertens F (eds) *WHO Classification of Tumours: Pathology and Genetics of Tumours of Soft Tissue and Bone*. Lyon: IARC Press, pp. 264–270

Roberts P, Chan D, Grimer R, Sneath R & Scales J (1991) 'Prosthetic replacement of the distal femur for primary bone tumours' *Journal of Bone and Joint Surgery (Br)* 73-B: 762–769

Rounseville C (1992) 'Phantom limb pain; the ghost that haunts the amputee' *Orthopaedic Nursing* 11(2): 67–71

Salisbury J & Byers P (1994) 'Osteoblastic and cartilaginous neoplasms' *in*: Salisbury J, Woods C & Byers P (eds) *Diseases of Bones and Joints*. London: Chapman & Hall, pp. 315–334

Schwartz C, Constine L, Putnam T & Cohen H (1993) 'Paediatric solid tumours' *in*: Rubin P (ed.) *Clinical Oncology* (7th edn). Philadelphia: W.B. Saunders Co., pp. 282–288

Scully S, Ghert M, Zurakowski D, Thompson R & Gebhardt M (2002) 'Pathologic fracture in osteosarcoma: prognostic importance and treatment implications' *Journal of Bone and Joint Surgery (Am) 84-A* (1): 49–57

Sensky T (1996) 'Eliciting lay beliefs across cultures: principles and methodology' *British Journal of Cancer 74* (suppl. XX1X): S63–S65

Sloper P (1996) 'Needs and responses of parents following the diagnosis of childhood cancer' *Child Care Health and Development 22*(3): 187–202

Souhami R & Tobias J (eds) (1986) 'Bone and soft tissue sarcomas' *in*: *Cancer and its Management*. London: Blackwell Scientific, pp. 433–452

Spears N (1994) 'In vitro growth of oocyte' *Human Reproduction 9*(6): 969–976

Stoker D, Cobb J & Pringle J (1991) 'Needle biopsy of musculoskeletal lesions' *Journal of Bone and Joint Surgery (Br) 73-B*: 498–500

Taylor J & Muller D (1995) *Nursing Adolescents*. Oxford: Blackwell Science Ltd.

Tebbi C & Erpenbeck A (1996) 'Cancer' *in*: Rickert V (ed.) *Adolescent Nutrition*. New York: Chapman & Hall, pp. 479–502

Tow B & Tan M (2005) 'Delayed diagnosis of Ewing's sarcoma of the right humerus initially treated as chronic osteomyelitis: a case report' *Journal of Orthopaedic Surgery 13*(1): 88–92

Uchida A, Araki N, Shinto Y, Yoshikawa H, Kurisaki E & Ono K (1990) 'The use of hydroxyapatite ceramic in bone tumour surgery' *Journal of Bone and Joint Surgery (Br) 72-B*: 298–302

Unwin P, Cannon S, Grimer R, Kemp H, Sneath R & Walker P (1996) 'Aseptic loosening in cemented custom-made prosthetic replacements for bone tumours of the lower limb' *Journal of Bone and Joint Surgery (Br) 78-B* 1: 5–13

Ushigome S, Mochinami R & Sorenson P (2002) 'Ewing's sarcoma/primitive neuroectodermal tumour (PNET)' *in*: Fletcher C, Unni K & Mertens F (eds) *WHO Classification of Tumours: Pathology and Genetics of Tumours of Soft Tissue and Bone*. Lyon: IARC Press, pp. 298–300

von Essen L & Enskar K (2003) 'Important aspects of care and assistance for siblings of children treated for cancer: a parent and nurse perspective' *Cancer Nursing 26*(3): 203–210

Wallace W & Brougham M (2005) 'Subfertility in adolescents with cancer: who is at risk and what can be done?' *in*: Eden T, Barr R, Bleyer A & Whiteson M (eds) *Cancer and the Adolescent*. Oxford: Blackwell, pp. 133–154

Whelan J (2005) 'Advances in osteosarcoma' *in*: Eden T, Barr R, Bleyer A & Whiteson M (eds) *Cancer and the Adolescent*. Oxford: Blackwell, pp. 113–120

White C (1995) 'Life crises for children and their families' *in*: Carter B & Dearmun A (eds) *Child Health Care Nursing*. Oxford: Blackwell Science Ltd., pp. 116–129

White N, Maxwell C, Michelson J & Bedell C (2005) 'Protocols for managing chemotherapy-induced neutropenia in clinical oncology practices' *Cancer Nursing 28*(1): 62–69

Wicart P, Mascard E, Missenard G & Dubousset J (2002) 'Rotationplasty after failure of a knee prosthesis for a malignant tumour of the distal femur' *Journal of Bone and Joint Surgery 84-B*: 865–869

Wilson K (1993) 'Education for the hospitalised child' *Paediatric Nursing* (4): 24–25

Wittig J, Bickels J, Priebat D, Jelinek J, Kellar-Graney K, Schmookler B & Malawer M (2002) 'Osteosarcoma: a multidisciplinary approach to diagnosis and treatment' *American Family Physician 65*: 1123–1132

Woodgate R (2005) 'A different way of being: adolescents' experiences with cancer' *Cancer Nursing 28*(1): 8–15

Wu C, Cohen S, Richman J, Rowlingson A, Courpas G, Cheung K, Lin E & Liu S (2005) 'Efficacy of postoperative patient-controlled and continuous infusion epidural analgesia versus intravenous patient-controlled analgesia with opioids: a meta-analysis' *Anesthesiology 103*(5): 1079–1088

Yang Y & Damron T (2004) 'Comparison of needle core biopsy and fine needle aspiration for diagnostic accuracy in musculoskeletal lesions' *Archives of Pathology and Laboratory Medicine 128*: 759–764

Part 4

Radiotherapy

18

The Nature of Radiotherapy

Monica Hopkins

Introduction

Radiotherapy has traditionally been a poorly understood area of medicine, often linked in the public's mind and the media with harm. However, in the treatment of cancer in children and young people radiotherapy plays an important role. Its main function is to improve tumour control and overall survival in patients with brain, central nervous system and solid tumours, and is also part of the curative treatment of some lymphomas and leukaemias. Radiotherapy is also a useful tool in managing symptoms in patients at the palliative and end-of-life stage of their disease.

Radiotherapy can be a daunting experience for children, young people and their parents. Radiotherapy departments are often away from the principal treatment centre in a different hospital with new staff, equipment and procedures to get used to and a focus on stillness during treatment that is new and challenging.

The most valuable help that nurses (as well as other members of the wide multidisciplinary team involved in radiotherapy) can provide for children, young people and their families is to demystify some of this and decrease fear by providing accurate information and thus a sense of control. Patients and their families require preparation and ongoing support as well as specialised nursing care and observation. The aim of Part 4 is to introduce radiotherapy as a therapeutic treatment modality, describe how radiothery works, is administered and regulated, and outline the attendent nursing care for acute side effects (late effects are described in Chapter 21).

The medical evidence base of radiotherapy is almost entirely from studies involving adult patients (Wells, 1998; Faithfull, 1999; Donato et al., 2001; Olsen et al., 2001; Curry et al., 2005), the focus of this work is therapeutics and new administration methods, with little on the effects of radiotherapy to the patient (Selek et al., 2005; Merchant et al., 2006). Nursing research is similarly limited (Faithfull et al., 2002; Jordan et al., 2002), with very little from the perspective of children/young adults (Scott et al., 2002; Freeman et al., 2004), or the UK. What is available is predominantly commentary, with few pieces to guide nursing practice (Scott et al., 2002, Faithfull et al., 2002). The work that is available for nursing to base its care on often concerns the efficacy of radiotherapy in studied neoplasms (St Clair et al., 2004; Buwalda et al., 2005; Nag & Tippin, 2003), dose-toxicity studies (Howard et al., 2005; Dorr et al., 2006; Reddick et al., 2006) and late effects (Reiling et al., 1999; Grill et al., 1999; Bassal et al., 2006). Descriptions of

Cancer in Children and Young People   Edited by Faith Gibson and Louise Soanes
© 2008 John Wiley & Sons, Ltd

appropriate nursing care in this chapter are taken from such work and the experiences of practitioners in the field. Issues such as appropriate mouth care in children are not well sourced in the nursing research literature. In addition, although skin care has become a more popular focus in the adult literature, current research on this topic remains scant and poorly disseminated in practice (Campbell & Lane, 1996; Naylor & Mallet, 2001). These issues and other pertinent aspects of nursing care will be outlined in Part 4 and include an analysis of the literature concerning patient preparation and family support.

Indications for the use of radiation in the care of children with cancer

Although used for over a century, understanding the use of radiation in the treatment of childhood cancer continues to evolve. Radiotherapy can be used as the sole mode of therapy or in conjunction with surgery, chemotherapy, or both, as a multi-modal approach to treatment. Radiotherapy can be used both as a curative intervention for radiosensitive tumours or as palliation to control distressing symptoms of advanced disease such as pain, obstruction, compression and bleeding. It may also be used to treat oncological emergencies to give temporary relief from a life-threatening complication of tumour growth until definitive treatment can be commenced, for example, superior vena cava syndrome or spinal cord compression.

The childhood malignancies most commonly treated with radiotherapy are:

- *brain tumours and CNS tumours*: primary treatment for many brain and CNS tumours neuroblastoma; part of the multi-modal therapy used to treat residual, bulky, unresectable, metastatic disease or disseminated disease and in emergency situations, i.e. spinal cord compression;
- *Ewing's sarcoma*: used for localised control for tumours in bones that are indispensable (hence surgery is not an option), inoperable and metastatic;
- *rhabdomyosarcoma*: treatment for inoperable, metastatic tumours and local control where surgical resection is not possible;

- *Hodgkin's disease*: part of the multi-modal therapy for Hodgkin's disease;
- *non-Hodgkin's lymphoma*: used in emergency situations, i.e. spinal cord compression, superior vena cava syndrome.
- *Wilms' tumour*: local control in stage III disease, and whole lung irradiation in stage IV with lung metastates;
- *leukaemia*: reserved for central nervous system and testicular relapse (ALL) and total body irradiation pre-bone marrow transplant in relapsed patients (ALL and AML).

The nature of radiation

For a significant part of modern medical history, radiation has been used as a valuable investigative tool in diagnosis, and one of the most widely recognised medical images is the X-ray, which has served modern medicine well since its inception nearly over 100 years ago, and continues to do so. Since the late nineteenth century, medicine has also been aware of the therapeutic potential of radiation in treating cancer (Iwamoto, 1994). However, to understand how this power is harnessed, it is essential that the source of this energy and its characteristic behaviours are understood.

All matter is made up of atoms. It was thought that these were the smallest material entities, but in recent times it has been discovered that atoms are actually made from a number of different particles (Figure 18.1). The nucleus of an atom is made up of uncharged particles (neutrons) and positively charged particles (protons). Orbiting the nucleus are negatively charged particles (electrons), these are usually equal in number to the protons and hence balance the positive charge of the nucleus (Adamson, 2003). This is the situation in a stable atom. However, atoms can lose or gain electrons, to become ions, the physical process of converting an atom into an ion is called ionisation. Ions occur naturally such as sodium, potassium, calcium. These and other ions play an important role in the cell, particularly at the cell membrane. Ionisation can also occur if enough energy is given to an electron for it to escape its orbit of the nucleus (Adamson, 2003).

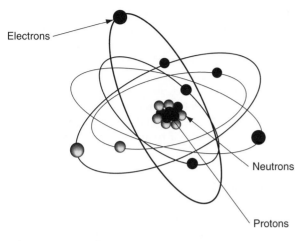

Electrons

Neutrons

Protons

Figure 18.1 A stable atomic structure.

Electrons discarded from an atom carry their energy with them. This movement of energy is called radiation. The radioactivity emitted can be manifested in a number of forms, commonly, electrons travelling at high speed, or electromagnetic radiation waves, such as gamma rays. This radiation energy is the destructive force used in radiotherapy to damage or destroy diseased cells.

Radiation is the transfer of energy from one point to another. Waves of energy can be of varying size, and the distance between one point on a wave and its identical position on the wave following is called the wavelength (Figure 18.2). Wavelengths can be short, and therefore the frequency or number of waves per unit of time is greater, or may be long, and slower in frequency. The greater the number of waves passing through a distance per unit of time, the greater the amount of energy that is passing through that space.

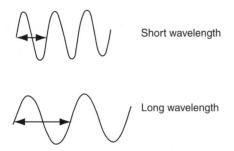

Short wavelength

Long wavelength

Figure 18.2 Short and long wavelengths.

A form of electromagnetic wave energy that is extremely familiar is light. Light is made up of radiation energy waves of lots of different lengths, some short, some long, that bundle together to become visible light. Separately, however, they are all different types of radiation wave energy and cover a wide spectrum of wavelengths. The longer wavelength (and therefore lower energy waves) are the infra-red and radio waves. The spectrum continues right through visible light to its other end, where the waves are of the shortest length, the highest frequency and therefore the greatest energy. These are called X-rays and gamma rays. X-rays and gamma rays have energies ranging from a few thousand volts (kilovolts, kV) to several million volts (megavolts, MeV). Energy of this form moves in bundles and a bundle of X-radiation is described as a photon.

The greater the energy of a photon, the greater its penetration into tissue (Iwamoto, 1994). This is important when planning clinical treatment, as tumours are obviously at different depths beneath the skin surface. Conversely, some forms of particulate radiation (i.e. streams of high-speed electrons) can penetrate the skin but often decline in energy quickly thereafter and so deliver their maximum radiation dose superficially. Recent experimentation with another form of particulate radiotherapy, protons, indicates that these can penetrate deep tissues but, unlike electrons, the radiation tails off sharply after reaching the target, leaving no exit dose (Taylor, 2003a). This would mean that the amount of tissue affected by radiation would be smaller and so hopefully reduce morbidity.

Artificial production of radiation for clinical use

Both gamma and X-ray radiation are used in clinical practice though X-rays are more commonly used (although similar to the X-rays used in imaging, the X-rays described here have a higher frequency and are more penetrating). X-rays are produced by firing high-speed electrons at a target of densely packed atoms. Some of the energy of the fast-moving electrons is converted into waves of energy of the X-ray form; the higher the kilovoltage of the electrons fired, the greater the X-ray energy. The machine used in production of such radiation is called a linear accelerator.

Radiation can be gained and used directly from a decaying isotope. This radiation is concentrated by holding a large quantity of radioactive material in specially constructed machinery that is able to direct energy as needed. There are many naturally occurring sources of radioactive elements, but for convenience and safety, radiotherapy departments use radiation energy produced artificially exploiting the principles of natural atomic decay. Non-radioactive substances or elements are used and their nuclei are destabilised on purpose, resulting in radioactive material. Common radioactive elements artificially produced are the radioactive forms of cobalt (Co) and caesium (Cs) (Co^{60} and Cs^{137}). Caesium produces gamma rays of relatively low energy levels compared to cobalt, which is able to produce gamma rays of very high energy, known as megavoltage radiation.

With all these materials, the quantity of radioactivity derived from an unstable atom reduces with time. A term referred to as half-life or T½ is used to determine how much radioactivity has decayed. The half-life is the time it will take for the intensity of the energy released to decrease to half its original amount (Table 18.2) and is different for each element.

This information has implications for the handling, storage and replacement of materials in a radiotherapy department. All radiotherapy units or oncology wards where radioactive isotopes are used must implement policies that are based on the current Department of Health guidelines on the handling and storage of radioactive matter (DoH, 2000).

An important characteristic of radiation energy (whatever form) is that its intensity decreases as it travels away from its source (Bomford, 2003). As a consequence in the therapeutic use of raidotherapy, the distance the radiation beam must travel to its target must be carefully calculated to ensure the required radiation intensity reaches the tumour, so when a beam of radiotherapy is aimed at a target through a wide field (i.e. skin) the contours of the body it traverses must be considered to ensure uniformity of dose across the field and the target.

For example, a beam that takes in the shoulder will travel a greater distance through tissue to a deep-seated target than a beam a few centimetres higher directed through the base of the neck. For these reasons the energy level of the beam travelling the shorter distance in tissue needs to be attenuated by special material to ensure equal intensity with the beam that travels further. These radiation attenuators are called compensators and are made from a wide variety of materials such as copper, brass or lead (Coleman, 2004). Their use results in a uniform intensity of treatment across the field.

Radiation dose

The international unit of dose is a Gray (Gy) or one-hundredth of a Gy, the Centigray (cGy). The dosages recorded in current clinical trials for childhood tumours are recorded in Gys or cGys. Standardisation allows effects from varying dosages to be compared. This is evident in the research to investigate the late effects of radiation dose (25Gy versus 35Gy) to the posterior fossa in children, particularly IQ (Grill *et al.*, 1999).

Effect of ionising radiation on human tissue

The damage to a cell caused by X-rays occurs in two ways; direct or indirect action. Radiation may deliver energy to the atoms of the cell's DNA,

Table 18.1 Factors contributing to cell radiosensitivity

- Type of cell
- Phase of the cell cycle the cell is in; cells that are resting and not actively producing DNA for cell division are less susceptible to the fatal effects of radiation
- Rate of division of the cell type; tissues made of cells that divide more rapidly are likely to have more cells in the dividing phase of their cell cycle and therefore are more radiosensitive, e.g. bone marrow, mucosa of gastrointestinal lining
- Degree of differentiation of the cell type; poorly differentiated cells are more radiosensitive as they are more likely to replicate
- Oxygenation; the greater the oxygen content of a cell, the more molecules there are to bind to hydroxyls and form resistant radicals which are influential in promoting cell death

Source: McMillan (2003).

changing its chemical structure and causing abnormal function (Adamson, 2003). However, the most important method of cell destruction is indirect action by the ionisation of water within the cell. Following radiation interaction, water molecules produce hydrogen ions and destructive hydroxyl radicals. These unstable hydroxyl radicals damage the nucleus of the cell by causing breaks in the DNA. Single strand breaks may be repaired and the damage overcome, however, a double strand break is harder to repair, and often results in cell death. There is almost immediate cell death if the chromosomal damage is irreparable as the cells cannot then form their essential proteins. However, many cells survive this initial onslaught, as the damage at first does not appear to be excessive, simply an aberration in the linkage of the DNA strand. However, the delayed effect is fatal, as the cell is unable to divide successfully at mitosis due to the number of chromosomal aberations that have been inadequately repaired (McMillan, 2003).

There are some cells within the body that are more sensitive to the effects of ionising radiation and these are termed radiosensitive. This can influence both the efficacy of radiotherapy as a choice of treatment and the extent to which healthy cells are damaged (Table 18.1) (McMillan, 2003).

Table 18.2   Half-life for some of the more common radioactive materials used in radiotherapy

Radioactive isotope	Half-life (T $\frac{1}{2}$)
Caesium[137]	30 years
Cobalt[60]	5.3 years
Iodine[131]	8.1 days
Iridium[192]	74 days
Strontium[85]	64 days
Radium[226]	1620 years
Technetium[99]	6 hours
Yttrium[90]	64.2 hours

Source: Ball & Moore (1980).

Hazards to healthy tissue during radiotherapy

Non-cancerous cells can be injured by radiation, just as they often are with the use of chemotherapy. However, one of the guiding principles of radiotherapy is to keep the death/damage rate of healthy tissue to a minimum, and so reduce adverse side effects on the body. It is to the body's advantage that healthy non-cancerous cells are able to repair their chromosomal tissue, after ionisation, far more effectively than malignant cells. This is often termed the therapeutic ratio of a radiotherapy regimen. Unfortunately, even healthy tissue can only tolerate so much radiation injury without complications, despite the ability to self-repair and this is referred to as the tolerance dose (Kunkler, 2003). This dose varies with the tissue, the volume irradiated, the form of radiation and finally the fractionation schedule.

As previously described, all forms of therapeutic radiation, waves or particles, produce their biological effect by ionisation of important intracellular macromolecules. Damage to DNA directly or through the utilisation of free radicals is most often the case. The adverse effects of such an onslaught on the cell structure and function are delayed in slower-dividing cells (i.e. organ tissue). Radiation injury can actually be repaired over as little as four to six hours in healthy tissue. Consequently, radiotherapy that is given in small frequent doses has a less damaging effect than a single large dose; this allows the same total dose to be given to the tumour. The process of breaking up therapeutic radiation into smaller doses is called fractionation (Adamson, 2003).

Fractionated radiation must be planned to facilitate a therapeutic ratio that allows efficient repair of radiation damage in healthy tissue and an efficient level of death in tumour cells (Taylor, 2003b). Factors influencing the therapeutic ratio are:

- radiation dosage per fraction;
- total dose of radiotherapy given;
- total treatment time.

These factors are manipulated to minimise long- and short-term toxicity and to maximise local tumour control, based on the tumour type and the tolerance of the tissues surrounding it. The ability to repair sub-lethal damage is greater in non-dividing cells (slow-growing healthy tissue) than in rapidly dividing cells (tumour cells, bone marrow, gastrointestinal mucosa and skin). Thus, smaller fractions, given over a shorter period, arguably result in more cumulative damage to tumour tissue (Habrand *et al.*, 2004a). This is of proven benefit in total body irradiation (TBI) (Veys & Rao, 2004), but not as yet in the treatment of brain tumours, where it is hoped it will make some considerable difference in reducing treatment neural toxicity (Skowronska-Gardas, 1994). Research into hyperfractionated radiotherapy, where a smaller dose of radiation is given more than once per day (at least 6 hours apart), is under way.

Proton radiotherapy

Protons are the positively charged particles that make up the nucleus of any atom alongside neutrons. When extracted from an atom and formed into an energy stream they can be used in a cytotoxic manner.

Protons can deposit their energy at a set depth of tissue with virtually no exit dose. Therefore, their use may reduce the volume of healthy tissue exposed to radiation after the beam has hit its intended target (Taylor, 2003a). Proton radiotherapy has the potential to deliver a stable planned dose of ionising radiation to the tumour volume while reducing the level of radiation delivered to adjacent tissues. Studies have demonstrated how the therapeutic ratio can be improved for CNS tumours by delivering a uniform dose of radiation to the target but little other tissue. Clinical experience in children remains limited, however, Mirabell *et al.* (2002) maintain that there is significant potential for reducing the risk of secondary malignancy in children if proton therapy is used for children with medulloblastoma (St Clair *et al.*, 2004) or even rhabdomyosarcoma.

At present there is little clinical evidence to support the theory for the beneficial use of proton therapy in children (Taylor, 2003a). Another factor is that protons are about 2.5 times more expensive to produce than photons, and there are currently no machines in the UK (at least not one that can penetrate beyond skin level). Although it is known to spare normal tissue and decrease treatment-related complications, there is yet to be a robust body of evidence to say it can guarantee better or even equivocal tumour control (Saran, 2004).

Conclusion

It is evident that there has been considerable development in the forms of therapeutic radiation available to use within the clinical setting. Work continues in the understanding of the biological effects of radiation on healthy tissue, and the consequences for the body of repeated exposure. It is this dichotomy between efficacy of treatment and toxicity that is driving developments in technology to improve the therapeutic ratio and administering radiation to the target alone, avoiding healthy tissue wherever possible. The following chapter will expand on the technological expansion in this field and the impact this is having on treatment and treatment sequelae.

References

Adamson D (2003) 'The radiobiological basis of radiation side effects' *in*: Faithfull S & Wells M (eds) *Supportive Care in Radiotherapy*. Edinburgh: Churchill Livingstone, pp. 71–95

Ball JL & Moore AD (1980) *Essential Physics for Radiographers*. Oxford: Blackwell Science Publications

Bassal M, Mertens AC, Taylor L, Neglia JP, Greffe BS, Hammond S, Ronckers CM, Friedman DL, Stovall M, Yasui YY, Robison LL, Meadows AT & Kadan-Lottick NS (2006) 'Risk of selected subsequent carcinomas in survivors of childhood cancer: a report from the Childhood Cancer Survivor Study' *Journal of Clinical Oncology* 24(3): 476–483

Bomford CK (2003) 'The physics of radiotherapy' *in*: Bomford CK & Kunkler IH (eds) *Walter and Miller's Textbook of Radiotherapy: Radiation Physics, Therapy and Oncology* (6th edn). Edinburgh: Churchill Livingstone, pp. 141–252

Buwalda J, Freling NJ, Blank LE, Balm AJ, Bras J, Voûte PA, Caron HN, Schouwenburg PF & Merks JH (2005) 'AMORE protocol in pediatric head and neck rhabdomyosarcoma: descriptive analysis of failure patterns' *Head & Neck* 27(5): 390–396

Campbell J & Lane C (1996) 'Skin care protocol for radiotherapy patients' *Professional Nurse* 12(2): 105–108

Coleman AM (2004) 'Radiotherapy procedures' *in*: Washington CM & Leaver D (eds) *Principles and Practice of Radiation Therapy* (2nd edn). St Louis, MO: Mosby, pp. 171–193

Curry WT, Cosgrove GR, Hochberg FH, Loeffler J & Zervas NT (2005) 'Stereotactic interstitial radiosurgery for cerebral metastases' *Journal of Neurosurgery* 103(4): 630–635

Department of Health (2000) *The Ionising Radiation Regulations*. London: HMSO

Donato V, Bonfili P, Bulzonetti N, Santarelli M, Osti MF, Tombolini V, Banelli E & Enrici RM (2001) 'Radiation therapy for oncological emergencies' *Anticancer Research* 21(3C): 2219–2224

Dorr W, Kost S, Keinert K, Glaser FH, Endert G & Herrmann T (2006) 'Early intestinal changes following abdominal radiotherapy comparison of endpoints' *Strahlenther Onkol.* 182(1): 1–8

Faithfull S (1999) 'Randomised trial, a method of comparisons: a study of supportive care in radiotherapy nursing' *European Journal of Oncology Nursing* 3(3): 176–184

Faithfull S, Hilton M, Booth K, Fielding P, Hindley A, Dickson R, Harrison P, Abraham M, Jackson M, Johnson J & Smith M (2002) 'Survey of information leaflets on advice for acute radiation skin reactions in UK radiotherapy centres: a rationale for a systematic review of the literature' *European Journal of Oncology Nursing* 6(3): 176–178

Freeman K, O'Dell C & Meola C (2004) 'Childhood brain tumors: parental concerns and stressors by phase of illness' *Journal of Pediatric Oncology Nursing* 21(2):87–97

Grill J, Renaux VK, Bulteau C, Viguier D, Levy-Plebois C, Sainte-Rose C, Dellatolas G., Raquin MA, Jambaque I & Kalifa C (1999) 'Long term intellectual outcome in children with posterior fossa tumors according to radiation doses and volumes' *International Journal of Radiation Oncology Biology Physics* 45(1): 137–141

Habrand JL, Abdulkarum B & Roberti H (2004a) 'Radiotherapeutical innovations in pediatric solid tumors' *Pediatric Blood & Cancer* 43(6): 622–628

Habrand JL, Abdulkarim B & Bernard A (2004b) 'Clinical applications of paediatric radiotherapy' *in*: Pinkerton R, Plowman N & Pieters R (eds) *Paediatric Oncology* (3rd edn). London: Arnold, pp. 129–141

Howard JP, Maris JM, Kersun LS, Huberty JP, Cheng SC, Hawkins RA & Matthay KK (2005) 'Tumor response and toxicity with multiple infusions of high dose 131I-MIBG for refractory neuroblastoma' *Pediatric Blood & Cancer* 44(3): 232–239

Iwamoto, R (1994) 'Radiation therapy' *in*: Otto SE (ed.) *Oncology Nursing* (2nd edn). St Louis, MO: Mosby

Jordan L, Beaver K & Foy S (2002) 'Ozone treatment for radiotherapy skin reactions: is there an evidence base for practice?' *European Journal of Oncology Nursing* 6(4): 220–227

Kunkler IH (2003) 'Effects of radiation on normal tissues' *in*: Bomford CK & Kunkler IH (eds) *Walter and Miller's Textbook of Radiotherapy: Radiation Physics, Therapy and Oncology* (6th edn). Edinburgh: Churchill Livingstone, pp. 296–306

McMillan TJ (2003) 'Principles of radiobiology' *in*: Bomford CK & Kunkler IH (eds) *Walter and Miller's Textbook of Radiotherapy: Radiation Physics, Therapy and Oncology* (6th edn). Edinburgh: Churchill Livingstone, pp. 286–295

Merchant TE, Kiehna EN, Kun LE, Mulhern RK, Lic C, Xiong X, Boop FA & Sanford RA (2006) 'Phase II trial of conformal radiation therapy for pediatric patients with craniopharyngioma and correlation of surgical factors and radiation dosimetry with change in cognitive function' *Journal of Neurosurgery* 104(2 Suppl.): 94–102

Mirabell R, Lomax A, Cella L & Scheider U (2002) 'Potential reduction of the incidence of radiation induced second cancers by using proton beams in the treatment of pediatric tumors' *International Journal of Radiation Oncology, Biology, Physics* 54(3): 824–829

Nag S & Tippin DB (2003) 'Brachytherapy for pediatric tumors' *Brachytherapy* 2(3): 131–138

Naylor N & Mallett J (2001) 'Management of acute radiotherapy induced skin reactions: a literature review' *European Journal of Oncology Nursing* 5(4): 221–233

Olsen DL, Raub W, Bradley C, Johnson M, Macias JL, Love V & Markoe A (2001) 'The effect of aloe vera gel/mild soap versus mild soap alone in preventing skin reactions in patients undergoing radiation therapy' *Oncology Nursing Forum* 28(3): 543–547

Reddick WE, Shan ZY, Glass JO, Helton S, Xiong X, Wu S, Bonner MJ, Howard SC, Christenson R, Khan RB, Pui CH & Mulhern RK (2006) 'Small white matter volumes are associated with larger defects in attention and learning among long term survivors of acute lymphoblastic leukaemia' *Cancer* 106(4): 941–949

Reiling M, Rubnitz J, Rivera G, Boyett J, Hancock M, Felix C, Kun L, Walter A, Evans W & Pui C (1999) 'High incidence of secondary brain tumours after radiotherapy and antimetabolites' *Lancet* 354(9172): 34–37

Saran F (2004) 'New technology for radiotherapy in paediatric oncology' *European Journal of Cancer* 40(14): 2019–2105

Scott L, Langton F & O'Donoghue J (2002) 'Minimising the use of sedation/anaesthesia in young children receiving radiotherapy through an effective play preparation programme' *European Journal of Oncology Nursing* 6(1): 15–22

Selek U, Ozyar E, Ozyigit G, Varan A, Buyukpamukcu M & Atahan IL (2005) 'Treatment result of 59 young patients with nasopharyngeal carcinoma' *International Journal of Pediatric Otorhinolaryngology* 69(2): 201–207

Skowronska-Gardas A (1994) 'Hyperfractionated radiotherapy for brain stem tumours in children' *Radiotherapy Oncology* 33(30): 259–261

St Clair WH, Adams CMD, Bues M, Fullerton BC, LaShell S, Kooy HM, Loeffler MD & Tarbell N (2004) 'Advantage of protons compared to conventional X-ray or IMRT in the treatment of a pediatric patient with medulloblastoma' *International Journal of Radiation Oncology, Biology, Physics* 58(3): 727–734

Taylor R (2003a) 'Proton radiotherapy for paediatric tumours: potential areas for clinical research' *Clinical Oncology* 15(1): S32–36

Taylor R (2003b) 'Paediatric oncology' *in*: Bomford CK & Kunkler I (eds) *Walter and Miller's Textbook of Radiotherapy: Radiation Physics, Therapy and Oncology* (6th edn). Edinburgh: Churchill Livingstone, pp. 583–596

Veys P & Rao K (2004) 'Allogeneic stem cell transplantation' *in*: Pinkerton R, Plowman N & Pieters R (eds) *Paediatric Oncology* (3rd edn). London: Arnold, pp. 513–537

Wells M (1998) 'What's so special about radiotherapy nursing?' *European Journal of Oncology Nursing* 2(3): 162–168

19

Administration of Radiotherapy

Monica Hopkins

Introduction

Having discussed the basic science underpinning radiotherapy, it is important to take this forward into a discussion on how radiotherapy is given to patients. This chapter outlines the routes of administration, the forms of treatment, the advantages and disadvantages of each, planning, dosage and implications for the care of the child or young person.

There are three main routes by which radiation can be delivered to tumour cells:

- externally, in a beam produced by a source external to the body (teletherapy);
- internally, by a radioactive source that has been implanted surgically (brachytherapy);
- by attaching a radioactive isotope to a metabolite or even an antigen-specific antibody (unsealed source).

Each of these will now be discussed in turn. This area of knowledge is rapidly increasing and has been positively affected by the growth in digital technology in medicine leading to more complex planning and administration that can more accurately target tumour tissue while sparing healthy cells surrounding it.

External beam therapy (teletherapy)

By far the most common method of delivery is external beam therapy or teletherapy. A beam of radiation energy is produced in either particulate or wave form. It is then focused for accuracy of target, depth and radiation intensity at a predetermined field of tissue. The energy contained within the beam is such that it causes the maximum degree of ionisation in tissues at a planned depth, i.e the tumour. This ensures minimal skin and superficial tissue damage. However, should skin or superficial tissue be the target, the intensity of radiation is altered accordingly, to a level that can be absorbed as soon as it reaches the skin. This may be done by positioning the child far away from the source or by placing a barrier between the skin and the machine to decrease intensity of the beam at that particular site and thus allow the radiation to act on the identified tissues. This barrier may be made of wax, copper, brass, lead or a similarly dense material that can attenuate the beam (Coleman, 2004) and is called a compensator. Compensators can be in the form of complex polystyrene moulds filled with a compensating material that is then moulded to the exact contours of the body (Coleman, 2004).

Cancer in Children and Young People   Edited by Faith Gibson and Louise Soanes
© 2008 John Wiley & Sons, Ltd

The delivery of the external beam needs to be planned in every detail to ensure maximum cell kill of diseased tissue and minimum damage to surrounding areas (Adamson, 2003). For these reasons dose, intensity, direction of beam and target area must be absolutely accurate. Significant time must be spent on planning and ensuring that each fractionated dose enters the tissue with exactly the same accuracy as the first. Hence, positioning, marking and immobility of the child's body are vitally important.

Treatment planning

Integration of radiotherapy into multimodality treatment requires a basic understanding of radiation planning, the influence of fractionation on tumour death and normal cell recovery, and the effect on the body of radiotherapy, including its effects when combined with surgery and chemotherapy. In the past there were usually only two or three fields, regularly shaped and symmetrical. The tumour had to be assumed to be regularly and compactly shaped, but it is agreed they are not. Nearby tissue had to be enclosed within the margins and protection for healthy tissue could only be afforded using shaped lead blocks or local shielding on the body. This was often inadequate and crude, exposing healthy tissue to unnecessary radiotherapy damage that led to significant late effects and possible tissue disfigurement (D'Angio, 1992), catastrophic to body image and quality of survival. Today technology has moved on significantly and so has planning.

Treatment planning involves making a number of different decisions on an individual basis. First, there must be accurate tumour imaging to outline the treatment field so that measurements can be collated to calculate the most appropriate form of radiotherapy. The angle of beam (e.g. anterior–posterior, lateral, oblique, rotating arcs) must be ascertained. In addition, there must be identification of vital structures that need to be shielded by shaping the beam in some fashion. Second, the dose of radiation energy required to reduce or obliterate the tumour load must be determined. This second consideration should be guided primarily by a designated protocol for the child's age and the histology of the tumour,

but also by clinical assessment. Third, the type of radiotherapy must be identified; X-rays, gamma rays or particulate radiation will deliver differing energy, remembering that the energy of the radiotherapy must reflect the depth of penetration required. Kilovoltage (kV) radiation has the lowest voltage and is used to treat very superficial lesions. Orthovoltage radiation has deeper penetration but still delivers quite high doses to the skin and is particularly well absorbed by bone. Megavoltage radiation allows the deepest penetration.

Linear accelerators, cobalt units and certain cyclotrons are capable of emitting megavoltage radiation (Taylor, 2003). The volume of tissue to be treated consists of the tumour (GTV – gross tumour volume) plus an area of healthy tissue, or margin, around it (CTV – clinical target volume). These clear margins must be identified to account for microscopic tumour extension.

There are other considerations, however, before the final area is identified: limitations of imaging investigation, characteristics of the movement and scatter of the form of radiation being used, and slight daily changes in body positioning and organ movement, might all increase the risk of missing the tumour if they have not been properly considered. Hence the planning target volume (PTV) is the CTV plus an extra margin again. Depending on the histology of the tumour, adjacent or regional lymph nodes may also be included in the tissue volume to be treated.

When planning the shape and angle of the beam of radiation, it is vital that these factors are simulated with a diagnostic radiographic machine equipped with a fluoroscopic unit. These machines simulate the path of the beam of radiation, but for more complex situations a specialised CT scanner simulation may also be utilised, where simultaneous scanning can identify the path of the beams and the tissue likely to be caught in the beams.

There is now an armoury of imaging available for planning and verification. Not all of these are available in every centre, due to resource difficulties (finances and appropriately trained personnel) and speed of technological advancement outstripping evidence of improved clinical outcomes (Munro, 2003). Until this time, the cutting edge of radiation technology will continue to be led by the advancement in the accuracy of imaging modalities, their ability to combine and define the target as well as evaluation of the efficacy of conformal therapies and the rise in sophisticated 3-D planning software.

The imaging modalities currently available in some UK centres are:

- *CT – Computerised Tomography* uses X-rays to outline the anatomy of the field and the target.
- *MRI – Magnetic Resonance Imaging* uses a magnetic field and its interaction with tissue to identify targets.
- *PET – Positron Emission Tomography* looks at chemical metabolism in cells and so gives metabolic data to aid identify target and possible spread.
- *SPECT – Single Photon Emission CT* uses radionucleotides to scan the body but then presents resulting data in a computerised tomography format to give a 3-D image of the body.
- *MRS – Magnetic Resonance Spectrometry* is a magnetic resonance image that tracks chemical signals within the body and therefore outlines a chemical map of the body.

Access to all these modalities will lead to better anatomical mapping of complex areas such as the brain, and identification of the position of critical structures for planning as well as identifying gross tumour volume (GTV) more effectively (Soomal & Saran, 2004). Functional imaging (PET, MRS) may help identify microscopic disease spread and therefore define the clinical tumour volume (CTV) better, perhaps helping to reduce the significant margins that had to be planned in the past when knowledge of such spread was poor. The future will see further progression in multimodal imaging, i.e. improvements in the technology of functional imaging and access to it, and its fusion with improved anatomical imaging (Saran, 2004). Many fusion techniques, however, have so far only been recommended within the intracranial cavity as there is little organ movement between the individual scans taken, so the fusion of images from different modalities is more successful. Other cavities have significant organ movement and therefore the data are harder to combine (Soomal & Saran, 2004). It may soon be possible for centres in the UK to have access to treatment machines with CT mounted upon them so when a patient has been planned and is ready to be treated, they can produce a high-resolution CT to check internal soft and bony anatomy for position prior to each fraction. These positions change daily with decrease in tumour volume itself and alterations in tissue integrity within the same cavity (Court *et al.*, 2005).

Close monitoring of critical structure and tumour position may be made even more effective by the advent of an automatic CT-guided adaptive technique (ART) to modify the beam shape (Court *et al.*, 2005). This is a very new technique whereby a daily CT image detects subtle changes in target position and critical structure position and thereby modifies the machine set-up accordingly. ART detects inter-fraction changes and corrects the beam, thereby enabling dose distributions within various tissues to remain close to those originally planned.

The planning process can be complicated when a child has had surgery or chemotherapy prior to radiation. In these cases it is often difficult to identify the true position and volume of the original tumour bed (prior to any therapy) and so determine possible areas of microscopic residual disease. For this reason, collaboration between surgeons and clinical oncologists before surgery is vital to fully evaluate and document the extent of the disease at its presentation.

After the target tissue volume is set and the fields to be irradiated have been identified, thought needs to be given to the total dose of radiation and the number of fractions into which it should be divided (although these considerations may already have been dealt with in a national treatment protocol). There is a considerable effort to be made in balancing the positive and negative effects of prolonging treatment by dividing doses (Cosset *et al.*, 1994). The larger the dose per fractionation, and the larger the total dose in a shorter period of time, the more significant the risk of late effects, such as fibrosis or necrosis (Kunkler, 2003; Tarbell *et al.*, 2006). These forms of tissue damage are caused by insufficient cell repair between each dose fraction, thereby allowing significant cell damage to occur in healthy tissue that is not always visible for some time if the tissue is slow growing (Habrand *et al.*, 2004b). Delayed tissue damage may be evident only after some length of time as it may take many mitotic cycles before cell death occurs, especially in slow-growing tissues. This is in addition to the time taken for the full effect of acute inflammatory changes to be evident within a tissue (Haustermans & Withers, 2004). Late effects are a result of the combined effect of vascular endothelial damage and the damage sustanined by parenchymal stem cells in the irradiated tissue (Tarbell *et al.*, 2006).

In addition, increased fractionation in prolonging total treatment time not only promotes healthy tissue repair but also allows for re-oxygenation of hypoxic tumour tissue, and therefore increases its radiosensitivity (Lutterbach & Guttenberger, 2000; McMillan, 2003). This can be useful where the tumour has a hypoxic centre due to its large size outstripping the blood supply. The outer margins of the mass are destroyed by earlier fractions allowing time for the more resistant central cells to become better oxygenated and therefore more radiosensitive.

However, protracted courses of small doses of radiation, though reducing acute effects, may actually allow tumour re-growth, or re-population, as it does in healthy tissue, because malignant cells have also been allowed time to repair (Adamson, 2003). This is also the argument for not recommending pauses in treatment once a regimen has started. As cell death occurs during radiation, there is actually a stimulus for cells currently in G^0, the resting stage of the cell cyle, to enter the cycle to replace lost tumour cells (Adamson, 2003). Consequently there may be a stimulous for tumour growth once radiotherapy commences that must be countermanded with continued cytotoxic therapy.

Treatment planning by manual methods is long gone; modern centres have highly sophisticated hardware and software for planning radiotherapy. Three-dimensional (3-D) planning systems are now in use that can link a CT scanner simulator to the therapy beam generator. The complex anatomical data from the scanner are transmitted directly to the administration device. Software will recommend the size and shape of the field and the professional can adapt these to the individual patient and tumour location with an instant feedback image to demonstrate the effects of any modifications they make to the recommended plans (Bomford, 2003). These 3-D plans create a considerable amount of data and require considerable skill to use. Accurate treatment is

dependent on detailed anatomical data from CT or CT/MRI fused images, with the possible addition of functional data (PET, MRS). Portal images (those taken by radiotherapy machines through the same aspect as the beam pathway) are essential to confirm beam accuracy, using pre-determined markers and for day-to-day positioning of the patient. They also identify positions of any shields or compensators, and this process serves to verify the dose each tissue receives on a daily basis (Bomford, 2003).

Methods for improving the accuracy of administration to tumour while avoiding healthy tissue

Conformal radiotherapy

As previously mentioned, modern advances in computer technology have led to significant advances in the imaging available to the oncology team, thereby enabling an increased level of complexity to be attained in radiotherapy planning (Bucci *et al.*, 2005). Gone are the days of 2-D images and manual calculations. Oncologists and radiographers have been working with 3-D images and computer calculations for almost 10 years and 4-D planning, i.e. data that change over a time-line (Bomford, 2003), is on the horizon.

Conformal radiotherapy is a method that aims to deliver a homogeneous dose to all tumour tissue, without unnecessary toxicity to the patients' healthy tissue (Habrand *et al.*, 2004a). In essence, it is the shaping of a high-dose beam to match more closely the shape and volume occupied by the disease itself. This can also be seen as conformal avoidance – where the beam is shaped to maximise the amount of healthy tissue it avoids.

Conforming the beam to the shape of the tumour or tumour tissue is achieved using devices such as collimators and wedges and it is essential to improve target accuracy. It brings the planning target volume (PTV) closer and closer to the clinical target volume (CTV) and also aims to ensure the beam avoids critical structures or even previously treated non-tumour tissue. 3-D conformal radiotherapy has made definite improvements to the quality of radiotherapy available to patients (Khatua & Jalali, 2005).

This 3-D planning calculates beam instructions that are translated to the beam by means of positioning of shields called multi-leaf collimators attached to the linear accelerator delivering the photons. The computer linked to the machine moves the collimators rapidly and automatically to the specifications of the plans. Multi-leaved collimators (MLC) are moveable rectangular tungsten leaves that allow dynamic beam shaping. Each leaf can move independently under digital control. They are placed in front of the beam as it exits the source. There are many of them lined up in rows, and they can be of varying sizes. As each is moved into its own unique position, a serrated shadow is cast across the field. This shadow should outline the desired shape of the beam to affect the child's plan. The smaller the leaves, the more detailed and complex the shadow can be. The longer it stays in position the more dose it will absorb and in so doing protects a defined portion of the field and any tissue in it. In conformal radiotherapy the collimators are left in position for the full fractionated dose.

However, leaves can be manipulated while the beam is on; this is called dynamic collimation, whereby some parts of the field will receive more radiation than others. This concept, which serves to further increase the conforming process, will be developed further in the section on intensity modulated radiotherapy (IMRT).

Photon energy reacts differently with various tissues so planners can input the different tissue interactions into the computer to predict tissue penetration and dose distribution. Finally, when any form of conformal radiotherapy has taken place, high-intensity CT can be used to verify the delivered dose. As with all radiotherapy techniques, conformal radiotherapy is only as effective or safe as the quality of the imaging, planning, localisation and immobilisation. Conformal planning in all its forms demands highly trained and skilled professionals to deliver these complex treatment plans from start to finish.

Intensity modulated radiotherapy (IMRT)

Technology is developing whereby collimator blades can be moved during the duration of the beam (dynamically) to produce the optimal dimensions of the beam at each different depth so as to get closer to the treatment plan (Bilsky et al., 2001). (IMRT) is a method that optimises the shape and size of the beam as it penetrates the tissues to and through the target to meet the dose demands of the target tissues while avoiding critical doses to nearby structures (Nutting et al., 2000). To do this requires advanced imaging, planning, verification and delivery, all in a 3-D manner.

IMRT is an advanced conformal technique that delivers non-uniform doses across a field while avoiding critical tissue (even when it is wrapped around a target) and at the same time escalating the dose to particular areas of the target (Saran, 2004). The intensity of each beam is modulated according to the needs for a high dose to the target and a low dose to critical structures in the way. Multiple beams, all modulated, create sharp dose gradients across the field, consequently only a fraction of any dose is delivered to the tissues adjacent to the tumour.

The use of IMRT is facilitating significant strides forward in accuracy and safety of radiation oncology. It is a very new technology but extremely promising and indeed exciting (Hong et al., 2005). Evidence on clinical outcomes is scarce at present and confined to areas such as head and neck, prostate and para-spinal lesions in adult therapy (Zelefsky et al., 2002). The use of IMRT could have a profound effect on decreasing ototoxicity and xerostomia in children and adults (Saran, 2004).

The planning required for IMRT is inductive, in that the plan starts with data being entered on maximum and minimum doses for all structures in the field, especially critical structures, and tumour. It then works backwards to a beam that is conformed throughout with multi-leaf collimators changing dynamically in shape (under computer control) as the beam traverses the depth of tissue. Therefore it calculates the tissue dosages, beam shapes and beam angles to derive the treatment directives (Krasin et al., 2004b; Saran, 2004).

Clinical oncologists are now able to conform beams to very irregular tumours such as those which have concave areas that are filled with healthy tissue (Saran, 2004). As well as affecting dose distribution to spare healthy tissues (Krasin et al., 2004a), it can also be used to fire a higher dose to high-risk areas.

This offers good target coverage and the possibility of dose escalation while simultaneously keeping critical structures (eyes, ears, hypothalamus axis, cord, etc.) within pre-determined dose levels. However, there are disadvantages, as this technique may lead to a greater volume of healthy tissues getting a small dose of radiation which can increase the secondary malignancy risk (Saran, 2004).

Fusing the data from imaging techniques such as MRI and CT has been very successful in accurately targeting CNS tumours but merging anatomical imaging with functional techniques such as PET would help to define targets so that margins of the tumour could be identified more accurately and so decrease the clinical target volume (gross tumour volume plus margin for microscopic spread). At present there is evidence of the efficacy of fusing CT and PET in the treatment of brain tumours but no other sites (Saran, 2004). There will always be inherent difficulties in treating tumours in the chest and abdomen as inspiration, cardiac output and peristalsis cause considerable tissue movement. For this reason breathing techniques during imaging have been explored in the past but now the idea of 4-D computerised tomography that can isolate images that show the movement of organs over time may be a more useful avenue of future research in overcoming these challenges (Keall, 2004). For the present, IMRT planned with image fusion (CT and MR) results in outstanding local control despite using greatly reduced margins (Wolden *et al.*, 2005).

The final stage of the planning process, prior to commencement of treatment, is often carried out on a machine called a simulator, which has been structured to mimic the geometry of the treatment machine or, as in the case of some more recent models in the US, built onto the treatment machine itself. The simulator uses diagnostic rather than therapeutic doses of radiation to simulate the treatment field in terms of size, shape, angle and volume. The radiographs obtained from this procedure are used to demonstrate adequate coverage of tumour volume and the reproducibility of the treatment field. In order to obtain a satisfactory treatment plan it may be necessary to simulate multiple fields, approaching the tumour from different positions. Families often worry that during such a delay in starting treatment the tumour may be progressing; therefore constant support and reassurance must be undertaken by the named nurse in preparing the family for these

procedures, and full explanations should be given as to their necessity and benefit. The child and the family should be allowed to voice their concerns over delay in treatment but they should be reassured that this period has been anticipated within the treatment plan.

Maintaining accuracy of treatment (immobilisation)

Once the beams have been planned, it is necessary to take steps to ensure that the angles of the beam can be maintained throughout therapy. Radiation energy decreases as it travels over a given distance (Bomford, 2003). The decrease in energy follows a uniform path, i.e. it is possible to calculate the intensity of the radiation at a given point away from the source. This is important for clinical use, as the distance the child is from the radiation source has implications for the intensity of the radiation or dose to which the child's tissue will be exposed. As the dose must be accurately replicated daily, identical body positioning is maintained for, and during, each dose. For critical accuracy, such as when treating the brain or head and neck tumours, a shell is made for each individual to immobilise their head. This shell must be an exact fit, so that even the smallest movements are restricted to prevent alterations in the treatment field. More extreme versions of immobilisation used for stereotactic radiotherapy, where frames, cradles and body vacuum packs can be used, will be discussed later in the chapter (Bomford, 2003).

Moulds are made using plaster of Paris to take an impression of the child's head. Plaster of Paris dries in less than a minute, and the cast is filled with plaster to form a reproduction of the area. The plaster reproduction is then used to make a perspex shell and this is then checked for comfort and accuracy. Once the shell is deemed to fit well, the rough edges are filed and markings for alignment of beams can then be made. The shell is then used at each treatment to hold the postion of the area to be treated. Other techniques and materials to make these shells quicker and with less discomfort to the child are now available, such as the orfit mould. This is a sheet of mesh-like plastic which, when warmed, can be moulded around any body part. The material cools quickly to a rigid structure able to restrict movement.

A shell is not always required. In the treatment of many peripheral areas the radiographers will align the treatment field by means of laser lights on the radiotherapy machine (Bomford, 2003). This alignment is then checked using anterior and posterior markers and can be confirmed by portal imaging or simultaneous scanning. Radiotherapy only takes a few minutes but much time is often spent beforehand in positioning the child so that treatment can be given to the exact area required. Very small children may require a general anaesthetic for planning and treatment if they are unable to comply with the planning and delivery of radiotherapy, though the skills of hospital play specialists in a structured programme may enable children as young as 3 years of age to comply.

In order that the machinery can be aligned accurately, markings are made around the target treatment field; these are not easily removed. The child's position must then be held throughout the dose of radiation. If a shell is to be used for treatment, the marks will be placed on this. If a shell is not used, the child will have the ink marks drawn on their skin, to define the exact treatment field. This is referred to as 'marking up' and special marker pens are used by the radiographers to do this. The marks must remain in place for the duration of treatment. In the event of fading, the radiographers may need to re-draw the lines. Should the marks start to fade while on weekend leave, the family should be asked to redraw over the marks with a felt tip pen, which must be a different colour from the one used by the radiographers, so that they can distinguish between the two. The marks should not be washed off during the course of the treatment.

Occassionally, due to tissue damage and consequent oedema or severe weight loss/gain, the shell may no longer fit and a new one will need to be cast. This can be time-consuming and distressing to the child and the family.

Nursing care issues in the planning process

Parents often voice their concerns and fears that their child will be 'radioactive' after receiving radiotherapy treatment, and fear that their child's skin, clothing, urine and stools may be contaminated following treatment. They may also worry that the treated child may be a danger to other members of the family. During preparation for treatment, it is therefore important to reinforce that the child is not radioactive at any time, and no radiation safety precautions are necessary following teletherapy treatment. Precautions are only required when sealed or unsealed sources are used, such as brachytherapy or ^{131}ImIBG (metaiodobenzylguanidine) treatment.

When considering all these factors, it can be seen that the efficacy of radiotherapy lies in the accuracy of the planning. Nursing care of the child while undergoing this experience is critical to ensure that planning is precise and successful in its goals, but also that the child is able to cooperate through understanding and awareness rather than fear and insecurity. The family obviously plays a major part in helping the child to feel safe and protected while preparing for therapy. For this experience to be positive and not cause psychological disturbance, the child and family need to be well informed of every stage and of its significance. At the same time, they should be involved as partners, planning how best to deal with each experience with the knowledge they have of their own child. It is therefore imperative that nurses have a clear understanding of the planning process itself, in order to be able to prepare the child and family as effectively as possible. Iwamoto (1994) outlines the main teaching priorities in preparing a family for external beam therapy:

1. A step-by-step route through all the events that will lead up to treatment, e.g. planning and simulation, moulds and shielding devices, daily treatment schedules, ongoing clinical evaluation through therapy, access to advice and support, follow-up and assessment.
2. Time factors: length of time in planning, daily visit and treatment times, length of course.
3. The radiotherapy environment, the unit, mould room, treatment room and machinery.
4. Specific effects and toxicities.
5. What happens, why it happens, when it will happen and how long it will last.
6. Reassurance must be given that the child/ young person is not radioactive.

7. Explanation of what measures the child and family can take to minimise or even prevent side effects.
8. Discussion of possible delayed or late effects and the resources available for care, support and advice.
9. Provision and nature of follow-up for the child/young person and their family.

These guidelines were developed for the care of adult patients but form a useful framework for use with children/young people. However, the format and educational strategies utilised in dealing with children or young people and their families may need to be tailored to suit individuals. Written information is helpful and there must be time to answer questions. However, the cognitive ability to utilise abstract information about an unknown subject is not developed until mid-adolescence. Children and young people who have not yet aquired this cognitive process, therefore, require visual and sensory information to understand what is to happen. Photographs, models, touching and examining machinery at close quarters, walking around a radiotherapy suite and playing with mould room materials are all vital components of an effective teaching plan.

Play preparation for radiotherapy in younger children is often based upon the concept of desensitisation (Slifer et al., 1994) founded upon established methods of reducing children's anxiety (Warzak et al., 1991) and teaching behavioural control through operant conditioning (Slifer et al., 1993). Desensitisation is a behavioural therapy technique used for decreasing fear and/or anxiety about an identified object or situation (Slifer et al., 1994). The child who is to undergo radiotherapy requires desensitisation to the equipment, staff and routine of planning and treatment prior to commencement. Children who are too young to be able to identify the source of their fears respond to those of their parents and family, and feel the sense of impending separation. Children can be supported significantly by involving parents in the desensitisation process (Lew & La Valley, 1995). Desensitisation includes step-by-step rehearsals of the stages of planning and treatment, first, through experiential play and model equipment and then through exploration of the actual radiotherapy

suite. Constant positive reinforcement each time the child manages to touch, hold, manipulate and practise with equipment or a routine is absolutely essential (Slifer et al., 1994). After desensitisation children can go on to learn motion control, again through keeping still for photographs for longer and longer periods, with the use of constant positive feedback (Cooper et al., 1987), gradually resulting in an ability to tolerate therapy without sedation. These techniques have proved to be extremely effective in preparing children for radiotherapy and avoiding anaesthesia (Scott et al., 2002).

The role of the play specialist cannot be underestimated in this situation, he or she is perfectly placed to coordinate and lead a team approach to meeting these preparatory needs. The play specialist is highly skilled in strategies and current techniques in play preparation and has the necessary knowledge of child development and resources to create a preparation plan to suit any individual.

Preparing a young person for radiotherapy may need to address different issues, often using different perhaps more abstract strategies. This age group may have better control over their own body positioning but can be equally as anxious and distressed about the prospect of radiation therapy. They not only worry about the efficacy of treatment but also the side effects, especially those that leave a negative cosmetic effect, as has been so evident in surgical studies in this age group (Stewart et al., 1994). Open honest discussion of the need for radiotherapy and the consequences for them must be the starting point. There are no formal studies into the needs of young people during radiotherapy but literature on their coping with illness and therapy in other specialities should help to influence our practice (Burkhart & Rayens, 2005; Justus et al., 2006). The checklist advocated by Iwamoto (1994) discussed earlier has resonance with this group. Involving young people in all discussions, empowering them to explore and question procedures as well as the long-term consequences of treatment may go some way to reducing anxiety and promoting a positive locus of control that facilitates coping in these young people (Burkhart & Rayens, 2005). A positive approach to education, communication and self-exploration can improve a young person's self-concept and feeling of inclusion in care, both of which are widely held to be positive indicators of self-care in young people with chronic disease (Justus *et al.*, 2006). Inherent in this approach is ensuring a positive respect for independent thought and action.

In preparing the child/young person and the family for planning and therapy, it is essential that they understand that he/she will be alone in the machine room for the duration of the treatment fraction. However, this is for a short period of time and the child will be observed constantly by staff and the family on a video monitor, and can communicate through the intercom. Favourite toys or blankets may be comforting at these times, in addition to favourite music or an audio story. However, honesty and information often are the most useful ways to decrease the young person's/child's fear and anxiety. It may be possible for the play specialist to devote time and experience to accompanying certain children on their first visits to the radiotherapy suite for planning, mould room and treatment, until the child and radiotherapy staff have become familiar with each other.

Should preparation be unsuccessful due to the child's age, developmental immaturity or extreme psychological distress, the child can be sedated or even anaesthetised with a short-acting medication, such as profonol or an appropriate alternative under the care of a paediatric anaesthetist. However, the aim of nursing interventions is to avoid this wherever possible (Scott *et al.*, 2002). Bucholtz (1992) and Oski *et al.* (1990) point out possible concerns about the use of sedation in treating children. First, it is possible that sedation may disrupt a child's daily activity, growth and development. Second, it is difficult to guarantee that sedation will always be successful and for how long. Timing sedation to coincide with a tightly timed radiotherapy slot can be problematic and, if unsuccessful, another course of action needs to be considered. It is a significant nursing challenge to negotiate appropriate sedation, time its administration and monitor the child for physical response before, during and after therapy (Bucholtz, 1992).

Scott *et al.* (2002) suggest that each child should be thoroughly assessed before considering sedation or anaesthesia. Age, developmental level, physical state, previous experience of therapy and anxiety levels should all be taken into account. The ultimate goal is to prevent the child from moving while in the radiotherapy suite but this must be balanced against the possible trauma to the child and the fact that children require close monitoring throughout. Should anaesthesia prove necessary, an anaesthetist must be present to monitor the child. Even when children have been considered suitable for anaesthesia, it is always important to ensure that they are assessed daily for contraindications such as respiratory dysfunction, infection and altered states of consciousness.

It must also be remembered that all children in this country are treated in units that predominantly care for large numbers of adult patients and they have very busy schedules worked around the speed with which adults can be prepared and treated. Children and their required preparation take up an enormous amount of time in these busy departments. The need for sedation or anaesthesia places considerable strain on the department for the extra time and resources to accommodate such a child within a room. If the child is sedated, then accuracy of timing cannot be guaranteed and the room may be left waiting for a child that is not quite sedated enough. If anaesthesia is required then extra staff and resources are necessary to prepare, monitor and recover the child in safety. Improved play preparation not only reduces the necessity for sedation and anaesthesia but also means that the child can be helped to cooperate with treatment to such an extent that the radiotherapy rooms are not left unused for large portions of the day while staff attempt to assist a child who is experiencing distress and difficulty in maintaining a position for treatment.

Brachytherapy

Internal delivery or brachytherapy is a method of delivering radiation that is quite rare in treating childhood cancers, but is useful where surgery or external beam radiotherapy may have devastating consequences for the surrounding tissue. Radioactive material can be placed either interstitially, intracavitarily within an applicator, or placed permanently within selected tissue. Significant local control and fewer late effects should make this form of therapy advantageous in paediatrics (Fontanesi *et al.*, 1994). Athough at present brachytherapy does not play a role in paediatric protocols, there are some case reports and small series studies describing a number of different tumours types in which it has been used; head and neck (Buwalda *et al.*, 2004, Buwalda *et al.*, 2005); brain tumours (Beutler *et al.*, 2005; Larson *et al.*, 2004; Mayr *et al.*, 2002); soft tissue sarcomas (Nag *et al.*, 2003; Merchant *et al.*, 2000); Wilms' tumours (Ghandi *et al.*, 2005); the eye (Shields *et al.*, 2004), as well as in previously treated recurrences. There is currently no nursing literature on the care of these children during their treatment and so it must be extrapolated from adult guidelines.

Radioisotopes may be sealed or unsealed, temporary or permanent, and they can have variable dose rates – low, medium, high or even pulsed (Martinez-Monge *et al.*, 2006). Sealed is when the isotope is either contained within an applicator at placement or loaded into the applicator after it has been placed in the required position (afterloaded); these sources are removed and therefore are called temporary sources. They are housed in a small carriage or applicator and are made to measure to fit the specific cavity by mould room technicians. To ensure a perfect fit, the mould may need to be formed within the cavity with the child possibly under sedation or anaesthesia. It therefore follows that preparation by experienced nursing staff is essential for all concerned.

Many unsealed sources are pieces of radioactive material in the form of seeds or wires that are inserted permanently into a tissue and left to decay down into inert matter. Dose rates range from <2 Gy/hr at a low rate, through 2–12 Gy/hr at a medium dose rate to >12 Gy/hr at a high dose rate. Finally, the brachytherapy may be pulsed, i.e. a vehicle for the source is placed within a cavity or tissue and then it is remotely afterloaded for a few minutes at a time and then remotely removed or unloaded again. Dose rates for pulsed treatments are usually 1–2 Gy every 1–4 hours for a period of days (Martinez-Monge *et al.*, 2006). Sealed sources may be used in conjunction with any of the other treatment modalities, especially teletherapy or on their own.

In addition to these methods, there is also a radiosurgical method where an intra-operative single exposure of high-dose rate source is given during a surgical procedure. The isotope used is determined by the dose rate required, the tissue penetration necessary and whether they are to be temporary or permanent placements. A significant advantage to this method as a high-dose rate can be used and yet critical structures adjacent and in danger of toxicity can be moved out of the way for a short period.

There may be many possible advantages to this method of radiotherapy delivery that have yet to be highlighted in outcome studies. There does not have to be any allowances made for organ or body movement, or set-up error in defining the planning target volumes, so far less tissue needs to be treated. The energy level of the source, which influences penetration through tissue, can be minimised as the dose emanates from the centre of the tumour and therefore need not penetrate healthy tissue beyond that. Finally, treatment is quicker, often measured in minutes or days rather than weeks, and consequently it may be fitted into a complex chemotherapy schedule better.

The most common brachytherapy technique is low-dose rate therapy with Iridium 192 which is afterloaded into a previously placed vehicle, an applicator or catheter. This is removed after therapy is completed. This would be better done remotely but then the patient is severely restricted as they are emitting still quite high doses of radiation and so must spend significant periods alone. Higher-dose pulsed treatments may be more useful for children needing constant supervision and companionship. The source is afterloaded remotely but only left in place for very short periods and can then be retracted into a safety device till the next pulse. The source can be retracted to allow carers to enter the room and be with the child or for nursing/medical interruptions (Martinez-Monge *et al.*, 2006). Iodine 125 can and is commonly used to beneficial effect in minimising risk to care-givers as it has far less penetration through tissue, but also as it can be used to treat tumours adjacent to radiosensitive tissue such as gonadal tissue. When children or young people are treated with this source, lead aprons or mobile lead shields are sufficient protection for carers. Yttrium 90, Gold 198 and phosphorous 32 can be obtained in liquid form and can be injected into cystic lesions such as craniopharyngiomas. In occular brachytherapy, a plaque is made containing the source and placed upon the surface of the eye for retinoblastoma. Plaques themselves are usually made of a shielding material and the source attached is often Iodine 125.

The plaque is left in place for 2–4 days with a total dose of 35–55 Gy to the immediate tumour which equates to about 0.3–0.6 Gy/hr.

Where an applicator or catheter has been inserted, there must be a process of verification similar to teletherapy before afterloading can take place. If there has been surgical intervention to accomplish this, especially interstitial placement, then loading should occur after 3–5 days to allow for healing and the reduction of swelling in the area. Intracavitary placements that occur after the surgical excision of an original tumour has healed can be loaded straightaway. Where Iodine 125 has been used in an unsealed form, as seeds interstitially, then patients do not require admission as the low-energy source does not penetrate beyond the tumour bed.

All of this is still considerably rare in children with few pockets of expertise such as the AMORE group in The Netherlands. Consequently, there are no agreed guidelines for care or protocols to follow for efficacious therapy (Martinez-Monge et al., 2006).

Despite the seemingly positive benefits of the theory, in practice, toxicity is evident in high-dose rate regimens. Some adjacent tissues have exhibited both acute and late toxicity but the results are encouraging in the limited nature of the toxicity and the smaller volumes of healthy tissue affected. As previously mentioned, the literature is the work of a handful of institutions, with small numbers of often previously treated children, so it is hard to draw conclusions for the future. However, its use in areas that are already pre-treated or in inaccessible positions is attractive, as is the possibility of reducing growth retardation and second malignancy rates by reducing the planning target volume.

The risk to staff and the family in caring for the child with a sealed radiation source depends upon the dose rate emitted by the source at any given time. Dose rate is the rate at which ionising radiation is delivered to the tissues from its source (Hassey-Dow, 1992). In many cases the radiation will not penetrate more than the depth of the tissue in which it has been placed and the child should not emit any radiation. However, this is not always the case. This situation should, therefore, always be discussed in advance with the radiation protection adviser within the hospital and care

planned accordingly. Should the radiation from the source extend beyond the body, the child should be nursed alone in a cubicle with their own washing and toilet facilities. Nurses and the family should limit contact with the child to approximately 30 minutes per day until the radiation protection officer indicates otherwise or the source is removed.

Information on the care of children in this situation is principally as that described for the child with an unsealed radiation source; however, each institution has its own written information for patients and carers that detail all radio-protection precautions and the facilities available to cope with these. If the child has had a sealed radiation source placed within a cavity with an external orifice, care must be taken to ensure it is not dislodged. Should this occur, the source should be retrieved with long-handled forceps and placed in a lead container (Maguire, 1993).

Use of unsealed sources (intravenous radioactive materials)

[131]ImIBG (metaiodobenzylguanidine) is a radioactive material currently used in the UK for the treatment of stage IV neuroblastoma. Metaiodobenzylguanidine (MiBG) with I^{131} radio isotope was reported to concentrate in >90% of neuroblastomas and is a sensitive and specific indicator for this tumour. It can be a tumour-targeting vehicle for delivering therapeutic doses of radiation (Hoefnagel, 1999). The original idea for its use was to avoid excessive drug therapy, and its associated toxic effects and possible resistance. In more recent times it has been used as a treatment option in high-risk patients.

MiBG contains a specific radioactive isotope of iodine. It is made artificially and then bound to a synthetic form of a chemical called guanethidine that neuroblastoma cells absorb (Brophy et al., 2005). Neuroblastoma and other adrenal gland tumours take up [131]ImIBG in a similar way to the transport of noradrenaline in these cells. This affinity for a radioactive chemical allows radiation to be taken directly to tumour cells without damaging the surrounding healthy tissue (Brophy et al., 2005). Work continues to refine the methods of administration, dose, the timing alongside chemotherapy and the exact number of courses for best effect (Howard *et al.*, 2005). The radioactive chemical is given intravenously under protective conditions. Taking oral iodine for a defined period of time before, during and after treatment prevents uptake of the radioactive isotope by the thyroid gland, which would lead to its destruction (UKCCSG, 2006).

As ^{131}ImIBG is given intravenously, all body tissues become radioactive, and the only exit for this material is through excretion. Therefore, all bodily fluids must be handled as radioactive waste and disposed of in the cubicle (Maguire, 1993). As most of the compound collects in the urine, this is by far the most hazardous waste and must be treated very carefully, particularly accidental spillages (Brophy *et al.*, 2005). Special facilities are required for the administration of such therapy as the child becomes radioactive and those caring for them, as well as other visitors, require personal protection equipment when nursing or caring for the child. Visiting should be restricted to adults only and no pregnant women should attend. Nurses and the family have limited contact with the child for a defined period per day and must wear a radioactivity monitoring strip. Staff who have contact with the child during this period must also carry a radioactivity monitoring device to calculate cumulative doses over the set number of days. It follows from these data that all bodily fluids or matter lost by the child must be carefully collected and disposed of, in keeping with government guidelines on the disposal of radioactive waste (Department of Health, 2000a) and the ionising radiation regulations (Department of Health, 2000b). These guidelines are actioned by the radiation protection adviser (Gibbs, 1991) within a given institution.

Facilities that allow constant supervision of the child while maintaining minimal physical contact are therefore essential. In addition, all the child's needs must be met within the room as nothing may leave the room until the radioactivity has decreased when isotope decay and excretion occur. As far as possible, all material objects required for the duration of the child's stay in the room should be disposable.

During infusion (which lasts approximately 30 minutes to one hour) and for the first four hours afterwards, the child must be monitored closely for signs of allergic reaction to the radioactive agent.

This may necessitate frequent monitoring of vital physical signs, as often as every five minutes. For the safety of nursing staff the child should be monitored electronically for pulse, respiration and blood pressure, so that results may be displayed on a monitor outside the room; this would preclude the necessity of continuous direct contact with the child for the first few hours after infusion. However, the use of a mobile shield within the room can also be beneficial for nurses and carers alike.

The child will need to be isolated in hospital for approximately 7–10 days after the infusion, due to the radioactive emissions from all body tissues, and from vulnerable family members for a few more weeks thereafter. The exact length of stay is dependent on the readings of the emissions assessed daily. When the emissions have decreased considerably, the child may leave isolation and return home. Unfortunately, in some cases it may still be some days after this before the child can be in the same building as other children or pregnant women. Siblings may need to be cared for by relatives and friends until the radiation protection adviser has determined the child to be no risk to the family environment. Discharge usually occurs when the child has been measured at or below 30 Bq for a family with young children at home, or 150 mega bequerels (mBq) if the child is returning to an environment of adults only.

Given the need for such minimal staff contact, only the immediate physical needs of the child can be attended to using a mobile shield where possible, although they should be monitored visually throughout this period, preferably by use of closed circuit television. Or as in the case of some purpose-built units where the room is sub-divided by lead-lined half-doors that block emissions from a small child or a larger one playing on the floor This situation would obviously be intolerable for a small anxious child, therefore it can be necessary to sedate such children during the isolation period, until the level of radiation is low enough that parents/carers can spend prolonged periods of time with the child. Oral sedation is used to sedate the child, therefore a nasogastric tube is passed to allow administration of sedation and other drugs once the child is asleep, the child is usually kept nil by mouth during sedation to avoid vomiting, and potential aspiration, and IV fluids used to maintain hydration. [131]ImIBG may cause considerable feelings of nausea and at times vomiting may ensue; this vomit is potentially very dangerous radioactive material and in the sedated child there is also the risk of aspiration. It is recommended that thought be given to the administration of effective antiemetic cover during the first 2–3 days. The sedated child will need to have their position changed every four hours to prevent pressure points and chest infections, at these times other care is also carried out, i.e nappy changes, hygiene and mouth care, to avoid prolonged exposure for staff.

The room in which the child is nursed should be designed for the use of radioactive materials, with protective walls, and ensuite bathroom. A Geiger counter should be kept within the designated cubicle to monitor the emissions from the treated child. Their decrease in magnitude must be recorded accurately and, indeed, all items of equipment and materials required in the child's care must be assessed before disposal or removal from the room once treatment has commenced. All this equipment may be anxiety-provoking for both the child and the family; it is therefore essential that the family be prepared for these measures with clear and accurate information beforehand and ongoing support and advice throughout the treatment.

The parents and members of the child's family may find the separation and possible sedation of the child extremely distressing. It can be anxiety-provoking to think of one's own child being so dangerously radioactive that such extreme safety measures are needed. As a consequence, nursing care must respond to the need for information, reassurance and support throughout this difficult time. Encouraging the parents to choose clothing or advise on positioning for the sedated child promotes a sense of protection. For the child who is awake during this time, telephone, webcam and video links are invaluable, where protected visual contact cannot be maintained. Choosing games or DVDs and preparing favourite foods also help to maintain caring contact, essential to the child and the parents or siblings. Each therapeutic site has written information for staff and families to prepare them for the experience and explain the radioprotective measures.

Is the efficacy of this treatment sufficient to warrant this level of intensive care and distress to the child and family? Past experience has revealed MiBG to have 30–50% response rate in phase I/II trials including a study in the UK. Primary toxicity was reversible myelosuppression – severe thrombocytopenia and moderate neutropenia (Lashford et al., 1992). Studies have varied the number of courses administered: it has not been indicated if there is a toxicity link with multiple courses. Howard et al. (2005) carried out a retrospective review of patients at one US centre and found multiple course achieved improved responses but myelo-toxicity, especially in platelets, was dose-limiting. They concluded it was prudent to administer MiBG courses with stem cell support. However, this may preclude children with bone marrow involvement. It was noted that there was some delayed response to treatment which may have affected good results on infusions thereafter. Non-haematological toxicity, e.g. nausea, vomiting, hypertension, anorexia, pruritis, dry mouth and asymptomatic hypothyroidism, did not increase with multiple infusions. It is of note that although common haematological toxicity did not lead to toxic death, there was prolonged thrombocytopenia even with stem cell support. The future of this therapy lies only in a robust evaluation of MiBG plus chemotherapy without pre-treatment, results and toxicity profiles may then be quite different.

Radioactive isotopes bound to tumour-specific antibodies

This is a relatively new and extremely experimental form of radiation therapy. Antibodies are identified that are specific to surface antigens being presented on the tumour cell surface. These are then bound to radioactive particles of relatively low energy and given intravenously to the patient. This is an extremely complicated procedure as tumour antigens must be identified, monoclonal or polyclonal antibodies must then be developed and produced in sufficient quantities (usually in mice or rabbits), and then they must be successfully combined with a radioactive source. Radiation dosing at a micro level of α-emitting drugs is obviously advantageous. Radio-immunotherapy can reduce the organ toxicity associated with external beam therapy. Although the radioactive load in this therapy is much lower than [131]ImIBG therapy, protective care of children involved should follow the same government guidelines until their emitted radioactivity is below safe contact levels. This timeframe will depend entirely on the half-life of the radioactive isotope attached to the antibody (Coons, 1995). It may be useful in radiosensitive paediatric tumours using either intravenous or intrathecal vehicles. Modak and Cheung (2005) argue that radio immunotherapy is still in viable development though it has struggled for many years to overcome biological barriers (Pizer *et al.*, 1991). They feel it has a valuable role to play in offsetting treatment failure due to lack of control of minimal residual disease (MRD). Due to the sustained attack on a child's immune system during conventional therapy, their highly immuno-compromised state makes it possible to repeatedly administer radio-labelled monoclonal antibodies for specific tumour antigens without induction of a host antibody response. However, there are no studies in children, hence there is a complete lack of safety and efficacy profiles.

Currently tumour antigen radio-immunological therapy for specific embryonal tumours is being investigated. However, it is a long and complex process and may not be successful as it is hard to comply with current drug development laws. There is not only a great need for rapid development of more radio-labelled monoclonal antibodies, but also to improve targeting and the reduction of adverse immunological responses. Few antibodies are currently available as not many children's tumour antigens have been identified and there has been a lack of phase 1 or phase 2 studies in this area (Modak & Cheung, 2005).

Administration of alternative radiotherapy techniques

Stereotactic radiation

Stereotactic methods were originally used for precise neurosurgery, and they have proved to be the ultimate immobilisation and location tool. The method was then adapted for radiotherapy to exploit the two essential properties of patient positioning and target identification. Stereotactic radiotherapy is a highly conformal type of radiation therapy exposing very little healthy tissue to therapy in addition to its target, as it is able to use tight margins effectively. Stereotactic radiotherapy merges stereotactic surgery with conventional fractionated radiotherapy (Lew & La Valley, 1995). This method of radiation delivery is utilised when a small intracranial area of cancerous tissue adjacent to highly sensitive organs (or heavily pre-treated tissue) requires radiotherapy. It allows the delivery of maximum tumourcidal doses of radiation while limiting the damaging dose to surrounding tissue. A three-dimensional approach is taken to locate and fix the target for therapy and, indeed, for the guidance of therapy (Dunbar & Loeffler, 1994). Limited in its use initially, it has grown from single fraction to multi-fraction use and moved on from surgically attached frame to non-invasive frames (using individual bite grips to reproduce its position) and body cradles (Saran, 2004).

A stereotactic frame is constructed to the exact measurements of the child's anatomy. As mentioned, it rarely requires surgical fixation, except in radiosurgery, as it can be constructed with a fixed bite block so that when this is in the correct position within the mouth all other points are identically located on the skull. This frame is used to guide an external beam of radiation to the precise point of disease. All frames should be non-invasive, re-locatable and immobilising to ensure accurate reproducible positioning throughout planning and treatment (Kooy, 1993). Stereotactic radiotherapy is now also conformal and the two most popular methods for immobilisation should be reviewed. The first is a lightweight paediatric frame-based system with individualised mouth bite and head-rest and this usually ensures only 1.0 1.5mm variability. In the second type, children may be encased in a customised Perspex shell that can be bolted to the table, in addition to a moulded bag of polystyrene beads individually shaped then made rigid by vacuum, to hold the head and upper body in place. These last two maintain a 1.5mm–2.5mm variability (Saran, 2004). In comparison, a traditional mask has a 4–5mm variability. Non-invasive stereotactic frames rely on using bony pressure points and fixed CT localisation points to guide the radiotherapy beam. Whole-body stereotactic frames are less well developed in this country than in the US.

The radiotherapy is then given in fractionated doses to attain the most effective tumour control with minimal late effects (Brell *et al.*, 2006). As mentioned, in recent years the technique has moved on to conformal fractionated stereotactic radiotherapy. New developments have added considerably to the potential uses of the stereotactic method. Yamada *et al.* (2005) describe how IMRT can be used stereotactically for high-dose radiation to lesions adjacent to the spinal cord, successfully avoiding damage to this sensitive structure. IMRT is delivered with a non-invasive body frame for multifractional stereotactic radiotherapy. These body frames have been developed as immobilising devices specifically for stereotactic spinal IMRT, where marked points on the frame, as well as the bony prominences that they are fixed onto, are used as locating points for the therapy.

This method of conformal radiotherapy, again benefits from using fused CT/MR imaging in paediatric neuro-oncology. These can be very useful in slow-growing well-demarcated tumours. The CT gives excellent information on calcification points, tissue density and bony anatomical data for location and penetration planning. It can be a very useful way to deliver a uniform dose to a non-spherical lesion. Multiple fixed fields shaped using MLCs (multi-leaf collimators), micro MLC or lead shields planned carefully to avoid critical structure can treat tumour volumes with aggressively smaller margins. This is made possible because of excellent locating and positioning which means late effects should be decreased. For thoracic tumours it may also be necessary to utilise an active breathing control device. This controls the delivery of radiation during a standard breath hold. It can decrease markedly the volume of heart and lung unnecessarily exposed, but it does need active support from the child. Advanced preparation of the child, to practise breath holding can be extraordinarily beneficial, in these rare circumstances.

Stereotactic radiosurgery

This is where a single ablative fraction is administered using a stereotactic frame. This is akin to surgery, and can have significant late effects. The necessary radiation dose can be produced by adapted linear accelerator or a gamma knife (a cobalt 60 machine). There is a rapid fall-off of dose after the beam hits the target. With this being a single high-dose fraction, immobilisation is normally a pinned frame placed under general anaesthetic. All planning, simulation, verification and treatment are carried out at one session to minimise distress to the child or adolescent. The dosage is usually sufficiently high to cause immediate cell death to the targeted tumour bed, mirroring radical surgical removal (Marcus *et al.*, 2005).

There has, in the past, been a need for at least 3cm of safe distance from a vital organ so its use was restricted in small children. However, this technique can also be combined with IMRT as a new development which may broaden its use in children and decrease its toxicity to adjacent critical structures.

Total body irradiation in the treatment of leukaemia

As leukaemic cells are well oxygenated and highly proliferative, they are extremely radiosensitive. However, they are difficult to locate and identify for therapy. Total body irradiation (TBI) is a procedure in which the entire body is exposed at one time to gamma radiation (Dreifke & DeMeyer, 1992). The goals of TBI are to eradicate the leukaemic cell count, in addition to immunosuppressing the child so that they can receive a donor marrow without mounting an immune response. In summary, the goals of TBI are:

1. to attain sufficient immunosuppression to allow engraftment of a foreign donor marrow for allogeneic bone marrow transplant;
2. to remove or reduce residual disease;
3. to provide sufficient space for the new donor marrow to grow.

(Silverman & Goldberg, 1996)

Removal of the child's bone marrow and circulating leukaemic cells involves administering a homogeneous dose of radiation to all body tissues. The radiation given is of a lower dose and intensity than a beam directed at a localised area (Iwamoto, 1994). The dose is usually within the 8–14 Gy range (depending on fractionation), although it can be given as a single dose, the toxicity profile associated with that is markedly increased from a fractionated regime.

This form of preparation for transplant was first attempted in 1925, although the concept had first been discussed almost 20 years earlier (Dudjak, 1992). Until 1979, most regimens of TBI were single-fraction (Dudjak, 1992), fractionated doses were then introduced in an attempt to decrease late-onset toxicity without an adverse effect on efficacy (Goolden *et al.*, 1983). It was then found that fractionation worked more efficiently even when given in very small doses (Storb, 1989). The total dose given is sufficient to be lethal to the bone marrow tissue. Stem cells within the marrow are destroyed and so regrowth is impeded. A hyper-fractionated regimen (twice daily) is followed over 3 to 5 days to allow healthy tissue throughout the body to repair itself. Complex calculations need to be made to ensure effective yet safe doses are given equally throughout the varied tissues of the body. Positioning of the child may need to be altered during a fractionated dose to facilitate this. A lower dose of radiation is aimed at the lungs to offset unnecessary fibrosis; this is accomplished by using the arms as a shield for each lung or using shields made from pieces of radiation-attenuating material.

TBI can only be carried out with the child positioned quite some considerable distance from the radiation source, so as to ensure small doses are given accurately to all sections of the body, and to get the field to be as large as possible. Although small doses are recommended when treating the whole body, care must be taken as too low a dose rate may allow only sub-lethal damage to occur. This may result not only in leukaemic cells surviving TBI, but also the other cells of the child's own immune system, which could then attack the donor marrow. In contrast, too high a dose rate can cause irreversible organ damage, for example, to the lung tissue. Positioning is therefore an extremely important variable in TBI. It can be manipulated to control the energy of the beam when it enters the child, the homogeneity of the dose and the protection of critical organs. Dose rate fractions and treatment distance vary considerably centre to centre and protocol to protocol. However, there are some more common elements from the literature:

- The regime usually lasts 3–4 days, often on a hyper-fractionated or twice-daily schedule.
- It is a small daily dose of 1.5–2 Gy split between the two fractions.
- Children and adolescents should lie on their side, turning half-way through each fraction to maintain homogeneity.

This form of conditioning may cause a variety of acute (and chronic) side effects, many more than a chemotherapy-only regime, and therefore these children require intensive preparation and support throughout their treatment. Although TBI is given in fractionated doses to reduce some of these toxicities, they may still cause considerable problems to children treated in this manner. The possible side effects of TBI are summarised in Table 19.1.

Locatelli *et al.* (1993) highlight that the majority of late effects from bone marrow transplant are due to this form of conditioning, although hypothyroidism is usually only seen with single-fraction doses. Cataracts (Calissendorff *et al.*, 1991), lachrymal gland dysfunction and endocrine dysfunction are particularly worrying side effects which may account for the interest in alternative forms of conditioning over the years.

What does the future hold for radiotherapy?

The next decade of development in radiotherapy is likely to be one of consolidation (Soomal & Saran, 2004). That is the rapid advance in digital technology that has driven recent advances in 3-D planning, the ability to fuse images and the dynamic collimation of beams based upon real-time computerised tomography data now need to be fully integrated into paediatric practice across the UK. In parallel, enhanced target definition must continue to advance in line with success so far and bring about the targeting data essential for the most effective planning. High quality anatomical imaging is a resource that oncologists currently depend upon; this will in the future be the case for functional imaging also. The final stage of this development is the perfecting of techniques and software to allow fusion of images from many different modalities both within and without the CNS.

Table 19.1 Possible side effects of TBI

System	Side effect	Time from TBI to symptoms
Gastrointestinal	Nausea and vomiting	Immediately to 24 hours
	Stomatitis	Within a few days
	Diarrhoea	Immediately to a few days
	Loss of appetite	Immediately to a few days
	Pain or swelling in salivary glands	Immediately to 24 hours
	Dry mouth	Immediately to a few days
	Thick saliva	Immediately to a few days
Skin	Redness	Within a few hours
	Itching/tingling	Within a few hours
	Darkening of skin	2–3 weeks
	Hair loss (all of body)	7–10 days
Reproductive	Sterility	Immediately
	Premature menopausal symptoms	Months to years
Miscellaneous	Cataracts	1.5–5 years
	Fatigue	Sudden or gradual
	Fever	Within a few hours
	Bone marrow failure	7–10 days
	Abnormal growth	Months to years

Source: Dreifke & DeMeyer (1993).

Between these two goals of improving target definition and accurate dose delivery lies the way forward to the most effective tumour eradication and decrease in treatment morbidity. Particulate therapy advances are exciting in terms of the use of protons in paediatric oncology but the huge investment necessary to set up one such unit in this country seems hard to imagine in the current political and financial climate. However, valuable research into the outcome of proton therapy in children will continue (Kirsch & Tarbell, 2004; St Clair et al., 2004) outside the UK and this is to be welcomed in developing an evidence base that will be highly useful in the more distant future.

Consolidation too could be used to describe the goal of clinical research for the immediate future. Evidence of clinical effectiveness in these new therapies and planning processes is vital for continued growth in their use. Studies into efficacy of a new technology for a named site or specific histology will only be significant when the majority of CCLG centres have the resources to deliver these new highly conformal techniques and alternative fractionation schedules. The evidence to support the hoped-for improvements in care in terms of reduced toxicity with equal if not better tumour control may be even longer in coming to fruition. Late effects studies are protracted and complex in analysis, but after many years of data collection in a changing health-care context it becomes harder to make comparisons in clinical outcome. So many variables have materialised in these long time frames; changes in surgical and diagnostic techniques, improvements in rehabilitation strategy and access, educational support strategies and finally the attitude of patients and carers themselves to self-determined care and survivorship.

Radiotherapy has an important part to play in the management of children with cancer. Specialisation among clinical oncologists and therapeutic radiographers is recognised as important in providing high quality care (NICE, 2005), as is the need for anaesthesia and play specialist support for very young children during radiotherapy treatment. The *Improving Outcomes in Children and Young People with Cancer* report (NICE, 2005) recommends that centres providing radiotherapy to children and young people should comply with a defined set of requirements, these relate to staffing, age-appropriate facilities, adherence to national standards and participation in clinical trials. The guidance goes on to suggest that high-risk/complex radiotherapy, i.e. TBI, or biologically targeted radio-isotope treatments, take place in agreed supra-regional centres. Bringing services into line with these recommendations will require resources and collaborative working across England, and how this will affect services in the rest of the UK remains to be seen.

In conclusion, radiotherapy advances are complex and expensive but extremely interesting to those involved in the care of children or young people with cancer. There is, however, a dilemma, in that the evidence of its improved patient outcome will only come after massive capital investment in the technologies themselves and the people to operate them, yet how can we justify such outlay without proof of its worth? Basic science and associated research in adult cancers will have to suffice as a foundation until the numbers in case reports and small series add up to clinical evidence that can be relied upon.

References

Adamson D (2003) 'The radiobiological basis of radiation side effects' in: Faithfull S & Wells M (eds) Supportive Care in Radiotherapy. Edinburgh: Churchill Livingstone, pp. 71–95

Beutler D, Avoledo P, Ruebic JC, Mehecke HR, Müller-Brand J, Merlo A & Kühne T (2005) 'Three year recurrence-free survival in a patient with recurrent medulloblastoma after resection, high dose chemotherapy and intrathecal Yttrium-90-labelled DOTAO-D-Phe1-Tyr3-octreotide radiopeptide brachytherapy' Cancer 103(4): 869–873

Bilksy MH, Yenice K, Lovelock M, Yamada J. (2001) 'Stereotactic intensity-modulation radiation therapy for vertebral body and paraspinal tumors' Neurosurgy Focus 11(6): e7–9

Bomford CK (2003) 'The physics of radiotherapy' in: Bomford CK & Kunkler IH (eds) Walter and Miller's Textbook of Radiotherapy: Radiation Physics, Therapy and Oncology (6th edn). Edinburgh: Churchill Livingstone, pp. 141–252

Brell M, Villà S, Teixidor P, Lucas A, Ferrán E, Marín S & Acebes JJ (2006) 'Fractionated stereotactic radiotherapy in the treatment of exclusive cavernous sinus meningioma: functional outcome, local control, and tolerance' Surgical Neurology 65(1): 28–33

Brophy P, Schmus C & Balistreri L (2005) 'Meeting the nursing challenges in treating children with 131I-MIBG' Journal of Pediatric Oncology Nursing 21(1): 9–15

Bucci MK, Bevan A & Roach M (2005) 'Advances in radiation therapy: conventional to 3-D, to IMRT, to 4D, and beyond' Journal of Clinical Cancer 55(2): 117–134

Bucholtz JD (1992) 'Issues concerning the sedation of children for radiotherapy' Oncology Nurses Forum 19(4): 649–655

Burkhart PV & Rayens MK (2005) 'Self concept and health locus of control: factors related to children's adherence to recommended asthma regimen' Pediatric Nursing 31(5): 404–409

Buwalda J, Blank LE, Schouwenburg PF, Copper MP, Strackee SD, Voute PA, Merks JH & Caron HN (2004) 'The AMORE protocol as salvage treatment for non-orbital head and neck rhabdomyosarcoma in children' European Journal of Surgical Oncology 30(8): 884–892

Buwalda J, Freling NJ, Blank LE, Balm AJ, Bras J, Voûte PA, Caron HN, Schouwenburg PF & Merks JH (2005) 'AMORE protocol in pediatric head and neck rhabdomyosarcoma: descriptive analysis of failure patterns' Head & Neck 27(5): 390–396

Calissendorff B, Bolme P & el Azazi M (1991) 'The development of cataracts in children as a late effect of bone marrow transplantation' Bone Marrow Transplant 7(6): 427–429

Coleman AM (2004) 'Radiotherapy procedures' in: Washington CM & Leaver D (eds) Principles and Practice of Radiation Therapy (2nd edn). St Louis: Mosby, pp. 171–193

Coons T (1995) 'Monoclonal antibodies: the promise and the reality' Radiologic Technology 67(1): 39–64

Cooper CO, Heron TE & Heward WL (1987) Applied Behavioral Analysis. Columbus, OH: Bobbs-Merrill

Cosset JM, Socie G, Dubray B, Girinsky T, Fourquet A & Gluckman E (1994) 'Single dose versus fractionated total body irradiation before bone marrow transplantation' International Journal of Radiation, Oncology, Biology, Physics 30(2): 177–192

Court LE, Dong L, Lee AK, Cheung R, Bonnen MD, O'Daniel J, Wang H, Mohan R & Kuban D (2005) 'An automatic CT-guided adaptive radiation therapy technique by online modification of multileaf collimator leaf positions for prostate cancer' International Journal of Radiation Oncology Biology, Physics 62(1): 154–163

D'Angio GJ (1992) 'An overview and historical perspective of late effects of treatment for childhood cancer' in: Green DM & D'Angio GJ (eds) Late Effects of Treatment for Childhood Cancer. New York: John Wiley & Sons, Ltd, pp. 3–11

Department of Health (2000a) The Protections of Persons against Ionising Radiation Arising from Any Work Activity London: HMSO.

Department of Health (2000b) *The Ionising Radiation Regulations*. London: HMSO

Dreifke L & DeMeyer E (1992) 'Information guide for patients receiving total body irradiation before bone marrow transplantation' *Cancer Nursing* 15(3): 206–210

Dudjak L (1992) 'Alteration in dose fractionations and treatment volumes' *in*: Hassey-Dow K & Hilderley LJ (eds) *Nursing Care in Radiation Oncology*. Philadelphia, PA: WB Saunders & Co

Dunbar SF & Loeffler JS (1994) 'Stereotactic radiation therapy' *in*: Mauch PM & Loeffler JS (eds) *Radiation Oncology: Technology and Biology*. Philadelphia, PA: WB Saunders & Co.

Fontanesi J, Rao BN, Fleming ID, Bowman LC, Pratt CB, Furman WL, Coffey DH & Kun LE (1994) 'Pediatric brachytherapy: the St Jude Children's Research Hospital experience' *Cancer* 74(2): 733–739

Ghandi S, Meech SJ, Puthawala MA, Fergusson WS, Cardarelli GA & Dupuy DE (2005) 'Combined computer tomography – guided radiofrequency ablation and brachytherapy in a child with multiple recurrences of Wilms' tumour' *Journal of Pediatric Hematology & Oncology* 27(7): 377–379

Goolden AW, Goldman JM, Kam KC & Dunn PA *et al.* (1983) 'Fractionation of whole body irradiation before bone marrow transplantation of patients with leukaemia' *British Journal of Radiology* 56: 245–250

Habrand JL, Abdulkarum B & Roberti H. (2004a) 'Radiotherapeutical innovations in pediatric solid tumors' *Pediatric Blood & Cancer* 43(6): 622–628

Habrand JL, Abdulkarim B & Bernard A (2000b) 'Clinical applications of paediatric radiotherapy' *in*: Pinkerton R, Plowman N & Pieters R (eds) *Paediatric Oncology* (3rd edn). London: Arnold, pp. 129–141

Hassey-Dow K (1992) 'Principles of brachytherapy' *in*: Hassey-Dow K & Hilderley LJ *Nursing Care in Radiation Oncology*. Philadelphia, PA: WB Saunders & Co

Hoefnagel CA (1999) 'Nuclear medicine therapy of neuroblastoma' *Qualitative Journal of Nuclear Medicine* 43(4): 336–343

Hong TS, Ritter MA, Tomint WA & Harari PM (2005) 'Intensity modulated radiation therapy: emerging cancer treatment technology' *British Journal of Cancer* 92(10): 1819–1824

Howard JP, Maris JM, Kersun LS, Huberty JP, Cheng SC, Hawkins RA & Matthay KK (2005) 'Tumor response and toxicity with multiple infusions of high dose 131I-MIBG for refractory neuroblastoma' *Pediatric Blood & Cancer* 44(3): 232–239

Iwamoto, R (1994) 'Radiation therapy' *in*: Otto SE (ed.) *Oncology Nursing* (2nd edn). St Louis: Mosby

Justus R, Wilson J, Walther V, Wyles D, Rode D, Lim-Sulit N (2006) 'Preparing children and families for surgery: Mount Sinai's multidisciplinary perspective' *Pediatric Nursing* 32(1): 35–40

Keall P (200) '4 dimensional computerised tomography imaging and treatment planning' *Seminars in Radiation Oncology* 14(1): 81–90

Khatua S & Jalali R (2005) 'Recent advances in the treatment of childhood brain tumours' *Pediatric Hematology and Oncology* 22(5): 361–371

Kirsch DG & Tarbell NJ (2004) 'New technologies in radiation therapy for pediatric brain tumours: the rationale for proton radiation therapy' *Pediatric Blood & Cancer* 42(5): 461–464

Kooy HM (1993) 'Three dimensional treatment planning for stereotactic radiosurgery of intra-cranial lesions' *International Journal of Radiation Oncology, Biology, Physics* 21: 683–693

Krasin MJ, Crawford BT, Zho Y, Evans ES, Sontag MR, Kun LE & Merchant TE (2004a) 'Intensity-modulated radiation therapy for children with intra-ocular retinoblastoma: potential sparing of the bony orbit' *Clinical Oncology* 16(3): 215–222

Krasin MJ, Hudson MM & Kaste SC (2004b) 'Positron emission tomography in pediatric radiation oncology: integration in the treatment-planning process' *Pediatric Radiology* 34(3): 214–221

Kunkler IH (2003) 'Effects of radiation on normal tissues' *in*: Bomford CK & Kunkler IH (eds) *Walter and Miller's Textbook of Radiotherapy: Radiation Physics, Therapy and Oncology* (6th edn). Edinburgh: Churchill Livingstone, pp. 296–306

Larson DA, Suplica JM, Chang SM, Lamborn KR, McDermott MW, Sneed PK, Prados MD, Wara WM, Nicholas MK & Berger MS (2004) 'Permanent iodine 125 brachytherapy in patients with progressive or recurrent glioblastoma multiforme' *Neuro-oncology* 6(2): 119–126

Lashford LS, Lewis IJ, Fielding SC, Flower MA, Meller S, Kernshead JT & Ackery D (1992) 'Phase I/II study of 131 metaiodobenzylguanidine in chemoresistant neuroblastoma: a UKCCSG study' *Journal of Clinical Oncology* 10(12): 1889–1896

Lew CM & La Valley B (1995) 'The role of stereotactic radiation therapy in the management of children with brain tumours' *Journal of Pediatric Oncology Nursing* 12(4): 212–222

Locatelli F, Giorgiani G, Pession A & Bozzola M (1993) 'Late effects in children after bone marrow transplantation: a review' *Haematologica* 78(5): 319–328

Lutterbach J & Guttenberger M (2000) 'Anaemia associated with decreased local control of surgically treated squamous cell carcinoma of glottic larynx' *International Journal of Radiation Oncology, Biology, Physics* 48(5): 1345–1350

Maguire P (1993) 'Radiation therapy' *in*: Foley GV, Fochtman D & Mooney KH (eds) *Nursing Care of the Child with Cancer* (2nd edn). Philadelphia, PA: WB Saunders, pp. 117–130

Marcus KJ, Goumnervoa L, Billet AL, Layally B, Scott RM, Bishop K, Xu R, Young Poussaint T, Kieran M, Kooy H, Pomeroy SL & Tarbell NJ (2005) 'Stereotactic radiotherapy for localized low-grade gliomas in children: final results of a prospective trial' *International Journal of Radiation Oncology, Biology, Physics* 61(2): 374–379

Martinez-Monge R, Cambeiro M, San-Julian M & Sierrasesumaga L (2006) 'Use of brachytherapy in children with cancer: the search for an uncomplicated cure' *The Lancet Oncology* 7(2): 157–166

Mayr MT, Crocker IR, Butker EK, Williams H, Cotsonis GA & Olson JJ (2002) 'Results of interstitial brachytherapy for malignant brain tumors' *International Journal of Oncology* 21(4): 817–823

McMillan TJ (2003) 'Principles of radiobiology' *in*: Bomford CK & Kunkler IH (eds) *Walter and Miller's Textbook of Radiotherapy: Radiation Physics, Therapy and Oncology* (6th edn). Edinburgh: Churchill Livingstone, pp. 286–295

Merchant TE, Parsh N, del Valle PL, Coffey DH, Galindo CR, Jenkins JJ, Pappo A, Neel MD & Rao BN (2000) 'Brachytherapy for pediatric soft tissue sarcoma' *International Journal of Radiation Oncology, Biology, Physics* 46(2): 427–432

Modak S & Cheung NK (2005) 'Antibody-based targeted radiation to pediatric tumors' *Journal of Nuclear Medicine* 46 (suppl. 1): 157S–163S

Munro AJ (2003) 'Challenges to radiotherapy today' *in*: Faithfull S & Wells M (eds) *Supportive Care in Radiotherapy*. Edinburgh: Churchill Livingstone, pp. 17–38

Nag S, Tippin D & Ruymann FB (2003) 'Long-term morbidity in children treated with fractionated high-dose-rate brachytherapy for soft tissue sarcomas' *Journal of Pediatric Hematology Oncology* 25(6): 448–452

National Institute for Clinical Excellence (2005) 'Guidance on cancer services: cancer in children and young adults' *in*: NICE *The Manual: Improving Outcomes in Children and Young People with Cancer*. London: NICE, pp. 45–50

Nutting C, Dearnaley DP & Webb S (2000) 'Intensity modulated radiation therapy: a clinical review' *British Journal of Radiology* 73(869): 459–469

Oski FA, DeAngelais CD & Feigin RD (1990) *Principles and Practice of Pediatrics*. Philadelphia, PA: JB Lippincott & Co

Pizer B, Papanastassiou V, Hancock J, Cassano W, Coakham H. & Kemshead J (1991) 'A pilot study of monoclonal antibody targeted radiotherapy in the treatment of central nervous system leukaemia in children' *British Journal of Haematology* 77(4): 466–472

Saran F (2004) 'New technology for radiotherapy in paediatric oncology' *European Journal of Cancer* 40(14): 2019–2105

Scott L, Langton F & O'Donoghue J (2002) 'Minimising the use of sedation/anaesthesia in young children receiving radiotherapy through an effective play preparation programme' *European Journal of Oncology Nursing* 6(1): 15–22

Shields CL, Meadows AT, Leahey AM & Shields JA (2004) 'Continuing challenges in the management of retinoblastoma with chemotherapy' *Retina* 24(6): 849–862

Slifer KJ, Bucholtz JD & Cataldo MD (1994) 'Behavioural training of motion control in young children undergoing radiation treatment without sedation' *Journal of Paediatric Oncology Nursing* 11(2): 55–63

Slifer KJ, Cataldo MF & Cataldo MD (1993) 'Behaviour analysis of motion control for pediatric neuroimaging' *Journal of Applied Behavioral Analysis* 26: 469–470

Soomal R & Saran F (2004) 'Recent advances in radiotherapy' *in*: Pinkerton R, Plowman N & Pieters R (eds) *Paediatric Oncology* (3rd edn). London: Arnold, pp. 609–620

St Clair WH, Adams CMD, Bues M, Fullerton BC, LaShell S, Kooy HM, Loeffler MD & Tarbell N (2004) 'Advantage of protons compared to conventional X-ray or IMRT in the treatment of a pediatric patient with medulloblastoma' *International Journal of Radiation Oncology, Biology, Physics* 58(3): 727–734

Stewart EJ, Algren C & Arnold S (1994) 'Preparing children for a surgical experience' *Today's OR Nurse* 16(2): 9–14

Storb R (1989) 'Bone marrow transplantation' *in*: DeVita VT, Hellman S & Rosenberg SA (eds) *Cancer: Principles and Practice of Oncology*. Philadelphia, PA: JB Lippincott, pp 427–439.

Tarbell NT, York T & Kooy H (2006) 'Principles of radiation oncology' *in*: Pizzo PA & Poplack DG (eds) *Principles and Practice of Pediatric Oncology* (5th edn). Philadelphia, PA: Lippincott, Williams & Williams, pp. 421–432

Taylor R (2003) 'Paediatric Oncology' *in*: Bomford CK & Kunkler I (eds) *Walter and Miller's Textbook of Radiotherapy: Radiation Physics, Therapy and Oncology* (6th edn), Edinburgh: Churchill Livingstone, pp. 583–596

UKCCSG/PONF Mouthcare Group (2006) *Mouth Care for Children and Young People with Cancer: Evidence-based Guidelines*. Guideline Report. Version 1.0 February 2006

Warzak WJ, Engel LE, Bischoff, LG & Stefans VA (1991) 'Developing anxiety reduction procedures for a ventilator dependent pediatric patient' *Archives of Physics, Medicine and Rehabilitation* 72(7): 503–507

Wolden SL (2005) 'Radiation therapy for non-rhabdomyosarcoma soft tissue sarcomas in adolescents and young adults' *Journal of Pediatric Hematology Oncology* 27(4): 212–214

Yamada Y, Lovelock DM, Yenice KM, Bilsky MH, Hunt MH, Zatcky J & Leibel SA (2005) 'Multi-fractionated image guided and stereotactic intensity modulated radiotherapy of paraspinal tumors: a preliminary report' *International Journal of Radiation Oncology, Biology, Physics* 62(1): 53–61

Zelefsky MJ, Fuks Z, Hunt M, Yarnada Y, Marion C, Ling CC, Arnols H, Venkatraman ES & Liebel SA (2002) 'High dose intensity modified radiation therapy for prostate cancer; early toxicity' *International Journal of Radiation Oncology, Biology, Physics* 53(5): 1111–1116

20 Tumours and Radiotherapy Treatment

Monica Hopkins and Cornelia Scott

Radiotherapy retains a significant role in the treatment of many childhood cancers, haematological and solid tumours alike. Many tumours are radiosensitive: rhabdomyosarcoma, Ewing's sarcoma, retinoblastoma, lymphoma, neuroblastoma, but perhaps the group most associated with this modality are the central nervous system (CNS) tumours. This chapter will begin by examining radiotherapy in children with CNS tumours.

Brain tumours

Radiotherapy is used to varying degrees in many brain tumour regimens. A true intracranial germinoma is curable with radiotherapy alone and is treated with such, whereas medulloblastoma is treated with some chemotherapy but is not curable without radiotherapy. The main radiosensitive brain tumours are:

1. germ cell tumour (pure germinoma – highly radiosensitive);
2. glioma (low-grade, optic glioma, astrocytoma);
3. high-grade and brain stem glioma (improved survival but rarely curative);
4. ependymoma;
5. pinealblastoma;
6. medulloblastoma (cranio-spinal dose of RT can be reduced in standard risk medulloblastoma);
7. primitive neuroectodermal tumour (PNET);
8. craniopharyngioma.

Tumours that are considered low-grade, and where at least 95 % of the mass can be removed, may in some instances require no further therapy. These children will be followed up closely by imaging surveillance and clinical examination. Where the tumour is high-grade or anaplastic and fast-growing, it is considered malignant and always requires further therapy after surgery (Shiminski-Maher & Wisoff, 1995).

In the past 15 years or so, the addition of chemotherapy in the use of the more traditional radiotherapy has increased the survival rate of children with certain brain tumours (Blaney *et al.*, 2006). Individual tumour growth, position and clinical consequences must be explained when discussing the possible future morbidity and prognosis with the family (Shiminski-Maher, 1993).

However, research into tumours, such as the germ cell tumours, PNETs and medulloblastomas, now is underway to establish the optimum dose and fractionation of radiotherapy required. For all tumours, the decision on the most appropriate therapy must be made on radiobiological data. The decision to treat the tumour by radiotherapy alone is usually reserved for tumours that do not metastasise outside the brain or seed the CSF. Combined modality of chemotherapy and radiotherapy may be efficacious in these cases.

Brain tumours with the potential for neuroaxis spread or which have already metastasised at diagnosis are tumours such as medulloblastomas/PNETs or intra-cranial germ cell tumours. The current CCLG/SIOP protocols recommend cranio-spinal radiotherapy if the child is over the age of 3 years. Infants with medulloblastoma/PNET receive chemotherapy first, followed by focal radiotherapy to the tumour site.

The use of chemotherapy in the past two decades in randomised controlled trials in the UK, Europe and North America, has allowed a reduction in the dose of radiotherapy to the cranio-spinal axis (Freeman et al., 2004). This development appears to have brought about better disease-free and overall survival. Children with standard risk medulloblastoma are entered into a PNET protocol where the 'standard arm' delivers a reduced dose of cranio-spinal radiotherapy followed by repeated cycles of maintenance chemotherapy. The 'experimental' arm of the protocol uses alternatively fractionated radiotherapy (e.g. HFRT) followed by maintenance chemotherapy. HFRT, in twice-daily fractions, delivers a higher overall dose to the cranio-spinal axis, the posterior fossa and the tumour bed than in the standard arm. Hyperfractionation has the potential to increase the anti-tumour effect without an equivalent increase in CNS late effects. The dose–response relationship for medulloblastoma is well known and it seems that increasing the dose, without increasing the late effects on CNS tissue, might also improve local and regional tumour control (HIT-SIOP PNET 4, 2004).

Children with high-risk medulloblastoma/PNET or with metastatic disease at diagnosis are currently entered into a protocol with hyperfractionated radiotherapy as standard treatment. This is a hyperfractionated accelerated radiotherapy regimen delivered twice daily over five weeks, thus delivering a higher dose of radiotherapy than in previous regimens. The radiotherapy will be followed by repeated cycles of maintenance chemotherapy. Combined-modality therapy is a significantly more prolonged regimen and will require many visits to both the radiotherapy centre and the principal treatment centre, which in most treatment centres are at two different hospitals. Children may need to stay in hospital for prolonged periods due to infections. This has social and financial implications for the family and emotional implications for the child. One parent/carer will need to be with the hospitalised child. Parents/carers may not be able to continue working and the family's home and social life will be affected. The child receiving treatment may not be able to attend school for days or weeks at a time and may lose contact with peers, causing further distress and isolation.

Chemotherapy for these tumours includes extremely myelosuppressive agents and some children have limited bone marrow reserve, which may mean delays in administering the chemotherapy or having to abandon it altogether towards the end of the planned treatment. Chemotherapy regimens for children under the age of 3 and protocols for children with a pinealblastoma or a secreting germinoma, which precede local or cranio-spinal radiotherapy, may cause delays to radiotherapy schedules while bone marrow recovery is awaited, especially if the child has an infection. These children may also require increased blood product support and GCSF (granulocyte colony stimulating factor) during and sometimes even after their radiotherapy. Future developments in this field include the use of stereotactic radiotherapy, IMRT and targeted radiotherapy using monoclonal antibodies (Modak & Cheung, 2005) as well as the use of proton beam radiotherapy (Taylor, 2003a).

Adverse effects of radiotherapy in the treatment of brain tumours

Localised radiation to the brain may cause significant morbidity to surrounding tissue. The immediate acute side effects of this form of radiotherapy are documented in Table 20.1.

As a result of these effects, the parents and the child will require honest informative preparation to allow them to feel that they have made an active, informed decision. The acute symptoms may be extremely distressing, in addition to the experience of receiving therapy every day. The nursing role is undoubtedly one of preparation and support

Table 20.1   Acute side effects of radiotherapy

Site of radiotherapy	Tumour group	Side effect	Nursing care
Brain	CNS prophylaxis for ALL Brain tumours (astrocytoma, glioma, craniopharyngioma, brain metastases)	Cranial meningeal irritation Headache Cerebral oedema Nausea and vomiting Skin sensitivity Somnolence Fatigue Alopecia	Assess for symptoms of meningitis and neuro dysfunction Pain control Monitor for signs of raised intra cranial pressure Anti-emetics and possible i.v. fluids Skin care teaching Preparations for somnolence Encourage rest and adequate nutrition Preparation for hair loss
Spinal	Medulloblastoma Primitive neuroectodermal tumour (PNET) CNS prophylaxis for ALL	Nausea and vomiting Headache Fatigue Somnolence Alopecia Myelosuppression Tracheal irritation Oesophagitis Skin sensitivity	Anti-emetics and possible i.v. fluids Pain control Rest, encourage diet and fluids Preparation for somnolence Preparation for hair loss Monitor blood counts, assess for signs of infection, anaemia and bleeding. Cough linctus Pain control and fluids Skin care teaching
Head and neck	Nasopharyngeal carcinomas Paramenigeal mescenchymal tumours Hodgkin's disease	Skin – chemotherapy recall reactions Orbital inflammation Mucositis Xerostomia Taste alteration Oesophagitis	Skin care teaching Pain control and saline eye care Rigorous oral assessment and mouth care. Clean nares with warm water and saline nose drops Baseline dental and ENT assessment Nutritional advice Soft, non-irritant foods and encourage fluids
Eye	Retinoblastoma	Conjunctivitis Skin sensitivity Reduced tear production Minimal alopecia	Saline eye care Skin care teaching Artificial tears Preparation for hair loss
Chest	Neuroblastoma Lymphoma Pulmonary metastases PNET	Pneumonitis Oesophagitis Myelosuppression	Monitor respiratory status closely Pain control, nutritional assessment and support. Monitor blood counts, assess for signs of infection, anaemia and bleeding.
Abdomen (including para-arotic nodal fields)	Hepatoblastoma Neuroblastoma Wilms' tumour Rhabdomyosarcoma Soft tissue sarcomas PNET	Abdominal cramping and diarrhoea Nausea and vomiting Mucositis Anorexia Infertility - girls Myelosuppression Skin sensitivity	Antispasmodics, anti-diarrhoeals and pain control. Personal assessment and peri-anal care Antiemetic cover and possible I.V fluids Rigorous oral assessment and mouth care. Nutritional assessment and support Possible oophoropexy for girls Monitor blood counts, assess for signs of infection, anaemia and bleeding. Skin care teaching
Pelvis	PNET Rhabdomyosarcoma	Abdominal cramping and diarrhoea Cystitis Proctitis	Antispasmodics, anti-diarrhoeals and pain control. Personal assessment and peri-anal care Monitor genitourinary discomfort and monitor for signs of infection – encourage fluids and administer pain control. Topical relief for anal discomfort. Personal hygiene education

Table 20.1 (Continued)

Site of radiotherapy	Tumour group	Side effect	Nursing care
		Mucositis	Rigorous oral assessment and mouth care.
		Alopecia	Preparation for hair loss
		Skin recall reactions	Skin care teaching and regular skin care
Extremities	Ewing's sarcoma Rhabdomyosarcoma	Functional limitation	Loose comfortable clothing, passive exercises with physiotherapy supervision
		Skin recall reactions	Monitor skin condition and treat accordingly
		Increased risk of fracture	Health education and avoidance of trauma

throughout therapy. In addition, it is imperative that there is sensitive assessment for alterations in neurological status, discomfort due to pain, fatigue or nausea, fear and anxiety and altered nutritional status. Diligent skin care must be performed at the entry and exit site and daily assessment of tissue viability made.

In some treatment protocols up to five fields will be irradiated together; it is therefore essential to monitor children closely for any evidence of skin injury, especially if the fields have overlapped at any point as in the treatment of the cranio-spinal axis, where head and spinal fields join. The occurrence of such overlap may precipitate small areas of skin erythema or even desquamation, as well as that which may arise from the point of the localised beam to the tumour bed. It must also be a priority to observe the child's original surgical wound site for signs of tissue damage.

Radiotherapy to the brain requires the use of immobilisation devices, i.e. wearing a mask or mould; some children need to lie in a prone position for access to the spinal fields. These positions and immobilisation devices may cause distress and anxiety in some children and their preparation should reflect such an awareness (see Chapter 21 for more details).

Acute lymphoblastic leukaemia with CNS involvement

Cranial radiotherapy in acute lymphoblastic leukaemia (ALL) is only given to patients who have CNS disease at diagnosis or a CNS relapse of their leukaemia. In patients who have CNS involvement at diagnosis, a dose of 24 Gy will be given after the consolidation phase and before the first maintenance phase. Children who present with a CNS relapse are more likely to receive radiotherapy at a later stage. If they are to receive a bone marrow transplant (BMT), cranial radiotherapy will be administered just prior to total body irradiation (TBI) and the total dose received by the brain will not exceed 24 Gy.

Current leukaemia protocols warn of the use of thiopurines (mercaptopurine and thioguanine) during cranial irradiation as this may predispose to the occurrence of brain tumours. Both thiopurines and radiation damage DNA and their combined use have been demonstrated to cause a higher incidence of brain tumours in heavily treated patients (Reiling *et al.*, 1999) as would be the case in a child with relapsed disease. Thiopurines should therefore not be given during cranial radiotherapy.

Children presenting with CNS disease are rare and those with high white cell counts will be transferred to a high-risk protocol with the possibility of transplant. Therefore it may be that very few nurses will care for a child with ALL who requires craniospinal radiation. When this does occur, the family is often extremely vulnerable as they are aware that they have been placed in a poorer prognosis grouping, i.e. a high white cell count or established progressive disease. They have also learned that their child could potentially suffer many more late effects than any other child with leukaemia. Paediatric nurses caring for the child and the family must ensure that the interdisciplinary plan of care that they coordinate reflects the needs of the whole family.

Craniospinal radiotherapy may result in many unpleasant immediate effects, including stomatitis, myelosuppression and some degree of somnolence. This combination of effects can cause the child to be severely compromised nutritionally and to suffer considerable discomfort as it is often difficult to assess oral cavity status and the need for pain relief in a somnolent child. Nursing care should reflect this awareness in child and family preparation, and in oral cavity care.

Tumours of the head and neck

Post-nasal space and parameningeal sites of soft tissue sarcomas (including rhabdomyosarcomas) require irradiation to the head and neck regions which presents a host of nursing challenges due to the severe acute side effects observed with these treatments. Radiotherapy to these sites must be carefully planned in order to avoid excessive field sizes as there is major morbidity from bone and soft tissue hypoplasia in this area (Taylor, 2003b). Radiotherapy to the primary site is given at week nine of the protocol with concurrent chemotherapy. Radio-sensitising chemotherapy agents have to be omitted during radiotherapy and should be re-introduced gradually, in order to prevent a 'recall reaction' with extreme soreness of the external skin and internal mucosa.

The possibility of a prolonged treatment period in children with Stage IV mesenchymal disease may also lead to an increased risk of mucosal and skin breakdown if sufficient respite is not allowed for these tissues to repair themselves. There must be a break in therapy if larger doses of radiation are planned.

Radiotherapy treatment of post-nasal space tumours may cause considerable mucosal damage within the nasal passages, buccal cavity and pharynx (Carli et al., 2004). Tissue breakdown, as well as causing discomfort and pain, may be a significant cause of systemic infection. The salivary glands may also be damaged and therefore unable to produce saliva for lubrication, host defence and preliminary digestion.

An aspect of care which may be overlooked is that of nutritional status. Prolonged radiotherapy to this area, plus the time that recovery of such an area requires, may cause the child's nutritional status to be compromised for some time. Many children have their nutritional requirements met nasogastrically throughout radiotherapy treatment but this may be difficult with nasopharyngeal tumours. There is therefore increasing interest and exploration into the use of percutaneous gastrostomies (PEG) and some oncology centres choose to insert a PEG prior to radiotherapy, particularly in very young patients. There is significant research interest in this topic in the joint working groups of PONF/CCLG.

Retinoblastoma

Hurwitz et al. (2006) identify that radiation therapy plays an important role in the control of multifocal tumours and tumours situated near the optic nerve or macula. In the treatment of retinoblastoma the inclusion of the entire retina in the field whilst ensuring protection of the lens have always represented a challenge to the radiation oncologist. However, brachytherapy and lens-sparing external beam radiotherapy have developed with some success for the use in selected lower-risk patients. Indeed, the advent of the lens-sparing technique of radiotherapy has enabled the whole eye to be treated without irreparable damage to the retina thus maintaining useful vision in a proportion of patients (Shields et al., 2004). Unfortunately the recurrence rate is still a concern in these patients up to four years post end of therapy.

There exist many conservative treatments such as cryotherapy for peripheral and very small tumours with no seeding, laser photocoagulation for small tumours with no vitreous seeding and chemotherapy for very small tumours away from the retinal vasculature without seedings (Hurwitz et al., 2006). These methods are used to spare the eye and can be very effective in well-selected tumours where there is no evidence of disease in the other eye or metastasis elsewhere. If there is recurrence after such modalities, it is usually treated with plaque radiotherapy.

External beam radiotherapy is used to treat the whole eye, in the case of advanced disease to spare the eye (without sight) or the whole orbit after enucleation when there has been extension in the optic nerve. Currently, only two centres in the UK provide a specialist retinoblastoma service: Birmingham Children's Hospital and Great Ormond Street Hospital for Children, London.

Education for the child and the family includes eye hydration, prosthesis care, skin care and discussion of late effects on occular function and ophthalmic follow-up. Any discussion about late effects must also include information about possible long-term bone deformities and connective tissue damage from radiation injury around the orbit.

As chemotherapy for retinoblastoma has become so successful, fewer children are receiving radiotherapy. Children who do require it receive radiotherapy of a relatively low dose of approximately 40 Gy post-enucleation or 20 Gy lens sparing technique in less advanced disease. A number of children who suffer from an orbital rhabdomyosarcoma, will continue to require radiotherapy and they too will be at risk of hypoplasia of the orbit and chronic dry eye (Wexler et al., 2006).

Non-Hodgkin's lymphoma

Radiotherapy for NHL in childhood is rarely given (Taylor, 2003b). Therapy for NHL is based on multiagent chemotherapy with CNS prophylaxis with intrathecal chemotherapy and cure rates are in the region of 80 %. However, children with T cell NHL may be considered for BMT with TBI in the event of multiple relapse.

Hodgkin's lymphoma

The management of Hodgkin's lymphoma in children/young people in the UK in recent years has not included radiotherapy as a modality for primary treatment other than in stage I disease. However, evidence from the current North European Trial suggests a consistently better overall survival rate (above 95 %) by combining risk-adjusted chemotherapy and radiotherapy for all stages of disease (UKCCSG, 2005). In light of this evidence, as well as concerns about the number of relapses/progression for stage II and stage IV patients, radiotherapy is now part of recommended treatment plans for even moderate disease.

Patients are stratified into three treatment groups depending on the stage of their disease. All three groups will receive initial courses of chemotherapy before reassessment with CT/MRI scan and additionally a PET (positive emission tomography) scan. A PET scan shows areas of active cancer metabolism rather than 'abnormal' anatomical areas such as scar tissue. The result of the PET scan will determine the need for additional treatment which will include radiotherapy. Patients who are found to be PET negative and had minimal disease at diagnosis will stop all treatment, PET positive patients receive radiotherapy. In all other groups, all patients, whether PET positive or negative, receive further courses of chemotherapy and those with a positive PET scan will receive radiotherapy after chemotherapy.

Radiotherapy should be started as soon as possible after completing chemotherapy. Radiotherapy should be given to all initially involved sites with a 1.5–2 cm margin at a dose of 20 Gy in 10 fractions and a boost may be necessary to poor responding or bulky residual disease at 10 Gy in 6 fractions. The dose per fraction given may be reduced to 1.5 Gy for very young children or for large volumes. Care must be taken when treating the mediastinum, and lateral margins should thus be determined on post-chemotherapy rather than initial diagnostic imaging. If the spine is in the treatment field, it must be treated symmetrically in order to avoid scoliosis in later life.

Where disease is situated in the cervical or mandibular regions, radiotherapy fields must be planned with care to minimise adverse reactions. The mandibles and clavicles are shielded where possible to prevent serious growth retardation in these bones which, in turn, leads to severe deformity and body image difficulties. A mask made of a thermoplastic material may be required for immobilisation and to keep the chin/jaw out of the treatment field. Thyroid function is an area of concern after involved field radiotherapy treatment and must be monitored, with full endocrine follow-up into adulthood.

The possible adverse effects of radiotherapy to the cervical region and pharyngeal area have been highlighted elsewhere. However, skin changes which may cause discoloration following erythema, in conjunction with weight loss due to nutritional deficits, may result in significant alterations to a young person's body image which must be addressed. It is also imperative, in view of possible thyroid dysfunction, that investigation of hormonal function is carried out regularly and that the family is kept informed of the significance of such results. Thyroxine replacement therapy should be instituted promptly, if required, as it is essential for continued growth and development. Young people are one of the main age groups affected by this particular malignancy and their preparation needs may be different from younger children. These young men and women may already have established views on the advantages and disadvantages of nuclear radiation, as well as many concerns about bodily insult and the effects on the hormonal system so important to their burgeoning sexuality. They will also need to be aware of the potential damage to their cardio-vascular system after mediastinal radiotherapy and be discouraged from smoking.

Radiotherapy for abdominal tumours

This field of treatment is often used for the irradition of hepatoblastoma, Wilms' tumour and neuroblastoma. Full abdominal radiation is much rarer in the treatment of children. Flank radiotherapy is a more commonly desired field. Any abdominal field carries a risk of temporary or possibly even chronic enteritis, with consequent malabsorption problems. These issues must be anticipated and explained to families so that a full multidisciplinary nutritional plan can be prepared for each eventuality during and post radiotherapy. When caring for children undergoing therapy for these forms of cancer there will be a considerable number of very young children undergoing radiotherapy. There is therefore a need for effective preparation to elicit some degree of cooperation and, more importantly, to decrease fear and anxiety.

Malignant mesenchymal tumours such as rhabdomyosarcoma

For treatment purposes, children with mesenchymal tumours are often assessed on the extent of their disease, the position of the tumour and histology. They are then placed in one of three

risk groups: low, medium or high. In general, children with low-risk disease are not randomised to receive radiotherapy, whereas children with high-risk non-metastatic disease require localised therapy. Children with metastatic disease may receive radiotherapy to both the primary site plus sites of metastatic disease. The most common tumours in this group treated in paediatric units are rhabdomyosarcomas and these are treated on a number of different protocols, depending on their site, stage and histological subtype. Non-rhabdoid tumours are treated on the basis of their histology, chemosensitivity and post-surgical stage.

Decisions about radiotherapy may be taken following rigorous periods of chemotherapy, surgery and anxiety-provoking re-assessment scans. Preparation for radiotherapy must be sensitive to the fact that the child and the family may have recently received information that there remains residual disease after initial therapy, and they may therefore be extremely distressed. Radiotherapy post-surgery requires acute nursing observation for (and a research-based response to) possible tissue injury at the wound site.

Radiotherapy is offered as a treatment option for many children with tumours of Stage IV classification. Treatment may be extensive and a short rest may be needed during the treatment episode to allow for mucosal regeneration at any point along the gastro-intestinal tract. In situations where the child has metastatic disease, both primary and metastatic sites can be treated simultaneously. Treating multiple sites highlights the need for pro-active care to minimise side effects. This must be discussed thoroughly with the family at treatment planning and be considered by nursing staff when they are observing the child for adverse responses.

Wilms' tumour

In the child with a Wilms' tumour, post-operative radiotherapy to the flank of the body is indicated in high-risk disease in dosages and fractions dependent on histology. Tumours found to have favourable histology receive about a 30% lower dose than those with unfavourable histology. Treatment fields will extend medially to include the full width of the spinal column to ensure symmetrical growth retardation in this area. In the case of lung metastases, radiotherapy is also included for disease containment. The lungs can be irradiated from the apex to T11/T12.

Whole abdominal radiotherapy is indicated for diffuse intra-abdominal disease or gross tumour rupture before or during surgery. If lung radiotherapy is to be given at the same time, care must be taken to match the two fields to avoid any overlap. As children are given chemotherapy in addition to radiotherapy, it must be considered that drugs such as dactinomycin and doxorubicin may enhance skin and lung injury in some children.

Although the spinal column is always included in the radiation field to ensure symmetry of growth, unilateral exposure of ribs and flank muscles can cause some degree of atrophy on the affected side. This, in turn, presents the child with the potential for quite severe body image difficulties later in life. The family of such a child must be informed of this risk so that they can prepare their child in later life. Lung irradiation, with its attendant morbidity, must be fully explained to the parents and the child so that their experiences postradiotherapy will not leave them feeling bewildered at the degree of morbidity their child in may experience.

Neuroblastoma

In the treatment of extensive or high-risk neuroblastoma all three modalities of therapy are part of current treatment protocols. Radiotherapy will be given to all patients to the pre-operative extent of the primary tumour after myeloablative chemotherapy with stem-cell transplant. Radiotherapy should commence after an interval of 60 days post transplant due to the risk of busulphan-enhanced radiotoxicity. This may be delayed for up to 30 days to allow for recovery from transplant-related toxicities. A dose of 21 Gy in 14 daily fractions is currently prescribed.

The planning of radiotherapy using CT scans and radiation simulators takes time and patience with young children, and children under the age of 4 years benefit from being anaesthetised in order to allow for treatment accuracy. Furthermore, the pre-operative tumour volume plus associated nodes and a 2 cm safety margin may

constitute a fairly large area to be treated. This extensive field may include vital structures, especially bone, with attendant growth failure risks. The family should receive all possible information before treatment so that active participation in long-term decisions can be maintained.

Previous protocols attempted to compare the efficacy of using a radioactive isotope – mIBG – in a therapeutic manner in the first-line treatment of children with advanced disease with standard treatment but with no conclusive evidence found with initial methodologies. However, the current national neuroblastoma protocol uses this isotope only in the diagnosis and re-staging of the disease. It may still be an option for salvaging resistant disease but few centres in the UK have the necessary facilities such as a Radionuclide Therapy Suite to enable the safe nursing care of children treated with radioactive materials (see Chapter 19). Many children with neuroblastoma are under the age of 5 years and may not comply very easily with the restriction of being isolated for at least five days and might need interventions such as sedation and/or catheterisation.

Pelvic irradiation

Rhabdomyosarcoma and other soft tissue sarcomas may also be found in the lower abdomen and pelvis. Irradiation of this area of the body results in many acute and distressing side effects (see Table 20.1). Localised tissue changes may produce pain and disruption (possibly permanent) to elimination of faecal matter and urine if the area includes the bladder or the bowel. The parents and the child should be fully aware of potential problems that may arise after such therapy, although they may not occur in all children. This will serve to reduce anxiety and distress should symptoms present. The parents should have sufficient knowledge to recognise symptoms at home during and after treatment so that they can contact the unit and not become distressed at the thought that the symptoms may be due to advancing disease.

Due to the need for wide-field irradiation for some pelvic tumours, the child/young person will become myelo-suppressed. Blood product transfusions as well as GCSF injections may become necessary during radiotherapy. Nursing staff will need to monitor blood counts and instigate such interventions in line with local radiotherapy guidelines.

Extensive radiotherapy to the pelvic area may lead to particular problems in maintaining skin integrity due to the difficulty in keeping clothing loose and reducing shearing forces in underwear. In addition, areas of irradiated skin may rub against one another as the child moves, causing pain and further skin trauma. This discomfort may discourage the child from moving about and so decrease their self-care abilities. Older children and young people may find the position of the radiation injury a source of considerable embarrassment when skin integrity assessment is carried out by nursing staff or when extensive skin care interventions are necessary. This embarrassment may lead to a reluctance to permit observation. Careful discussion and negotiation must be undertaken by nursing staff with the child or young person, to determine levels of observation and physical contact. These should be both psychologically comfortable for the child and appropriate for the safe maintainance of skin integrity and prevention of tissue breakdown. Furthermore, if the pelvic radiotherapy has the potential for severe side effects on the reproductive organs, issues such as fertility and sexuality must be discussed in advance of therapy with the parents of a young child as well as the young person themselves.

Some children/young people may require another form of radiation, brachytherapy. This method delivers a higher dose of radiation to a defined area by means of radioactive wires or capsules (see Chapter 19) inserted straight into a body cavity or tissue area. The radiation is delivered over a number of days and the patient may need to be nursed in a specially protected room with minimal staff contact to avoid excessive exposure of staff to radioactive materials. This treatment has been used in recurrent vaginal rhabdomyosarcoma to gain local control of the disease with minimal damage to healthy tissues through insertion of a radioactive irridium source.

Extremity radiation

Rhabdomyosarcoma and bone tumours may present at distant sites, i.e. arm or leg, hence the treatment may cause restrictions in mobility or function and the resulting loss of mobility may have social implications (Table 20.1).

All children who receive radiotherapy to their limbs must be protected from unnecessary trauma to the bone/muscle until the tissue is healed. This means that health education about avoiding traumatic contact that may damage the bone/muscle must be stressed, for example, some sports or social interests. It may also be the case that the child undergoes surgery either before or after radiotherapy; tissue viability must be a primary concern in these situations. A bone which has received radiotherapy may also be more prone to injury such as a fracture and in a young child, growth in the treated bone will be reduced, leading to a shorter and narrower limb. Muscle bulk may also be reduced in the affected limb, which in turn will also affect function and movement in that limb.

Conclusion

Across the speciality there is diversity in approach despite a shared academic knowledge on advances in radiotherapy techniques and toxicity evaluations. There is no literature that documents any analysis of this phenomenon but it does seem evident that there are some countries focusing on radiotherapy as a central aspect of care and others that appear to wish to reduce its role in curative therapy. It may be proposed that within Europe, Germanic-derived protocols appear to highly value the curative advantage of higher doses of radiotherapy despite the consequent and significant toxicity associated. However, in sharp contrast, in French-led trials, the emphasis is most obviously on reduction of treatment toxicity by using therapeutic journeys that minimise radiotherapy input. The UK appears to sit somewhat closer to the French approach than the German approach in this matter, but the situation is dynamic and changes with the challenges faced in improving cure rates in certain highly malignant tumours.

Medical philosophy and the prevailing quality of survival culture within a country are part of the complex conclusions drawn. The balance between the needs for cure versus those for quality of survival in children and young people, with brain tumours most particularly, are weighted uniquely to each health care context. In contrast, many US units are in the enviable position of being able to take full advantage of the recent advances described in Chapter 22. This translates into more radiotherapy for younger children than is normally considered on this side of the Atlantic. Indeed, it appears that far more aggressive treatment is possible for all due to the access to highly conforming techniques such as IMRT, or alternative radiation sources such as protons.

References

Blaney SM, Kun LE, Hunter J, Rorke-Adams LB, Lau C, Strother D & Pollack IF (2006) 'Tumours of the central nervous system' *in*: Pizzo PA & Poplack DG (eds) *Principles and Practice of Pediatric Oncology* (5th edn). Philadelphia, PA: Lippincott, Williams & Williams, pp. 786–864

Carli M, Cecchetto G, Sotti G, Allaggio R & Stevens MC (2004) 'Soft tissue sarcomas' *in*: Pinkerton R, Plowman N & Pieters R (eds) *Paediatric Oncology* (3rd edn). London: Arnold, pp. 339–371

Freeman K, O'Dell C & Meola C (2004) 'Childhood brain tumors: parental concerns and stressors by phase of illness' *Journal of Pediatric Oncology Nursing* 21(2): 87–97

HIT-SIOP PNET 4 Protocol (2004) Final version. UKCCSG/SIOP

Hurwitz RL, Shields CL, Shields JA, Chevez-Barrios P, Hurwitz MY & Chintagumpala MM (2006) 'Retinoblastoma' in: Pizzo PA & Poplack DG (eds) *Principles and Practice of Pediatric Oncology* (5th edn).

Philadelphia, PA: Lippincott, Williams & Williams, pp. 865–886

Modak S & Cheung NK (2005) 'Antibody-based targeted radiation to pediatric tumors' *Journal of Nuclear Medicine* 46 (suppl. 1):157S–163S

Reiling M, Rubnitz J, Rivera G, Boyett J, Hancock M, Felix C, Kun L, Walter A, Evans W & Pui C (1999) 'High incidence of secondary brain tumours after radiotherapy and antimetabolites' *Lancet* 354(9172): 34–37

Shields CL, Meadows AT, Leahey AM & Shields JA (2004) 'Continuing challenges in the management of retinoblastoma with chemotherapy' *Retina* 24(6): 849–862

Shiminski-Maher T (1993) 'Physician–patient–parent communication problems' *Paediatric Neurosurgery* 19(10): 104–108

Shiminski-Maher T & Wisoff JH (1995) 'Pediatric brain tumours' *Critical Care Nursing Clinics of North America* 7(1): 159–169

Taylor R (2003a) 'Proton radiotherapy for paediatric tumours: potential areas for clinical research' *Clinical Oncology* 15(1): S32–S36

Taylor R (2003b) 'Paediatric oncology' *in*: Bomford CK & Kunkler, I (eds) *Walter and Miller's Textbook of Radiotherapy: Radiation Physics, Therapy and Oncology* (6th edn). Edinburgh: Churchill Livingstone, pp. 583–596

UKCCSG/PONF Mouthcare Group (2006) *Mouth Care for Children and Young People with Cancer: Evidence-based Guidelines*. Guideline Report. Version 1.0 February 2006

Wexler LH, Meyer WH & Helman LJ (2006) 'Rhabdomyosarcoma and the undifferentiated sarcomas' *in*: Pizzo PA & Poplack DG (eds) *Principles and Practice of Pediatric Oncology* (5th edn). Philadelphia, PA: Lippincott, Williams & Williams, pp. 971–1001

21 Acute and Sub-acute Side Effects of Radiotherapy

Monica Hopkins and Cornelia Scott

Introduction

Healthy tissues can be divided into two types for the purposes of anticipating reactions to ionising radiation. There are those which proliferate rapidly, for example skin, gut, bone marrow and hair follicles. These are known as acute reacting tissues. There are also tissues that proliferate slowly, if at all, and these include lungs, brain and kidneys. These tissues express radiation damage at a later stage. In each case cellular injury occurs by the same process but is not expressed until the cell attempts division. The severity of acute damage is influenced by a number of factors:

- the treatment field;
- radiation fraction interval (hence the increase in acute toxicity with hyperfractionation);
- dose per radiation fraction;
- duration of treatment;
- radiosensitivity of the tissue;
- type of machine and energy of the radiation.

In contrast, sub-acute and late reactions depend on time, dose factors and total dose.

Acute reactions in healthy tissue

Both healthy and malignant cells attempt to repair themselves within six hours after exposure to radiation (Tarbell *et al.*, 2006). However, malignant cells may be far less effective in their attempt to recover (Hilderley, 1992a, b). Healthy tissues which proliferate rapidly, unfortunately, can still sustain damage which, though often reparable, does temporarily affect function. The more proliferative tissues, such as skin, gastrointestinal mucosa, bone marrow, and hair follicles, will demonstrate effects of radiation quite rapidly, usually during the course of treatment. In addition, some of the less proliferative tissues in the body can express acute trauma when directly targeted with radiotherapy. Acute reacting tissues may, as a result of their injury, proceed to demonstrate chronic and long-term dysfunction often due to fibrotic post-inflammatory changes within the tissue itself or its vascular bed (O'Donoghue, 2004).

Cancer in Children and Young People   Edited by Faith Gibson and Louise Soanes
© 2008 John Wiley & Sons, Ltd

Skin

Radiotherapy causes biochemical changes within cells, and the DNA molecules are susceptible to radiation damage during mitosis. The surface layer of the skin, the epidermis, consists of stratified squamous cells that are renewed by constantly dividing basal cells that lie adjacent to the dermis. Radiation treatment results in the impairment of cell re-population (Zimmerman *et al.*, 1998; Kunkler, 2003), and therefore affects the integrity of the upper dermis layer (Hopewell, 1990). The cell renewal time of the epidermis is 2–3 weeks, and skin reactions may take this time to become fully apparent and may continue for a similar period once treatment is complete (Owens *et al.*, 2004).

Clinical signs that may be observed are:

- *Initial redness or erythema*. This is usually seen within seven days of the onset of radiotherapy. The characteristic redness is due to dilation of the capillaries in response to radiation damage (Kunkler, 2003). As erythema progresses, increased vascularity and inflammatory obstruction of the capillaries develop.
- *Dry desquamation*. This is caused when there is cell death in the upper layers of the skin. The decreased ability of the epidermal basal cells to replace the surface cells leads to desquamation. The sweat and sebaceous glands are also damaged and are dysfunctional, causing extreme dryness. This often begins approximately 2–4 weeks after therapy commences.
- *Moist desquamation*. This clinical presentation is seen as doses approach the limits of skin tolerance. Moist desquamation is a result of extreme damage to the epidermis allowing the dermis to be exposed and serous fluid to leak from the tissue (Lawton & Twoomey, 1991). The area is now at risk of infection and, in cases of widespread damage, fluid loss (McDonald, 1992). This is a potentially serious situation that may even lead to a break in therapy to allow the tissue to heal.

At the end of treatment, the remaining basal cells will repopulate the tissue. However, if the tolerance dose has been exceeded, the basal cells will have been killed, resulting in ulceration (McDonald, 1992) and possibly leading to tissue necrosis (Barkham, 1993).

Adverse reactions to radiotherapy in healthy tissue are often graded as to their severity as part of an overall toleration assessment. Grading is normally based on how severely the radiotherapy damage affects quality of life. In the past, the use of varied systems for recording integumentary system damage were confusing as they often combined different manifestations of injury in the same tissue. Sitton (1992) maintains that adherence to local skin management regimens, as well as innate individual differences, may account for varying skin responses to radiotherapy. Campbell and Lane (1996) maintain that as skin cannot repair itself until radiotherapy is completed, nursing care must focus upon the relief of discomfort and the promotion of a good healing environment. At all times the priority should be to minimise the injury caused to the skin by prevention of the excessive dryness that follows erythema, as this can lead to skin breakdown. Doing so prevents further trauma and, at the same time, treating the skin gently at all times decreases friction and erosion of epidermal cells. It should also be stressed that no skin agent other than moisturisers should be used on wounds unless a substantial case can be made as to its contribution to wound healing.

Nursing care varies around the country and indeed practice needs to be confirmed through research as advocated by Barkham (1993). There appears to be little consensus over identification of the levels of skin injury. Topical agents range from simple moisturisers to steroid preparations, zinc oxide cream, powders and silicon compounds and a myriad of dressings are utilised in practice with little rationale as to choice. The literature in the UK has little to offer in terms of research-based interventions, but examination of practice and wound care research from other areas of practice has contributed to a growing knowledge base. Core principles now seem to be consistent in many commentaries on radiotherapy care. The aim of care should be to relieve discomfort and symptoms until radiotherapy has taken its full effect. In this way, nurses are able to prevent further trauma and infection and so promote prompt healing after therapy is complete. These core principles had originally been brought together in a skin care policy developed by Campbell and Lane (1996). This policy has been superseded by a skin care guideline policy by Owens *et al.* as set out by the Cookridge Hospital (Figure 21.1).

Cookridge Hospital Skin Care Policy

Key recommendations

1. A patient's skin should be assessed for predictive factors prior to radiotherapy commencing.
2. Those assessing the skin should be able to demonstrate appropriate knowledge as outlined in the guidelines.
3. All patients/carers should receive written information about skin care prior to commencing radiotherapy.
4. The modified RTOG grading scale should be used to assess skin on commencement of radiotherapy.
5. Preventing damage to the skin through friction should be advised.
6. Aqueous cream should be used to maintain optimum skin condition whilst the skin is intact.
7. If the skin becomes broken, the use of aqueous cream should be stopped and the appropriate foam dressing applied.
8. Patients with an RTOG scale of 2.5 or above at the end of radiotherapy should be referred on to the appropriate health care professionals.

1   Introduction

The majority of patients receiving external beam radiotherapy are expected to develop a skin reaction (Olsen *et al.*, 2001). However, skin care guidelines are not intended to prevent the reaction but to avoid exacerbation of the damage (Porrock & Kristjanson, 1999; Walker, 1992).

1.1   Scope

Radiotherapy is delivered within the cancer centre. However, it is recognised that care of children and young people, receiving radiotherapy impacts across the cancer centre, shared care units and primary care teams.

These guidelines are intended for the use of all health professionals, who care for patients who will have, are having or have had radiotherapy.

1.2   Aim

To ensure that radiotherapy patients receive consistent, evidence-based advice and care in the management of any skin reactions through:

- promoting an optimum healing environment;
- minimising patient distress and discomfort;
- accurate and consistent assessment and documentation of the nature and severity of skin reactions;

- increasing multidisciplinary knowledge and awareness across the cancer centre, care units and primary care teams.

2   Education and training

It is recommended that all health professionals who are responsible for assessing, managing and documenting a patient's skin pre-radiotherapy, during and post-radiotherapy, have the following knowledge:

- ability to differentiate skin reactions according to the RTOG scale;
- knowledge of the predictive factors;
- ability to advise patients and provide evidence for this advice;
- knowledge of the current recommended management of skin care reactions as recommended in these skin care guidelines.

3   Pre-radiotherapy management

Prior to radiotherapy commencing, a baseline assessment of the skin and its potential to develop a reaction should be recorded on the patient's radiotherapy treatment card (College of Radiographers, 2000). Assessment should continue throughout the patient's treatment and for an agreed period post radiotherapy.

3.1   Skin assessment

Skin assessment and grading in the literature are most commonly undertaken using Cox *et al.*'s (1995) abbreviated version of acute radiation scoring criteria (RTOG), developed by the Radiation Therapy Oncology Group in 1985. In current practice within radiotherapy departments, routine grading and recording of skin reactions is not common (College of Radiographers, 2000). A consistent approach to skin assessment is required where the skin status is recorded and graded by an appropriately trained member of the multidisciplinary team (COR, 2000). Though observer ratings do not account for the subjective aspects of skin damage, such as pain and discomfort, the agreed scoring criteria such as the RTOG (Table 21.1) is recommended (COR, 2000). If the skin reaction is causing pain, refer to the Paediatric Acute Pain Guidelines (Leeds Teaching Hospital, 2002).

3.2   Predetermining skin reaction intensity

Predetermining the nature and severity of skin reactions can be difficult as radio-sensitivity of skin varies between individual skin structures and a number of predictive factors identified by Porrock *et al.* (1998).

Figure 21.1   Cookridge Hospital skin care policy (2003)

Table 21.1 RTOG Grading System

RTOG grading	Description
RTOG 0	No visible change to skin
RTOG 1	Faint or dull erythema
RTOG 2	Tender or bright erythema
RTOG 2.5	Patchy moist desquamation (breakdown of the epidermis)
RTOG 3	Confluent, moist desquamation
RTOG 4	Ulceration, haemorrhage and necrosis

It is recommended that consideration be given to predictive factors (Table 21.2) prior to radiotherapy commencing. These factors may influence the information given to the patient relating to the intensity of their skin reaction. It will also underpin the information given to health professionals upon transfer of care from the cancer centre to shared care units and primary care.

3.3 Frequency of assessment

Assessment of skin reactions forms a part of the routine patient review during radiotherapy. The RTOG score will be recorded on the radiotherapy treatment card at the following times:

- pre-radiotherapy by the clinician;
- on the first day of treatment by a radiographer or CNS in oncology.

Radiographers will then check the skin on a daily basis and record any change on the treatment card. Once an RTOG score of 2.5 is reached or anticipated, they will refer on to the appropriate inpatient or outpatient nursing staff. Patients with an RTOG score of 2.5 or above upon completion of treatment should be referred onto the relevant nursing team by the appropriate health-care professional.

4 Patient information

To enable patients to consent to radiotherapy they must be fully informed (www.doh.gov.uk/consent). Patient information is integral to the consent process and patients should continue to be informed throughout their treatment programme. The content of patient information may vary. This may be influenced by the presence of predictive factors in the initial assessment. Patients should be given accurate and, where possible, evidence-based advice in relation to caring for their skin during and after radiotherapy. Current advice is outlined in Table 21.3.

Table 21.2 Predictive factors

Factor	Description
Trauma	Caused by increased skin to skin contact. E.g. - Axilla, infra-mammary fold, groin and buttocks as well as skin to clothing contact will increase the skin reaction and shorten the onset from the commencement of radiotherapy. Patients should be advised to pat the skin dry with a soft towel and wear loose clothing.
Previous damage	The presence of previous damage such as surgery may increase the intensity of the skin reaction e.g. scar.
Radiotherapy treatment modality	If a 'boost' – i.e. an additional dose of radiotherapy is given to a specific area the intensity of the skin reaction will increase.
Energy of radiotherapy	The higher the energy, the lesser the skin reaction.
Radiotherapy dose	The higher the dose, the greater the skin reaction.
Bolus	The presence of bolus, (a tissue equivalent material) increases the skin reaction. The thicker the bolus, the greater the skin reaction.
Age	Some very young children have a decrease in subcutaneous fat and a thinning of the dermis and epidermis (Dellafield 1986), and are thus likely to experience a greater reaction.
Nutrition	Malnourished patients or those on a poor diet will have a greater skin reaction.
Chemotherapy	Some chemotherapy drugs are radio sensitising (e.g. 5 Flurouracil (5FU) and Actinomycin D) and as such, will increase the skin reaction (Duchese, 1988).
Anxiety	Anxiety and stress have a negative effect on the immune system and healing and so increase the skin reaction, prolonging the time it takes to heal (Pediana, 1992).
Lifestyle	Smoking and alcohol abuse restrict capillary blood flow and increase the skin reaction (Porrock et al., 1998).
Infection	The presence of infection will increase the skin reaction and prolong the time it takes to heal.
Radiosensitive chronic illness	The presence of illnesses such as lupus will increase the skin reaction, prolonging the healing time.

Figure 21.1 (Continued)

Table 21.3 Patient advice relating to skin care

Advice	Action	Evidence
Prevent friction on the skin in the treated area	Wear soft, loose clothing with no tight straps/waist bands, collars etc. Omit shaving or shave using an electric shaver as this reduces the chance of cutting the skin. Avoid the use of hot water bottles. Avoid rubbing the skin. Wash gently and pat dry.	Radiation impairs cell re-population and integrity of the upper dermis layer (Sitton, 1992: Zimmermann, 1998: Hopewell, 1990). Additional friction or damage will further impair viability of the skin.
Sun protection	Exposing the treated area to direct sunshine for at least the first year following treatment should be avoided or a total sun block (minimum of factor 45) should be applied to that area.	There is no conclusive research to support this. Therefore consensus of opinion has been collated.
Swimming	Once a skin reaction occurs (RTOG 1 onwards), swimming should be avoided due to the additional trauma of drying and risk of infection if skin integrity is compromised. The loss of skin marks should also be avoided.	There is no literature to evidence advice on swimming.
Washing and personal hygiene	Treated area may be washed using normal soap and water. If skin stings or is irritated then a milder soap should be sought. Pat skin dry rather than rub to avoid friction. Avoid perfumed creams, fragrances and deodorants in the affected area. Hair can be washed normally. However, hot hairdryers should be avoided.	There is no significant difference between washing with water alone and washing with soap and water (Campbell and Illingworth, 1996).

5   Management of skin reactions

5.1   Reactions graded RTOG 0–2.5

It is recognised that there is a paucity of literature relating to the effectiveness of creams in relation to skin reaction for patients receiving radiotherapy (Porrock & Kristjanson, 1999). Indeed, there has been a multitude of products suggested for use on radiotherapy reactions but little real evidence of their evaluation.

The report from the College of Radiographers makes recommendations for a robust evaluation of the creams used for topical application. From the evidence available a consensus has been agreed that aqueous cream should be given to all patients on commencing radiotherapy. Aqueous cream has been described as helping to maintain optimum skin condition during radiotherapy (Spencer, 1988). In addition, there is no significant evidence to suggest that there is any advantage to using an oil-based moisturiser as opposed to aqueous cream (Porrock & Kristjanson, 1998). The use of lanolin-based creams is contraindicated due to the potential for increased skin sensitivity, which has implications for skin traumatisation (Linnit, 2000; COR, 2000).

5.2   Use of aqueous cream

Aqueous cream (unfragranced) should be supplied to patients at the start of treatment. Care should be taken with children with eczema in the treatment field as a recent study suggested adverse skin reactions with the use of this emollient (Cork et al., 2003). Therefore, it is recommended that the cream be used under the supervision of the clinical oncologist and a patch test be done before treatment starts.

Application of cream is recommended at least twice per day in the treated area though treatment marks should be avoided. More frequent application is advisable as skin reaction increases until there is skin breakdown (i.e. RTOG >2.5: see RTOG Grading), when the cream should be stopped. The use of E45 moisturising cream is not recommended as it contains lanolin that can cause increased sensitivity in some patients.

5.3   Use of other topical skin agents

The following soothing agents may be used in addition to the moisturising creams: Pure Aloe Vera, Evening Primrose Oil (Gamma Linoleic Acid, GLA) and topical Vitamin C (if the patient so chooses). However, the carrier creams of these products should be checked for metal-based compounds as these should not be used. There is still no conclusive evidence to support the use or avoidance of other topical agents (Halperin et al., 1993).

5.3.1   Talcum powder should be avoided in the treated area

Talc absorbs moisture and can block hair follicles and pores, thus causing more irritation. Such a drying and blocking effect

Figure 21.1   (Continued)

Table 21.4 Guideline summary for the management of radiation-induced skin reactions

Presentation	Aim	Intervention	Advice/education
RTOG 0 No visible change to skin	To promote hydrated skin To maintain skin integrity	Ensure aqueous cream is applied at least twice per day. Please refer to 5.2 for recommendations on the use of aqueous cream for children with eczema	Generalised advice. Avoid excess extremes of heat - i.e., hot water bottles and ice packs.
RTOG 1 Faint or dull erythema, mild tightness of skin and some itching Decreased sweating Epilation	To promote hydrated skin To maintain skin integrity	Advise frequency of applications of aqueous moisturiser (3 to 4 times daily).	Wash with regular products, changing to a milder brand if irritation occurs. Pat gently dry after washing. Do not rub.
RTOG 2 Tender or bright erythema, itchy, irritating areas of skin	To retard skin breakdown	Continue moisturising with aqueous cream. Use 1 % Hydrocortisone cream **sparingly** for acute itching only.	Avoid use of perfumed products i.e. deodorant, perfumes, creams, etc. Do not use talc on treated area, except sparsely over skin marks. Wear natural fibres against skin rather than synthetics.
RTOG 2.5 Patchy/moist desquamation (broken skin with exudate) Moderate oedema	To prevent infection To attain optimum conditions for wound healing	Use aqueous moisturiser on unbroken skin only. Withdraw the use of hydrocortisone. Use foam dressings e.g. Allevyn over areas of broken skin.	Keep area covered, avoiding exposure to direct sunshine. Maintain balanced dietary intake and increased fluid intake.
RTOG 3 Confluent moist desquamation (broken skin with exudate), pitting erythema	To prevent infection To attain optimum conditions for wound healing	Withdraw the use of moisturising cream. Use foam dressing e.g. Allevyn on affected areas. This should only be replaced on strike through. If exudate is green and odorous or patient is pyrexial, swab for C & S and treat with antibiotics if infection present.	Swimming should be avoided when reactions become evident due to increased skin trauma. (i.e. RTOG 1 onwards)
RTOG 4 Ulceration, bleeding	To prevent infection To attain optimum conditions for wound healing To control bleeding	Use foam dressing e.g. Allevyn on affected area. This should only be replaced on strike through. Use Kaltostat for haemorrhage. For ulceration and necrosis use a Hydrocolloid, i.e. granuflex or Hydrogel, i.e. aquaform. If exudate is green, has an offensive odour, or if patient is pyrexial, swab for C & S and treat with antibiotics if infection present.	Soothing agents such as Aloe Vera & Evening Primrose Oil can be used if the patient choses.

Figure 21.1 (Continued)

contradicts the optimum conditions required for maintenance of healing of skin (Campbell & Illingworth, 1992; Spencer, 1988).

5.3.2   Gentian Violet (crystal violet) should not be used as it is carcinogenic, especially on mucous membranes and open wounds (BNF 38, 1999, p. 528).

5.3.3 1% Hydrocortisone Cream

Should only be applied sparingly for severe pruritis, twice per day following moisturising with aqueous cream. It should be discontinued if any break occurs in the skin (i.e. at RTOG >2.5). Though steroids reduce inflammatory response they also make the skin more friable and may reduce capillary blood flow which can delay healing (Campbell & Lane, 1996). All patients should receive information from their radiotherapy treatment centre on recommendations for skin care during and after therapy.

5.4   Treatment of skin reactions RTOG 2.5–4

Moist desquamation occurs when the inflamed epidermis blisters and sloughs leaving an exposed and painful area of dermis that may exude serum (Campbell, 2000). The aim is to promote patient comfort through control of the exudate, maintain pain control and prevent infection (Table 21.4). The use of aqueous and hydrocortisone cream must cease when the skin becomes broken.

5.4.1   Use of dressings

A foam dressing (e.g. Allevyn, Mepilex) is recommended where broken skin is present (RTOG 2.5–3), as it fulfils the characteristics of an ideal dressing (Morgan, 1993). Foam dressings should only be replaced when strike-through occurs. Kaltostat is currently recommended (LTH Trust wound care guidelines) for use on bleeding reaction sites for its haemostatic properties. If the reaction site is ulcerated or necrotic, an appropriate hydrocolloid dressing (i.e. granuflex) or a hydrogel (e.g. aquafoam, Trudgian, 2000) should be used.

5.4.2   Use of antibiotics

Antibiotics should not be routinely administered. If an infection is suspected, i.e. green exudate, an offensive odour or if the patient is pyrexial, a swab of the area should be taken for culture and sensitivity. Antibiotics should be prescribed if an infection is isolated. Each reaction will vary in the length of time it takes to heal. In general most skin reactions graded 2.5–3 can expect to take up to six weeks after radiotherapy has finished to heal. If there appears to be no improvement in the reaction site, further advice should be sought from a radiotherapy nurse specialist or radiographer specialist. Reactions of RTOG 4 are uncommon, it is not possible to estimate healing times for such reactions. If a patient does present with a grade 4 reaction, the patient's medical team/Clinical Nurse Specialist/ Macmillan Radiographer should be contacted for further advice.

6   Post-radiotherapy management

Following completion of treatment:

> Week 1–2: Acute skin reaction may become more marked.
> Week 2–3: Reaction will begin to settle.

Children and young people with severe skin reactions should be seen regularly in the outpatient review clinic. They and their families should be encouraged to continue with the advice given for treatment until the skin reaction has settled, then return to their normal skin care routine. For advice or information, patients, carers or health professionals can contact the radiotherapy department during office hours.

Figure 21.1   (Continued)

As described above, a formal assessment tool for assessing skin integrity before instigating care is now available in the UK literature through the RTOG scale, which has been devised with adults in mind by the Radiation Therapy Oncology Group. The Department of Health in Scotland has also produced a 'Best Practice Statement on Skincare of Patients Receiving Radiotherapy', which is available on the Internet (www.nhshealthquality.org/nhsqis/files). As with the Cookridge Guidelines, their practice has been guided by, among others, experienced specialist nurses in radiotherapy, therapy radiographers and tissue viability nurses. Although recommendations for assessment methodology can thus be proposed, it is important that this assessment tool is validated in its use with children. Issues to consider in daily skin observation are:

1. The total radiation field must be fully described and identified on the child's care plan. It is imperative that the nurse caring for the child is fully aware of the treatment angles in order to be cognisant of the exact treatment field. It is possible to have a significant skin reaction at the exit site of the treatment field, therefore this area also requires close observation.
2. Preventative measures should be instigated from the day of treatment to keep the affected area of skin well moisturised.

3. Daily assessment should be made in conjunction with the child and the family for the presence and severity of erythema, moisture level of skin, and evidence of breaks in skin integrity. It must be remembered that radiation skin injury is cumulative and will extend for some weeks after therapy ends.

4. All areas of erythema and desquamation must be documented and preferably drawn, with accurate dimensions, in the child's assessment documentation and care plan.

5. All teaching and guidance given, in addition to actual intervention, must be documented in detail and adhere to the recognised policy of the unit to prevent confusion and inconsistency of care. It is recommended that to aid consistency of approach in grading skin damage, visual aids are preferable to written description alone. Clear colour photographs of each stage can promote increased staff awareness and expertise in recognition of each stage. This can only aid consistency of approach in care and family education. These photographs may be displayed in teaching rooms within the unit, or in a learning package within the treatment area for ease of referral for assessment of a child.

Once the skin area has been assessed, a pro-active plan of care needs to be negotiated to assist the child in caring for their skin, and to prevent further trauma. Nurses must also be aware of the most effective measures for dealing with skin breakdown should it occur during or after therapy. The principles of skin care for radiotherapy injury are summarised in the previously described policy (Table 21.3). All relevant aspects of skin care such as hygiene, moisturisation, wound healing and health promotion have been discussed and give both the nurses looking after a child and family research-based evidence of how to care for a child with a radiotherapy skin reaction (Owens et al., 2003).

In addition to the physical nursing care of skin injury, the psychological consequences must also be considered. Skin injury is an outwardly visible reminder of the disease and its treatment, a constant reflection of the loss of body integrity during treatment. Children and young people may find this very distressing and suffer body image difficulties at this time and thereafter. It is vitally important to generate an awareness of these difficulties with relevant personnel and seek to allow expression of feelings and emotions around this subject without platitudes and dismissals. Concerns about tissue integrity must be dealt with promptly, honestly and with appreciation of the social implications of body image to the child.

The gastrointestinal tract

The replacement time of cells in the gastrointestinal tract is approximately three to six days. Cell loss and denuding of the mucosa can, therefore, occur within a few days of starting treatment. Damage to the mucosa of the oropharynx is a significant management issue in caring for children receiving radiotherapy to the head and neck area. These treatments can have a variety of effects on the involved mucosa, from mild inflammation to ulcerated, bleeding tissues (Dodd et al., 2004). Dodd advocates that significantly more work should be directed at the recognition, diagnosis and treatment of oral radiotherapy injury in patients receiving head and neck radiotherapy. There is at present no paediatric literature specifically related to this issue. In general, nursing research has focused on the child receiving chemotherapy or combined modality therapy, however, principles of oral assessment for acute damage apply to each situation and goals of care are largely transferable, except for the addition of chronic damage only seen in radiotherapy.

Mouth

Trotti et al. (2003) and Sciubba and Goldenberg (2006) discuss the effect of radiation on the oral cavity. Radiation stomatitis is the injury that occurs when the rate of mucosal cell death exceeds the rate of tissue repair, resulting in the mucosa becoming thin and inflamed. Stomatitis is an early sign of radiation damage and occurs within 7–14 days of the onset of treatment (Dodd et al., 2004) when the oral cavity is within the treatment field, for example when receiving craniospinal radiation or a head and neck field.

Sciubba and Goldenberg (2006) estimate that 90–100 % of patients whose radiation fields include the oral cavity will develop some degree of oral complications as a result of their treatment. Stomatitis may last up to three weeks after the end of treatment and, in severe cases, can last for much longer after therapy completion. When receiving TBI, the oral cavity will be within the treatment field and here, too, mucosal damage is significant. Zerbe *et al.* (1992) argue that those patients who receive TBI as part of their conditioning treatment for transplant have significantly more severe stomatitis than those transplant patients who do not.

Radiation stomatitis can be a serious problem. Actively proliferating cells of the mucosa are killed and regeneration is suppressed throughout treatment. In addition, salivary glands may also be irradiated and damage can occur to such an extent that secretion of saliva is precluded. This is usually a temporary effect but can be permanent (Iwamoto, 2001). As a result of this tissue trauma, inflammation causing pain and distress is often prevalent. Erythema develops as dead mucosal cells are sloughed with cleansing, leading to mucosal tenderness, altered taste sensations and some degree of dryness (Dodd *et al.*, 2004). As erythema increases in severity, so does the associated sensation of pain and an understandable decrease in motivation to eat, to maintain oral hygiene and even to communicate. The damage to the mucosa will continue to progress throughout the treatment period and will often appear to be most severe after the completion of therapy; at which time the slightest trauma to the mucosa will result in bleeding, ulceration and extreme pain (Holmes, 1986).

If infection of this damaged tissue can be prevented or minimised, and the child receives adequate nutrition to produce new tissue, then these acute effects will heal quickly (Little, 1996). These two conditions are pivotal nursing aims that can only be addressed if the child is pain-free and is adequately supported psychologically throughout this emotionally debilitating period. Radiotherapy for nasopharyngeal tumours presents some of the worst examples of severe stomatitis. However, in the past, preventative measures have been considered that can compromise local control and the decision still lies with the radiation oncologist. It has been suggested that the greater degree of conformity in modern techniques will lead to a decrease in the amount of severe toxicity experienced in the buccal cavity without compromising tumour control in head and neck tumours.

Radiotherapy damage to the salivary glands is due to an alteration in their vascular supply brought about by irradiation. Ductal and acinar cells of the glands, which produce the required combination of enzymes and bactericidal serous fluid, respectively, subsequently degenerate and salivary output is both decreased in volume and altered in composition (Kostler *et al.*, 2001). Initially, saliva becomes more viscous and lubrication is decreased; as the salivary gland damage progresses, the mouth becomes increasingly dry so that chewing and swallowing become difficult. In addition to the acutely painful stomatitis and consequent psychological distress such symptoms can sometimes elicit, it must be remembered that certain analgesics and antidepressants can also dehydrate the oral mucosa (Fox *et al.*, 1986). Therefore, it may be necessary to increase fluid intake with these pharmacological agents. Saliva has the function of controlling bacterial growth by the lubrication of the buccal cavity with bacteriostatic enzymes and so aids the motility of food and debris out of the cavity and into the gut (Carl, 1983). McDonald and Marino (1992) state that saliva also prevents the cavity being subjected to extremes of temperature when food and fluid are being ingested, in addition to the remineralisation of teeth with calcium and the facilitation of taste by presenting the buds with particulate matter in fluid. Should saliva production be reduced, dental decay and an increased potential for oral infection will ensue. Preparations of artificial saliva, which come as sprays, may relieve the symptoms of a dry mouth as will the chewing of sugar-free gum. Both these interventions are recommended in the recent Mouth Care Guidelines produced by the Mouth Care Working Group of the CCLG/PONF (Mouth Care Guideline Report, 2006; available on the web at www.ukccsg.org). For further discussion of mouth care, see Part 1 of this book.

Oral candida is the most significant infective agent associated with severe stomatitis. However, other infective agents may be found if saliva production has decreased or is absent. Where this is the case, food debris adheres to the tissue surfaces by becoming trapped around teeth, and then decomposes. Tooth decay can be enhanced by this situation as well as demineralisation of the tooth enamel (Little, 1996). All these conditions can cause the breath to become foul-smelling which is embarrassing and emotionally distressing for all age groups.

Knowledge of all these potential problems has assisted oncology nurses in identifying the primary objectives of mouth care for the child receiving radiotherapy to the oral cavity (Feber, 1995):

1. Relief of the pain and discomfort of mucosal and salivary injury.
2. Removal of food debris from the teeth and oral cavity before decomposition occurs.
3. Facilitation of the maintenance of nutritional and fluid intake, as well as communication.
4. Prevention of oral infection (although some children will not be immunocompromised).

All four objectives will help to promote the rapid healing of mucosal and salivary injury while optimising comfort and psychological well-being. These objectives should be addressed simultaneously and within an assessment/evaluation framework, for consistent and effective care.

Oral hygiene and the prevention of infection

All children/young people who receive radiotherapy to the head and neck area need to have their oral state assessed prior to, during and after radiotherapy. The 2006 Mouth Care Guidelines, produced jointly by the CCLG and PONF, favour the oral assessment guide by the GOSH Oral Care Working Party (2004) (Gibson *et al.*, 2006) with the central tenet of intervention being the removal of food debris from the mouth, essential to prevent further tissue damage and infection.

In the above mouth care guidelines, the authors propose that teeth should be brushed at least twice a day with a fluoride toothpaste. They further advise the use of a small, soft toothbrush, if the child has a sore mouth, as brushing the teeth is the most effective way of maintaining oral hygiene. This may be extremely difficult for the child when their mouth is already sore and in this case, parents should be instructed on how to clean the mouth with oral sponges instead. A regular mouth

care regimen is therefore vital for these children (Gibson & Nelson, 2000) to prevent mucositis. The main aims of oral hygiene are to achieve and maintain a healthy, clean and moist oral cavity, to prevent infection and to promote healing and patient comfort. Strong commercial mouthwashes are not advised as they can cause dryness and irritation (Campbell, 1987). Consequently, alternative regimens may be utilised to relieve the discomfort caused by the mucosal damage and clean the buccal cavity. Gentle syringing of water or normal saline can be used to remove food debris when stomatitis is particularly severe (Campbell, 1987). Effervescent soda water is also recommended in the literature for loosening food debris without irritating the mucosa (Little, 1996). Some radiotherapy units use normal saline washes regularly as a means of removing debris from the buccal cavity and in the presence of decreased salivary output to moisten the mucosa and so decrease friction and mucosal trauma (Iwamoto, 2001). Feber (1995) argues that normal saline is non-irritating, palatable and does not cause injury to the new epithelial cells, and is therefore the solution of choice when a toothbrush is no longer tolerable (Campbell, 1987). Care should be taken with the use of normal saline as the child may swallow it, causing thirst and even vomiting which may negate the intervention. It may also be perceived to have an unpleasant taste to some children. It may be better in some cases to use water which will be just as effective if moisture is required.

According to the CCLG/PONF Mouthcare Guidelines, a number of other products and treatments have been shown to be potentially beneficial in the prevention of mucositis in adult populations only. Their use in children can only be considered within randomised controlled trials. Gelclair, a mucosal coating agent, has more recently been used for comfort. It forms a protective barrier over the inside of the mouth to soothe oral mucositis pain by shielding exposed nerve endings. It comes in single dose sachets or pump bottles and needs to be washed around the mouth (BNF, 2005). Studies in the adult population have found Gelclair to offer good pain relief and a new study is being piloted in four centres to look at the efficacy of Gelclair in the paediatric/young people population.

It is a widely held tenet (Coleman, 1995; Feber, 1995) that the single most important variable in the healing of mucosal damage, irrespective of the methods used, is the frequency of mouth care, resulting in improved oral hygiene. Removing food debris and moisturising the mucosal tissue are the most important issues as only then can nutritional intake have its effect on mucosal regeneration. Therefore, as radiation stomatitis becomes more severe, mouth care must increase in frequency.

It is essential that children have a full dental assessment, as well as ongoing dental support, prior to head and neck radiotherapy (Bentzen & Overgaard, 1995). Ideally, all children embarking on any cancer treatment should have an initial assessment of their oral cavity by a dentist affiliated to the paediatric oncology centre (UKCCSG/PONF, 2006). Radiation-induced dental decay has long been a recognised hazard of treatment to the head and neck (Iwamoto, 2001). This is due to the increased risk of caries following treatment to this area. It is therefore important that children are told of the importance of taking great care of their teeth for the rest of their lives. Significant dental problems are caused by a combination of decreased salivary fluid, alterations in oral microflora, decreased buccal lubrication and changes in the salivary pH. Should children complain of tooth pain or report changes in tooth appearance, further consultation with a dentist should be sought immediately.

Promotion of nutritional intake

Nutrition can often pose a major problem for children and in particular for those children receiving treatment for CNS or head and neck tumours. Good nutrition is vital for cell repair, resistance to infection, maximising a child's ability to tolerate therapy (Iwamoto, 2001) and ultimately improving a child's or young person's quality of life (Ladas et al., 2005). Those children and young people who receive therapy to the aforementioned areas may suffer severe damage to many areas involved in the ingestion and indeed digestion of nutritional food and drink. In addition to the damage caused to the digestive tract, enjoyment of food may also be compromised. The pain and discomfort of stomatitis are in addition to the damage caused to the salivary glands, the cause of mucosal

dryness and poor taste sensation. This lack of salivary fluid prevents lubrication of food, making it extremely difficult to swallow. The salivary glands may recover to some extent after completion of treatment, but it is important to inform the parents and the child/young person that if the glands were in the field, then it could continue to be a problem for the rest of his/her life.

As mentioned, alteration in taste may also be experienced, which can result in dislike of many common and previously favourite foods, and may, in some cases, even lead to anorexia. The irradiation of the buccal cavity damages the child's taste cells, and taste buds simply atrophy and die (Dodd et al., 2004). Taste sensation can be lost temporarily which decreases the child's motivation to eat. This effect can last for many months post-treatment and in some cases it is permanent (Young, 1988). The child may also experience dysphagia if the oesophagus is in the treatment field. This may mean communication is impaired, which can lead to a sense of isolation and may precipitate further emotional distress.

The importance of adequate nutrition cannot be underestimated when caring for the child undergoing radiotherapy. Malnutrition is a common complication of cancer treatment and can have a profound effect on energy levels and consequently quality of life (Ladas et al., 2005). However, as continued growth and development are desired throughout treatment and the fact that children differ from adults in their metabolic needs (Picton, 1998), it is of paramount importance in paediatric oncology. Many studies confirm that children and young people undergoing radiotherapy ingest lower amounts of nutrients than age-based standards before the issues of malabsorption in abdominal fields are even taken into consideration.

Weight should be closely monitored throughout therapy and calorie supplements should be utilised earlier rather than later. A 10 % weight loss since diagnosis should be the absolute maximum a child or young person should experience before significant support measures are instigated; however, even before weight loss nutritional support and surveillance should be a priority. In the case of head and neck tumours, early intervention at the start of therapy is vital as the child may be able to tolerate only liquids towards the end of treatment due to pain and inflammation, when mouth and pharynx have been included in a field. This may continue for about two weeks. Adequate pain control should be the first step in encouraging a child to place food and drink in their mouth; it is imperative to break the association of oral intake with pain and discomfort. A diet that is visually attractive, with enticing aromas and tastes to the individual, should also be a primary objective. However, food must also be nutritionally appropriate, with additional calories and protein to ensure adequate resources for cell repair. Small, frequent meals are often more acceptable to a child/young person with a diminished appetite. They should be allowed as much time as possible to eat meals, as discomfort, altered taste sensation and decreased salivary output may make chewing and swallowing difficult. Extra fluids should be encouraged, particularly with meals and snacks (sauces and gravies are often useful). In addition, it may be necessary to inform the child and the family that spicy and citrus foods can cause considerable pain. This may be an area of concern for the family whose daily diet contains high proportions of these ingredients, and in this case, dietetic support can be invaluable.

Where oral intake is no longer possible, supplemental enteral feeding must be explored. Nasogastric tube placement can be extremely effective with a convenient feeding schedule, of either bolus or extended infusion feeding, at curtailing weight loss and supplementing nutritional intake to offset malnutriton. In certain circumstances the condition of the nasopharyngeal mucosa may not permit nasogastric feeding. The use of percutaneous endoscopically guided gastrostomy tubes (PEG) in patients receiving radiation therapy to a tumour of the head and neck area is a relatively new concept that is gaining in popularity in children's units across the country. Saunders *et al.* (1991) report from a study of 126 adult patients that results have been very positive. The patients were able to maintain full nutritional intake throughout radiotherapy without any additional inpatient episodes for nutritional support. Only 1 % of the sample experienced a localised wound infection and no other placement complications were witnessed. Flietkau *et al.* (1991) have also experimented with this device in patients who were quite severely nutritionally compromised prior to therapy. They suggest that nutritional status can actually be improved during therapy by the use of this gastrointestinal access. There is limited paediatric literature related to this subject as yet. Barron *et al.* (2000), looked at the efficacy and safety of PEGs in the paediatric oncology/haematology population of The Hospital for Sick Children in Toronto over a four-year period. They concluded that retrograde tube placement was safe and gastrostomy feeding effectively reversed malnutrition and prevented weight loss in this patient population. In the UK, many individual units are using PEGs in children with nasopharyngeal tumours and increasingly for children with medulloblastoma/PNET as both these groups of children have difficulties in eating/swallowing during radiotherapy, caused by mucositis. Additional nursing care of a PEG includes care of the entry site and prevention of infection. Education and preparation for children and their families are required and are usually provided by the dietician as well as the nurse, in order that the device can be used safely and effectively at home. Vigilance for signs and symptoms of wound infection will have to be maintained in hospital and at home; paediatric oncology outreach nurse specialists and community children's nurses can help to facilitate this. Audits currently undertaken by the CCLG CNS division's nutritional subgroup will inform the format of prospective nutritional sub-studies for future CNS tumour trials.

Pain control

Protocols for oral pain control must be based upon a consistent oral assessment. The child's perception of their oral pain should be assessed on a regular and frequent basis alongside the status of their mucosa so that appropriate analgesics can be administered and mouth care and nutritional intake are facilitated. Opiates are most often the drugs of choice with severe stomatitis pain. However, experience in this area has also led to the use of certain topical agents such as Gelclair (see earlier). Pain control should be dealt with promptly and where possible prophylactically, as once the child has made the link between pain and eating it is exceptionally hard to break this association. Medications should be offered which will help to soothe the pain experienced in the mouth and throat, in particular, prior to mealtimes. This should help to facilitate eating as far as possible.

Paracetamol Mucilage is one of the most beneficial products to use (this is a preparation from the Christie Hospital in Manchester). However, children sometimes have problems because of its lack of palatability. Gels containing local anaesthetics, such as mucaine or lignocaine, can also be extremely useful (Little, 1996). Alternatives may be found within the range of soluble aspirin compounds. However, these must be used with caution in children aged under 12 years, and then never in the presence of a low platelet count. Finally, there are local anaesthetic sprays and rinses, such as Difflam, but care needs to be taken as many of these are drying to the mucosa (Fox et al., 1986). Artificial saliva sometimes helps to relieve dryness, but many children find the available preparations unpalatable.

Small intestine

The gastrointestinal tract has a tolerance for treatment lower than that of the skin. Abdominal discomfort and diarrhoea may therefore occur with abdominal radiotherapy as a result of a widespread inflammatory response to tissue destruction in the bowel. Husebye et al. (1994) identified that enteropathy was a serious and acute side effect of abdominal radiotherapy which is poorly diagnosed and treated. These authors argue that in severe cases it can present with symptoms of malnutrition, poor small bowel motility or intestinal obstruction. Work by Meric et al. (1994) at the Children's Hospital of Philadelphia, sought to prevent the problem. This team has experimented with an absorbable pelvic mesh sling, to pull the small bowel out of the field of aggressive pelvic radiotherapy. They reported no significant complications in seven children; however, one child experienced a post-operative ileus, and a further child had a temporary small bowel obstruction. Although the team succeeded in preventing radiation enteritis, significant surgical care was necessary to overcome complications and although this technique has been utilised in the UK, it is by no means widespread. Pelvic radiotherapy can also have devastating consequences for the large bowel (Sedgewick et al., 1994), and the rectum may be particularly affected. Excessive diarrhoea is often experienced, with pain on defecation and incontinence in severe cases.

Although abdominal radiation is rare in treatment for children in the UK, possible side effects must be borne in mind for the occasional situation where a paediatric oncology nurse is called upon to care for such a child. The child may be particularly weakened by such side effects, and with acute enteritis, this may be enough to temporarily prevent continuation of therapy. Children require close observation throughout these episodes, as dehydration and acute electrolyte imbalances may occur very quickly. These children may be in considerable distress due to the pain associated with the inflammatory process, and may require intensive pain management with opiates. As the wall of the bowel may become ulcerated at any point, extreme care must be taken in assessing all symptoms to ensure that any breach in the bowel wall is quickly identified. Close observation of vital signs, including changes in abdominal appearance, and the loss of bowel sound, is required, in addition to the monitoring of fluid and electrolyte status. A high standard of perianal care is also needed, as profuse diarrhoea is likely to cause anal excoriation and possibly fissures, which can then become a focus for infection. If the radiation field extends to include the perianal area, as in extensive pelvic tumours, the skin may already be friable from radiation erythema and therefore even more susceptible to breakdown.

Children with profuse and often distressing diarrhoea require a low residue or even elemental diet, antispasmodics and occasionally medication to thicken stools. All stools should be observed for evidence of bleeding within the bowel from ulceration and documented accordingly. Hygiene, nutrition and pain control are the primary caring objectives in addition to maintenance of homeostasis.

In the long term, such manifestations of inflammation may lead to adhesions within the pelvic or abdominal cavity and these must be considered when symptoms are prolonged. Nausea and/or vomiting may also be induced if the lining of the stomach, small intestine or brain is involved in the treatment field. The effect on these sites can cause irritation of the chemoreceptor trigger zone, and the vomiting centre, by 5HT binding to receptor sites within the vagus nerve (Pervan, 1993). In addition, raised intracranial pressure due to cerebral oedema following brain irradiation can also precipitate extreme nausea (Dunne-Daly, 1994). On assessment it may be necessary to give antiemetic medication before therapy. In children who receive spinal and/or abdominal radiotherapy, sickness can be a refractory problem. Giving a $5HT_3$ receptor antagonist half an hour prior to treatment has been found to be effective (Sullivan et al., 1992; Zoubek et al., 1993). Dexamethasone may also be added to the $5HT_3$ antagonist to enhance its effect.

TBI can cause severe nausea and vomiting, especially following emetogenic chemotherapy (Pervan, 1993), however, it can be treated to good effect with ondansetron and dexamethasone.

Bone marrow

Normal bone marrow is essential for life, since the cells it produces are responsible for the transportation of oxygen and carbon dioxide, for clotting and for the maintenance of the body's defence system. This bodily system, with its rapidly proliferating cell population, is extremely radiosensitive (McMillan, 2003). Destruction of the bone marrow will therefore have significant and far-reaching effects on the whole body.

Treatment fields involving small areas of bone marrow will not have a significant effect on blood counts. Abdominal or thoracic irradiation includes 15–25% of the active bone marrow in children and therefore a drop in blood counts will be obvious. More than 25–30% of a child's active bone marrow is located in the extremities, and this then concentrates in the central bones at adolescence (Chamley et al., 2005). Consequently, if large areas of the bone marrow are involved in the treatment field, haematopoiesis will be affected and peripheral blood counts will need careful monitoring during and after treatment. Irradiation of these sites should be considered myelosuppressive. Bone marrow failure is complete after total body doses of 5–10 Gy (Kun & Moulder, 1993). Poor red cell production can often be sustainable without intervention for several weeks, due to the long lifespan of the red blood cell in the peripheral system (120 days). However, the radiotherapist may decide to maintain haemoglobin levels above 10 gm/l, as it is considered by some that therapy may not be as effective if it is given when the haemoglobin is below this level. Ionising radiation, as previously noted, is potentiated in its clinical effect by the availability of oxygen, aiding the production of free radicals to cause cell damage. Radiotherapy is far more effective if tissues are well oxygenated. Low haemoglobin levels, therefore, can compromise the efficacy of therapy. Since leukocytes play a major role in the body's resistance to infection, a decreased white cell count significantly increases the risk of infection. A fall in the white blood cell count can occur within the first week of radiotherapy treatment (Plowman, 1983). This is due primarily to the fact that the large marrow reserve of already differentiated cells compensates for the initial loss of proliferating cells. In addition, white blood cells generally spend a much shorter part of their lifespan in the peripheral system. Neutropenia may then follow which leaves the child at an increased risk of systemic infection, which is no less serious than that caused by chemotherapy. Lymphopenia occurs most frequently in patients receiving craniospinal radiotherapy or widespread nodal therapy (Kun & Moulder, 1993), due to a large area of the marrow and lymphatic system being treated. The lymphocytes are affected more quickly than the neutrophils as they are more radiosensitive (Plowman, 1983). If the child does become lymphopenic, they should receive prophylaxis against opportunistic infections, particularly pneumocystis infections, which can prove fatal. In many cases GCSF may be started to support marrow repopulation and offset serious infection. Repopulation of the marrow in the treated areas may take several weeks and it may be necessary to continue to monitor blood counts closely and for some time after therapy has been completed.

Nursing intervention to prepare and educate the child and the family about how to recognise and avoid infection are comparable to those implemented for myelosuppression caused by chemotherapy. The cell turnover of platelets is particularly rapid in the peripheral system when prevention of bleeding is required or when they reach the end of their normal lifespan. They are extremely vulnerable to ionising radiation and thrombocytopenia may be the first sign of bone marrow suppression (Kun & Moulder, 1993). A fall in the platelet count can occur within seven days of starting treatment. Again, the large marrow reserve compensates for the initial loss of proliferating cells, but as the platelets themselves survive in the blood for only approximately nine days, this reserve is soon depleted. Blood product support is fundamental to the care of the child, but perhaps more important is the advice and support given to the family to facilitate their avoidance of trauma and prompt identification of petechiae and bruising. Severe thrombocytopenia is a criterion for interrupting and maybe even halting a radiotherapy course altogether in some CNS protocols.

Cytomegalovirus precautions will be necessary in potential bone marrow transplant recipients. Craniospinal radiotherapy affects a large area of bone that contains functional marrow. During this form of treatment, in particular, the blood counts will need to be closely monitored. It may be possible to check the blood counts twice a week initially, but as the blood counts begin to fall it is necessary to check them, on occasion, as frequently as daily. It is also necessary to check counts prior to radiotherapy treatment, as the treatment may be delayed if the patient is neutropenic, or if the platelet count is too low (less than 25 000/ml). This may be the case where the child has previously received chemotherapy.

Hair follicles

Hair follicles renew themselves rapidly and are therefore easily susceptible to radiotherapy if within a treatment field. As many children are receiving 'combination therapy', they may already have significant alopecia from their chemotherapy, but for those receiving cranial irradiation alone there may be only sporadic hair loss within the field that is being treated (Strohl, 1990). This may actually cause more problems than the widespread alopecia that accompanies chemotherapy as it is more straightforward to wear a wig or present a fashionable bald look. Hair loss due to chemotherapy is most often a temporary state and it will grow back several weeks after completion of treatment, but the proportion of those who sustain permanent hair loss is higher in children who have undergone radiotherapy. Some children experience permanent thinning, whereas others may

have areas where there is no new growth at all. This is usually dependent on the dose of radiotherapy given. Temporary hair loss occurs if the child receives up to 30 Gy; however, the loss is permanent at doses above 55 Gy (McDonald, 1992). Hair re-growth normally begins about two to three months post-treatment and continues for up to a year post-irradiation. When re-growth occurs, the hair may be a slightly different colour and texture (Dunne-Daly, 1994).

Care of the scalp is as for any other skin area and therefore the guidelines described earlier can be used. The scalp may be far too sensitive to wear a wig during and immediately after radiotherapy. Soft cotton scarves, bandanas or baseball caps are therefore recommended. The prophylactic use of moisturising creams on the scalp is essential to prevent significant skin trauma. The effect on body image of this hair loss depends on the individual and the permanence of the loss. It is most important that the child is prepared for this adverse effect and, although accuracy of predictions of permanent loss is not very high, this issue will need to be introduced with older children.

Fatigue

This symptom, so often described by patients after undergoing any form of radiotherapy, is often attributed to myelosuppression, somnolence in cases of brain irradiation, or the adverse effects of pain and poor nutrition. Indeed, Tiesinga et al. (1996) suggest that fatigue is a complex, multidimensional and non-specific subjective phenomenon, for which no definition is widely accepted. Their extensive literature review unfortunately only discusses adult literature from the 1980s and confirms general feelings of malaise that are poorly attributed in cause. There is a considerable amount of literature concerning the experience of fatigue while receiving treatment for cancer (Piper, 1988; Winningham et al., 1994), but little to describe the effect of radiotherapy alone (Haylock & Hart, 1979; King, 1985). There appears to be no paediatric literature on the subject except in discussion of nutrition or myelosuppression in radiotherapy. Tiesinga et al. (1996)

do acknowledge that continued fatigue can be psychologically compromising. Winningham *et al.* (1994) recommend that patients and their families require preparation for fatigue and continued support throughout treatment.

Gibson *et al.* (2005) investigated cancer-related fatigue in children and young people. Most healthcare professionals acknowledged that children and young people suffered from fatigue, as did carers themselves, however, few knew how to address the problem. Although it is often a recommended strategy to encourage frequent rest periods between daily activities, or to reduce levels of activity, this advice may actually contribute to further debilitation in the older child, especially if this is for prolonged periods (Winningham, 1992). Young children will often take naps as and when they feel the need, but for older children it may be more useful to promote strategies such as gentle exercise or a change of activity to one that interests and distracts the individual (Graydon *et al.*, 1995). Physical activity helps to maintain energy levels, whereas enforced immobility or resting may lead to a cycle of increased fatigue, i.e. the less the individual does, the more fatigued they feel and the less they feel able to do. Winningham (1992) proposes that this may be enhanced by the structural and biochemical changes that take place when skeletal muscle is inactive for prolonged periods. Gentle exercise, frequent changes of activity and interesting distractions may all increase feelings of well-being and also increase activity tolerance (Bloom *et al.*, 1990).

Brain

Acute toxicity is possible in children after whole or partial brain irradiation. The mechanisms of the acute reactions are inflammation, oedema and increased intracranial pressure (Berger, 1992). This acute damage results in symptoms of headache, nausea and vomiting (Moore, 1995). Iwamoto (2001) highlights the fact that symptoms may also progress to visual disturbances, seizures, motor function difficulties, slurred speech and altered states of consciousness. Medical management is based on antiemetic and steroid therapy. The role of the nurse is to provide education and

support to the family to help cope with these distressing symptoms. The prompt instigation of antiemetic support or as a prophylactic measure prior to radiotherapy is required and ondansetron is the first drug of choice (Sullivan *et al.*, 1992; Zoubek *et al.*, 1993). Other antiemetics may need to be added as per local guidelines. Pain control, as per unit protocol, is required for moderately severe and possibly debilitating headaches. Subacute damage to the brain can manifest itself several weeks after therapy due to damage to the oligodendroglial cells which results in inhibition of myelin formation and a transient demyelinisation of brain tissue (Berger, 1992). In children, the main presenting reaction is somnolence syndrome. This may manifest as extreme drowsiness (William & Karlson, 1977) or, in some severe cases, dysphasia, fever and ataxia (Bleyer, 1981).

Research studies have concentrated mainly on children who have reported experiencing this condition when receiving prophylactic cranial radiation for lymphoblastic leukaemia (Littman *et al.*, 1984; Mandell *et al.*, 1989). There is no literature describing its prevalence in children receiving TBI or with brain tumours, but what has been described and documented is generalised fatigue rather than the more debilitating symptoms of somnolence. Studies which have aimed to estimate the cause and effect of this condition have shown a wide variety of results. There have also been a number of criteria used to diagnose it (Faithfull, 1991). Although some studies have used EEG readings to try to determine criteria for diagnosis, Littman *et al.* (1984) argued that they had established clinical criteria based on the subjective interpretations of the observing researcher. The internal and external validity of such studies could be called into question.

Faithfull (1991) therefore undertook a qualitative study whereby adult patients kept a radiotherapy diary. Although the subjects were adults and the study utilised a distinctly different methodology, the results were remarkably similar to the earlier studies in children mentioned above. Descriptions of feeling exhausted, that any effort would be a struggle, in addition to sensory changes, impaired hearing and limb weakness, were all documented by patients. In common with many other research samples the patients complained that the experience had left them afraid that something was 'dreadfully wrong' and that they had relapsed. This study concluded, in keeping with previous literature, that more education and preparation should be undertaken with patients and their families prior to anticipated somnolence. Symptoms of somnolence have been consistently described as being less severe in those children who received cranial radiation as a prophylactic leukaemic measure than in those who were treated, with whole brain radiotherapy for a brain tumour (Faithfull, 1991). In addition, there has been some work to suggest that the incidence of somnolence in children receiving prophylactic cranial radiation can be reduced by giving concurrent doses of steroids (Mandell *et al.*, 1989). Many texts argue that somnolence is only a minor side effect, which will pass quickly (Moore, 1995). However, experience has taught health professionals not to be complacent about it. It is extremely important to ensure that the parents and the child are aware of the potential effects of somnolence. Young people may find it devastating to their social interactions which are so vital for their well-being. It is true, however, that some children will experience very little in the way of symptoms, so much so that they may not realise they have even had any degree of somnolence. However, it can be the cause of a great deal of concern and distress for their family. The child may sometimes sleep around the clock and carers often become concerned about the lack of fluid and dietary intake they are able to manage. Occasionally, the effects experienced can be very similar to those experienced at diagnosis and can place the family under a great deal of stress (Freeman *et al.*, 1973).

The nutritional and hydration status of the child should be monitored at clinic visits and, indeed, through education of the parents to observe for signs of dehydration and nutritional deficit. The parents must be reassured by staff that this is a temporary effect of treatment and the child will become more and more alert. A dietetic referral may be required if there is a prolonged weight loss associated with decreased nutritional intake. Supplements to oral intake or to 'top up' nasogastric feeds may be indicated in the younger child. However, most children are able to maintain their intake by small, high-calorie meals and frequent fluids when awake.

Pneumonitis

Radiation pneumonitis is an acute side effect of irradiation of the chest and lungs (Strohl, 1992). This acute pneumonitis is characterised by oedema and sloughing of endothelial cells in the smaller vessels, which allows fluid to accumulate in the interstitial tissues. The cells lining the alveoli are also affected and the swelling and sloughing of these cells also causes excess exudate (Strohl, 1992). Fibrosis and vascular changes contribute to decreased lung compliance and volume. The pneumonitis begins to subside when the exudate is finally absorbed and regeneration of cells begins. Fibrosis may remain after cellular repair and forms the basis of the late-occurring effects.

The child suffers from dyspnoea, cough and fever, which generally subsides after two to three months. With larger doses of radiation, symptoms can present within two to three weeks (Moss & Cox, 1989). Pneumonitis can occur with doses above 7.5 Gy, even as a cumulative fractionated dose (Van Dyk *et al.*, 1981). The child requiring radiotherapy that includes the lung fields requires observation for signs of respiratory distress and compromise. Admission for respiratory monitoring, support and anti-inflammatory medication may be necessary, although this is a rare complication in paediatric oncology as care is taken when irradiating the chest, keeping the dose to a minimum. The child and the family must be adequately informed of this potential side effect and must be prepared for its occurrence. They need to know what symptoms to look for and when they should contact the unit if they are at all concerned. Paediatric oncology outreach nurse specialists and community children's nurses will be able to offer ongoing advice and support in the community.

Cystitis

In aggressive radiation therapy to the pelvic area in children and young people, often to treat rhabdomyosarcoma, the bladder receives significant doses of radiation. General symptoms of acute inflammation or cystitis are common, such as dysuria, decreased bladder capacity, frequency, urgency and nocturia (Iwamoto, 2001). Assessment and monitoring of symptoms are a primary nursing objective. An increased fluid intake should be encouraged and analgesic and antispasmodic medications may be required to relieve dysuria (McCarthy, 1992). In combination with myelosuppression from chemotherapy, infection risk is high and symptoms should always be assessed with this in mind; urinary tract infections require prompt antibiotic treatment.

Preparation of the child and parents is a primary objective in nursing care. Advice on maintaining fluid intake, despite frequency and nocturia, is essential, as is the use of highly acidic fluids, such as cranberry juice, which can decrease bacterial growth within the bladder by preventing bacteria from adhering to it (Lowe & Fagelman, 2001). In older children, items such as coffee, tea, alcohol and tobacco should be discouraged as they further irritate the lining of the bladder. Loose cotton underclothing and trousers are also thought to have some positive effect. Acute effects on the bladder subside within two to eight weeks.

Conclusion

The immediate effects of treatment can be distressing, painful and perhaps life-threatening and nurses play a pivotal role in the prompt identification of symptoms. Good preparation of the child and the family before therapy helps to alleviate some of the anxiety and trauma engendered by such symptoms. It is essential that nurses caring for children undergoing radiotherapy are aware of and understand the basis of the radiation injury and the most appropriate evidence-based care. It is clear that the literature on research-based care in this area is scant and much more is needed. In the meantime, care must be based on a sound theoretical rationale using reflective experiential learning.

Although this chapter has sought to highlight some of the acute toxicity associated with intensive radiotherapy, it must be borne in mind that each child is an individual and may experience all or none of the symptoms mentioned. It is worth remembering that much of the literature relied upon today has been written after observation of children receiving radiotherapy over the past 10–15 years prior to recent developments in radiotherapy techniques. It is hoped, and indeed expected, from theoretical abstraction that many of the more severe effects can be reduced, if not avoided altogether, with increasing conformal techniques, better, more responsive supportive care and improved familial preparation for good nutrition, skin care and infection control.

References

Barkham A (1993) 'Radiotherapy skin reactions and treatments' *Professional Nurse* 8(11); 732–736

Barron MA, Duncan DS, Green GJ, Modrusan D, Connolly B, Chait P, Saunders EF & Greenberg M (2000) 'Efficacy and safety of radiologically placed gastrostomy tubes in paediatric haematology/oncology patients' *Medical Pediatric Oncology.* March, 34(3): 177–182

Bentzen SM & Overgaard M (1995) 'Actual versus ideal treatment time in radiotherapy for head and neck cancer' *International Journal of Radiation Oncology, Biology, Physics* 31(3): 687–688

Berger B (1992) *Neurologic Aspects of Pediartrics.* Boston: Butterworth-Heinemann

Bleyer WA (1981) 'Neurologic sequelae of methotrexate and ionising radiation: a new classification' *Cancer Treatment* 65: 89–98

Bloom JR, Gorsky RD & Fobair P et al. (1990) 'Physical performance at work and at leisure' *Journal of Psychosocial Oncology* 8(1): 49–63

BNF (2005) *British National Formulary.* London: British Medical Association and the Royal Pharmaceutical Association.

Campbell IR & Illingworth MH (1992) 'Can patients wash during radiotherapy to the breast or chest wall? A randomised controlled trial' *Clinical Oncology* (Royal College of Radiologists) 4: 78–82

Campbell J (2000) 'Skin care for patients undergoing radiotherapy' *in:* Feber T (ed.) *Head and Neck Oncology Nursing.* London: Whurr Publishers, pp. 219–228

Campbell J & Lane C (1996) 'Skin care protocol for radiotherapy patients' *Professional Nurse* 12(2): 105–108

Campbell S (1987) 'Mouth care in cancer patients' *Nursing Times* 22(83): 59–60

Carl W (1983) 'Oral complications in cancer patients' *American Family Physician* 27: 161–170

Coleman S (1995) 'An overview of the oral complications of adult patients with malignant haematological conditions who have undergone radiotherapy and chemotherapy' *Journal of Advanced Nursing* 22: 1085–1091

College of Radiographers (2000) *Treatment of Radiotherapy-induced Acute Skin Reactions: A Clinical Guideline for Use by the College of Radiographers.* London: College of Radiographers

Cork J, Timmins J, Holden C, Carr J, Berry V, Tazi-Abini R & Ward S (2003) 'An audit of adverse drug reactions to aqueous cream in children' *The Pharmaceutical Journal* 271: 72–77, 747–748

Cox J, Stetz J. & Pajak T (1995) 'Toxicity criteria of the radiation therapy oncology group (RTOG) and the European Organisation for Research and Treatment of Cancer (EORTC)' *International Journal of Oncology, Biology, Physics* 31(5): 1341–1346

Dodd M, Miaskowski C & Paul S (2004) 'Immediate side effects of large fractionation radiotherapy' *Clinical Oncology* 9: 96–99

Dunne-Daly CF (1994) 'Nursing care and adverse reactions of external radiation therapy: a self learning module' *Cancer Nursing* 17(3): 236–256

Faithfull S (1991) 'Patients' experiences following cranial radiotherapy: a study of the somnolence syndrome' *Journal of Advanced Nursing* 16(8): 930–946

Feber T (1995) 'Mouth care for patients receiving oral irradiation' *Professional Nurse* 10(10): 666–670

Flietkau R, Iro H, Sailer D & Sauer R (1991) 'Percutaneous endoscopically guided gastrostomy in patients with head and neck cancer' *Recent Results in Cancer Research* 121: 269–282

Fox PC, van der Verv PF, Baum BJ & Mandel ID (1986) 'Pilocarpine for the treatment of xerostomia associated with salivary gland dysfunction' *Oral Surgery* 3: 243–248

Freeman J, Johnston P & Voke K (1973) 'Somnolence after prophylactic cranial irradiation in children with acute leukaemia' *British Medical Journal* 4(891): 523–525

Gibson F, Cargill J, Allison J, Cole S, Stone J, Begent J & Lucas V (2006) 'Establishing content validity of the oral assessment guide in children and young people' *European Journal of Cancer* 42: 1817–1825

Gibson F & Eden T (2005) 'Efficacy of Gelclair in reducing the pain of oral mucositis in children and young people with cancer: a new study' *Contact Magazine*, www.ukccsg.org.uk/contact

Gibson F & Nelson W (2000) 'Mouthcare of children with cancer' *Paediatric Nursing* 12(1): 18–22

Graydon JE, Bubela N, Irvine D & Vincent L (1995) 'Fatigue-reducing strategies used by patients receiving treatment for cancer' *Cancer Nursing* 18(1): 23–28

Halperin EC, Gaspar L, George S, Darr D & Pinnel S (1993) 'A double blind, randomised prospective trial to evaluate topical vitamin C solution for the prevention of radiation dermatitis' *International Journal of Radiation Oncology, Biology, Physics* 26(3): 413–416

Haylock PJ & Hart LK (1979) 'Fatigue in patients receiving localised radiation' *Cancer Nursing* 2: 161–167

Hilderley L (1992a) 'Radiation oncology: historical background and principles of teletherapy' *in*: Hassey-Dow K & Hilderley LJ (eds) *Nursing Care in Radiation Oncology.* Philadelphia, PA: WB Saunders & Co

Hilderley L. (1992b) 'Pain and fatigue' *in*: Hassey-Dow K & Hilderley LJ (eds) *Nursing Care in Radiation Oncology.* Philadelphia, PA: WB Saunders & Co

Holmes S (1986) 'Radiotherapy: planning nutritional support' *Nursing Times* 829(160): 26–29

Hopewell J (1990) 'The skin, its structure and response to ionising radiation' *International Journal of Radiation Biology* 57(4): 751–773

Husebye E, Hauer-Jensen M, Kjorstad K & Skar V (1994) 'Severe late radiation enteropathy is characterised by impaired motility of proximal small intestine' *Digestive Disease Science* 39(11): 2341–2349

Iwamoto R (2001) 'Radiation therapy' *in*: Otto SE (ed.) *Oncology Nursing* (3rd edn). St Louis: Mosby

King KB (1985) 'Patients' descriptions of the experience of receiving radiation therapy' *Oncology Nurses Forum* 12(4): 55

Kostler WJ, Henjna M, Wenzel C & Zielinski CC (2001) 'Oral mucositis complicating chemotherapy +/or radiotherapy: options for prevention and treatment' *CA Cancer Journals Clinical,* 51(5): 290–315

Kun LE & Moulder JE (1993) 'General principles of radiotherapy' *in*: Pizzo PA & Poplack DG (eds) *Principles and Practices of Pediatric Oncology* (2nd edn). Philadelphia: JB Lippincott & Co

Kunkler IH (2003) 'Effects of radiation on normal tissues' *in*: Bomford CK & Kunkler IH (eds) *Walter and Miller's Textbook of Radiotherapy: Radiation Physics, Therapy and Oncology* (6th edn). Edinburgh: Churchill Livingstone, pp. 296–306

Ladas EJ, Sacks N, Meacham L, Henry D, Enriquez L, Lowry G, Hawkes R, Dadd G & Rogers P (2005) 'A multidisciplinary review of nutritional considerations in the pediatric oncology population' *Nutritional Clinical Practice* 20(4): 377–393

Lawton J & Twoomey M (1991) 'Breast care: skin reactions to radiotherapy' *Nursing Standard* 6(10): 53–54

Linnit N. (2000) 'Skin management in lymphoedema' *in*: Twycross R, Jenns K & Todd J (eds) *Lymphoedema.* Oxford: Radcliffe Medical Press

Little J (1996) 'Head and neck cancer: oral care during radiotherapy' *Nursing Standard* 10(22) 39–42

Littman P, Meadows A, Polgar G, Borns PR & Rubin E (1984) 'Pulmonary function in survivors of Wilms' tumour' *Cancer* 32: 2773–2776

Lowe FC & Fagelman E (2001) 'Cranberry juice and urinary tract infections: what is the evidence?' *Urology,* 57: 407–413

LTH (2002) Adult Acute Pain management Guideline, Leeds Teaching Hospitals NHS Trust http://nww.lhp.leedsth.nhs.uk/common/guidelines/detail.asp?ID=180 accessed July 3 2003

Mandell L, Walker W, Steinhez P & Fuks Z (1989) 'Reduced incidence of the somnolence syndrome in leukaemic children with steroid coverage during prophylactic cranial radiation therapy'. *Cancer 63*: 1978–1988

McCarthy CP (1992) 'Altered patterns of elimination' *in*: Hassey-Dow K & Hilderley L (eds) *Nursing Care in Radiation Oncology*. Philadelphia, PA: WB Saunders, pp. 317–322

McDonald A (1992) 'Altered protective mechanisms' *in*: Hassey-Dow K & Hilderley LJ (eds) *Nursing Care in Radiation Oncology*. Philadelphia, PA: WB Saunders

McDonald E & Marino C (1992) 'Dry mouth: common but treatable' *Geriatric Medicine* 22(6): 43

McMillan TJ (2003) 'Principles of radiobiology' *in*: Bomford CK & Kunkler IH (eds) *Walter and Miller's Textbook of Radiotherapy: Radiation Physics, Therapy and Oncology*. (6th edn). Edinburgh: Churchill Livingstone, pp. 286–295

Meric F, Hirschi RB, Mahboubi S, Womer RB, Goldwein J, Ross AJ (3rd) & Schnaufer L (1994) 'Prevention of radiation enteritis in children, using a pelvic mesh sling' *Journal of Paediatric Surgery* 29(7): 917–921

Moore IM (1995) 'Central nervous system toxicity of cancer therapy in children' *Journal of Pediatric Oncology. Nursing* 12(4): 203–210

Morgan D (1993) *Formulary Wound Management Products* (6th edn). Chichester: Media Medica

Moss W & Cox J (1989) *Radiation Oncology; Rationale, Technique and Results*. (6th edn). St Louis: C.V. Mosby & Co

O'Donoghue JA (2004) 'Radiation biology' *in*: Pinkerton R, Plowman N & Pieters R (eds). *Paediatric Oncology* (3rd edn). London: Arnold, pp. 115–128

Olsen DL, Raub W, Bradley C, Johnson M, Macias JL, Love V & Markoe A (2001) 'The effect of aloe vera gel/mild soap versus mild soap alone in preventing skin reactions in patients under going radiation therapy' *Oncology Nursing Forum* 28(3): 543–547

Owens J, Copelan L, Marshall S, Miller C, Stocks K & Waters D (2003) *Radiotherapy Skin Care Guideline*. Available from the Regional Radiotherapy Centre, Cookridge Hospital, Leeds

Pervan V (1993) 'Understanding anti-emetics' *Nursing Times* 89(10): 36–38

Picton SV (1998) 'Aspects of altered metabolism in children with cancer' *International Journal of Cancer* (suppl. 11): 62–64

Piper B (1988) 'Fatigue in cancer patients: current perspectives on measurement and management' *in*

American Cancer Society (ed.) *Nursing Management of Current Problems; State of the Art. Proceedings of the 5th National Conference of Cancer Nursing*. New York: American Cancer Society

Plowman PN (1983) 'The effects of conventionally fractionated, extended portal radiotherapy on the human peripheral blood count' *International Journal of Radiation Oncology, Biology & Physics* 9: 829–839

Porrock D & Kristjanson L (1999) 'Skin reactions during radiotherapy for breast cancer: the use and impact of topical agents and dressings' *European Journal of Cancer Care* 8: 143–153

Porrock, D, Kristjanson L, Nikoletti, S, Cameron, F. & Pedler P (1998) 'Predicting the severity of radiation skin reactions in women with breast cancer' *Oncology Nursing Forum* 25(6): 1019–1029

Saunders JR, Brown MS, Hirata BW & Jaques DA (1991) 'Percutaneous endoscopic gastrostomy in patients with head and neck malignancies' *American Journal of Surgery* 162(4): 381–383

Sciubba JJ & Goldenberg D (2006) 'Oral complications of radiotherapy' *The Lancet, Oncology* 7(2): 2311–2318

Sedgewick DM, Howard GC & Fergusson A (1994) 'Pathogenesis of acute radiation injury to the rectum: a prospective study in patients' *International Journal of Colorectal Diseases* 9(1): 23–30

Sitton E (1992) 'Early and late radiation-induced skin alterations. Part II: Nursing care of irradiated skin' *Oncol Nurs Forum* 19: 907–912

Spencer T (1988) 'Dry skin and skin moisturisers' *Clinician Dermatology* 6:3

Strohl RA (1992) 'Ineffective breathing patterns' *in*: Hassey-Dow K & Hilderley L (eds) *Nursing Care in Radiation Oncology*. Philadelphia, PA: WB Saunders

Sullivan MJ, Abbott GD & Robinson BA (1992) 'Ondansetron antiemetic therapy for chemotherapy and radiotherapy induced vomiting in children' *New Zealand Medical Journal, 105*(942): 369–371

Tarbell NT, York T & Kooy H (2006) 'Principles of radiation oncology' *in*: Pizzo PA & Poplack DG (eds) *Principles and Practice of Pediatric Oncology* (5th edn). Philadelphia: Lippincott, Williams & Williams, pp. 421–432

Tiesinga LJ, Dassen TWN & Halfens RJG (1996) 'Fatigue: a summary of the definitions, dimensions and indicators' *Nursing Diagnosis* 7(2): 51–62

Trotti A, Bellm LA, Epstein JB, Frame D, Fuchs HJ, Gwede CK, Komaroff E, Nalysnyk L, Zilberberg MD (2003) *Mucositis*

Trudgian J (2000) 'Investigating the use of aquafoam hydrogel in wound management' *British Journal of Nursing* 9(14): 943–948

UKCCSG/PONF Mouthcare Group (2006) *Mouth Care for Children and Young People with Cancer: Evidence-*

based Guidelines. Guideline Report. Version 1.0 February 2006

Van Dyk J, Keane TJ, Kan S, Rider WD & Fryer CJH (1981) 'Radiation pneumonitis following single dose irradiation: a re-evaluation based on absolute dose to lung' *International Journal of Radiation Oncology, Biology, Physics 11*: 461–467

Walker VA (1992) 'Skin care during radiotherapy' *Nursing Times* Dec. 8: 2068–2070

William R & Karlson I (1977) *Sleep Disorders, Diagnosis and Treatment*. New York: John Wiley Medical

Winningham ML (1992) 'How exercise mitigates fatigue: implications for people receiving cancer therapy' *in*: Carroll-Johnson RM (ed.) *The Biotherapy of Cancer*. Pittsburgh: Oncology Nursing Press, pp, 761–768

Winningham ML, Nail LH, Burke MB & Brophy L *et al.* (1994) 'Fatigue and the cancer experience: the state of knowledge' *Oncology Nurses Forum 21*: 23–36

Young M (1988) 'Malnutrition and wound healing' *Heart and Lung 17*(1): 60

Zerbe MB, Parkerson SG, Ortlieg ML & Spitzer T (1992) 'Relationships between oral mucositis and treatment variables in bone marrow recipients' *Cancer Nursing 15*(3): 196–205

Zimmerman J, Budach W & Dorr W (1998) 'Individual skin care during radiotherapy treatment' *Strahlentherapie und Onkologie, 174*(suppl. III): 74–77

Zoubek A, Kronberger M, Puschman G & Gadner H (1993) 'Ondansetron in the control of chemotherapy induced and radiotherapy induced emesis in children with malignancies' *Anticancer Drugs* (suppl. 2): 17–21

22 The Role of Radiotherapy in Palliative Care

Monica Hopkins

Radiotherapy can be an extremely effective palliative measure (Davies & de Vlaming, 2006; Wolfe & Sourkes, 2006). The requirement for palliation could be to treat the consequences of an oncological emergency, i.e. spinal cord compression in relapsed patients where cure is no longer achievable. Radiotherapy may also be part of a package of end-of-life care to minimise distressing symptoms and maximise quality of life, as in the control of bone pain. This chapter will explore both pathways for radiotherapeutic treatment and highlight the challenges for nursing patients and their families during these significant points in their cancer journeys.

The decision to use radiotherapy in the palliative care of children

It is often asserted that much of the radiotherapy administered in the care of people with cancer is delivered with palliative intent. This fact does, of course, refer to adults who may require several courses.

In children, radiotherapy has proved itself extremely useful in the treatment of many neoplasms, when the aim of care is to cure. It can also be a useful tool in the palliation of distressing symptoms of advancing disease in the pre-terminal child (haemoptysis, mediastinal obstruction, bleeding, pain and raised intracranial pressure).

Palliative radiotherapy can be used in many situations where radiation would not be considered a useful modality for cure, i.e. with apparently radio-resistant tumours. These neoplasms may be thought incurable by standard dose radiotherapy, but palliative radiotherapy may be able to control the tumour sufficiently to relieve the symptoms (Wolfe & Sourkes, 2006).

Despite this testimony to its efficacy, the use of radiotherapy must be considered very carefully in caring for a child in the terminal and pre-terminal stages of disease, as this modality of treatment has its costs. The child and the parents must be active members of the treatment decision (Timmermans *et al.*, 2005), and be in full possession of all the facts about its use, efficacy and adverse consequences in terms of comfort, freedom and the loss of precious time at home with loved ones (Spinetta, 1989; Paulino, 2003). They must be aware, as should all professionals involved, that this is not a last attempt at cure, but a palliative measure, that although it may convey symptom relief for a period of time, it is not a permanent measure. The child and the family should not be

Cancer in Children and Young People   Edited by Faith Gibson and Louise Soanes
© 2008 John Wiley & Sons, Ltd

offered this therapy in order to create hope in a desperate situation (Maher *et al.*, 1993).

The tumour may indeed respond in a significant manner to radiotherapy, but it will not put the child into a state of remission. It must be clear to all involved that the expenditure in time, travelling, effort and discomfort will be worth the possible benefits (Wolfe & Sourkes, 2006). In addition, the possibility of failure must also be considered, as even a radiosensitive tumour may be so large that it may not shrink sufficiently to alleviate the symptoms. Thankfully, significant tumour shrinkage is not always required to remove discomfort, for example, it is the cellular changes induced in bone tissue that decrease the excruciating pain of bone metastases (Kirkbride, 1995).

In many cases the use of palliative radiotherapy entails only short courses of therapy at relatively low doses, but the healthy surrounding tissue may still be damaged, especially where there may be insufficient time for conformal planning that would facilitate the sparing of healthy tissue. Ethically one must be sure that radiotherapy will not add to pain and discomfort such as when the buccal mucosa is involved in a radiation field, or by the induction of severe vomiting by irradiating the upper abdomen (Kunkler, 2003).

The symptoms that are considered to respond most effectively to radiotherapy will now be discussed in detail.

Radiotherapy in oncological emergencies

Spinal cord compression

Spinal cord compression may be caused by either an extradural or intradural lesion, or perhaps a combination of both. It may be due to an extension of a primary lesion, such as an ependymoma or an astrocytoma (Baines, 2002), or metastases from a non-CNS tumour that has developed extradurally to the cord (Hoskin *et al.*, 2003), such as neuroblastoma, primitive neuroectodermal tumour, rhabdomyosarcoma, Ewing's sarcoma or a non-Hodgkin's lymphoma. After extensive investigation which should include MRI (Jacobs & Perrin,

2001) and the commencement of corticosteroids (Haut, 2005; Rheingold & Lange, 2006), palliative radiotherapy can be extremely effective in radiosensitive tumours (Donato *et al.*, 2001; Davies & de Vlaming, 2006).

The literature has always been extremely positive about the use of radiotherapy to relieve this difficult situation (Rheingold & Lange, 2006). Yet there is a growing school of thought that recommends the use of new, more effective surgical techniques in certain circumstances; where the compression is progressing rapidly; where the cause is a radio-resistant tumour; where the child has already received maximal tolerated doses of radiotherapy; where neurological deterioration continues throughout therapy (Jacobs & Perrin, 2001; Patchell *et al.*, 2005) or where the child has an unstable bony spine (Loblaw *et al.*, 2005). Decompressive surgery followed by radiotherapy was advocated recently as being even more effective than radiotherapy alone (Patchell *et al.*, 2005) for a positive functional outcome. However, almost all of this debate is in the adult literature and more individual decisions need to be made in the acute setting of paediatrics.

The nature of emergency radiotherapy requires some discussion as there are many considerations to be made before a schedule of adminsitration can be agreed upon. Fractionated radiotherapy is recommended to prevent compromising oedema that may result from a larger single dose. However, the exact dose and number of fractions are debated in the literature. In general, a short course of 20–30 Gy over 5–10 fractions is most common with no significant difference in outcome between either schedule, but a one-off dose of 8 Gy can also be recommended (Maranzano *et al.*, 2005) if neurological recovery is not anticipated and pain relief is paramount, especially if the patient is in the terminal stages of their illness. This can possibly be achieved without significant morbidity but all these data are for older children and adults.

Whatever the fractionation, a single posterior field is suggested that extends the length of the compression plus one verterbral body above and below as margins (Kunkler (2003) advocates two if MRI images are not available). There may need to be a 1–2 cm lateral margin and in addition vital structures anterior to the cord must be protected.

Conformal, stereotactic and IMRT methods may have significant roles to play in protecting delicate structures including the cord and may possibly be discussed in relation to any child's treatment.

Prognosis for neurological recovery is dependent on the speed of diagnosis and commencement of treatment. Children who are still mobile at the time of treatment have a better chance of being able to walk again following treatment (Kunkler, 2003). Care of the child and family is principally concerned with support through such frightening symptoms and intensive investigation. This must be coupled with detailed and accurate neurological assessment throughout the experience, including movement, sensation, bowel and bladder control (Schafer, 1994; Haut, 2005). Care must be taken to ensure respiratory function is closely monitored and supported, depending on the position of the compression, especially in the first few days of therapy when oedema may precipitate complications. It is well to remember that these children may be receiving large doses of steroid and will need careful monitoring for side effects and promptly instigated weaning once any crisis is over. In addition, pain control should be accurately assessed and documented and the necessary prophylactic measures taken to relieve discomfort; as well as care to avoid the complications of prolonged immobility (Schafer, 1994).

Superior vena cava obstruction

This is a serious, though fortunately rare, complication of a large tumour load, which constitutes a significant oncological emergency in any child. An upper mediastinal or neck tumour of any histology can potentially lead to compression of this vessel but T cell non-Hodgkin's lymphoma is most often the cause in children (Rheingold & Lange, 2006). It can also be caused, however, by thoracic neuroblastoma, Hodgkin's lymphoma and Ewing's sarcoma. This condition is often accompanied by other symptoms, such as dysphagia and stridor (Neal & Hoskin, 2003). Obstruction may signal the beginning of the child's distress, but thrombosis will inevitably follow and may become life-threatening (Neal & Hoskin, 2003). Clinical signs and symptoms are described below:

Signs are:

- oedema of face, neck and upper thorax;
- peri-orbital oedema, with or without protrusion of the eye;
- subconjuctival haemorrhage;
- plethora of the face;
- increased pressure of the jugular veins;
- dilation and prominence of the collateral vessels of the neck and upper thorax;
- inspiratory wheeze;
- tachycardia.

Symptoms are:

- swelling of the face and upper limbs;
- breathlessness, dry cough, stridor (wheeze);
- headache;
- visual disturbances and dizziness;
- bloodshot eyes;
- hoarseness (rare);
- chest pain (rare);
- swelling of the fingers/hands.

(Henman, 2001)

Following diagnosis using radiography and CT scanning, treatment is initiated as quickly as possible. Although chemotherapy is often the treatment modality of choice, especially if the causal lesion is a lymphoma (Pinkerton et al., 1994; Neal & Hoskin, 2003), radiotherapy is also very effective when the disease is acute and a rapid response is needed (Donato et al., 2001; Henman, 2001; Davies & de Vlaming, 2006). A combination of modalities may be used, with the dose of radiotherapy being dependent upon:

- tumour type;
- tumour size;
- condition of the child.

Acute observational skills are needed by nurses to recognise respiratory and cardiac compromise before, during and immediately after therapy. The child and the family require explanations and reassurance about the progress of the condition and the rationale for treatment. The child should be helped to find the most comfortable position for ease of breathing; nurses should encourage chest expansion and deep breathing (Haut, 2005). Oxygen may be prescribed and requires administration in a controlled and humidified form through either nasal cannulae or a mask, depending on the flow rate and the child's preference. Oxygen saturation monitoring should be undertaken as gaseous exchange may be compromised due to vena cava congestion.

The cardiovascular system must also be observed, as obstruction may be affecting venous return to the heart (and thus stroke volume) even in the period immediately after therapy while the mass is still present. This may lead to compromise of the peripheral vascular system and the child should be assessed for levels of perfusion and signs of peripheral shutdown. There is the potential for alteration in cerebral perfusion as evidenced by an altered state of consciousness, which should be assessed at each interaction and carefully documented (Schafer, 1994).

The child should be monitored closely for fluid and electrolyte destabilisation when there is a risk of tumour lysis syndrome (Yamazaki et al., 2004). Large amounts of fluid may be infused to irrigate the kidneys, which requires careful monitoring, and blood biochemistry should also be assessed frequently. Following therapy, as the mass decreases, observation for respiratory and cardiovascular compromise can be less frequent. However, kidney function and skin integrity assessments must be maintained and carefully documented for alterations in status.

In general, there is considered to be no difference in efficacy between schedules of 20 Gy over 5 fractions or 30 Gy over 10 (Donato et al., 2001). There are no national ganecdotaluidelines and even the predominantly adult literature is anecdotal. Hence treatment decisions in this emergency lie with the experience of the medical staff caring for this child.

Radiotherapy in end of life symptom management

Control of bone pain

It is not truly understood why it is that metastases in the bone tissue cause such severe pain, nor why the cellular changes induced by radiotherapy relieve it. The area around the lesion is typically tender on palpation, and in more severe cases,

in which the response to radiotherapy is greatest, pain is unable to be controlled by normal palliative measures. Pain relief, however, once attained, is usually durable for long periods of time (Sze et al., 2006). Painful bone metastases are most common in solid tumours such as neuroblastoma.

Control of bone pain is probably the most common use of palliative radiotherapy and, indeed, is where the most significant amount of evaluatory research has been carried out (Wu-Jackson et al., 2004; Szumacher et al., 2005; McQuay et al., 2006). In the past, the literature repeatedly quotes the same response statistics, i.e. that 55–66% of patients will receive total relief from their pain with radiotherapy and 90% will experience some partial relief of symptoms (Kirkbride, 1995). However, a recently published Cochrane Review has not found this to be the case in the randomisd trials they reviewed (McQuay et al., 2006). Only 25% of patients achieved complete relief. Only half of these achieved this within four weeks, with the majority within 12 weeks. In fact, they found only 41% achieved a significant level of relief overall.

The method of administration is where the most controversy lies. The argument for a benefit in any form of fractionation is weak but there are caveats to the one-off treament option. The re-treatment rate for single fraction therapy was significantly higher then for fractionated schedules, as was the fracture rate (McQuay et al., 2006), these are significant concerns and maybe require careful consideration. Where bone pain arises from the vertebral column, however, many practitioners are concerned about giving such high doses (8 Gy) as usual in single fraction therapy, near to the spinal cord. However, with the increasing use of steroetactic and conformal techniques, this reservation may be overcome.

This evidence does appear to be influencing UK practice but there are no published studies in children to reflect this, it is anecdotal knowledge to the author. The situation has also been unclear internationally, indeed, a Canadian working party was set up to devise evidence-based guidelines on the use of radiotherapy for painful bone metastasis in adults (Wu-Jackson et al., 2004). They recommended that in previously non-irradiated sites, where the goal is pain relief, then a single 8 Gy treatment at the appropriate target volume is recommended. It is pertinent that in a study of patients' views on this subject by Szumacher *et al.* (2005), most preferred a single fraction for many practical and family considerations.

Extensive fractionation is thought to be of use, however, in the prevention and treatment of pathological fractures in lytic lesions. This is used to greatest effect when in conjunction with orthopaedic surgery to fixate the fracture internally. Prevention of such a problem is far more successful than trying to seal the bone after a fracture. It must therefore be remembered that before irradiating large destructive bone metastases, it is strongly recommended that an orthopaedic consultation is sought.

Whatever the course of radiotherapy, the role of the nurse is in the accurate assessment of pain before, during and after therapy. The child and the family are likely to be distressed and will require information, honest reassurance and support throughout the experience of palliative radiotherapy. Returning to a department previously associated with curative treatment may be stressful for the family and confusing for the child, especially if attempts have already been made to prepare the family for the eventual death of the child.

Control of bleeding

Radiotherapy will control bleeding from widespread malignant ulceration, as in soft tissue sarcomas such as rhabdomyosarcoma. External beam radiotherapy will also control haemoptysis in most cases where conventional haemostatic agents have not proved effective. Unfortunately, most of the information available on the use of radiotherapy for this problem is anecdotal and research in this area is not immediately evident. Haematuria has also been treated effectively with radiation and single fractions are used in such situations. The child who is not yet in the terminal stages of disease may also be treated to prevent haemorrhage due to tumour erosion, e.g. epithelial haemangioma (Kirkbride, 1995), when conventional wound care is insufficient.

Bleeding is one of the most frightening and distressing symptoms, however small the actual blood loss. Here, the role of the nurse is in speed of recognition of symptoms and reassurance to the family. The form of radiotherapy to be used in these circumstance is low-energy beams in order to deliver the dose as superficially as possible.

Metastases

Radiotherapy has a significant role to play in alleviating troublesome brain metastases that are causing unacceptable cerebral signs in a pre-terminal child. These lesions can be responsible for such disabling symptoms as headache, nausea, seizures and neurological impairment. Cranial radiation is most often the answer as the source of these problems is predominantly raised intracranial pressure. Use of a short course of radiation to reduce the lesion causing this may mean it is possible to reduce the dose of steroids in use.

Lung metastases from any primary tumour, but especially from bone tumours, can lead to bronchial obstruction which can cause premature and extremely distressing respiratory impairment. Sometimes it may be appropriate to use single-dose therapy to relieve such a symptom.

Other distressing symptoms of advancing disease that can be treated by the use of radiotherapy are liver metastases causing pain from a stretched liver capsule, thoracic or pleuritic pain from mediastinal masses and metastatic lung deposits (Kunkler, 2003). There is also a role for radiotherapy in the control of bleeding from either a fungating or ulcerating lesion on the skin surface or perhaps an eroding bronchial mass or for the relief of actual obstruction in the chest or abdomen (Wolfe & Sourkes, 2006).

Palliative therapy should aim for simplicity in procedure, for the quick relief of symptoms, and to prevent complications that can lead to discomfort, pain or distress. Dosages and fractionation schedules are usually determined by the oncologist in response to the child's condition and the needs of the family. The concurrent use of steroids with single radiation doses to reduce associated oedema is also a clinical decision to be made by the oncologist, depending on the child's status. It is beyond the remit of this chapter to cover all the psychosocial aspects of good palliative care (see the West Midlands Paediatric Macmillan Team, 2005). Radiotherapy is merely a tool to be used to relieve physical discomfort so that the child can resume living a dignified life. Many of the symptoms described previously are disabling and visible to the child, and nurses should be cognisant of the issue of body image, especially at this difficult time. Accepting one's personal identity is part of making sense of existence and this can be a necessary step in working positively towards death.

Preparation and nursing care for the child undergoing palliative radiotherapy should be similar to the standards set in curative therapy although time may be short. Consequently, flexibility is required in caring for these children and their families. It may be beneficial to have the primary palliative care nurse accompany the child and the family to the unit so that continuity of care is maintained while the child is within the radiotherapy suite. The parents will then have a supportive professional present who can also be an advocate with intimate knowledge of the child's status and the family's wishes.

References

Baines MJ (2002) 'Spinal cord compression: a personal and palliative care perspective' *Clinical Oncology* 14(2): 135–138

Davies D & deVlaming D (2006) 'Symptom control at the end of life' *in*: Goldman A, Hain R & Lieben S (eds) *The Oxford Textbook of Palliative Care for Children*. Oxford: Oxford University Press, pp. 497–513

Donato V, Bonfili P, Bulzonetti N, Santarelli M, Osti MF, Tombolini V, Banelli E & Enrici RM (2001) 'Radiation therapy for oncological emergencies' *Anticancer Research* 21(3C): 2219–2224

Haut C (2005) 'Oncological emergencies in the pediatric intensive care unit' *AACN Clinical Issues in Advanced Practice Acute Critical Care* 16(2): 232–245

Henman R (2001) 'Superior vena cava syndrome' *Clinical Excellence for Nurse Practitioners* 5(2): 85–87

Hoskin PJ, Grover A & Bhana R (2003) 'Metastatic spinal cord compression: radiotherapy outcome and close fractionation' *Radiotherapy Oncology* 68(1): 175–181

Jacobs WB & Perrin RG (2001) 'Evaluation and treatment of spinal metastases: an overview' *Neurosurgical Focus* 11(6): 10

Kirkbride P (1995) 'The role of radiation therapy in palliative care' *Journal of Palliative Care* 11(1): 19–26

Kunkler IH (2003) 'Effects of radiation on normal tissues' *in*: Bomford CK & Kunkler IH (eds) *Walter and Miller's Textbook of Radiotherapy: Radiation Physics, Therapy and Oncology* (6th edn). Edinburgh: Churchill Livingstone, pp. 296–306

Loblaw DA, Perry J, Chambers A & Laperriere NJ (2005) 'Systematic review of the diagnosis and management of malignant extradural spinal cord compression: the Cancer Care Ontario Practice Guidelines Initiatives neuro-oncology disease site group' *Journal of Clinical Oncology* 23(9): 2028–2037.

Maher EJ, Timothy A & Squire CJ (1993) 'Audit: the use of radiotherapy in NSCLC in the UK' *Clinical Oncology* 5: 72–79

Maranzano E, Bellavita R, Rossi R, De Angelis V, Frattegiani A, Bagnoli R, Mignogna M, Beneventi S, Lupattelli M, Panticelli P, Biti G. & Latini P (2005) 'Short course versus split course radiotherapy in metastatic spinal cord compression: results of a Phase III, randomised multicenter trial' *Journal of Clinical Oncology* 23(15): 3358–3365

McQuay HJ, Collins SL, Carroll D & Moore RA (2006) 'Radiotherapy for the palliation of painful bone metastases' The Cochrane Database of Systematic Reviews, issue 1. The Cochrane Collaboration. London: John Wiley & Sons Ltd

Neal AJ & Hoskin PJ (2003) *Clinical Oncology: Basic Principles and Practice* (3rd edn). London: Arnold

Patchell RA, Tibbs PA, Regina WF, Payne R, Sans S, Kryscio RJ, Mohiuddin M & Young B (2005) 'Direct decompressive surgical resection in the treatment of spinal cord compression caused by metastatic cancer: a randomised controlled trial' *Lancet* 366(9486): 643–648

Paulino AC (2003) 'Palliative radiotherapy in children with neuroblastoma' *Pediatric Hematology & Oncology* 20(2): 111–117

Pinkerton CR, Cushing P & Sepion B (1994) *Childhood Cancer Management: A Practical Handbook*. London: Chapman Hall Medical

Rheingold SR & Lange BJ (2006) 'Oncologic emergencies' *in*: Pizzo PA & Poplack DG (eds) *Principles and Practice of Pediatric Oncology* (5th edn). Philadelphia: Lippincott, Williams & Williams, pp. 1202–1230

Schafer SL (1994) 'Oncologic complications' *in*: Otto S (ed.) *Oncology Nursing*. St Louis: Mosby, pp. 406–439

Spinetta P (1989) *Living with Childhood Cancer*. St Louis: CV Mosby

Sze WM, Shelley M, Held I & Mason M (2006) 'Palliation of metastatic bone pain: single fraction versus multi-fraction' The Cochrane Database of Systematic Reviews, issue 1. The Cochrane Collaboration. London: John Wiley & Sons Ltd

Szumacher E, Llewellyn-Thomas H, Franssen E, Chow E, DeBowe G, Danjoux, C, Hayter C, Barnes E & Andersson L (2005) 'Treatment of bone metastases with palliative radiotherapy: patients' treatment preferences' *International Journal of Radiation Oncology, Biology, Physics* 61(5): 1473–1481

Timmermans LM, van der Maazen RW, Verhaak CM, van Roosmalen MS, van Daal WA & Kraaimaat FW (2005) 'Patient participation in discussing palliative radiotherapy' *Patient Education and Counselling* 57(1): 53–61

West Midlands Paediatric Macmillan Team (2005) *Palliative Care for the Child with Malignant Disease*. London: Quay Book MA Healthcare Limited

Wolfe J & Sourkes B (2006) 'Palliative care in a child with advanced cancer' *in*: Pizzo PA & Poplack DG (eds) *Principles and Practice of Pediatric Oncology* (5th

edn). Philadelphia: Lippincott, Williams & Williams, pp. 1531–1555

Wu-Jackson SY, Wong RKS, Lloyd NS, Johnston M, Bezjak A & Whelan, T (2004) 'Radiotherapy fractionation for the palliation of uncomplicated painful bone metastases – an evidence based practice guideline' *BMC Cancer* 4(1): 71–73

Yamazaki H, Hanada M, Horiki M, Kuyama J, Sato T, Nishikubo M, Ishida T & Inoue T. (2004) 'Acute tumor lysis syndrome caused by palliative radiotherapy in patients with diffuse large B-cell lymphoma' *Radiation Medicine* 22 (1): 52–55

Part 5

Late Effect of Cancer Therapies

23

Overview of Long-Term Follow-Up

Susan Mehta

Since the 1960s, great advances in the treatment of childhood cancer have improved survival rates; in contrast to a five-year survival rate of 10 % for children with leukaemia in the 1960s, the survival rate had increased to 80 % by the mid-1990s in the UK (Stiller *et al.*, 2004). This improvement in the treatment of cancer is reflected in the majority of paediatric cancers. In Northern Europe, 3 in 4 children who have had cancer survive longer than 5 years after their treatment (Gatta *et al.*, 2003), this time point can often be taken as an indicator of cure due to the greatly reduced risk of recurrence after this time. This success now equates to a growing number of adult survivors. In 1971, there were 1400 adult survivors of childhood cancer in the UK, of whom only 100 had survived to the age of 30 years. However, by the turn of this century, the number had increased to 15,000 adult survivors, including 7000 aged over 30 years (Stiller *et al.*, 2004). It is predicted that by the year 2010 about 1 in 250 adults will be a survivor of childhood cancer (Wallace & Green, 2004). The term 'survivor' has been in use since the 1970s, and its use in paediatric oncology has been somewhat controversial. Strictly speaking, the term 'survivor' may be used to describe any person diagnosed with cancer who is alive. With problems in early stages of diagnosis being very different from those in the long

term, Meadows (2003) offers a practical definition of a long-term childhood cancer survivor as a patient who has survived at least five years from the last indication of disease and is at least two years from the end of therapy. Most specialists accept this definition or slight variations of it when defining long-term survivors of childhood cancer.

Interest in long-term follow-up began in the 1970s as a result of improving survival rates for childhood cancer. Long-term follow-up aims to optimise the quality of life for survivors of childhood cancer. Although many children treated for childhood cancer will be free of complications and live completely healthy lives, a significant minority suffer long-term physical and psychological damage from their treatment. Paediatric oncologists and haematologists in the UK currently recommend that children treated for cancer should be followed-up for life (Scottish Intercollegiate Guidelines Network (SIGN), 2004). This ensures that any adverse effects can be detected and treated early and, additionally, information can be gathered to influence treatment protocols of the future (Wallace *et al.*, 2001).

However, as more children survive, the numbers who suffer adverse effects also increase (Wallace *et al.*, 2001). Acute and late effects commonly occur

---

because of the non-specific nature of cancer treatment. The effects can be static or progressive and they can appear at the time of treatment or many years later. Acute problems such as myelosuppression, mucositis and alopecia, which emerge during treatment, last for a short period of time and usually resolve soon after the completion of chemotherapy or radiotherapy. On the other hand, after completion of therapy, longer-term problems may emerge. Chemotherapy with multiple drugs, radiotherapy and surgery can cause long-term problems and the challenge is to identify and manage the delayed consequences of cancer treatment (Ganz, 2001). The risks of long-term effects are related to the treatment given, the dose of chemotherapy or radiotherapy, the extent and site of surgery, the child's age at the time of treatment and gender.

Future challenges

The survivors of childhood cancer need effective management in order to meet their varying needs and ensure the best possible future for them. Currently in the UK the long-term follow-up service is led by medical teams but this is not sustainable given the escalation in the numbers of survivors. Specialist oncology nurses with expertise in late effects can take over the routine monitoring of a great many of the survivors; this leaves the medical teams to focus on survivors with more complex problems. A model for this approach already exists in the USA (Gibson & Soanes, 2001), and recent research in the UK has enabled the voices of young people who have survived childhood cancer to contribute their views on how the service should be developed in the future (Gibson *et al.*, 2005).

To guide this follow-up, the National Institute for Clinical Excellence (NICE, 2005) has recommended that a key worker should be assigned to each patient. This model of care was the preferred choice when young people were given the opportunity to voice their own opinions about long-term follow-up (Gibson *et al.*, 2005). The Department of Health (DoH) and the Royal College of Nursing (RCN) have published policy documents on transitional care and its implementation *Transition: Getting it Right for Young People*

(DoH, 2006) and *Adolescent Transition Care* (RCN, 2004) respectively. These policy documents recognise the need for health-care professionals to begin planning for the transfer of adolescent patients to appropriate adult care. Within the long-term follow-up service it is recognised that it is inappropriate to continue monitoring young adults in the paediatric setting. Transitional care is a challenge and it is recognised that young people should be cared for in age-appropriate facilities (NICE, 2005). Adult services need to be provided and nurse specialists are able to plan and implement the transition process (RCN, 2004).

Long-term effects of cancer treatment

The long-term effects of chemotherapy and radiotherapy may be classified in a number of ways; they can be discussed by cancer type, by treatment protocols or by the body system affected. In Part 5, the late effects are discussed according to the body system affected since the treatment protocols for various cancers evolve and change.

The discussion of adverse effects is arranged as follows:

- endocrinopathies (including gonadal dysfunction and fertility);
- liver;
- neurological;
- eyes;
- craniofacial and dental;
- skin;
- musculoskeletal;
- hearing;
- gastrointestinal;
- cardiac;
- renal and bladder;
- pulmonary complications;
- second malignancies, including breast care and meningiomas.

The nursing role

The nursing role is becoming increasingly important in long-term follow-up and is discussed later in this section. Young people need to know about their past disease and treatment. They need to take responsibility for their own health as they become young adults. The United Kingdom Childhood Cancer Study Group (UKCCSG), now the Childhood Cancer and Leukaemia Group (CCLG), has produced the *After Cure* booklet and treatment-related fact sheets (Griffiths, 2005). Using these resources, each patient should receive a treatment summary, including total doses of chemotherapy, radiotherapy, details of surgery and any anticipated late effects they might develop (NICE, 2005). The nurse with expert knowledge about late effects can play an important role in providing this information by completing the *After Cure* treatment summary card (Griffiths, 2005) in collaboration with the young person.

Young people with busy lives need to understand the benefits for their future health if they are going to continue attending long-term follow-up clinics long after their treatment has been completed. Compliance is a problem and innovative ways need to be developed to monitor young people. Some cancer centres are extending the length of time between clinic visits by sending an annual health questionnaire or offering telephone support.

Health education

Encouraging healthy lifestyle choices cannot prevent late effects, but may minimise long-term problems, as outlined in Chapter 26. Education of the patient gives them ownership over their own health care, providing information on their health risks and what action they would be advised to take. The patient can be offered the *After Cure* booklet (Griffiths, 2005) which gives them information on many issues such as why they need to be seen, healthy living, fertility, insurance, employment, travel and disability. The booklet is accompanied by a treatment card, which summarises the patient's own treatment details, and factsheets on specific late effects.

The role of nurses as health educators is particularly important. With increasing concerns for the general population about obesity, smoking, alcohol and drug abuse, the specialist nurse has a golden opportunity to target this group of young people, helping them to make healthy lifestyle choices.

Conclusion

Having achieved success in the treatment of childhood cancer we now face the challenge of improving the quality of life in the long term and Chapter 27 discusses quality of life issues in depth.

References

Department of Health (2006) *Transition: Getting It Right for Young People: Improving the Transition of Young People with Long Term Conditions from Children's to Adult Health Services.* http://www.dh.gov.uk/ accessed April 2007

Ganz P (2001) 'Late effects of cancer and its treatment' *Seminars in Oncology Nursing* 17: 241–248

Gatta G, Corazziari I, Magnani C, Peris-Bonet R, Roazzi P & Stiller C (2003) 'Childhood cancer survival in Europe' *Annals of Oncology* 14 (suppl. 5): 119–127

Gibson F, Aslett, H, Levitt, G & Richardson A (2005) 'Developing alternative models of follow-up care in the young adult survivor of childhood cancer' *CLIC Sargent Final Report*, November 2005

Gibson F & Soanes L (2001) 'Long-term follow-up following childhood cancer: maximizing the contribution from nursing' *European Journal of Cancer* 37: 1859–1868

Griffiths A (ed.) (2005) *After Cure.* Leicester: Childhood Cancer and Leukaemia Group (CCLG)

Meadows A (2003) 'Pediatric cancer survivors: past history and future challenges' *Current Problems in Cancer* 27(3): 112–126

National Institute for Clinical Excellence (2005) *Improving Outcomes of Children and Young People with Cancer.* London: NICE

Royal College of Nursing (2004) *Adolescent Transition Care: Guidance for Nursing Staff.* London: RCN

Scottish Intercollegiate Guidelines Network (2004) *Long Term Follow-up of Survivors of Childhood Cancer.* Edinburgh: Scottish Intercollegiate Guidelines Network publication No. 76

Stiller C, Quinn M & Rowan S (2004) 'Childhood cancer' *in*: ONU, *The Health of Children and Young People.* London: Office for National Statistics, pp. 1–16

Wallace WH, Blacklay A, Eiser C, Davies H, Hawkins M, Levitt GA & Jenney ME (2001) 'Developing strategies for long term follow-up of survivors of childhood cancer' *British Medical Journal* 323 (7307): 271–274

Wallace WH & Green D (2004) 'Introduction' *in*: Wallace WHB & Green D (eds) *Late Effects of Childhood Cancer.* London: Arnold, pp. 1–2

24 Potential Physical Issues Following Cancer Treatment

Ruth Elson and Susan Mehta

Endocrinopathies

Endocrine abnormalities are the most common complications of cancer therapy in childhood. They have a negative impact on growth, body image, sexual function and quality of life (Darzy et al., 2004). The endocrine system is composed of a group of glands, which control many body functions including growth, pubertal development, urine production and stress responses. The glands include the pituitary, hypothalamus, thyroid, parathyroid, adrenal, pancreas, ovaries and testes. The pituitary and hypothalamus glands have a major role in the endocrine system as they produce hormones that influence the other endocrine glands. Hormones are chemical messengers produced by the glands, carried to the rest of the body in the blood. Hormones have to be in balance to maintain several bodily functions such as growth, development and regulation of the body's metabolism. Hypopituitarism is when there is a lack of one or more of the pituitary hormones. If a patient lacks three or more pituitary hormones, they are said to have panhypopituitarism.

The pituitary hormones and their functions are:

- *Growth hormone (GH)* – stimulates the growth of bone and other tissues.

- *Adrenocorticotrophic hormone (ACTH or corticotropin)* – stimulates the adrenal glands to produce cortisol (hydrocortisone). Cortisol has major effects on glucose, protein and lipid metabolism as well as the immune system and enables the body to deal with physical stress such as illness, fever and trauma.
- *Thyroid-stimulating hormone (TSH)* – stimulates the thyroid gland to produce thyroxine.
- *Reproductive hormones (gonadotrophins)* – including luteinising hormone (LH) and follicle stimulating hormone (FSH), stimulate the testes and ovaries to produce testosterone, oestrogen and progesterone.
- *Anti-diuretic hormone (ADH)* – controls water balance in the body by controlling urine output.
- *Prolactin* – controls milk production when women are breast-feeding.

Multi-pituitary hormone deficiency (hypopituitarism) is caused by damage to the hypothalamic-pituitary axis (HPA). The following treatments or conditions can cause damage to the HPA:

- brain tumours
- cranial radiation
- cranio-spinal radiation
- nasopharyngeal radiation

Cancer in Children and Young People   Edited by Faith Gibson and Louise Soanes
© 2008 John Wiley & Sons, Ltd

- oropharyngeal radiation
- radiation to the orbit or eye
- radiation to the ear
- infratemporal radiation
- total body irradiation
- surgery to the brain
- infections in the brain
- trauma to the brain
- surgical removal of or impaired development of the pituitary gland.

(Skinner & Wallace, 2005;
Children's Oncology
Group (COG), 2006)

Thyroid gland

Potential problems

Abnormalities in structure and function of the thyroid gland may occur after childhood cancer and its treatment. The thyroid gland may be damaged itself or be affected by damage to the HPA (SIGN, 2004). Chemotherapy-only bone marrow transplant conditioning regimes using busulphan have been implicated in causing thyroid dysfunction (Shalet & Brennan, 2002). However, the principal cause of thyroid morbidity is irradiation. Direct and indirect radiation to the thyroid gland may lead to thyroid dysfunction and predispose to thyroid tumours. Radiation damage to the thyroid gland commonly includes hypothyroidism and thyroid tumours, although there is a possibility of hyperthyroidism (Spoudeas, 2004).

Risk factors for thyroid dysfunction include:

- radiotherapy to a field including the thyroid gland, this includes neck, spine, mantle, mediastinum and total body irradiation;
- I-MIBG (metaiodo-benzyl guanidine) treatment for neuroblastoma;
- bulsulphan-based conditioning.

Thyroid cancer as a secondary primary cancer is rare but a highly significant potential long-term problem following childhood cancer treatment (SIGN, 2004). The risk of thyroid tumours following neck irradiation is dose related (Shalet & Brennan, 2002). Doses as low as 0.3 Gy have been associated with thyroid cancer (Spoudeas, 2004). The period between radiation to the neck and the clinical presentation of a thyroid tumour may be many years after treatment. Risk of malignant change is thought to be increased, if TSH is elevated (Skinner & Wallace, 2005). Increased risk factors for tumour development in an irradiated gland are female sex, young age, thyroid irradiation dose and duration of raised TSH levels (Spoudeas, 2004).

Assessment

Thyroid dysfunction can occur during treatment or decades after treatment (Sign, 2004). At each long-term follow-up clinic the patient's neck should be palpated for signs of thyroid nodules or masses and if found these will need further investigation. A clinical history may also reveal signs of hypothyroidism such as fatigue, dry skin, reduced concentration, constipation and weight gain (Griffiths, 2005). However, abnormal thyroid function tests (TFTs) may occur in the absence of any clinical signs and symptoms. Survivors who have had radiotherapy to the neck, spine or brain should have TFTs including tetraiodothyronine (T4) and TSH levels on completing therapy and annually thereafter (Skinner & Wallace, 2005).

Management

Young people who have received any of the risk factor treatments should be advised to read the *After Cure* fact sheet about the thyroid gland which includes advice about secondary thyroid cancer and thyroid dysfunction (Griffiths, 2005). Education on the recognition of the signs of potential thyroid dysfunction can be undertaken by specialist nurses and should include signs and symptoms of potential problems. Medical attention should be sought if a neck mass is detected (SIGN, 2004). Urgent referral to an endocrinologist and specialist thyroid surgeon is required if the thyroid gland palpation is abnormal. Ultrasound of the neck will be required and a fine needle biopsy of the lump undertaken. Tumours are usually papillary in nature and have a good prognosis if effectively treated with total thyroidectomy.

Treatment should be undertaken in a recognised centre of excellence (Spoudeas, 2004).

If a patient's thyroid function tests are abnormal they should be discussed with or referred to an endocrinologist. Thyroid hormone replacement therapy is safe and effective. Treatment with thyroxine is indicated if the TSH is raised on two successive occasions, whether or not the T4 is low, to suppress the TSH. This treatment is given as the risk of malignant change to the thyroid gland is increased if the TSH is elevated (Skinner & Wallace, 2005).

Hypothalamic pituitary axis

Potential problems

- deficiency of one or more anterior pituitary hormones has been described following cranial irradiation for primary brain tumours;
- tumours involving the HPA;
- nasopharyngeal tumours;
- tumours of the base of the skull;
- solid tumours of the face and neck;
- cranial irradiation in acute lymphoblastic leukaemia;
- total body irradiation in bone marrow transplant;
- isolated growth hormone deficiency is the most common manifestation of radiation to the HP axis.

(Darzy et al., 2004)

There is a strong correlation between total radiation doses and schedule and the development of pituitary hormone deficits. Low doses of radiation (18–50 Gy given in small fractions of 1.8–2.5 per day) result in isolated growth hormone deficiency. Early panhypopituitarism or multipituitary hormone deficiency is caused by high-dose radiation (greater than 60 Gy) (Darzy et al., 2004).

Pituitary hormones are lost in sequential order of

1. growth hormone (GH);
2. luteinising hormone (LH) and follicle stimulating hormone (FSH);
3. adrenocorticotrophic hormone (ACTH or corticotropin);
4. thyroid-stimulating hormone (TSH).

The risk of loss of hormones increases, not only with radiation dose but also with time from treatment (Skinner & Wallace, 2005). In girls, radiotherapy to the HPA may result in delayed puberty, the risk increasing with higher doses (30–40 Gy). Lower doses (less than 24 Gy) are more commonly associated with precocious puberty in young girls (Skinner & Wallace, 2005). Girls and boys treated for brain tumours with high doses of radiation (25–50 Gy) may develop early puberty (Darzy et al., 2004). Survivors of childhood cancer may have impaired growth before, during and after their cancer treatment. Many factors are responsible, including the disease process, complication of treatment, e.g. infection, direct effects during treatment such as nutrition which may have been depleted by anorexia or vomiting and direct or indirect late effects caused by the therapy. Cranial radiation can cause growth hormone deficiency and growth retardation. This can be compounded by other pituitary hormone deficiencies particularly adrenocorticotrophin (ACTH), FSH, LH and TSH (SIGN, 2004).

Localised tumour treatment can adversely affect growth and function of individual organs, e.g. spinal growth is affected by spinal radiation and can result in skeletal disproportion. Sex hormone deficiencies can also be caused by abdominal surgery or radiotherapy; this can lead to impaired growth and pubertal development. These patients can have an attenuated pubertal growth spurt. Risk of growth impairment to any survivor depends upon the cancer type, treatment given and age at presentation.

Risk factors include:

- radiation to HPA, including CNS, spinal and TBI;
- brain tumours even in absence of radiotherapy;
- bone marrow transplantation patients who have received total body irradiation (TBI) conditioning after previous cranial radiotherapy are at the highest risk.

(Skinner & Wallace, 2005)

Assessment

All children who have survived cancer should have their growth assessed regularly until final height has been achieved and puberty completed. Six-monthly height and weight measurements should be recorded accurately on the appropriate growth charts. It is essential for recipients of TBI or abdominal radiotherapy to have sitting heights to determine any skeletal disproportion. Tanner pubertal staging should be undertaken at least six-monthly and in boys should include a testicular volume assessment using an orchidometer. Height velocity and annual bone age measurements should also be undertaken to determine any discrepancy in age and bone maturation (Skinner & Wallace, 2005).

Management

Referral to an endocrinologist should be considered in the following circumstances:

- abnormal growth, i.e. growth falling below or rapidly crossing the growth percentiles for that child;
- height velocity is below the 25th percentile;
- evidence of puberty at less than 9 years for girls and 10 years for boys;
- TBI or radiation doses greater than 30 Gy to the HPA;
- height is less than the 10th percentile;
- discrepancy between their pubertal stage and growth rate.

(Skinner & Wallace, 2005)

Dynamic pituitary testing needs to be undertaken to prove growth hormone and or cortisol (hydrocortisone) deficiency. The insulin tolerance test (ITT) is the gold standard test to detect these. Cortisol deficiency may be caused by direct adrenal gland damage from surgery or radiotherapy or may be caused by HPA abnormalities; it can also be suppressed by long-term or high-dose steroid therapy. If a child is found to be cortisol-deficient, they should have replacement corticosteroid therapy, plus advice about corticosteroid treatment for intercurrent illness and be advised to wear a medical alert device. This advice should be given to the patient, their family and schools or other agencies caring for them.

Final height below the target height in childhood cancer survivors is common, due to:

- growth hormone deficiency;
- precocious puberty;
- spinal irradiation.

A target height range should be calculated for each patient, so that their growth can be monitored against personal family data. Growth hormone treatment should be considered for children who fail to achieve a peak growth hormone response greater than 20 mu/L during an ITT (NICE, 2005). Pre-pubertal height gain has an effect on final height and can be optimised by growth hormone treatment. Final height is achieved at the end of puberty when bones have matured and epiphyseals fused. A child with precocious puberty has a reduced time available for growth hormone to help them grow as their bones will mature and their epiphysis fuse at an earlier age. It may be necessary to treat with a gonadotrophin-releasing hormone (GnRH) analogue to delay puberty while they have growth hormone treatment to maximise their height (Darzy et al., 2004). Growth hormone therapy is safe and there is no evidence of increasing risk of relapse, recurrence or de novo malignancies in children treated with growth hormone (Skinner & Wallace, 2005).

At the end of growth, growth hormone treatment should be stopped and the young adult's HPA retested. There is evidence to suggest that growth hormone replacement is important to maintain normal bone mineral density, body composition, cardiovascular lipid profile as well as quality of life in adulthood (Skinner & Wallace, 2005). Growth hormone may need to be continued in adulthood, in line with NICE guidance (NICE, 2005). Growth hormone can be restarted in a young adult if they have a peak growth hormone response less than 9mu/L during an ITT. This treatment should be continued until they have achieved 'peak bone mass', usually around 25 years of age. They undertake further testing and quality of life assessments.

Gonadal dysfunction

Normal pubertal development needs to be recognised and understood by teams caring for children who have undergone treatment for childhood cancer, so that they can diagnose any hormonal deficiencies early. Table 24.1 outlines the stages of pubertal development in girls.

Table 24.1 Girl's pubertal development

Tanner stage	Breast development	Pubic hair
Stage 1	Pre-adolescent: elevation of papilla only.	Pre-adolescent: The vellus over the pubes is not further developed than that over the abdominal wall, i.e. no pubic hair.
Stage 2	Breast bud stage: elevation of breast and papilla as small mound. Enlargement of areola diameter.	Sparse growth of long, slightly pigmented downy hair, straight or slightly curled, chiefly along labia.
Stage 3	Further enlargement and elevation of breast and areola, with no separation of their contours.	Considerably darker, courser and more curled. The hair spreads sparsely over the junction of the pubes.
Stage 4	Projection of areola and papilla to form a secondary mound above the level of the breast.	Hair now adult in type, but the area covered is still considerably smaller than in the adult. No spread to the medial surface of the thighs.
Stage 5	Mature stage: projection of papilla only, due to recession of the areola to the general contour of the breast.	Adult in quantity and type.

Source: Marshall & Tanner (1969). Reproduced with permission of *Archives of Disease in Childhood*.

The onset of normal female puberty is characterised by the appearance of breast buds (breast stage 2). This can happen from as early as 8.4 years to as late as 13.5 years. Girls with breast buds before 8 years are described as having precocious puberty, girls with no breast development until after 13.5 years are said to have delayed puberty. Both these conditions need referral to a paediatric endocrinologist for assessment. It will take an average of 2 years from the onset of puberty to menarche. The attainment of breast stage 4 is a prerequisite for the onset of menstruation (Skinner & Wallace, 2005).

Boy's pubertal assessment (Table 24.2) should include Tanner staging of secondary sexual characteristics and measuring testicular volume, using a Prader orchidometer. The pre-pubertal testis measures approximately 2ml in volume. A boy's puberty begins with enlargement of their testes to 4ml volume, at an average age of 11.5 years.

A boy's growth spurt starts when their testis is 8ml and reaches its maximum rate when testicular volume is approximately 12ml. A normal adult testis measures 15 to 25 ml. Azoospermia is likely if the adult testis measure 10ml or less (Skinner & Wallace, 2005).

Table 24.2 Boy's pubertal development

Tanner stage	Genital development	Pubic hair
Stage 1	Pre-adolescent: testes, scrotum and penis are of about the same size and proportion as in early childhood.	Pre-adolescent: The vellus over the pubes is not further developed than that over the abdominal wall, i.e. no pubic hair.
Stage 2	Enlargement of the scrotum and testes. Skin of scrotum reddens and changes in texture. Little or no enlargement of the penis at this stage.	Sparse growth of long, slightly pigmented downy hair, straight or slightly curled, chiefly at the base of the penis.
Stage 3	Enlargement of the penis, which occurs at first mainly in length. Further growth of testes and scrotum.	Considerably darker, courser and more curled. The hair spreads sparsely over the junction of the pubes.
Stage 4	Increased size of penis with growth and breadth and developing glans. Testes and scrotum larger; scrotal skin darkened.	Hair now adult in type, but the area covered is still considerably smaller than in the adult. No spread to the medial surface of the thighs.
Stage 5	Genitalia adult in size and shape.	Adult in quantity and type.

Source: Marshall & Tanner (1970). Reproduced with permission of *Archives of Disease in Childhood*.

Potential problems

- delayed or arrested puberty;
- precocious puberty;
- impaired fertility;
- adverse pregnancy outcome;
- early menopause;
- erectile dysfunction.

Risk factors

- In girls, radiotherapy to any field including the ovaries or uterus, this includes: TBI, spinal, abdominal or flank irradiation.
- In boys, radiotherapy to the testes, including TBI.
- Chemotherapy from the following agents:

  - Alkylating agents
  - BCNU
  - Busulphan
  - CCNU
  - Chlorambucil
  - Cyclophosphamide
  - Ifosphamide
  - Melphalan
  - Mustine
  - Nitrogen mustard
  - Thiotepa
  - Cisplatin
  - Cytarabine
  - Dacarbazine
  - Procarbazine

- In girls of older age at time of BMT treatment
- In boys of younger age at time of BMT treatment.

(Skinner & Wallace, 2005)

High-dose radiotherapy (>24 Gy) to the HPA as given for the treatment of brain tumours may result in delayed puberty, whereas lower doses are associated with precocious puberty especially in young girls (Skinner & Wallace, 2005).

Radiation doses in excess of 50 Gy to the HPA may render a child gonadotrophin-deficient. The occurrence of gonadotrophin deficiency increases with time post irradiation of the brain. Gonadotrophin deficiency may range from subtle, i.e. only detected by a gonadotrophin-releasing hormone (GnRH) test, to severe impairment associated with low sex hormone levels (Darzy et al., 2004).

Factors affecting girls

Chemotherapy and radiotherapy may damage the ovaries resulting in oocyte depletion, loss of hormone production, uterine dysfunction and lead to premature menopause (SIGN, 2004). However, reproductive function is generally preserved following cancer in childhood treated by chemotherapy alone.

Total body irradiation, abdominal and pelvic radiotherapy can all cause impaired ovarian function and may affect uterine function. High-dose irradiation to the uterus can cause irreversible damage to the uterus's blood supply and prevents adequate growth. Abdominal radiation involving the pelvis, i.e. whole or in some cases flank radiation that extends into the pelvis and crosses the midline, is associated with low birth weight in offspring, early delivery and birth defects in offspring if they were treated with abdominal radiotherapy (Skinner & Wallace, 2005). Cranial irradiation may indirectly impair ovarian function by causing hypogonadotrophic hypogonadism (Critchley et al., 2004).

Factors affecting boys

Pre- and post-pubertal testes are susceptible to radiotherapy and alkylating agents. Sertoli cells (germ cells) are more susceptible than Leydig cells (hormone-producing cells). Direct irradiation to the testes causes permanently impaired spermatogenisis and Leydig cell dysfunction. However, most pre-pubertal boys undergoing bone marrow transplant who have conditioning which includes chemotherapy and fractionated TBI can expect to progress normally through puberty. TBI usually causes impaired spermatogenesis, but has a variable effect on Leydig cell function.

Decreased testicular volume in post-pubertal boys is associated with impaired spermatogenesis. As testicular volume is reduced in males with germ cell failure, it is not a good measure of pubertal development in post-transplant patients or any males who have had radiotherapy to their testes (Skinner & Wallace, 2005). Loss of Leydig cell function before or during puberty will result in failure to enter puberty or arrest puberty. Cytotoxic insult following normal secondary sexual characteristics can present as erectile dysfunction loss of libido and fatigue (Thomson & Wallace, 2004).

Assessment

- All patients should have pubertal staging every 6 months; this should include testicular examination, both texture and volume assessment in boys using an orchidometer. In females breast examination should be included.
- Measure and chart growth until normal pubertal spurt is established and continue until completion of puberty and growth.
- Measure sex hormones (testosterone and oestrogen), gonadatrophins (FSH and LH) and Inhibin B from approximately 8–10 years of age.
- When appropriate, discuss the need for contraception, even in the presence of impaired fertility.
- Semen analysis when appropriate for males.
- Enquire about menstrual history, menopausal symptoms and explain the risk of possible premature menopause for females.

(Skinner & Wallace, 2005)

Management

Refer to endocrinologist if there is concern about:

- growth (as previously discussed in HPA axis);
- delayed pubertal development/precocious puberty;
- Leydig cell or ovarian failure.

Boys will require androgen supplementation for induction and progression of puberty and testosterone treatment in adulthood. Girls require slowly increasing doses of oestrogen to encourage progression through puberty with normal breast development and to enhance secondary sexual characteristics. Girls will also need cyclical hormone replacement. Girls on hormone replacement may need a trial off therapy to assess possible ovarian recovery. Refer to reproductive medicine services as needed (Critchley et al., 2004; Skinner & Wallace, 2005).

Fertility

Radiotherapy and alkylating chemotherapy can damage male and female reproductive systems. The majority of children who survive cancer into adulthood are fertile but those whose fertility is impaired suffer physical and psychological late effects (Grundy et al., 2001).

Female fertility: potential problems

Concern over fertility has also been reported by survivors in several studies (Wasserman et al., 1987; Gray et al., 1992). The effects of cancer and its treatment on reproduction and fertility are well documented. Most survivors are fertile, with a small, but significant number of survivors at risk of infertility (Levitt & Jenney, 1998; Byrne et al., 2004a,b). Risk factors for infertility include gonadal irradiation and treatment with alkylating agents (such as cyclophosphamide). More recently, treatment with high dose (24 Gy) cranial irradiation before the age of 10 in boys (Byrne et al., 2004a), and cranial radiotherapy at any dose around the time of menarche in girls (Byrne et al., 2004b), have been reported as risk factors for infertility. Radiotherapy and chemotherapy damage the ovaries and can accelerate depletion of oocytes, risking the onset of premature menopause and reduced hormone production (Critchley et al., 2004).

Chemotherapy

Generally girls are likely to be fertile following chemotherapy but they are at risk of having an early menopause (Skinner & Wallace, 2005). The ovary is less susceptible to damage following alkylating chemotherapy than the testis (Levitt & Jenney, 1998; Brennan & Shalet, 2002). Ovarian function usually recovers after high-dose cyclophosphamide (200mg/kg) when used in conditioning regimes for bone marrow transplantation. However, recovery is unlikely when treatment with alkylating chemotherapy is combined with total body irradiation (Levitt & Jenney, 1998). Girls who have survived treatment for Hodgkin's disease are more likely than boys to retain their fertility but their reproductive life is likely to be shortened with a risk of early menopause (Skinner & Wallace, 2005).

Radiotherapy

Focused radiotherapy to the abdomen or pelvis can cause uterine dysfunction and ovarian impairment (Skinner & Wallace, 2005). When radiotherapy is given at a young age, pubertal uterine growth is affected and impaired blood perfusion can affect the outcome of a pregnancy, increasing the risk of nulliparity, early miscarriage and small-for-dates babies (Brennan & Shalet, 2002). The LD_{50} (radiation dose causing 50% death of cells) is <4 Gy for the human oocyte (Grundy et al., 2001). Gonadal damage from radiotherapy can result in either infertility or premature menopause in adult life. Cranial radiotherapy >24 Gy can cause pituitary damage and delay pubertal development and cranial radiotherapy <24 Gy can result in precocious puberty (Skinner & Wallace, 2005). Coming to terms with infertility or the possibility of an early menopause can cause psychological problems for young women and they will need support and advice about assisted reproductive techniques.

Assessment

Assessment of pubertal development should be monitored using the Tanner scale as described in the endocrine section. Normal pubertal development and onset of menarche with regular periods is predictive of relatively unimpaired fertility (Levitt & Jenney, 1998). Young women should be encouraged to give a menstrual history and discuss symptoms of early menopause such as hot flushes and dyspareunia caused by vaginal dryness (Skinner et al., 2005).

Management

Young women who are at risk of premature menopause or have impaired fertility should be referred to a specialist in reproductive medicine and receive advice on assisted reproduction and hormone replacement therapy. Women at risk of premature menopause should be clearly advised of this to enable them to make a decision to have children early. Irrespective of the degree of fertility impairment, women need appropriate advice about contraception (Skinner & Wallace, 2005).

Preservation of fertility before treatment

- Embryo freezing is more successful than mature oocyte preservation but is only possible for adult patients with partners.
- Mature oocyte collection and freezing is possible for post-pubertal women but the success rate for subsequent live births is low. The need for inducing super-ovulation delays the start of treatment (Critchley et al., 2004).
- The ovaries can be moved out of the field of radiotherapy to preserve ovarian function. This is a risky procedure and is rarely recommended in the UK (Levitt & Jenney, 1998).
- Ovarian tissue cryopreservation is still considered experimental although one live birth has been reported in Belgium (Singh, 2004). There is a risk of reintroducing malignant cells following this procedure. The procedure is considered experimental at present and is not widely available.

Male fertility: potential problems

The testes are susceptible to gonadotoxic chemotherapy and radiotherapy damage before and after puberty. The germinal epithelium where sperm are produced is more susceptible to toxicity from chemotherapy and radiotherapy than Leydig cells, which are involved in the production of testosterone (Levitt & Jenney, 1998). Therefore, pubertal development is rarely impaired but fertility is more likely to be affected.

- *Radiotherapy.* Azoospermia usually results after low-dose radiotherapy (> 1.2 Gy) to the testes but normal sex hormones are produced because Leydig cells are preserved at doses up to 12 Gy (Grundy et al., 2001).

- *Chemotherapy*. Alkylating chemotherapy is the most gonadotoxic of cytotoxic drugs and the effects are dose dependent. The cumulative dose of cyclophosphamide >7.5 g/m^2 is associated with a high risk of azoospermia, but with doses <3.5 g/m^2 fertility is likely to be preserved (Levitt & Jenney, 1998).
- *Surgery*. Surgery involving the pelvis can cause nerve damage resulting in impotence (Levitt & Jenney, 1998).

Assessment

Long-term follow-up assessment of pubertal development and fertility should include:

- Testicular volume and Tanner staging of secondary sexual development. Normal progression through puberty is likely even after bone marrow transplantation. Decreased testicular volume indicates impaired spermatogenesis and is likely after high doses of alkylating agents or testicular radiotherapy (SIGN, 2004).
- Hormone serum levels of luteinising hormone (LH), follicle-stimulating hormone (FSH) and testosterone. Raised LH indicates damage to the Leydig cells, which can result in abnormal testosterone production and affect sexual function. Raised FSH indicates damage to the germinal epithelium and impaired spermatogenesis.
- Semen analysis can be carried out when the young person is mature enough to produce an ejaculate. This is the best way to assess fertility status and will confirm a normal sperm count, oligospermia or azoospermia (SIGN, 2004).

Management

Young men who have impaired fertility may benefit from assisted reproduction techniques such as intracytoplasmic sperm injection (ICSI) and in-vitro fertilisation (IVF) by donor sperm or cryopreserved sperm (Grundy *et al.*, 2001). Those who have failed to enter puberty may need testosterone replacement therapy. Irrespective of the degree of fertility impairment, young men should be offered appropriate advice on contraception,

as even with a low sperm count they can father children naturally (Skinner & Wallace, 2005).

Preservation of fertility before treatment

Cryopreservation of spermatozoa should be offered to postpubertal males providing they can consent to the procedure themselves (Grundy *et al.*, 2001; SIGN, 2004). A semen sample would need to be produced; the nurse has a role in offering sensitive support and counselling during decision-making. Ideally this group of patients will be treated in a specialist adolescent centre where the procedure will be handled sensitively. The young person needs to be able to give consent to collection and storage of sperm and this is possible for young men around the age of 14 years who are Fraser-competent (SIGN, 2004). All young men and women need support and information if they are at risk of fertility problems and should be given the CCLG *After Cure* fact sheet (Griffiths, 2005) about either male or female fertility. It is also important to reassure young men and women who have not received gonadotoxic chemotherapy or radiotherapy that their fertility is likely to be normal.

Liver

Hepatic complications although uncommon are primarily observed as acute treatment toxicity from childhood cancer treatment. There is only limited information about the long-term outcomes of liver injury (Hudson, 2004).

Risk factors

- hepatic surgery;
- radiation to field including the liver;
- total body irradiation;
- chemotherapy:
  - Actinomycin-D
  - Busulphan
  - Methotrexate
  - Thiopurines especially thioguanine
- multiple blood transfusions.

(Skinner & Wallace, 2005)

Potential problems

Never intentionally give > 35 Gy hepatic radiation as tolerance = <35 Gy. Radiation doses over 35 Gy to the liver can cause hepatotoxicity. Other predisposing factors include young age at treatment, the use of actinomycin-D and doxorubicin in combination with partial hepatectomy (Hudson, 2004).

The following cytotoxic drugs can all cause hepatocellular toxicity; methotrexate, actinomycin-D, busulphan and thiopurine (Skinner & Wallace, 2005). However, most children have a complete recovery from acute hepatic injury when the causative agents are stopped (Hudson, 2004).

Hepatic veno-occlusive disease (VOD) presents with jaundice, right upper quadrant pain, hepatomegaly, liver dysfunction, ascites and thrombocytopenia, it can be mild or life-threatening with progressive hepatic failure. Hepatic veno-occlusive disease can be caused by both radiotherapy and chemotherapy. Treatment for VOD is largely supportive, full recovery has been reported but long-term sequelae of hepatic VOD is not yet known (Hudson, 2004).

The commonest cause of chronic liver disease in survivors of childhood cancer is chronic graft versus host disease following bone marrow transplant. Patients receiving blood transfusions before September 1991 are at risk of transfusion-acquired hepatitis. All blood products since September 1991 are tested for human immunodeficiency virus (HIV), hepatitis B virus (HBV), hepatitis C virus (HCV) and cytomegalovirus (CMV). Before September 1991 HCV testing was not included (Skinner & Wallace, 2005). Patients who had blood transfusions prior to September 1991 should be counselled and offered HCV screening. It has not yet been established what the long-term consequences of hepatic injury due to veno-occlusive disease (VOD), chronic GvHD or transfusion-acquired hepatitis are. Viral hepatitis B and C may result in chronic hepatic dysfunction, however, chronic hepatitis B and C do predispose to liver-related morbidity and mortality from cirrhosis, end-stage liver disease and hepatocellular carcinoma. Liver disease is accelerated if both viruses are present (Hudson, 2004).

Assessment

At long-term follow-up clinic patients with any of the risk factors should have a physical examination for:

- hepatosplenomegaly;
- spider angioma;
- palmar erythema;
- icterus;
- liver function tests (bilirubin, transaminase and alkaline phosphtase).

Management

Young people found to have HCV/HBV serology should be referred to an infectious disease specialist or hepatologist. If examinations or investigations reveal new or significant abnormalities, these should be investigated as appropriate and referred to a gastroenterologist or hepatologist (Skinner & Wallace, 2005). Patients with cirrhosis should have alpha-fetoproteins (AFP) measured as a screening tumour marker for neoplasms such as hepatocellular carcinoma and an utrasound scan undertaken.

Survivors with liver dysfunction should be counselled about at-risk behaviour such as excessive alcohol intake. Recommended daily units are stated in the health education chapter of this section. Immunisation against hepatitis A and B viruses is also recommended. Patients with chronic hepatitis should be advised how to reduce transmission of their infection to their household and sexual partners. Children and young people may benefit from antiviral therapy if they have chronic hepatitis (Hudson, 2004).

Neurological impairment

Long-term survivors of leukaemia, lymphoma and brain tumours who were treated during childhood and adolescence are at risk of neurocognitive and neuropsychological effects (Robison & Bhatia, 2003).

Neurological: potential problems

- peripheral neuropathy;
- ifosfamide encephalopathy;
- leukoencephalopathy;
- seizures;
- Moya Moya disease;
- intracranal aneurysms;
- radiation necrosis;
- radiation- or chemotherapy-induced myelopathy;
- benign and malignant central nervous system (CNS) tumours;
- migraine-like episodes.

Risk factors for neurological impairment include chemotherapy, radiotherapy and surgery (Table 24.3).

Table 24.3 Risk factors for neuropsychological impairment

All survivors but especially	<ul><li>Central nervous system tumours</li><li>Acute lymphoblastic leukaemia (ALL) treated with central nervous system (CNS) radiotherapy or intrathecal chemotherapy</li><li>BMT, especially those receiving total body irradiation at an early age</li></ul>

Peripheral neuropathy can be caused by vincristine, cisplatin dose greater than $300mg/m^2$ and thalidomide. It is dependent upon the dose and duration of therapy. Vincristine neuropathy is usually fully reversible when treatment is ceased; however, if a patient has an underlying peripheral neuropathy such as Charcot-Marie-Tooth disease, then vincristine peripheral neuropathy can be more severe (Duffner, 2004).

Chemotherapy-induced encephalopathy especially with ifosfamide presents with seizures, visual and auditory disturbances and acute confusion. It can progress to irreversible coma but more commonly resolves a few days after drug therapy has stopped. Exposure to the causative drug should be avoided in the future.

Leukoencephalopathy is treatment-induced most commonly as a consequence of cranial irradiation and/or methotrexate. On computerised tomography (CT) scan it appears as calcification with diffuse areas of white matter necrosis and widened subarachnoid spaces. Grading depends upon the extent of change seen on magnetic resonance imaging (MRI) (Duffner, 2004). Leukoencephalopathy is associated with memory loss, dementia, focal motor signs, seizures, ataxia and neuropsychological dysfunction. Radiation-induced leukoencephalopathy is usually dependent on dose, fraction and volume, age at treatment and time following treatment. Patients who receive greater than 70 Gy of radiation are more likely to develop leukoencephalopathy than those who receive less than 60 Gy (Duffner, 2004). Methotrexate-induced leukoencephalopathy may develop in the absence of either leptomeningial disease or cranial irradiation (Duffner, 2004). Leukoencephalopathy is the commonest cause of seizures, although they are associated with chemical meningitis as seen during acute lymphoblastic leukaemia (ALL) treatment or as a sign of secondary CNS tumour following cranial irradiation or bone marrow transplant.

There is an increased prevalence of CNS tumours after BMT. Meningiomas are being increasingly reported after cranial irradiation (Leiper, 2002). A high cumulative radiotherapy dose can cause secondary tumours. Children who were treated for a brain tumour with cranial irradiation and children who have received TBI with previous craniospinal radiotherapy for CNS prophylaxis (in previous ALL protocols) are at increased risk (Skinner & Wallace, 2005). These same doubly irradiated patients have been shown to exhibit 'soft' neurological signs predominantly of impaired co-ordination (Leiper, 2002).

Moya Moya disease is a late-onset form of vasculopathy consisting of basilar occlusive disease (Duffner, 2004). Patients present with a progressive syndrome of transient ischaemic attacks, frank strokes, seizures, motor weakness and dementia. It can occur between 7 and 24 years following cranial radiotherapy. Patients at highest risk are those whose hypothalamic area was irradiated with doses greater than 50 Gy or non-fractionated irradiation.

Intrathecal methotrexate and cytosine have been associated with a chemotherapy-induced myelopathy. This myelopathy is characterised by weakness or paralysis with loss of bowel and bladder function. The prognosis for recovery is very poor (Duffner, 2004). Radiation necrosis can occur up to two years following cranial irradiation at doses of greater than 60 Gy (Duffner, 2004). Vasculopathy, migraine-like episodes and strokes have been documented in cranially irradiated adults and children. Reduced brain perfusion has been shown to occur after treatment for acute lymphoblastic leukaemia, which did not include cranial irradiation.

Assessment

At the clinic, children and young people need a routine neurological assessment. They should be examined for signs of raised intracranial pressure and the cranial nerves assessed. Peripheral neuropathy is often diagnosed by observing an abnormal gait. A history should be taken and patients should be asked if they suffer from headaches. Any history of seizures or headaches may need referral for a neurology opinion (Skinner & Wallace, 2005).

Management

Drug treatment should be considered for painful neuropathy with referral to neurologists, physiotherapists and occupational therapists as required. Neuropsychological assessment may also be needed (Skinner & Wallace, 2005). The nurse specialist should provide the CCLG *After Cure* fact sheet (Griffths, 2005) on radiotherapy to the brain and second malignant tumours. Discussion about the possibility of these late problems requires sensitive discussion and the specialist nurse is in an ideal position to offer this support.

Neuropsychological

Potential problems

Functional impairment can affect activities of daily living, education and employment, while cognitive impairment can cause intellectual decline, attention deficits and memory deficits.

Young age at treatment

The effects of neuropsychological impairment on a patient's quality of life are discussed in Chapter 27, so will not be discussed here.

Children treated for ALL with cranial radiotherapy or intrathecal methotrexate and malignant brain tumour survivors are at risk of neurocognitive deficits. The risk is directly proportional to the aggressiveness of the CNS therapy received (Mulhern et al., 2004).

Many factors can contribute to the neurological problems associated with ALL and brain tumour treatments. These can include the age of the child at treatment; time elapsed from treatment; and socio-economic status. It is often difficult to separate the late neurological effects such as IQ loss and academic failure from non-biological factors. Loss of social and environmental stimulation and missed schooling which is associated with childhood illness can also have a negative impact (Mulhern et al., 2004).

Children treated for brain tumours before the age of 4 are exposed to neurotoxic agents when the brain and psychological development are at their greatest. Unlike children with ALL, children with brain tumour have multi-focal insults on their CNS, such as the space-occupying lesion itself, trauma of surgery, radiotherapy and secondary effects such as visual impairment and seizures. All these insults can have an adverse effect on the patient's psychological performance (Mulhern et al., 2004).

Neuropsychological dysfunction occurs more commonly in children under 3 years of age treated with BMT who have previously been treated with cranial irradiation. It is generally accepted that cranial radiotherapy and young age at treatment have an adverse effect on cognitive function, which becomes more apparent the longer the patient is followed up (Leiper, 2002).

Neurocognitive deficits tend to be progressive in nature (Robison & Bhatia, 2003). Survivors of leukaemia who were less than 6 years of age at the age of treatment may develop significant decline in IQ, affecting attention and non-verbal cognitive processing skills. These children have problems with expressive and receptive language, attention span and visual and perceptual motor skills. They commonly complain of difficulty in reading, language and mathematics (Robison & Bhatia, 2003).

Assessment

History and examination should be undertaken at the long-term follow-up clinic. Enquiries should be made regarding schooling and education and employment in young adults. Ability to perform activities of daily living and self-care should be assessed. Neurological deficits also need to be assessed, and this can be done initially by enquiring about memory, attention, intelligence, visual-spatial, verbal and fine motor function skills (Skinner & Wallace, 2005).

Management

Close liaison is needed with schools for all at-risk children. Referral to a neuropsychologist or educational psychologist may be required for patients experiencing difficulties. A statement of educational need or extra time in exams for any patient with difficulties should be considered. Community child health services need to be involved in planning care for any child with a disability, any young adult with a disability needs referral to the young adult with disability team. Social work referral may also be necessary if a patient requires help with benefits and housing, etc. (Skinner & Wallace, 2005).

Eyes

Potential problems

Each of the different tissues of the eyes can be affected by cancer treatments especially radiotherapy and steroids such as prednisolone or dexamethasone (Skinner & Wallace, 2005). Radiotherapy involving the eyes in the field of radiation including, total body irradiation pre-bone marrow transplant can all significantly impair vision (Skinner & Wallace, 2005).

The percentage of children developing cataracts after TBI has decreased dramatically now that the dose is given as a fractionated course.

Radiotherapy can also cause watery eyes because of the damage to the lacrimal duct or conversely dry eyes (xerophthalmia) because of damage to the lacrimal glands (Ober et al., 2004). Dry sore eyes can be a sign of inflammation of the cornea associated with chronic graft versus host disease (GvHD). Painless vision loss is a major symptom of both retinopathy and optic chiasm neuropathy due to radiation damage to the retina or the optic nerve. Enucleation of one or both eyes may be necessary in the treatment for retinoblastoma.

Assessment

A clinical history should include questions about visual disturbances. Cataracts may present as painless blurring of vision, sensitivity to light or double vision in one or both eyes and are common following TBI. Teachers may have noticed that children have difficulty reading or seeing in class, children and young people may complain of persistent irritation on the surface of their eye or eyelid. Eyes should be examined with an ophthalmoscope at each visit (COG, 2006). Children and young people treated with TBI, radiotherapy to brain, eye or orbit, or those complaining of vision problems should be referred to an ophthalmologist (Skinner & Wallace, 2005).

Management

In the case of cataracts, ophthalmologists will monitor the patients' vision over many years and will only recommend cataract surgery when it becomes necessary. Cataract surgery is commonly done as a day case and involves the removal of the lens from the eye and replacement with an artificial lens. Dry sore eyes are treated by instilling regular artificial teardrops. Patients who have undergone enucleation need advice on keeping their eye socket clean and infection free. They also need free access to ophthalmology services to replace prosthetic eyes as and when necessary and to enhance and protect the remaining vision in the other eye (COG, 2006). All patients should be advised to wear UV protection sunglasses in bright sunlight.

Craniofacial and dental

Craniofacial, dental development and oral health can be abnormally affected by treatment for childhood cancer, especially that involving radiotherapy to the head and neck (Leiper, 2002a, b). Chemotherapy and radiotherapy can both have significant effects on developing facial structure and dentition (Sonis, 2004). Asymmetric, irregular facial and skull development involving bone, teeth and soft tissues can lead to altered appearance which can result in physical and psychosocial morbidity (Sonis, 2004).

Risk factors

- cranial and facial radiotherapy;
- TBI;
- chemotherapy;
- treatment at a young age.

Potential problems

Abnormal facial appearance and growth. Craniofacial growth may not be proportional. Calvarial growth is almost complete by 5 years of age while nasomaxillary, mandibular and dentition growth continues into adolescence (Sonis, 2004). Suppression of bony orbital growth can be a life-long complication for children with bilateral retinoblastoma treated with external beam radiotherapy. Their appearance changes as they grow and they develop hollow temples, prominent brows, sunken orbits, shortening and narrowing of the midface along with a saddle nose shape (Ober *et al.*, 2004). Children treated with radiotherapy for nasopharyngeal rhabdomyosarcoma can also develop abnormal facial growth especially affecting their jaws. Mandibular growth is more sensitive to radiotherapy than maxillary growth (Skinner & Wallace, 2005). Children below the age of 5 years when treated with radiotherapy using doses of 24 Gy or above are at the greatest risk of developing facial skeletal abnormalities (Sonis, 2004).

Dental caries and periodontal disease

Dwarfism, enamel hypoplasia, root defects (absent or shortened roots), incomplete calcification, agenesis and eruption failure of teeth can all be caused by exposure to 4 Gy of radiation to developing teeth (Sonis, 2004). Chemotherapy given during dental development can also result in abnormal tooth development including tooth dwarfism, enamel hypoplasia and root anomalies (Sonis, 2004). Children receiving cancer therapy may be at a greater risk of dental disease owing to the adverse effects of therapy on the dental structures and salivary glands (Sonis, 2004). Susceptibility to dental caries increases when saliva production is compromised. Children receiving high-dose irradiation (40–60 Gy) to the head and neck are at an increased risk of dental caries secondary to salivary dysfunction. These radiation caries develop rapidly and can affect the entire crown of the tooth (Sonis, 2004). There may also be an increased risk of dental caries caused by sucrose-containing medication or fizzy drinks (Salis, 2004).

Following BMT, patients may complain of xerostoma. Decreased salivary secretion usually resolves within four years if patients have received chemotherapy alone as part of their conditioning regime. Studies have shown that their salivary secretion rates are then indistinguishable from healthy children (Dahlof *et al.*, 1997a). However, those receiving TBI as part of their conditioning continue to have decreased saliva secretion (Dahlof *et al.*, 1997b). Children with chronic graft versus host disease may display oral changes similar to those observed in adult patients. Symptoms may include mucosal lichenoid lesions, leukoplakia, erythemia mucoceles and ulceration. Treatment with cyclosporin may cause non-gingival tissue growth and require surgical excision (Sonis, 2004).

Assessment

Clinical examination should include an inspection of the mouth for any suspicious oral lesions and a clinical history should reveal any difficulty with swallowing or mastication. All childhood cancer survivors should undergo regular dental examination (Skinner & Wallace, 2005). Dentists need to be informed of the type of treatment patients have received (Griffiths, 2005).

Management

Good oral hygiene must be encouraged. Some children, especially those treated with high-dose radiotherapy, may require topical fluorides to make their teeth more acid-resistant (Salis, 2004). The *After Cure* fact sheet about teeth should be given to all at-risk young people (Griffiths, 2005). Regular dental examination should be encouraged with referral to a dental surgeon or orthodontist if treatment becomes necessary. Regular clinical photography should be considered to assist in possible facial reconstruction at a later date. Patients who require facial reconstruction should be referred to a maxillofacial surgeon during puberty to discuss their options (Skinner & Wallace, 2005).

Skin

Potential problems

Children and young people who have received any type of chemotherapy or radiotherapy have an increased risk of all skin cancers including melanoma, basal cell sarcomas and squamous cell cancer within the field of radiotherapy. Fibrosis of skin after radiotherapy and scleroderma caused by chronic GvHD cause thickened inflexible skin, which can lead to joint immobility (Benton & Tidman, 2004).

Assessment

All pigmented skin lesions should be inspected and monitored during long-term follow-up. Children and young people should be encouraged to inspect their skin regularly and be alert to changes on their skin. Moles that increase in size, thickness or change in pigmentation, become itchy or bleed should be referred to a dermatologist urgently (Skinner & Wallace, 2005).

Management

If skin cancer is suspected, an urgent referral to a dermatologist should be made because skin cancer is curable if treated early. Young people should be advised about protecting their skin in the sun and this is discussed in Chapter 26 under health education. Fibrotic skin needs regular moisturising and the underlying chronic GvHD has to be treated to improve scleroderma (COG, 2004).

Musculoskeletal

Musculoskeletal effects have a significant impact on the quality of life for childhood cancer survivors (Robison & Bhatia, 2003). They can affect facial appearance as discussed in the section about craniofacial and dental problems. Survivors of bone cancer may have undergone amputation or limb salvage surgery with endoprosthesis.

Potential problems

Skeletal effects are:

- avascular necrosis (AVN)
- osteochondroma (OC)
- osteoporosis
- reduced bone mineral density (BND)
- slipped epiphysis
- scoliosis, kyphosis
- endoprosthetic problems.

Muscular effects are:

- polymyositis
- weakness
- joint problems, sclerodermatous and joint contractures.

Bone, joints and muscles in radiation fields can develop fibrosis, stiffness, hypoplasia and deformities (Skinner & Wallace, 2005).

Second malignancies can develop within radiation fields.

Risk factors

Steroids, chemotherapy and radiotherapy including TBI, cranial and spinal radiotherapy are risk factors for musculoskeletal effects. Endocrinopathy, especially growth hormone deficiency or gonadal failure, is also a risk factor (Skinner & Wallace, 2004).

Avascular necrosis commonly occurs during cancer treatment but can also occur after treatment has been completed. Avascular necrosis is caused by a temporary or permanent interruption to the blood supply to the bone. It can occur in any bone but commonly affects the epiphysis of long bones such as the femur or humerus (COG, 2006). Femoral avascular necrosis occurs as a result of chemotherapy, particularly steroid treatment and as a consequence of TBI as well as more focal radiation (Levitt & Saran, 2004). Although the hip joint is most commonly affected by non-traumatic avascular necrosis in post-transplant patients, other joints can be affected and there may well be bilateral involvement (Leiper, 2002a, b).

Multiple osteochondromas are common after BMT, and can occur centrally or peripherally. They are associated with TBI but have also been associated with localised irradiation for other childhood malignancies. Osteochondromas can undergo malignant changes to present as osteosarcoma or osteochondrosarcoma, however this is very rare (Leiper, 2002a, b).

During childhood and young adulthood, normal bone formation occurs faster than bone loss enabling bones to grow and become denser. This process reverses in adulthood and bones slowly lose strength as part of the normal ageing process (COG, 2006). Osteoporosis or osteopenia results from too little bone formation or too much bone loss causing the bones to become weak. Minimal trauma can then cause fractures. Vertebral collapse may present as back pain, spinal curvature or loss of height (COG, 2006). Both underlying disease and chemotherapy affect bone turnover in childhood cancer patients and both contribute to reduced bone mass acquisition during treatment (Crofton, 2004). Steroids, especially prednisolone and dexamethasone, are a major component in the treatment acute lymphoblastic leukaemia and lymphoma in childhood. Dexamethasone is also used as an antiemetic and for tumour-associated oedema especially in brain tumour patients. Glucocorticoids enhance bone re-absorption and decrease bone formation, therefore decreasing bone mass

and increasing the risk of fractures (Brennan, 2004). High-dose methotrexate also impairs bone formation and enhances bone re-absorption (Crofton, 2004).

Irradiation indirectly causing growth hormone deficiency or sex steroid deficiency will also contribute to reduced bone mineral density (Brennan, 2004). Too much thyroid hormone can also result in osteoporosis (COG, 2006). Spinal deformity can be caused by radiotherapy. If the radiation field is symmetrical then the main effect will be a decrease in spinal height (a short back is often more evident when the patient is sitting). If the ephyseal plates are irradiated asymmetrically, then scoliosis, kyphosis or kyphoscioliosis may occur (Morgan & Conrad, 2004). Scoliosis and kyphosis can result from radiation to the trunk at doses of 20 Gy or greater (COG, 2006).

Young people and children who have had limb salvage surgery need follow-up for the rest of their lives. These patients may have had joint implants which only last approximately ten years and require future replacement surgery (Morgan & Conrad, 2004). A bone continues to grow throughout childhood and adolescence; patients often develop limb length discrepancies and need surgery to help correct them. Prosthetic loosening may arise, needing further surgery.

Assessment

At the long-term follow-up clinic, a history should be taken and patients questioned about diet and exercise. During physical examination, the spine should be observed for abnormal spinal curvature especially during pubertal growth spurts. Enquiries should be made about any back pain or fractures. Following bone marrow transplant, children and young people who have sclerodermatous joint contractures should be examined for other signs of chronic graft versus host disease (cGvHD). Dual-energy X-ray absorptiometry (DEXA) measurements are used to assess bone mineral density in the following patients:

- post-bone marrow transplant;
- those diagnosed with growth hormone deficiency;

- acute lymphoblastic leukaemia;
- medulloblastoma;
- clinical history of back pain or fractures.

(Skinner & Wallace, 2005)

Patients with signs or symptoms of avascular necrosis should have magnetic resonance imaging (MRI).

Management

All children and young people should be encouraged to take a diet rich in calcium and undertake weight-bearing exercise to improve their bone mineral density and bone strength. When a reduced bone mineral density is diagnosed referral to a specialist in bone disease is necessary. Patients with osteochondroma, slipped epiphysis, scoliosis or avascular necrosis should be referred to an orthopaedic surgeon. Treatment for avascular necrosis ranges from conservative treatment (involving pain relief, use of crutches to reduce weight bearing and physiotherapy exercises), to surgical treatment which may involve a bone graft, osteotomy wedge resection or arthroplasty (joint replacement). Scoliosis should be monitored and may need to be treated with a brace or surgery. Patients with musculoskeletal disease associated with cGvHD should have their immunosuppressive treatment reviewed.

Swelling or lumps which develop in the radiation field should be reported to a general practitioner immediately (Skinner & Wallace, 2005; COG, 2006). Children and young people who have endoprostheses need to have any bacterial infections treated promptly with antibiotics. All abscesses, boils, urinary tract infections and ingrowing toenails need treatment as bacteria can settle next to the metal bone replacement and start an infection. The signs of an infected metal bone replacement are pain and redness near the scar and/or development of stiffness and increased temperature in the limb. If not treated quickly, the metal replacement may need to be removed. Children and young people with such prostheses should also be told that it is imperative that they tell their dentist that they have metal bone replacement and they will need antibiotic cover for dental treatment (Griffiths, 2005).

Hearing

Potential problems

There are two types of hearing loss:

1. *Conductive hearing loss* due to a problem with transmission of sound through the outer and middle ear. This is caused by ear infections, if there is a build-up of ear wax, or if there has been damage to the ear drum or middle ear bones.
2. *Sensorineural hearing loss* caused by damage to the inner ear or auditory nerve. If the sensory hair cells have been damaged in the inner ear then the sound waves cannot be changed into nerve impulses and so the brain is unable to recognise sound. High and low-pitched sounds are processed by different sensory hair cells. The sensory hair cells which process high-frequency sounds are often damaged first and this may be the first indication of hearing loss. Sensorineural hearing loss is usually permanent whereas conductive hearing loss may improve over time (COG, 2006).

Risk factors

Hearing loss can be caused by:

- surgery to the brain or ear which affects the 8th cranial nerve (auditory nerve);
- platinum-based chemotherapy such as cisplatin (cumulative doses of cisplatin greater than $360mg/m^2$) increases the risk of auditory impairment);
- aminoglycoside antibiotics such as gentamicin or tobramycin;
- loop diuretics such as furosemide;
- radiation to any field involving the ear such as:

  - TBI
  - infratemporal
  - cranial
  - craniospinal
  - nasopharyngeal.

Radiation to the ear or brain can cause problems with ear wax, build-up of fluid in the middle ear, stiffness to the ear drum or middle ear bone damage. This damage can present as conductive hearing loss. Radiation can also damage the sensory hair cells in the middle ear causing sensorineural hearing loss (COG, 2006).

Assessment

A full history should be taken at the follow-up clinic. Children and young people may complain of tinnitus; however, more commonly parents say that their children have difficulty in hearing when spoken to especially if there is any background noise. Teachers may have also told parents that their child does not pay attention in class (Shearer, 2004). Audiograms should be performed at the end of patient's treatment and repeated at regular intervals if there are any signs of hearing loss.

Management

Hearing loss should be diagnosed promptly as it can affect children's speech development and education (Skinner & Wallace, 2005). Early referral to an audiologist for formal hearing assessment may be necessary. Children who cannot understand instructions during an audiogram may need to have their hearing tested using brainstem auditory evoked responses. Those with 'glue ear' need referral to an ENT surgeon for treatment. Patients with hearing problems may need referral to community healthcare consultants, educational psychologists and speech and language therapists to ensure appropriate needs are addressed (Skinner & Wallace, 2005).

Hearing should be protected by the early treatment of ear infections or excessive ear wax. Autotoxic drugs such as aspirin and gentamicin should be avoided. They should also be advised to protect their ears from very loud noises, both recreationally and occupationally, by wearing ear protection (COG, 2006).

Gastrointestinal

Long-term gastrointestinal complications of childhood cancer treatment can have a major detrimental effect on nutrition and growth. Chemotherapy, radiotherapy and surgery can all damage the gastrointestinal tract. Nutrition is compromised by the nausea and vomiting caused by these agents; however, most problems and side effects associated with chemotherapy are acute. Chemotherapy combined with radiotherapy may cause long-term effects.

The enterocyte has a life span of four days and is therefore affected by chemotherapy, especially alkylating agents, antimetabolites, vincristine and vinblastine. In acute stages of treatment, this is seen as mucositis, which may extend beyond the oral cavity (Meadows, 2004).

Factors which have equally important effects are:

- increased gastrointestinal permeability;
- mucosal damage;
- alteration of inflammatory response.

These are more likely to result in long-term complications; nutritional status and bowel flora may also influence the outcome.

Potential problems

Malnutrition can cause damage to the bowel resulting in malabsorption. Most gastrointestinal side effects from chemotherapy are acute and rarely result in long-term side effects. However, radiotherapy, surgery and chemotherapy in combination may produce chronic problems. Post-bone marrow transplant patients, who have needed long-term immunosuppression, may develop life-threatening infections caused by cryptosporidia or cytomegalovirus. Cytomeglovirus (CMV) can reactivate at any time causing CMV viremia, the virus can invade the gastrointestinal epithelium, causing secondary vasculitis and sub-mucosal ischaemia (Meadows, 2004).

Of all oncology treatments to the gastrointestinal (GI) tract radiotherapy is most likely to result in long-term complications. Radiation enteritis has three phases: early, delayed (months after treatment), and late (several years after treatment). Delayed and late radiation enteritis present with diarrhoea, vomiting, signs of obstruction such as abdominal distension and pain. Histopathology of the mucosa shows villous blunting with an increased plasma cell infiltration in the lamina propria. There can be full thickness fibrosis of the bowel wall, which can lead to stricture formation and result in ulceration of the mucosa and malabsorbtion (Meadows, 2004).

Adhesions and strictures present with symptoms of obstruction while blind loops present with diarrhoea (Meadows, 2004). A 'blind loop' is an area of the small intestine, which has poor motility and a profusion of bacteria. They are difficult to identify even with barium studies. Adhesions and blind loops can be caused by abdominal surgery and radiotherapy. Adhesions are diagnosed by plain abdominal X-ray and if possible barium studies. Strictures present with acute or subacute obstruction and patients may complain of increased pain on swallowing. A barium meal and follow-through is required to assess the extent of damage to the bowel (Meadows, 2004).

Chronic graft versus host disease of the gastrointestinal tract may present with difficulty in swallowing, retrostinal pain and anorexia, which results in severe weight loss. Barium swallow is again indicated to confirm diagnosis (Meadows, 2004).

Assessment

Gastrointestinal problems often present with failure to thrive (Meadows, 2004). Children and young people who have had radiotherapy or surgery to the GI tract should be asked if they have any difficulty swallowing, and questioned about their bowel habits. They should be examined for any signs and symptoms of malabsorption or intestinal obstruction. If symptoms are present they should be acted upon quickly and patients referred for further investigation (Skinner & Wallace, 2005).

Management

There needs to be a multidisciplinary approach to the management of long-term complications of the GI tract following childhood cancer treatment. Oncologists, gastroenterologists, surgeons and dieticians should work together as a team when gastrointestinal problems are diagnosed (Meadows, 2004).

Cardiac

Potential problems

Cardiotoxicity is a significant treatment-related late effect of chemotherapy (particularly with anthracyclines) and radiotherapy. The number of myocytes that comprise the myocardium of the heart are determined by six months of age. Cells that are damaged are not able to replicate but undamaged cells respond to increased demand by hyperplasia and hypertrophy (Levitt & Saran, 2004). Damage caused by radiotherapy or chemotherapy may impair this function especially at times of increased demand such as growth, strenuous activity such as weight lifting and pregnancy (Skinner & Wallace, 2005).

Risk factors for cardiotoxicity (Hinckle et al., 2004) include:

- high cumulative dose of anthracyclines (doxorubicin and daunorubicin) >250mg/m^2;
- younger age at the time of treatment;
- female gender;
- mediastinal radiotherapy used concomitantly with anthracycline treatment.

Dexrazoxane has been used with good effect for the prevention of cardiomyopathy in adults receiving high doses of anthracyclines (Hinckle et al., 2004). Although dexrazoxane has proved effective for reducing acute myocardial injury in children, long-term benefits have not yet been established. Radiotherapy can cause heart disease and affects all the layers of the heart, the pericardium, myocardium, valves and coronary arteries. Coronary artery disease caused by radiotherapy can result in sudden death many years after treatment has been completed and earlier than expected in the general population (Levitt & Saran, 2004).

Assessment

Cardiotoxic effects of anthracycline chemotherapy and radiotherapy treatment can occur during treatment, or immediately after treatment has been completed, or many years later. Young people should be monitored for signs of impaired function during treatment, at the end of treatment and then at regular intervals during adult life. Echocardiography is a non-invasive investigation; a reduced shortening fraction or ejection fraction indicates anthracycline cardiotoxicity (Hinckle *et al.*, 2004). In the UK it is recommended that after treatment with anthracyclines, asymptomatic patients should have echocardiograms every five years (Skinner & Wallace, 2005), more frequent assessment may be necessary if there is evidence of deteriorating function. Young people should be asked how they feel compared with their peers. At each visit to the long-term follow-up clinic a detailed health history may reveal signs indicative of cardiac impairment (Griffiths, 2005) such as:

- fatigue
- breathlessness
- chest pain
- palpitations
- fainting.

Management

Young people who have received cardiotoxic treatment should know about the long-term risks (Hinckle *et al.*, 2004); specialist nurses can undertake this education activity. Young people need to be advised how to recognise the warning signs of cardiotoxicity and report symptoms if they have concerns. Information is found on the CCLG *After Cure* fact sheet about the heart (Griffiths, 2005). Young people should be advised about the increased stress on the heart during pregnancy and during heavy weight lifting (Griffiths, 2005). The specialist nurse should advise obstetricians about the need for close monitoring and for cardiac assessment throughout the pregnancy. Young people should be encouraged to adopt a healthy lifestyle because it is known that risk factors for heart disease include:

- smoking;
- obesity;
- high blood pressure;
- inactivity (Hinckle *et al.*, 2004),

The nurse's role in health education is discussed in Chapter 26. There is more specific advice about smoking, weight control and exercise. Referral to a cardiologist becomes necessary if cardiac function is impaired (as evidenced by abnormalities on echocardiography or on clinical examination) (Skinner & Wallace, 2005). Angiotensin converting enzyme inhibitors (ACE inhibitors) are used to treat left ventricular function disorders and heart failure, but continuing deterioration may necessitate heart transplantation in extreme cases (SIGN, 2004).

Renal and bladder

Potential problems

Treatment for childhood cancer can cause nephrotoxicity, which can present acutely or it can develop over time. It may be progressive, reversible or irreversible (Skinner & Wallace, 2005).

Risk factors for renal impairment (Skinner & Wallace, 2005) include:

- pre-existing renal impairment;
- cancer affecting the kidney and requiring total or partial nephrectomy;
- ifosfamide administered to a child under 5 years in a cumulative dose > 80 g/m^2;
- dose of cisplatin > 40 mg/m^2 daily;
- radiation dose >12–20 Gy to the field that includes the kidney;
- previous or concurrent use of nephrotoxins (e.g. aminoglycoside antibiotics).

Ifosfamide and cisplatin are nephrotoxic and cause renal impairment in 30–60% of children. Chronic ifosfamide nephrotoxicity often leads to tubular damage, resulting in hypophosphataemic rickets or nephrogenic diabetes insipidus; glomerular damage may also occur (Sweetman, 2005). Methotrexate and nitrosoureas rarely cause severe problems. Carboplatin is less nephrotoxic than cisplatin but problems can develop in a similar way to those seen with cisplatin. Cisplatin causes damage to the renal tubules and can lead to hypomagnesaemia, hypocalcaemia, hypokalaemia and hyponatraemia (Skinner & Wallace, 2005).

The bladder can be damaged by:

- invasion of the bladder by the tumour;
- surgery involving partial or total removal of the bladder;
- metabolites of ifosfamide and cyclophosphamide are toxic to the bladder, but haemorrhagic cystitis and long-term damage are usually avoided by infusion of mesna with the chemotherapy;
- radiotherapy to a field that includes the bladder can cause acute problems followed by long-term fibrosis. Treatment at a young age as well as the volume of bladder irradiated increase the risk of bladder damage (Raney *et al.*, 2004).

Children who have received bone-marrow transplantation have a particularly high risk of developing late nephropathy or bladder problems because their treatment has often included nephrotoxic drugs and total body irradiation (Leiper, 2002a, b).

Assessment

Young people at risk of impaired renal function need to have regular measurement of their blood pressure, urinalysis for proteinuria and growth monitoring until final height has been reached. Serum urea, electrolytes and creatinine need checking every 5 years if renal function is normal at the end of treatment. Glomerular filtration rate (GFR) is monitored during treatment if nephrotoxic drugs are used and measurement only needs repeating if the serum creatinine is elevated or a previous GFR has been below 90ml/minute/1.73m^2 (Skinner & Wallace, 2005). Bladder damage may result in haematuria or urinary problems, which are revealed by taking a clinical history and carrying out routine urinalysis.

Management

Young people should understand the need to have their blood pressure checked annually either at the long-term follow-up clinic or by their GP if a kidney has been removed or if nephrotoxic treatment has caused renal impairment. They should

know that high blood pressure could develop years later (Griffiths, 2005).

Electrolytes may need to be supplemented according to serum biochemistry especially following treatment with ifosfamide, cisplatin or carboplatin (Skinner & Wallace, 2005). Children and young people with severe renal impairment need referral to a nephrologist. Children and young people who develop urinary symptoms may need referral to a urologist for further investigation. Young people with a history of chronic haemorrhagic cystitis are at a higher risk of second malignant tumours of the bladder (Skinner & Wallace, 2005). The specialist nurse should educate young people about the risk of developing late renal problems and inform them of the signs and symptoms of bladder complications. The *After Cure* fact sheet (Griffiths, 2005) about the kidney and bladder should be given to young people at risk of kidney or bladder problems.

Pulmonary

Potential problem

Chemotherapy, radiotherapy involving the lungs and thoracic surgery are all risk factors for developing late respiratory problems (Skinner & Wallace, 2005).

Chemotherapy

Busulphan, cyclophosphamide and carmustine are most often associated with pulmonary toxicity. The risk is higher in children younger than 5 years treated with carmustine. Bleomycin can cause severe toxicity in adults and studies by the CCLG and St Jude's Children's Research Hospital have sought to determine a safe dose of bleomycin for Hodgkin's disease and germ-cell tumours in children (Marina *et al.*, 2004).

Radiotherapy

Initially, radiotherapy involving the lungs can cause acute pneumonitis, injuring the type II pneumocytes, endothelial cells, fibroblasts and macrophages. The risk is dependent on the total dose of radiotherapy administered, volume of the lung irradiated and the dose of each radiation fraction. Children undergoing bone-marrow transplantation who receive total body irradiation together with chemotherapy with alkylating drugs are at a particularly high risk (Marina *et al.*, 2004).

Radiotherapy carried out at a young age with high doses and a larger treatment volume of the lung increases the risk of developing pulmonary toxicity (Skinner & Wallace, 2005). Growth of the ribs, sternum, muscles and cartilage can be impaired by radiotherapy at a young age and this might impair respiratory function during adulthood (Marina *et al.*, 2004). Clinical features of acute pnemonitis include cough, dyspnoea, chest pain, pleuritis and low-grade fever. Fibrotic changes follow the acute symptoms after about 2–4 months. Long-term deterioration can result from these fibrotic changes and usually becomes apparent within 1–2 years. Restrictive respiratory late effects may also present with chronic cough, dyspnoea and chest pain (Marina *et al.*, 2004).

Assessment

Assessment of individuals at risk of pulmonary toxicity should include history of exercise tolerance and they should be questioned about smoking. Baseline pulmonary function tests should be carried out at the end of treatment and if abnormal the tests should be repeated after a year. If the baseline tests are normal then assessment is based on symptoms of pulmonary impairment (Skinner & Wallace, 2005).

Management

Symptomatic patients with abnormal lung function should be referred to a respiratory specialist. Patients with lung disease are advised to be vaccinated against pneumococcal infection and have annual immunisation against influenza (Skinner & Wallace, 2005). The specialist nurse has a responsibility to educate young people about their risk of pulmonary toxicity and at-risk young people should be given the *After Cure* fact sheet about the lungs (Griffths, 2005). Even asymptomatic patients

may have a degree of lung damage and should be strongly advised to avoid smoking. Regular exercise will improve lung function. Chapter 26 gives more information about health education and smoking cessation programmes. Patient education about specific risks of treatment is important and those who have had bleomycin are at risk when receiving high oxygen concentrations and need to warn anaesthetists pre-anaesthetic (Griffiths, 2005).

Second malignancies

Potential problem

A second primary cancer is histologically different from the first one and develops later (Bhatia, 2004). A large UK-based cohort of patients who had survived childhood cancer for at least 3 years were followed up for up to 25 years and found to have a 4.2 % risk of developing a second malignant neoplasm (Jenkinson *et al.*, 2004). Patients who have survived childhood cancer treatment for hereditary retinoblastoma, Hodgkin's disease and soft-tissue sarcomas are at the greatest risk for developing second malignant neoplasms (Neglia *et al.*, 2001).

Radiotherapy

Exposure to radiotherapy at a young age increases the risk for developing a second malignancy. Radiotherapy combined with high doses of an alkylating agent also increases the risk (Jenkinson *et al.*, 2004). Following radiotherapy secondary bone tumours and sarcomas typically present after about 10 years (Bhatia, 2004). In the past, second malignancies occurred anywhere around the field of radiotherapy but now that radiation borders are defined better, second malignancies usually occur within the radiation field.

Patients who have received radiotherapy for Hodgkin's disease are at risk of developing breast cancer or thyroid cancer, depending on the radiotherapy field and dose (Bhatia, 2004). Bone tumours usually occur in young adults who have been treated for retinoblastoma, Ewing's sarcoma and other soft-tissue sarcomas. Cranial radiotherapy for brain tumours or for prophylaxis of central nervous system disease in leukaemia can lead to second gliomas and meningiomas in adulthood (Neglia *et al.*, 2001).

Chemotherapy

Epodophyllotoxins such as etoposide given at a young age increase the risk of developing acute-onset myeloid leukaemia; the risk increases with the dose given. Alkylating agents given in high cumulative doses to older children increase the risk of developing myelodysplasia about 46 years after such treatment (Bhatia, 2004).

Familial cancer syndromes

A number of familial cancer syndromes such as Li-Fraumeni syndrome, neurofibromatosis and Fanconi's anaemia predispose individuals to malignancies (Wallace *et al.*, 2001). Hereditary retinoblastoma also increases the risk for multiple second malignancies by as much as 69 % (Hawkins, 2004); the risk is higher when radiotherapy was part of initial treatment. Soft-tissue cancers often lead to second malignancies, especially if there is a strong history of cancer in the family (Bhatia, 2004).

Assessment

Long-term follow-up to specifically detect second malignancies is recommended for patients who are at high risk. Clinical examination within the radiation fields is particularly important. The skin should be examined for the appearance of pigmented naevi. A medical history and physical examination may reveal signs of a new primary tumour (Wallace *et al.*, 2001).

Management

Young people need to know about the risks of developing second malignancies. All young people need educating about the risks of their diagnosis and treatment. The CCLG has produced the *After Cure* fact sheet (Griffiths, 2005) relating to the risks

of radiotherapy and this should be given to all young adults who have had radiotherapy. A factsheet on second malignancies is also available. The specialist nurse can provide information and give advice about leading a healthy lifestyle, and avoiding smoking and exposure to the sun. Young people should be advised to watch out for features that might indicate the development of a malignancy. Any worrying signs should receive immediate medical attention.

In relation to pigmented naevi, young people should look out for changes in size, thickness, pigmentation, itching or bleeding (Skinner & Wallace, 2005); such changes require immediate referral to a dermatologist. Women who have received thoracic or mediastinal radiotherapy (particularly for Hodgkin's disease) should be advised to examine their breasts for lumps (see Chapter 26 for more detailed advice about self-breast examination). A formal programme for breast screening is advised in accordance with the Department of Health 2003 Directive (Skinner & Wallace, 2005). An annual MRI scan is advised for all women aged 25 to 29 years; thereafter, screening should continue by mammography according to the Department of Health directive (Skinner & Wallace, 2005).

References

Benton EC & Tidman MJ (2004) 'Cutaneous complications' *in*: Wallace WHB & Green D (eds) *Late Effects of Childhood Cancer*. London: Arnold, pp. 321–331

Bhatia S (2004) 'Epidemiology' *in*: Wallace WHB & Green D (eds) *Late Effects of Childhood Cancer*. London: Arnold, pp. 57–69

Brennan BMD (2004) 'Osteoporosis' *in*: Wallace WHB & Green D (eds) *Late Effects of Childhood Cancer*. London: Arnold, pp. 267–278

Brennan BMD & Shalet SM (2002) 'Endocrine late effects after bone marrow transplant' *British Journal of Haematology 118*: 58–66

Byrne J, Fears T R, Mills J L, Zeltzer LK, Sklar C, Meadows AT, Reaman GH & Robison LL (2004a) 'Fertility of long-term male survivors of acute lymphoblastic leukemia diagnosed during childhood' *Pediatric Blood Cancer. 42*(4): 364–372

Byrne J, Fears, TR, Mills JL, Zeltzer LK, Sklar C, Nicholson HS, Haupt R, Reaman GH, Meadows AT & Robison LL (2004b) 'Fertility in women treated with cranial radiotherapy for childhood acute lymphoblastic leukaemia' *Pediatic Blood Cancer* 42(7): 589–597

Children's Oncology Group (2006) *Long-Term Follow-up Guidelines.* Children's Oncology Group, CureSearch

Critchley HO, Thompson AB & Wallace WHB (2004) 'Ovarian and uterine function and reproductive potential' *in:* Wallace WHB & Green D (eds) *Late Effects of Childhood Cancer.* London: Arnold, pp. 225–238

Crofton PM (2004) 'Bone and collagen turnover' *in:* Wallace WHB & Green D (eds) *Late Effects of Childhood Cancer.* London: Arnold, pp. 279–292

Dahlof, G, Bagesund, M & Ringden, O (1997a) 'Impact of conditioning regimens on salivary function, caries associated micro-organisms and dental caries in children after bone marrow transplantation: a 4-year longitudinal study' *Bone Marrow Transplantation* 20: 479–483

Dahlof G, Bagesund M, Remberger M & Ringden O (1997b) 'Risk factors for salivary dysfunction in children 1 year after bone marrow transplantation' *Oral Oncology* 33: 327–331

Darzy KH, Gleeson HK & Shalet SM (2004) 'Growth and neuroendocrine consequences' *in:* Wallace WHB & Green D (eds) *Late Effects of Childhood Cancer.* London: Arnold, pp. 189–211

Duffner PK (2004) 'Long term neurologic consequences of CNS therapy' *in:* Wallace WHB & Green D (eds) *Late Effects of Childhood Cancer.* London: Arnold, pp. 5–17

Gray RE, Doan BD, Shermer P, FitzGerald A, Berry M, Jenkin D & Doherty M (1992) 'Psychologic adaptation of survivors of childhood cancer' *Cancer* 70(11): 2713–2721

Griffiths A (ed.) (2005) *After Cure.* Leicester: Childhood Cancer and Leukaemia Group (CCLG)

Grundy R, Gosden RG, Hewitt M *et al.* (2001) 'Fertility preservation for children treated for cancer (1): scientific advances and research dilemmas' *Archives of Diseases in Childhood.* 84: 355–359

Hawkins M (2004) 'Long term survivors of childhood cancers: what knowledge have we gained?' *Nature Clinical Practice Oncology* 1: 26–31

Hays DM, Landsverk J, Sallan SE, Hewett KD *et al.* (1992) 'Educational, occupational, and insurance status of childhood cancer survivors in their fourth and fifth decades of life' *Journal of Clinical Oncology* 10(9): 1397–1406

Hinckle AS, Proukou CB *et al.* (2004) 'Cardiotoxicity caused by chemotherapy' *in:* Wallace WHB & Green D (eds) *Late Effects of Childhood Cancer.* London: Arnold, pp. 85–100

Howell SJ, Radford JA, Smets EM & Shalet SM (2000) 'Fatigue, sexual function and mood following treatment for haematological malignancy: the impact of mild Leydig cell dysfunction' *British Journal of Cancer* 82(4): 789–793

Hudson M (2004) 'Hepatic complications' *in:* Wallace WHB & Green D (eds) *Late Effects of Childhood Cancer.* London: Arnold, pp. 170–175

Hudson MM, Mertens AC, Yasui Y, Hobbie W, Chen H *et al.* (2003) 'Health status of adult long-term survivors of childhood cancer: a report from the Childhood Cancer Survivor Study' *JAMA* 290(12): 1583–1592

Jenkinson HC, Hawkins MM, Stiller CA *et al.* (2004) 'Long-term population-based risks of second malignant neoplasms after childhood cancer in Britain' *British Journal of Cancer* 9: 1905–1910

Leiper AD (2002a) 'Non-endocrine late complications of bone marrow transplantation in childhood: part 1' *British Journal of Haematology* 118: 3–22

Leiper AD (2002b) 'Non-endocrine late complications of bone marrow transplantation in childhood: part 2' *British Journal of Haematology* 118: 23–43

Levitt GA & Jenney MEM (1998) 'The reproductive system after childhood cancer' *British Journal of Obstetrics and Gynaecology* 105: 946–953

Levitt GA & Saran FH (2004) 'Radiation damage' *in:* Wallace WHB & Green D (eds) *Late Effects of Childhood Cancer.* London: Arnold, pp. 101–113

Marina N, Sharis C & Tarbell N (2004) 'Respiratory complications' *in:* Wallace WHB & Green D (eds) *Late Effects of Childhood Cancer.* London: Arnold, pp. 114–122

Marshall WA & Tanner JM (1969) 'Variations in pattern of pubertal changes in girls' *Archives of Disease in Childhood* 44(235): 291–303.

Marshall WA & Tanner JM (1970) 'Variations in the pattern of pubertal changes in boys' *Archives of Disease in Childhood* 45(239): 13–23.

Meadows N (2004) 'The late effects of paediatric cancer treatment on the gastrointestinal tract' *in:* Wallace WHB & Green D (eds) *Late Effects of Childhood Cancer.* London: Arnold, pp. 162–169

Morgan H & Conrad EU (2004) 'Limb salvage and spinal surgery' *in:* Wallace WHB & Green D (eds) *Late Effects of Childhood Cancer.* London: Arnold, pp. 293–303

Mulhern RK, Phipps S & White H (2004) 'Neuropsychological outcomes' *in:* Wallace WHB & Green D (eds) *Late Effects of Childhood Cancer.* London: Arnold, pp. 18–36

National Institute for Clinical Excellence (2005) *Improving Outcomes of Children and Young People with Cancer.* London: NICE

Neglia P, Friedman D, Yasui Y, Mertens A, Hammond S, Stovall M, Donaldson SS, Meadow AT & Robison L (2001) 'Second malignant neoplasms in five-year survivors of childhood cancer: Childhood Cancer

Survivor Study' *Journal of the National Cancer Institute* 93(8): 618–629

Ober M, Beaverson K & Abramson D (2004) 'Ocular complications' *in*: Wallace WHB & Green D (eds) *Late Effects of Childhood Cancer*. London: Arnold, pp. 37–48

Raney RB, Zagone R & Ritchey M (2004) 'Bladder complications' *in*: Wallace WHB & Green D (eds) *Late Effects of Childhood Cancer*. London: Arnold, pp. 138–143

Robison LL & Bhatia S (2003) 'Late effects among survivors of leukaemia and lymphoma during childhood and adolescence' *British Journal of Haematology* 122: 345–359

Scottish Intercollegiate Guidelines Network (2004) *Long Term Follow up of Survivors of Childhood Cancer*. Edinburgh: Scottish Intercollegiate Guidelines Network publication No. 76

Shalet SM & Brennan BM (2002) 'Endocrine late effects after bone marrow transplant' *British Journal of Haematology* 118: 58–66

Shearer PD (2004) 'Hearing impairment' *in*: Wallace WHB & Green D (eds) *Late Effects of Childhood Cancer*. London: Arnold, pp. 49–54

Singh, D (2004) 'Live birth reported after ovarian tissue transplant' *British Medical Journal* 329: 761

Skinner R & Wallace WHB (2005) *Therapy Based Long Term Follow Up: A Practice Statement* (2nd edn). Leicester: United Kingdom Childhood Cancer Study Group

Skinner R, Wallace WHB & Levitt GA (eds) (2005) *Therapy Based Long Term Follow Up* (2nd edn). London: United Kingdom Children's Cancer Study Group

Sonis AL (2004) 'Craniofacial development, teeth and salivary glands' *in*: Wallace WHB & Green D (eds) *Late Effects of Childhood Cancer*. London: Arnold, pp. 176–185

Spoudeas HA (2004) 'Disturbance of the hypothalamic-pituitary thyroid axis' *in*: Wallace WHB & Green D (eds) *Late Effects of Childhood Cancer*. London: Arnold, pp. 212–224

Sweetman S (ed.) (2005) *Martindale: The Complete Drug Reference*. London: Pharmaceutical Press

Thomson AB & Wallace WHB (2004) 'Testicular function' *in*: Wallace WHB & Green D (eds) *Late Effects of Childhood Cancer*. London: Arnold, pp. 239–256

Wallace WH, Blacklay A, Eiser C, Davies H, Hawkins M, Levitt GA & Jenney ME (2001) 'Developing strategies for long term follow up of survivors of childhood cancer' *British Medical Journal* 323(7307): 271–274

Wasserman AL, Thompson EI, Wilimas JA & Fairclough DL (1987) 'The psychological status of survivors of childhood/adolescent Hodgkin's disease' *American Journal of Diseases of Childhood* 141(6): 626–631

25 The Role of the Nurse in Long-Term Follow-Up

Beverly Horne

The role of the nurse in long-term follow-up (LTFU) of childhood cancer survivors is a new and developing speciality. The LTFU nurse is the key worker for those who are 5 years and more from the end of their therapy and who live within the geographical area covered by their particular regional paediatric oncology unit. Information about the late effects of those treated for childhood cancer is constantly emerging and the ever-evolving knowledge base presents a challenge to the nurse.

The role of the LTFU nurse involves:

- assessment, planning, implementation and evaluation of programmes of care;
- support and advice;
- liaison and education;
- provision and facilitation of alternative models of care;
- research and audit;
- health promotion provision;
- participation in other specialist LTFU clinics.

Assessment, planning, implementation and evaluation of programmes of care

A patient who is referred to the clinic will require their treatment, physical and psychological complications and any other health issues summarised. From their individual summary the potential late effects of their treatment will be assessed using national guidelines (SIGN, 2004; Skinner & Wallace, 2005). A plan for the patient's follow-up will then be compiled and screening for the potential late effects organised. As the majority of the patients only attend once a year interventions will be implemented on the day of the clinic visit if possible. This helps to encourage attendance and means less time away from school or work. In the patient's plan, as well as screening for potential late effects, there should also be identification of possible health promotion target areas, e.g. for a woman who has had chest radiotherapy it would be appropriate to inform her about breast awareness due to her increased risk of breast cancer, compared to the general population (Bhatia et al., 1996). There are many issues involved in the planning of care for the LTFU patient with each plan being individually tailored to target the potential late effects of each patient. Implementation of the patient's care will occur through the investigations ordered from the nurse consultation session and from the medical review. During the nurse consultation session health promotion topics can be covered with adolescent and adult

Cancer in Children and Young People Edited by Faith Gibson and Louise Soanes
© 2008 John Wiley & Sons, Ltd

survivors (explored in further detail in Chapter 26). The patient can have a general health check, including measurement of body mass index (BMI), blood pressure, urinalysis and given the opportunity to discuss any issues that are important to them, covering subjects such as fertility, employment, insurance, second malignancies and psychological problems. Outcomes of recent investigations can be evaluated and a management plan for issues discussed and put into action, in consultation with the rest of the LTFU team, the relevant specialist or GP for continuing care as appropriate.

Support and advice

The LTFU nurse with specialist knowledge of potential late effects provides support and advice to the patient and other health professionals. Informing a patient of the possible risks can cause great anxiety and this may be lessened by the information being broached in a sensitive but appropriate way in order to induce a realistic awareness.

Psychological issues arise and the LTFU nurse is often the first port of call before a referral to the psychology services. Psychology input is sought when the problems stem from having had cancer and/or cancer treatment. All survivors of childhood cancer have the potential to suffer from psychological problems, and a significant number are likely to experience heightened anxiety over such issues as general health, relapse of disease or fertility (Zeltzer, 1993). All experiences are relevant and significant to the individual and there must be a conscious recognition of this on the part of the nurse. It is important not to compare patients' experiences and underestimate those who perhaps had minimal treatment and low-grade cancers. Referral to a psychologist who works with young people who have had cancer is desirable as skills and knowledge needed in helping this cohort of patients are quite unique. Understanding and empathy of their journey go a long way in developing a rapport with the childhood cancer survivors.

Patients and their families also have concerns about acute medical problems and whether these are connected with their cancer or treatment, concerns about whether they have relapsed and what to look out for, or if what they have heard in the media applies to them. Employment issues arise and one particular area that causes difficulties for the long-term follow-up patients are the armed services which are very reluctant to take cancer survivors. Insurance and employment will also be the subject of advice sought as some patients experience problems getting insurance, being asked to pay inflated premiums many years after the end of treatment. Referral to a social worker can help with educational or employment difficulties or for finding resources for the disabled survivor. Second malignancies are a potential risk, and advice is sought on symptomatology, risk and lifestyle choices. Lifestyle choices are an important area of focus at the LTFU clinic and health promotion forms part of the care.

Liaison and education

Liaison and education will form part of the LTFU nurse's role on a daily basis, providing specialist knowledge on late effects of childhood cancer treatment. The patient, service providers (GP, shared care centres, professional colleagues), members of the multidisciplinary team and other health professionals are among those who may require the expert knowledge that can be provided by the LTFU nurse.

Education of patients gives them ownership of their own health care, providing information on their health risks and what action they would be advised to take. The patient can be offered an *After Cure* booklet (Griffiths 2005) which gives them information on many issues such as why they need to be seen, healthy living, fertility, insurance, employment, travel and disability. The booklet is accompanied by a treatment card, which summarises the patient's own treatment details, and information sheets on specific late effects. These booklets are useful as the patient may have been too young to remember what their treatment or illness involved. Their parents may not be able to recall all the relevant details and perhaps asking their parents to relate what was a very difficult and painful time of their lives may be unacceptable for the patient. The LTFU nurse can fulfil this role by providing details of their previous cancer and its treatment and problems that may have occurred during the treatment or subsequently. Late effects of childhood cancer is a specialised field and one of the responsibilities of the LTFU nurse is in the education of other health professionals. There are only 22 regional paediatric oncology units across the UK and therefore late effects expertise is a rare but developing speciality.

Provision and facilitation of alternative models of care

There is great variety in the models of care that are in place within LTFU clinics. Traditionally childhood cancer survivors are never discharged and are given a medical review annually. However, a change in the way patients are followed up has had to come about in order to manage the growing number of LTFU patients. The majority of patients are still followed up in the traditional way but some have a low risk of late effects of their treatment and suggestions have been made regarding alternative ways (Table 25.1). The patients do not necessarily need a medical review once a year, some can attend every two years and the LTFU nurse can facilitate follow-up in between by post or telephone with a health status screening questionnaire (Figure 25.1). The purpose of this is to provide a point of contact with the patient and

to give an opportunity for them to inform the LTFU team of any problems that may have arisen in the previous year. They also provide a means of keeping track with GP changes, marital status, offspring, change of address, etc. These questionnaires have been found to be acceptable to the patient and prove a popular alternative to having to attend the hospital for an appointment (Horne, 2004). Ways forward for the future for those at low risk of late effects could include follow-up by e-mail or mobile phone text between their medical reviews. When consulted the childhood cancer survivors felt that a key worker was important to the LTFU service. A key worker whom they were able to develop and maintain a rapport with, who knew about their cancer and cancer treatment and who was able to communicate with them and support them and their parents (Gibson *et al.*, 2005).

In the USA there are established nurse-led LTFU clinics whereas in the UK this is not yet the norm. Certainly for the patients who are at low and moderate risk of late effects, it would seem appropriate for them to be followed up by LTFU nurse specialists. Nurse-led clinics that have evolved in the UK have been evaluated as cost effective, safe and acceptable to patients (Campbell *et al.*, 2000; Connor *et al.*, 2002; Cox & Wilson, 2003). Nurses taking a leading role in LTFU are one of the ways

Table 25.1 Proposed levels of follow-up

Level	Treatment	Method of follow-up	Frequency	Examples of tumours
1	Surgery alone	Post or telephone	1–2 years	Wilms' tumour stage I or II
	Low-risk Chemotherapy			Langerhans cell histiocytosis (single system disease) Germ cell tumours (surgery only)
2	Chemotherapy	Led by nurse or primary care doctor	1–2 years	Most patients (e.g. acute lymphoblastic leukaemia in first remission)
	Low-dose cranial irradiation (<24 Gy)			
3	Radiotherapy, except low-dose cranial irradiation	Medically supervised late effects clinic	Annual	Brain tumours
	Megatherapy			Post-bone marrow transplant Patients with stage IV tumours (any type)

Source: Wallace *et al.* (2001).

LONG-TERM FOLLOW-UP QUESTIONNAIRE

Name...

Date...

Hospital no....................................

Date of birth..................................

Date of next visit.............................

Please complete the following details:-

Address..

....

Telephone No...................................

GP + Address...................................

How is your health at the
moment?..

How has your health been since your last
visit to clinic?...............................

What medication, if any, are you taking?.......

What is your current educational/employment
situation?

(Please give details of courses, exams passed,
etc.)..

Have you had any major changes in your
domestic life?.................................

Is there anything else you would like us to
know about?....................................

PLEASE CONTINUE OVER THE PAGE IF
NECESSARY

Thank you, please return in the envelope
provided.

Figure 25.1 Postal questionnaire for long-term follow-up.

in which to manage the care of this ever-increasing cohort of patients (Gibson & Soanes, 2001) and also to fulfil the role of key worker which the survivors themselves have felt is important to the service (Gibson *et al.*, 2005).

Care can sometimes be carried out in primary and secondary settings as well as in the tertiary regional centre. Some LTFU clinics can be situated in shared care centres, they can be facilitated by the LTFU nurse and/or oncologist from the regional centre, or by the shared care team or by a collaboration of both. The advantage of this form of follow-up is that it is nearer to the patient's home, thereby increasing convenience and consequently the likelihood of attendance and also reducing travelling time. There is also the

possibility that some GPs may be willing to undertake the LTFU care under the direction of the LTFU team, and this may be instigated by the patient or the GP.

Transition of care to adult services at an appropriate age and level of development is theoretically an ideal way forward for childhood cancer survivors. However, the adult oncology services are stretched with patients of their own and the adult physician may not have the knowledge or experience of the paediatric protocols or the late effects these treatments may have had on the developing child. Unlike the paediatric team they would not gain from the increase in knowledge of late effects to inform their new treatment protocols. Therefore would there be enough benefit for the adult services to research as extensively as the paediatric services into the late effects of treatment? There is a danger that opportunities would be lost to add to the knowledge base of this speciality; thus the paediatric teams have a vested interest in maintaining a comprehensive and efficient service for the adult survivors of childhood cancer. With follow-up from the paediatric centre monitoring for late effects and gate-keeping for the referral to specialist adult services, the patient has the added advantage of still being in contact with their treatment centre.

Research and audit

Collaboration with and instigation of research are an important component of the LTFU nurse's role. It is only in the past 30 years that survival rates for childhood cancer have started to improve (Robertson *et al.*, 1994; Gatta *et al.*, 2003), therefore in medical terms this is a new speciality and one in which there are many areas to be explored. There is also a need to develop more evidence-based practice in caring for this cohort of patients that takes the risk/benefit ratio of continuing to attend the LTFU clinic into account. The protection and advocacy of the patient need to be actively pursued while undertaking the research, as they are a new and interesting group but consequently can be in danger of being over-researched. The types of research can include the exploration of medical, psychological and social late effects. LTFU, however, does need to be the subject of research in order to inform care and provide follow-up that is evidence-based (Hawkins, 2004).

Audit is essential in discovering if the patient is receiving efficient and appropriate interventions, looking at the needs of the patient and if they are being met. Are the patients satisfied with the service? How could it be improved? These are questions that audit can answer. It is important to ascertain the service users' views to provide a service that fulfils their requirements.

Health promotion provision

The LTFU clinic is an ideal place to provide health promotion. The patients already attend the clinic focusing on health issues and are likely to have built up a trusting relationship with the LTFU nurse. Childhood cancer survivors are at an increased risk of developing a second malignancy and also have other potential health risks due to their previous cancer treatments, therefore the lifestyle choices that they make can increase or reduce that risk (Hawkins, 2004). Consequently provision of health promotion can increase the quality of the care that the patient receives and this will be explored comprehensively in Chapter 26.

Participation in specialist LTFU clinics

Specialist clinics can add to the quality of the care that the patients receive. These can include fertility, neuro-oncology, bone marrow transplant and endocrine clinics. Neuro-oncology and bone marrow transplant clinics focus on a specific cohort of patients with the benefit of specialisation and consequently increased knowledge and experience. The endocrine and fertility clinics deal with late effects of the treatment. The LTFU nurse can be involved in all of these clinics and, certainly, in those run by other specialists the nurse can contribute with expertise of late effects of the particular treatment that the patient received. The nurse can also act as advocate and support for the patient in these situations.

Conclusion

The LTFU nurse is working in an ever-evolving field as treatment protocols change and to a certain extent potential late effects. Research is prolific targeting childhood cancer survivors so there is a need to keep up to date and anticipate the future needs of the service. For the nurse who has looked after acutely ill children with cancer it is uplifting to see those who are followed up long term going to university, gaining employment, getting married and having families. The role of the nurse in LTFU can be both challenging and rewarding.

References

Campbell J, German L, Lane C & Dodwell D (2000) 'Radiotherapy outpatient review: a nurse-led clinic' *Clinical Oncology* 12(2): 104–107

Connor CA, Wright CC & Fegan CD (2002) 'The safety and effectiveness of a nurse-led anticoagulant service' *Journal of Advanced Nursing* 38(4): 407–415

Cox K & Wilson E (2003) 'Follow up for people with cancer: nurse-led services and telephone interventions' *Journal of Advanced Nursing* 43(1): 51–61

Gatta G, Corazziari I, Magnani C, Peris-Bonet R, Roazzi P & Stiller C (2003) 'Childhood cancer survival in Europe' *Annals of Oncology* 14(suppl. 5): 119–127

Gibson F, Aslett H, Levitt G & Richardson A (2005) 'Developing alternative models of follow-up care in the young adult survivor of childhood cancer' *CLIC Sargent Final Report* November 2005

Gibson F & Soanes L (2001) 'Long-term follow-up following childhood cancer: maximizing the contribution from nursing'. *European Journal of Cancer* 37: 1859–1868

Griffiths A (ed.) (2005) *After Cure*. Leicester: Childhood Cancer and Leukaemia Group (CCLG)

Hawkins M (2004) 'Long-term survivors of childhood cancers' *Nature Clinical Practice Oncology* 1: 26–31

Horne B (2004) 'Postal follow-up of care for childhood cancer survivors' *Cancer Nursing Practice* 3(9): 26–28

Robertson CM, Hawkins MM & Kingston JE (1994) 'Late deaths and survival after childhood cancer: implications for cure' *British Medical Journal* 309(6948): 162–166

Scottish Intercollegiate Guidelines Network (2004) *Long Term Follow up of Survivors of Childhood Cancer*. Edinburgh: Scottish Intercollegiate Guidelines Network publication No. 76

Skinner R & Wallace WHB (2005) *Therapy Based Long Term Follow Up: A Practice Statement* (2nd edn). Leicester: United Kingdom Childhood Cancer Study Group

Zeltzer LK, Chen E, Weiss R, Guo, MD, Robison LL *et al.* (1997) 'Comparison of psychologic outcome in adult survivors of childhood acute lymphoblastic leukemia versus sibling controls: a cooperative Children's Cancer Group and National Institutes of Health study' *Journal of Clinical Oncology* 15(2): 547–556

26 Health Promotion for Long-Term Follow-Up Patients

Beverly Horne

Health promotion encompasses activities that address increasing levels of well-being and attempts to maximise a person's health potential (Pender, 1987). Risks to health can come from a number of factors, for example, genetic make-up, environment, health behaviours and exposure to infections. Reducing the risk of cancer is one of the most important reasons to carry out health promotion as cancer will affect one in three people within their lifetime, with the most common cancers being lung and breast (Department of Health, 2000a).

For a long-term follow-up (LTFU) patient, access to health promotion can improve the quality of the care that they receive. There is a risk in this cohort of patients of developing a second malignancy due to the carcinogenic potential of chemotherapy and radiotherapy given as treatment for the original cancer, along with the genetic predisposition in some individuals to develop tumours. Statistics from research looking at rates of second malignancies is retrospective as treatment protocols change, so it is very difficult to predict what each individual's risk of developing a second malignancy might be (Olsen *et al.*, 1993; Rosso *et al.*, 1994; de Vathaire *et al.*, 1999). Research, however, does tend to support the occurrence of second malignancies as a significant risk for childhood cancer survivors (Hawkins, 2004). Therapy

for childhood cancer can also have late effects on various body systems – heart, lungs, kidneys, etc. (see Chapter 24) – so by choosing to adopt adverse behaviours that risk their health, such as smoking or excessive alcohol consumption, they may be adding to a risk that they already have. Or conversely, by choosing to abstain from behaviours that risk their health, they will not be adding to that risk. Risk-taking behaviours of childhood cancer survivors can be influenced by health professionals, addressing any knowledge deficits, ensuring survivors know where their areas of vulnerability are and providing a health promotion intervention that is targeted to their particular circumstances (Hudson & Findlay, 2006). These health promotion interventions have been shown to be successful in changing risk-taking behaviours and increasing the motivation and perception of personal risk in this cohort of patients (Cox *et al.*, 2005).

There are a number of research studies comparing childhood cancer survivors with the general population as regards to health-risk-taking behaviours (Hollen & Hobbie, 1996; Bauld *et al.*, 2005). These studies have found either no difference between the two groups or that the childhood cancer survivors were at a lower risk of indulging in health-risk behaviours. Nevertheless as this cohort already have a propensity to potential health risks due to their treatment, they would still benefit from a health promotion intervention.

The purpose of primary health promotion is to encourage people to adopt a healthier lifestyle with secondary health promotion aimed at those who have a particular risk of developing a health problem (Webb, 1994). For LTFU patients both primary and secondary health promotion is important. When the patients attend a clinic, they are already focusing on their health, they will usually have developed a rapport with and have confidence in their LTFU nurse, therefore it is an ideal opportunity to talk to them about primary and secondary health promotion. Women have contact with health professionals and the benefit of primary health promotion at times when they seek contraceptive advice or when they become pregnant. For men, however, this opportunity does not always present itself, therefore to have the chance to focus on their health and issues that are important to them is one that should be taken advantage of in the LTFU clinic. Training in health promotion and keeping up to date with new developments may be facilitated through the public health resource facility with advice on what health promotion models might be useful in the relatively short time available with the LTFU patient. As the nurse gained experience, confidence in tackling sensitive subjects would develop. Resources could be made available for the patients such as leaflets, help-line numbers, web addresses as well as the discussion, information and advice around the relevant issues. The LTFU nurse has a responsibility to highlight areas that need secondary health promotion and this will be covered in more detail in the topics explored next. *The Long Term Follow Up Therapy Based Guidelines* (Skinner & Wallace, 2005), SIGN Guidelines (SIGN, 2004) and Children's Oncology Group (COG) Guidelines (COG, 2006) have been used to identify the following potential late effects of treatment.

Topics that can be covered within health promotion for LTFU patients are listed below but are by no means comprehensive as other issues may come to light within the nurse consultation session:

- smoking;
- alcohol consumption;
- recreational drug use;
- nutrition, physical activity and achieving a healthy weight;
- breast awareness;
- testicular self-examination;
- sexual health;
- sun protection.

These areas will be explored individually, however, it is the nurse's responsibility to keep up to date with new developments in each area and to develop close contact with the local public health resource library and training centre.

Smoking

A third of all cancers are caused by smoking – lung cancer predominantly but it is also a major cause of mouth, nasal passages, larynx, bladder and pancreatic cancers (Cancer Research UK, 2007a). Smoking is the biggest single cause of cancer in the world but smoking can also cause heart disease, stroke, bronchitis and emphysema (Cancer Research UK, 2007a). Smoking is addictive but most smokers would like to quit and there are positive health benefits to stopping smoking at any age (Perceval, 2002). There is a wealth of help available to assist those who would like to quit:

- NHS smoking cessation services.
- NHS smoking help-line.
- Nicotine replacement therapy – in the form of gum, patches, lozenges, nasal spray, inhalator and tablets – are available from the pharmacy and also on prescription. They work by giving fixed amounts of nicotine in each dose but without the harmful chemicals in tobacco smoke. They can help by reducing the cravings and break the habit so allowing the person to wean him or herself off smoking (Consumers Association, 2001).
- Zyban – a prescription-only medicine that is thought to work on parts of the brain that are involved in the addiction to nicotine. It is recommended starting Zyban 1–2 weeks before stopping smoking and taken for 7–9 weeks in total (Electronic Medicines Compendium, accessed April 2007).

People can also help themselves by adopting the following (Perceval, 2002):

- Making plans for coping with stressful situations.
- Plan for the date to stop, one that will be as stress-free as possible and stick to it.
- Think positively – concentrate on the good things about stopping smoking.
- Take one day at a time and congratulate themselves every day.
- Give up with a friend and support each other.
- Use nicotine replacement therapy or Zyban to help with the cravings.
- In the beginning avoid places where they know they will be tempted to smoke.
- Keep themselves busy and try and keep active.
- Add up all the money saved and spend it on themselves.
- Don't try 'just one' cigarette – it will make them start again.

The LTFU patients who will need secondary health promotion will be those who have had radiotherapy or surgery involving the lung or chemotherapy agents that can affect the lung such as bleomycin, busulphan or CCNU; also those who have received potentially cardiotoxic treatment such as radiotherapy involving the heart or chemotherapy agents such as the anthracyclines including daunorubicin, doxorubicin, epirubicin, mitozantrone.

Alcohol consumption

The risks from drinking more alcohol on a regular basis than the daily benchmarks are: liver damage, cirrhosis of the liver and cancer of throat and mouth. The risk of throat and mouth cancer increases in people who also smoke. Psychological problems including depression can also occur with over-indulgence of alcohol in the long term.

The daily benchmarks are:

- men – less than 3 to 4 units per day;
- women – less than 2 to 3 units per day.

Keeping to these recommended units would mean that there are no significant risks to health. Drinks vary in strength and size but some examples are:

- A half pint of ordinary strength lager, beer or cider = 1 unit
- 25ml measure of spirits = 1 unit
- Small glass of wine (9%abv) = 1 unit.

Sometimes people underestimate how much they drink and actually getting them to work out their intake in units can be enough to encourage them to cut down to an amount that is not going to do them long-term harm. For those people who are having trouble stopping, help will be available through their GP or Alcoholics Anonymous or other alcohol-related charities.

The LTFU patients who will need secondary health promotion will be those who have had liver tumours or surgery or radiotherapy that has included the liver and chemotherapy agents such as methotrexate; also those patients who have had any cancer involving the mouth or throat or any surgery or radiotherapy on those areas.

Recreational drug use

The risks from recreational drugs may be unexpected. Drugs that are sold on the 'street' may have been mixed with other substances so users can never be sure what they're getting. Users can also become tolerant to some drugs so that they need to take more to get the effect that they want. Users may also overdose where they take more than their bodies can handle and this can prove fatal (Health Education Authority, 1996a; Department of Health, 2002). Drugs have a variety of risks, as shown in Table 26.1.

The LTFU patients who need to be targeted for secondary health promotion will be dependent on the recreational drug being used. However, most of the recreational drugs have neuro-psychological effects and this could cause increased problems in those patients who have had brain tumours, radiotherapy to the central nervous system or chemotherapy treatment with intrathecal methotrexate or cytarabine.

Nutrition, physical activity and achieving a healthy weight

An unhealthy diet may be responsible for up to a third of all cancer deaths. A diet that is considered

Table 26.1 Classification of drugs

Drug	Classification	Risks
Cannabis	C	Affects short-term memory, co-ordination, ability to concentrate. Increases risk of respiratory problems. Can make users paranoid and anxious. Smoking cannabis with tobacco can lead to addiction to cigarettes.
Cocaine	A	Heart problems, chest pains, convulsions. May make users restless, confused and paranoid. Snorting cocaine can permanently damage the inside of the nose.
Crack	A	Can cause fatal heart problems, chest pains, convulsions, lung damage. The user can feel restless, nauseous and have problems sleeping.
Ecstasy	A	Tightening of the jaw, nausea, sweating, an increase in the heart rate, liver and kidney problems, possibly affecting brain chemistry. Users can feel tired and depressed afterwards.
Heroin	A	Dizziness and vomiting on first use. Can cause coma and death. Highly addictive drug with tolerances developing leading to the need for increasing amounts of the drug. Injecting can lead to damage of veins and gangrene, hepatitis and HIV.
LSD	A	Hallucinogenic effect called a 'trip', which once started cannot be stopped. Hallucinogenic effects may be extremely unpleasant and even terrifying. Users can feel paranoid and out of control. Users may experience flashbacks where parts of the trip are re-lived.
Magic mushrooms	A (when prepared)	Stomach pains, sickness and diarrhoea. Eating the wrong kind of mushroom can prove fatal. Can cause bad trips similar to LSD.
Speed	B	Tiredness, depression; can affect sleep, memory and concentration. Can cause heart problems and mental illness such as psychosis.

healthy is high in fruit, vegetables and cereals and low in salt, fat and sugar. People who eat at least five portions of fruit and vegetables a day are better protected against cancer and heart disease (Department of Health, 2007). Changing to a diet that's healthy should be done in small steps in order to maximise the potential of the changes being permanent. It can include changing the type and variety of foods eaten, when they are eaten, how much is eaten and how they are prepared (Department of Health, 2007).

Physical activity can bring about many physiological and psychosocial benefits – lower blood pressure, increased lung function, lower blood sugar, lower blood cholesterol, decreased mineral bone loss, decreased body fat and weight, improved flexibility, increased stamina, improved sleep quality, decreased stress levels, improved mood and self-esteem, to name but a few (Bomar, 1996). It is also thought to reduce the risk of certain cancers (Department of Health, 2000a). Becoming more physically active is possible for any age of person. Like dietary change, increasing activity should be done gradually in order to make the chance of sticking to a new routine more likely. It is important to choose an activity that is preferred

and fits in with their lifestyle and exercising with a friend can help with motivation as well as enjoyment. If undertaking strenuous exercise, it is advisable to warm up before and cool down afterwards, be aware of how the body feels and not to overdo it, this will help to reduce risk of injuries. Activities that would be suitable include brisk walking, cycling, swimming, gardening and dancing. The ideal amount of physical activity is 30 minutes of moderate exercise per day (Health Education Authority, 1996b).

Being overweight can lead to an increased risk of high blood pressure, heart disease, some cancers, gall bladder disease and osteoarthritis. A way of measuring body fat is the Body Mass Index or BMI; the way to calculate this is by dividing body weight in kilograms by the square of the body height in metres (Bomar, 1996). There are also charts available which makes the assessment of BMI easier especially when time with the patient is limited; the healthy range for BMI is between 19 and 25. To achieve a healthy weight, a healthy eating habit must be adopted or an increase in physical activity, but ideally a combination of both is usually the most effective (Health Education Authority, 1996b). The LTFU patients who may be targeted for secondary health promotion are those who have had acute lymphoblastic leukaemia especially females who have been found to be at an increased risk of obesity (SIGN, 2004).

Breast awareness

Breast cancer is the most common cancer in women (Department of Health, 2003) and breast awareness can help in finding a cancer at an earlier and more treatable stage (Austoker, 1994). Being breast aware means that a woman knows what her breast normally looks and feels like, knows what changes to look out for, will report changes to her GP straight away and will attend breast screening if over the age of 50 years (Austoker, 1994). Changes to be aware of are:

- a change in the outline, shape or size of the breast;
- puckering or dimpling of the skin on the breast;
- any lump in the breast or armpit or any area of thickening;
- any discharge from the nipple;
- any unusual pain or discomfort in the breast;
- any change in appearance of the nipple;
- constant pain in one part of the breast or in the armpit.

(Breast Cancer Care, 2005)

The LTFU patients who would need secondary health promotion of breast awareness are those who have received chest radiotherapy including the breast tissue (Bhatia *et al.*, 1996). It is important to target this group of patients in order to inform and encourage them to practise breast awareness (Horne, 2004). The Department of Health now classes childhood cancer survivors who have had this particular treatment as being at a higher risk of developing breast cancer than the general population and have put in place a high-risk screening programme for them (Department of Health, 2003).

Testicular self-examination

Testicular cancer is rare but it is the most common cancer in men who are under the age of 35. Like breast cancer, the earlier it is found, then the more successful treatment is likely to be (Department of Health, 2000b). Testicular self-examination is recommended as a way of early detection of testicular cancer. The following advice can be given (Department of Health, 2000b):

- Hold the scrotum in the palm of the hand and notice changes in the heaviness, shape or size of the testicles (it is normal for one testicle to hang lower than the other).
- Examine each testicle by using the hands to roll them between thumbs and fingers, they should feel smooth.
- Compare for any differences between the two testicles, there is little likelihood of something unusual being found in both.
- Other signs to look out for are a dull ache in the groin or abdomen, heaviness in the scrotum or pain in the testicle.

It is best for them to examine themselves in the bath or shower when the testicles are softer, making it easier to detect any changes. Testicular cancer is not the only cause of abnormalities though as the testicle can develop cysts or fluid collections, but an early review by the GP is essential to obtain a diagnosis. LTFU patients who need secondary health promotion addressing testicular self-examination include those who have had radiotherapy that has included the testes.

Sexual health

There is a risk of developing sexually transmitted diseases, including hepatitis B, HIV, chlamydia, genital warts and genital herpes for people who are sexually active, both homosexual and heterosexual. An extra risk for women is cervical cancer which has been linked to multiple sexual partners, early sexual activity or a history of sexually transmitted diseases (Nettina, 2006).

Having safer sex is recommended in order to reduce the likelihood of the risks of sexually transmitted diseases and also of unplanned pregnancies. Safer sex involves the use of condoms as barrier contraception (Department of Health, 2000b), and condoms still need to be used even if another contraceptive method is being used (Family Planning Association (FPA), 1995). Some Family Planning Association clinics and GP surgeries provide free condoms and the FPA has a helpline service that provides confidential information and advice on contraception and sexual health.

Sun protection

The main cause of skin cancer is the sun; most people do know about this but do not necessarily protect themselves from the risk (Department of Health, 2000a). People who are generally at risk are those with white skin, those who have lived in sunny countries and those with lots of moles. Also more specifically people with fair or freckled skin that doesn't tan; with red or fair hair and pale eyes; who have suffered from severe sunburn, especially in childhood; who have a personal or family history of melanoma; who have an outdoor job; or who have unusual moles – large, irregular and multi-coloured (Cancer Research UK, 2007b).

To protect the skin from the sun, the following advice is recommended (Cancer Research UK, 2007b):

- Take care not to burn.
- Avoid the sun between 11am and 3pm.
- Use a sunscreen all the time (SPF 15 or higher with UVA protection) even if tanned.
- Wear a wide-brimmed hat, UV protected sunglasses, tightly woven, loose-fitting clothing or keep in the shade.

A doctor should be consulted immediately if a mole or dark patch is getting larger or a new one is growing, if a mole has a ragged outline, if a mole has a mixture of different shades of black and brown. A doctor should be consulted within two weeks if the following signs have not resolved – inflammation of the mole or a reddish edge; bleeding, oozing or crusting mole, an itchy mole; or one that is noticeably larger than all the other moles. Patients attending the LTFU clinic who would need secondary health promotion of advice on sun protection are those that have received any radiotherapy as they are at a slightly increased risk of getting a skin cancer within the radiotherapy field.

Theoretical approaches and models

There are a number of theoretical approaches and models that can be used within health promotion. In caring for patients within a LTFU setting time is limited and the patients only return once a year so the practicalities need to be borne in mind for whatever approach and model adopted. A variety of topics are likely to be discussed and this may call for a range of approaches in any one session.

Approaches – examples (Naidoo & Wills, 2000):

- Behavioural change approach may be needed with a person who wishes to stop smoking.
- Educational approach may be used in guiding someone towards eating a healthier diet.
- Medical approach may be used in encouraging women to attend for cervical screening.
- Empowerment approach may be used with drug abusers.

There are also various models that could be used and just one example – the Health Belief Model – is explored below but others may be of use in this setting such as the Health Action Model which looks at issues of motivating factors and inhibitors to change behaviour (Tones & Tilford, 1994); or perhaps the Stages of Change model which describes behavioural change as pre-contemplation (not even considering changing behaviour), contemplation, action and maintenance of the change. Relapse is possible at any stage and the model stresses that realistic aims and commitment are essential for success (Katz & Perberdy, 1997).

Health Belief Model

In order to understand how a health professional might influence a LTFU patient to lead a healthier lifestyle, the Health Belief Model will be examined. The model is based on the assumption that a person must believe that they are at risk of developing a health problem in order for them to take action (Becker, 1974). The main circumstances that can influence behaviour are said to be: a person's perceived susceptibility to a disease; perceived severity of a disease; perceived costs and benefits of taking preventative action; perceived barriers to taking action; and cues to action. Cues to action encompass such situations as getting advice from peers, media campaigns, having a friend or family with an illness, or reading or hearing a news article relating to the problem (Becker, 1974).

Using a theoretical framework can help the health professional ascertain what might be useful in encouraging the LTFU patient to adopt a particular action, for instance, for those patients requiring secondary health promotion, the perceived susceptibility of a disease can be explored in relation to the previous cancer treatment. Perceived barriers can be explored for all the topics and advice may be able to be given that can help in overcoming these, for instance, one of the barriers to stopping smoking may be the fear of weight gain and this can be addressed by information on healthy diet and exercise. Each person will need to be individually assessed with regard to his or her health promotion intervention and information and advice given appropriately.

Conclusion

A realistic expectation of what can be achieved with health promotion in the LTFU clinic is needed as time with the patient is limited and infrequent but over the years hopefully a trusting therapeutic relationship will develop. The nurse will be able to re-visit what has been discussed previously, to explore progress on any behavioural changes planned and provide up-to-date information and advice on a variety of lifestyle choices. The quality of care that the LTFU patient receives will be enhanced by access to health promotion within a therapeutic setting.

References

Austoker J (1994) 'Screening and self-examination for breast cancer' *British Medical Journal* 309: 168–174

Bauld C, Toumbourou JW, Anderson V, Coffey C & Olsson CA (2005) 'Health-risk behaviours among adolescent survivors of childhood cancer' *Pediatric Blood & Cancer* 45(5): 706–715

Becker MH (1974) *The Health Belief Model and Personal Health Behaviour*. Thorofare, MJ: Charles B. Slack

Bhatia S, Robison LL, Oberlin O, Greenberg N, Bunin M, Greta M, Fossati-Bellani F & Meadows A (1996) 'Breast cancer and other second neoplasms after childhood Hodgkin's disease' *The New England Journal of Medicine* 334(12): 745–751

Bomar PJ (1996) *Nurses and Family Health Promotion*. Philadelphia, PA: WB Saunders Company

Breast Cancer Care (2005) *Breast Awareness* http://www.breastcancercare.org.uk Accessed April 2007

Cancer Research UK (2007a) *Smoking and Cancer – Beat the Addiction*. http://info.cancerresearchuk.org

Cancer Research UK (2007b) *Malignant Melanoma*. http://info.cancerresearchuk.org

Children's Oncology Group (2006) *Long-Term Follow-up Guidelines*. Children's Oncology Group, CureSearch

Consumers Association (2001) *Medicines to Help You Stop Smoking*. London: Consumers Association

Cox CL, McLaughlin RA, Raj SN, Steen BD & Hudson MM (2005) 'Adolescent survivors: a secondary analysis of a clinical trial targeting behavior change' *Pediatric Blood & Cancer* 45(2): 144–154

Department of Health (2000a) *The NHS Cancer Plan*. London: Department of Health

Department of Health (2000b) *Sexual Health for Men*. London: Department of Health

Department of Health (2002) *The Score: Facts about Drugs*. London: Department of Health

Department of Health (2003) 'Advice and support to be offered to women whose treatment for Hodgkin's disease may have increased their risk of breast cancer'. Press release 2003/0434, 10 November

Department of Health (2007) *How Much is Too Much? Drinking, You and Your Mates*. http://www.dh.gov.uk/ accessed April 2007

de Vathaire F, Hawkins M, Campbell S, Oberlin O, Raquin M, Schlienger J, Shamsaldin A *et al.* (1999) 'Second malignant neoplasms after a first cancer in childhood: temporal pattern of risk according to type of treatment' *British Journal of Cancer* 79(11/12): 1884–1893

Family Planning Association (1995) *Your Guide to Safer Sex and the Condom*. London: FPA

Hawkins M (2004) 'Long term survivors of childhood cancers: what knowledge have we gained? *Nature Clinical Practice Oncology* 1: 26–31

Health Education Authority (1996a) *A Parent's Guide to Drugs and Alcohol*. London: Health Education Authority

Health Education Authority (1996b) *Getting Active, Feeling Fit*. London: Health Education Authority

Hollen PJ & Hobbie WL (1993) 'Risk taking and decision making of adolescent long-term survivors of cancer' *Oncology Nurses Forum* 20: 769–776

Horne B (2004) 'Promoting breast awareness in childhood cancer survivors' *Cancer Nursing Practice* 3(6): 16–29

Hudson MM & Findlay S (2006) 'Health-risk behaviors and health promotion in adolescent and young adult cancer survivors' *Cancer* 197(7 suppl.): 1695–1701

Katz J & Perberdy A (1997) *Promoting Health Knowledge and Practice*. London: Macmillan

Naidoo J & Wills J (2000) *Health Promotion: Foundations for Practice*. Edinburgh: Bailliere Tindall

Nettina SM (2006) *The Lippincott Manual of Nursing Practice* (8th edn). Philadelphia, PA: Lippincott, Williams & Wilkins

Olsen JH, Garwicz S, Hertz H, Jonmundsson G, Langmark F *et al.* (1993) 'Second malignant neoplasms after cancer in childhood or adolescence' *British Medical Journal* 307: 1030–1036

Pender NJ (1987) *Health Promotion in Nursing Practice* (2nd edn). Norwalk: Appleton & Lange

Perceval J (2002) *Giving up for Life*. London: Department of Health

Rosso P, Terracini B & Fears TR (1994) 'Second malignant tumours after elective end of therapy for a first cancer in childhood: a multicenter study in Italy' *International Journal of Cancer* 59: 451–456

Scottish Intercollegiate Guidelines Network (2004) *Long Term Follow up of Survivors of Childhood Cancer*. Edinburgh: Scottish Intercollegiate guidelines network publication No. 76

Skinner R & Wallace WHB (2005) *Therapy Based Long Term Follow Up: A Practice Statement* (2nd edn). Leicester: United Kingdom Childhood Cancer Study Group

Tones I & Tilford S (1994) *Health Education, Effectiveness, Efficiency and Equity* (2nd edn). London: Chapman & Hall

Webb P (ed.) (1994) *Health Promotion and Patient Education: A Professional's Guide*. London: Chapman & Hall

27 Quality of Life in Long-Term Survivors of Childhood Cancer

Anthony Penn

In the past thirty to forty years, advances in the diagnosis, treatment and support as well as the centralisation of care of children with cancer have resulted in improved long-term survival. Between 70 and 75% of children and adolescents treated for cancer in the United States and Western Europe will achieve long-term survivorship (Gloeckler Ries *et al.*, 2003, Steliarova-Foucher *et al.*, 2004). Increased risk stratification aims to ensure that patients with good prognosis are not over-treated and put at risk for unnecessary late effects, and allows those with worse prognosis to have the best chance of cure. As a result, some children with cancer receive less intense treatment, while others with poorer prognoses receive more intense treatment than ever before. As more children are surviving cancer into adulthood and beyond, it has been recognised that the quality as well as the quantity of life is important when considering outcome in childhood cancer. Quality of life measures have become increasingly important in quantifying the burden of morbidity faced by children treated for childhood cancer. The Medical Research Council (UK) and the National Cancer Institutes (in the United States and Canada) insist that all clinical trials requiring sponsorship must include quality-of-life measures (MRC, 1996; Nayfield *et al.*, 1992).

Defining quality of life in the health-care setting?

Agreement on an acceptable definition of quality of life (QOL) has been difficult to attain. Bradlyn & Pollock (1996) suggested that it includes the social, physical and emotional functioning of the child or adolescent (and family), and that it is sensitive to the changes that occur throughout development. Quality of life is therefore multidimensional. It should take into account the survivor's ability to participate in everyday activities and where appropriate, family functioning. It is subjective, and measures of quality of life should always be made by the cancer survivor themselves, wherever possible.

It is important in the understanding of QOL that the same disease and/or treatment may not necessarily have an equal impact on each individual. The impact also depends on past experiences, lifestyle, hopes for the future, dreams and ambitions of the survivor and their ability to adapt to changes brought about by their illness and its treatment (Schipper *et al.*, 1996). For example, lower limb surgery for bone tumour may impact differently on different people. For a keen sportsman, loss of previous mobility may mean giving up dreams of

Cancer in Children and Young People   Edited by Faith Gibson and Louise Soanes
© 2008 John Wiley & Sons, Ltd

becoming a professional athlete as well as loss of access to previous social, sporting activities and friendships. For others, loss of mobility may not be so great and have little effect on their QOL.

Physical function

Physical late effects of treatment such as cardiomyopathy, endocrine disorders, obesity or physical defects due to surgery or radiotherapy can all affect the health status, physical functioning and QOL in survivors of childhood cancer. While there have been many reports on adverse physical late effects or outcome in survivors of childhood and adolescent cancer, little has been done to define the effects these physical disabilities have on quality of life.

Reports on physical function in childhood cancer survivors differ, depending on cancer type, treatment received and measures used to define physical health status. Generally survivors of childhood cancer report good physical health in comparison to normal controls, with the important exception of brain tumour, bone tumour and sarcoma survivors, who tend to score their physical health as being worse than other cancer survivors and/or normal controls (Apajasalo et al., 1996; Moe et al., 1997; Novakovic et al., 1997). This is despite the fact that approximately 65–75% of childhood cancer survivors are reported to have one or more physical late effects (Lackner et al., 2000; Oeffinger et al., 2000).

To date, the most relevant study addressing late effects, including physical function in long-term survivors of childhood cancer, is the large multi-institutional Childhood Cancer Survivor Study (CCSS). The group have produced some seminal work on health status, HRQL and other outcome measures in survivors of various types of childhood cancer (Gurney et al., 2003; Hudson et al., 2003; Nagarajan et al., 2004; Punyko et al., 2005). The study found that survivors were more likely than a randomly selected cohort of survivors' siblings, to report adverse heath status in the physical domains (Hudson et al., 2003). Predictably, adverse health status was more likely to be reported by survivors of brain tumours, bone tumours and sarcomas, due to aggressive multimodality treatment and its effect on areas of the body like the developing brain. A second report by

the CCSS on bone tumour patients found similar physical health and HRQL in amputee survivors compared with those who underwent limb-sparing surgery. Both groups of survivors reported excellent physical function and quality-of-life (Nagarajan et al., 2004).

Survivors report that treatment-related symptoms does not impact as negatively on QOL as long-term effects like aches, pain and fatigue (Zebrack & Chesler, 2002). Glaser et al. (1999) reported that pain affected approximately one-third of brain tumour survivors. Most studies of fatigue in survivors of cancer diagnosed in adulthood showed an increased reported incidence of fatigue (Holzner et al., 2003; Loge et al. 1999; Howell et al., 2000; Ruffer et al., 2003), with only a few finding no difference between survivors and controls (Smets et al., 1998). There is less published data on the prevalence of fatigue in the paediatric oncology population, and although some studies have shown excess fatigue in children undergoing or recently off treatment for cancer, the prevalence of fatigue in long-term survivors is not as clear. Langeveld et al. (2000) found fatigue to be a significant problem for some survivors. In contrast, a more recent report by the same group found no excess fatigue in survivors who had completed treatment an average of 15 years prior to there study (Langeveld et al., 2003). In a recent study by Meeske et al. (2004), children with brain tumours off treatment for more than a year (average 5.6 years without treatment) had significantly lower mean scores for fatigue than that in the normal population, suggesting increased fatigue in this population. Acute lymphoblastic leukaemia patients (average 6.5 years without treatment) scored in the normal range. Fatigue severity was inversely related to overall HRQL in this study (Meeske et al., 2004).

Psychological function

The incidence of psychological disturbance in survivors of childhood cancer has been well described, although findings vary. Some studies have found a significantly higher incidence of psychological problems compared to population norms and normal or sibling controls (Zeltzer et al., 1997; Zebrack & Chesler, 2002; Glover et al., 2003). In contrast, other studies reported no significant difference in psychological status between survivors and controls, with survivors being similar to the normal population or even doing better with regards to psychological function and QOL (Gray *et al.*, 1992; Apajasalo *et al.*, 1996; Elkin *et al.*, 1997; Eiser *et al.*, 2000). Gray *et al.*, (1992) found that survivors reported significantly more positive mood, less negative mood, higher intimacy motivation, more perceived personal control, and greater satisfaction with life than controls. However, the same study found that survivors were more likely than peers to have repeated years at school, be worried about issues of fertility, and to express dissatisfaction with important relationships

Post-traumatic stress disorder (PTSD), characterised by unwanted re-experiencing of a traumatic event, avoidance of reminders of the trauma and psychological arousal is increasingly being used to help explain the psychosocial consequences of having cancer as a child (Hobbie *et al.*, 2000, Kazak *et al.*, 2004, Langeveld *et al.*, 2004, Schwartz & Drotar, 2005). In order for a diagnosis of PTSD to be given, a person must have been exposed to an event defined as an imminent threat to life or a serious injury (in this case, cancer) and must manifest a psychological reaction (usually fear) to the event. Between 4.5 and 25% of survivors of childhood cancer have symptoms that meet the criteria for a diagnosis of PTSD, with additional survivors experiencing trauma symptoms, but not meeting the criteria for diagnosis of PTSD. The occurrence of PTSD in survivors appears to be associated with retrospective appraisal of threat to life at diagnosis, the degree to which the survivors' experience of the treatment was 'hard' or 'scary' as well as general anxiety, history of other stressful life events, female gender and lack of family or social support (Zebrack *et al.*, 2005). Interestingly, PTSD and post-traumatic stress symptoms seem to be more common in parents of survivors, than in the survivors themselves (Kazak *et al.*, 2004).

More recently the concept of post-traumatic growth (PTG) in survivors of childhood cancer has been introduced, suggesting that some survivors may not only 'survive', but also derive benefit or 'thrive' as a result of their difficult, life-threatening experience. Survivors who have a sense of purpose in life and perceive positive changes as a result

of cancer, report higher quality of life (Zebrack & Chesler, 2002). Some authors have suggested that such reports may be due to denial mechanisms on the part of the survivor (Apajasalo *et al.*, 1996, Elkin *et al.*, 1997), but Zebrack and Chesler (2001) showed that adolescents and young adults with cancer can experience positive self-images and outlook on life without necessarily denying their true condition or fears.

Cognition

Deficits in cognition, particularly in children treated with cranial irradiation and/or intrathecal methotrexate for brain tumour or leukaemia, may also adversely affect QOL in long-term survivors of childhood cancer. Cognitive deficit may affect academic achievement, limit occupational opportunities and contribute to difficulties in establishing independence and social integration in long-term survivors. Principal risk factors for children treated for brain tumours have been outlined in a recent paper (Grill *et al.*, 2004). Young age at diagnosis, neurofibromatosis type 1, hydrocephalus at presentation, surgical complications, increasing interval since treatment and importantly, the use of cumulative dose and volume of cranial irradiation were all described as certain risk factors for cognitive impairment.

Social function

Educational attainment, employment status, medical insurance, interpersonal relationships, marital status, parenthood and living situation have all been used to estimate differences in social integration between survivors and either the general population using population statistics, sibling controls or 'normal' non-cancer controls. The use of different outcome measures and different controls, as well as small numbers of survivors in some studies makes interpretation of the literature challenging. The hypothesis that survivors will do worse than the normal population in the above measures of achievement does not take into account that the cancer experience may change an individual's view on what is important in life, and that survivors' goals and ambitions may change as a result (Eiser

1998). Nevertheless, social integration is important, and does impact significantly on the QOL of childhood cancer survivors.

Education

Diagnosis of cancer and its treatment may affect school and education in many ways. Children may suffer cognitive deficits as a result of treatment. They may also miss a lot of school while hospitalised or recovering from treatment and as a result may fall behind their peers academically. Many studies have found little difference between survivors in general and either controls or population samples with regard to educational achievement (Allen *et al.*, 1990; Hays *et al.*, 1992; Dolgin *et al.*, 1999; Pastore *et al.*, 2001). However, subgroups of survivors who did not do as well with regard to educational achievement were identified. Hays *et al.* (1992) report decreased educational status in survivors of CNS tumours which is not surprising considering the aggressive multi-modal treatment used in some intracranial tumours, and the deleterious effect of cranial radiotherapy (CRT) on the developing brain.

Studies assessing academic achievement in survivors of acute lymphoblastic leukaemia (ALL) have revealed inconsistent results, although CRT, especially when given to young children does seem to play a major role (Mulhern *et al.*, 1992; Haupt *et al.*, 1994; Moe *et al.*, 1997; Kingma *et al.*, 2002). Kingma *et al.* (2002) found a significant difference in secondary education between survivors of ALL treated with CRT and siblings, with younger survivors fairing worse than those over 7 years of age. A recent large study from the CCSS by Mitby *et al.* (2003) found that survivors of all the major childhood cancer diagnoses were at increased risk of utilising special education services, with survivors of CNS tumours, ALL and Hodgkin disease at highest risk. The study also found that survivors of CNS tumours, leukaemia, non-Hodgkin's lymphoma and neuroblastoma were significantly less likely than siblings to complete high school. Time off school, limitations in participation in physical activities as well as experiencing a unique life-threatening event may also lead to social isolation from their peers and difficulties in establishing lasting meaningful relationships, as well as limiting future employment.

Employment and insurance

Independent living with the prospect of financial independence contributes to an individual's QOL (Jenney & Levitt, 2002). Some studies have reported job discrimination, decreased employment or decreased income in survivors of childhood cancer which in general seems to be most prevalent in survivors of CNS tumours (Mostow *et al.*, 1991; Dolgin *et al.*, 1998; Pui *et al.*, 2003). A large study by Pui *et al.* (2003) on long-term survivors of childhood ALL found that the rates of health insurance coverage and employment in survivors treated without CRT was similar to age and sex- adjusted national averages for the United States. Survivors may also have difficulties acquiring jobs or placements in the military services, either due to not fulfilling entry criteria, or as a result of history of cancer (Dolgin, *et al.*, 1999; Hays, 1993). Other studies found no difference in employment status or job discrimination between survivors and either controls or the general public (Evans & Radford, 1995; Pastore *et al.*, 2001; Boman & Bodegard, 2004).

Regarding insurance, many survivors report having had difficulties when applying for health or life insurance (for instance when applying for a mortgage) (Teta *et al.*, 1986; Hays, 1993; Vann *et al.*, 1995). Survivors may have to pay higher premiums, accept exclusion clauses, be refused certain types of insurance such as critical illness cover, or in some cases be refused health or life insurance altogether (personal communication with childhood cancer survivors). Increasing awareness of the prevalence of late effects and disability following childhood cancer may have the unfortunate effect of making it more difficult, or expensive for survivors to attain insurance in the future. A recent American study on the health care of young adult survivors of childhood cancer by Oeffinger *et al.* (2004) found a significant relationship between absence of health insurance and not reporting a general physical examination, a cancer-related visit, or a cancer centre visit which suggests that the presence or absence of health insurance may determine the extent of follow-up and health care in this potentially at-risk population.

Survivors also seem to worry about employment and insurance and this may affect QOL. Unemployed survivors report lower global self-worth scores than employed, and among survivors, predictors of negative self-concept included unemployment and believing that cancer treatment limited employability (Seitzman et al., 2004).

Interpersonal relationships and marriage

Problems with establishing and maintaining close interpersonal relationships have been reported among long-term survivors (Mackie et al., 2000). Prior social networks may not provide the type or kind of support that long-term survivors seek (Chesler & Barbarin, 1984). Specifically, adolescents and young adults report feeling that some friends are no longer able to relate to their life situation and get uncomfortable continuously talking with the patient about cancer, resulting in feelings of being 'different' and apprehensive about forming new friendships (Chesler et al., 1992). Consequently, many of these young people form (or would like to form) new friendship circles, often with other cancer patients and survivors with whom they feel can relate to their current life situation and past experience with cancer. National and international survivor meetings such as the International Confederation of Childhood Cancer Parents Organization (ICCCPO) Survivors' Conference allow fellow survivors to meet and discuss their experiences and feelings without feeling awkward and embarrassed, or worrying whether they will be understood. Such meetings also allow cancer survivors to learn about relevant, important issues such as late effects, long-term follow-up and life insurance.

With regard to interpersonal relationships, many studies have used marriage as a proxy for successful long-term relationships. Although some studies have found no difference in marital status (Dolgin et al., 1999), the majority of larger studies have found that survivors of childhood cancer are less likely to be married or to live as married than either normal controls, siblings or the general population

(Byrne et al., 1989; Nagarajan et al., 2003; Stam et al., 2005). When comparing tumour types, survivors of CNS tumours, particularly males, were less likely to have ever married and more likely to divorce or separate compared to those with other cancer diagnoses and the general US population. This once again emphasises the impact CNS disease and its treatment may have on QOL.

A recent Dutch study compared the course of life (attainment of developmental tasks and milestones) and socio-demographic outcomes in young survivors of childhood cancer with that of normal controls. Survivors achieved fewer milestones, or achieved them at an older age than their peers with regard to autonomy, social and psychosexual development (Stam et al., 2005). For example, survivors were found on average to have gone on holiday without their parents and experienced sexual intimacy at a later age than controls. Survivors also reported having fewer friends at secondary school than controls. Survivors were also found to differ from controls in some socio-demographic areas, including being less likely to be married or living with a partner, or be employed. The authors conclude, based on developmental psychology theory, that a course of life hampered by cancer and its treatment may lead to adjustment difficulties later in life, and that attention to specific deficits or gaps may assist health care providers in promoting favourable outcome for children with cancer both during and after treatment.

Conclusion

In summary, the literature available on quality of life in survivors of childhood cancer shows that while most survivors report a good quality of life, there is an important minority with physical and/or psychosocial lateeffects impacting negatively on their health status and quality of life. What has also become clear is that some survivors seem to experience a higher quality of life after their illness, as a result of their experience, than before. More research is needed to better define the variables both during and after treatment that may affect QOL in survivors, and to explain why some survivors thrive while others do not. This will help with the design of appropriate interventions and create support systems for children with cancer and their families to ensure good quality of life and promote post-traumatic growth for all childhood cancer survivors.

References

Allen A, Malpas JS & Kingston JE (1990) 'Educational achievements of survivors of childhood cancer' *Pediatric Hematology Oncology* 7(4): 339

Apajasalo M, Sintonen H, Siimes MA, Hovi L, Holmberg C, Boyd H, Makela A & Rautonen J (1996) 'Health-related quality of life of adults surviving malignancies in childhood' *European Journal of Cancer* 32(8): 1354–1358

Boman KK & Bodegard G (2004) 'Life after cancer in childhood: social adjustment and educational and vocational status of young-adult survivors' *Journal Pediatric Hematology Oncology* 26(6): 354–362

Bradlyn, AS & Pollock BH (1996) 'Quality-of-life research in the Pediatric Oncology Group: 1991–1995' *Journal National Cancer Institute* Monogram 20: 49–53

Byrne J, Fears TR, Steinhorn SC, Mulvihill JJ, Connelly RR, Austin DF *et al.* (1989) 'Marriage and divorce after childhood and adolescent cancer' *JAMA* 262(19): 2693–2699

Chesler MA & Barbarin O (1984) 'Difficulties of providing help in a crisis: Relationships between parents of children with cancer and their friends' *Journal of Social Issues* 40(4): 113–134

Chesler MA, Weigers M & Lawther T (1992) 'How am I different? Perspectives for childhood cancer survivors on change and growth' *in*: Green DM & D'Angio G (eds), *Late Effects of Treatment for Childhood Cancer*. New York: Wiley and Sons

Dolgin MJ, Somer E, Buchvald E & Zaizov R (1999) 'Quality of life in adult survivors of childhood cancer', *Social Work Health Care* 28(4): 31–43

Eiser C (1998) 'Practitioner review: long-term consequences of childhood cancer' *Journal of Child Psychology Psychiatry* 39(5): 621–633

Eiser C, Hill JJ & Vance YH (2000) 'Examining the psychological consequences of surviving childhood cancer: systematic review as a research method in pediatric psychology' *Journal Pediatric Psychology* 25(6): 449–460

Elkin TD, Phipps S, Mulhern RK & Fairclough D (1997) 'Psychological functioning of adolescent and young adult survivors of pediatric malignancy' *Medical Pediatric Oncology* 29(6): 582–588

Evans SE & Radford M (1995) 'Current lifestyle of young adults treated for cancer in childhood' *Archive Diseases of Childhood* 72(5): 423–426

Glaser A, Furlong W, Walker DA, Fielding K, Davies K, Feeny DH & Barr RD (1999) 'Applicability of the Health Utilities Index to a population of childhood survivors of central nervous system tumours in the U.K' *European Journal of Cancer* 35(2): 256–261

Gloeckler Ries LA, Reichman ME, Lewis DR, Hankey BF & Edwards BK (2003) 'Cancer survival and incidence from the Surveillance, Epidemiology, and End Results (SEER) program' *Oncologist* 8(6): 541–552

Glover DA, Byrne J, Mills JL, Robison LL, Nicholson HS, Meadows A & Zeltzer LK (2003) 'Impact of CNS treatment on mood in adult survivors of childhood leukemia: a report from the Children's Cancer Group', *Journal of Clinical Oncology* 21(23): 4395–4401

Gray RE, Doan BD, Shermer P, FitzGerald A, Berry M, Jenkin D & Doherty M (1992) 'Psychologic adaptation of survivors of childhood cancer' *Cancer* 70(11): 2713–2721

Grill J, Kieffer V & Kalifa C (2004) 'Measuring the neuro-cognitive side-effects of irradiation in children with brain tumors' *Pediatic Blood and Cancer* 42(5): 452–456

Gurney JG, Kadan-Lottick NS, Packer RJ, Neglia JP, Sklar CA *et al.* (2003) 'Endocrine and cardiovascular late effects among adult survivors of childhood brain tumors: Childhood Cancer Survivor Study' *Cancer* 97(3): 663–673

Haupt R, Fears TR, Robison LL, Mills JL, Nicholson HS, Zeltzer LK, Meadows AT & Byrne J (1994) 'Educational attainment in long-term survivors of childhood acute lymphoblastic leukaemia' *JAMA* 272(18): 1427–1432

Hays DM, Landsverk J, Sallan SE, Hewett KD *et al.* (1992) 'Educational, occupational, and insurance status of childhood cancer survivors in their fourth and fifth decades of life' *Journal of Clinical Oncology* 10(9): 1397–1406

Hobbie WL, Stuber M, Meeske K, Wissler K, Rourke MT, Ruccione K, Hinckle A & Kazak A (2000) 'Symptoms of posttraumatic stress in young adult survivors of childhood cancer' *Journal of Clinical Oncology* 18(24): 4060–4066

Holzner B, Kemmler G, Meraner V, Maislinger A, Kopp M, Bodner T, Nguyen-Van-Tam D *et al.* (2003) 'Fatigue in ovarian carcinoma patients: a neglected issue?' *Cancer* 97(6): 1564–1572

Howell SJ, Radford JA, Smets EM & Shalet SM (2000) 'Fatigue, sexual function and mood following treatment for haematological malignancy: the impact of mild Leydig cell dysfunction' *British Journal of Cancer* 82(4): 789–793

Hudson MM, Mertens AC, Yasui Y, Hobbie W, Chen H *et al.* (2003) 'Health status of adult long-term survivors of childhood cancer: a report from the Childhood Cancer Survivor Study' *JAMA* 290(12): 1583–1592

Jenney ME & Levitt GA (2002) 'The quality of survival after childhood cancer' *European Journal of Cancer* 38(9): 1241–1250

Kazak AE, Alderfer M, Rourke MT, Simms S, Streisand R & Grossman JR (2004) 'Posttraumatic stress disorder (PTSD) and posttraumatic stress symptoms (PTSS) in families of adolescent childhood cancer survivors' *Journal of Pediatric Psychology* 29(3): 211–219

Kingma A, Van Dommelen RI, Mooyaart EL, Wilmink JT, Deelman BG & Kamps WA (2002) 'No major cognitive impairment in young children with acute lymphoblastic leukemia using chemotherapy only: a prospective longitudinal study' *Journal of Pediatric Hematology and Oncology* 24(2): 106–114

Lackner H, Benesch M, Schagerl S, Kerbl R, Schwinger W & Urban C (2000) 'Prospective evaluation of late effects after childhood cancer therapy with a follow-up over 9 years' *European Journal of Pediatrics* 159(10): 750–758

Langeveld N, Grootenhuis MA, Voute PA, de Haan RJ & van den BC (2003) 'No excess fatigue in young adult survivors of childhood cancer' *European Journal of Cancer* 39(2): 204–214

Langeveld N, Ubbink M & Smets E (2000) ' "I don't have any energy": The experience of fatigue in young adult survivors of childhood cancer' *European Journal of Oncology Nursing* 4(1): 20–28

Loge JH, Abrahamsen AF, Ekeberg O & Kaasa S (1999) 'Hodgkin's disease survivors more fatigued than the general population' *Journal of Clinical Oncology* 17(1): 253–261

Mackie E, Hill J, Kondryn H & McNally R (2000) 'Adult psychosocial outcomes in long-term survivors of acute lymphoblastic leukaemia and Wilms' tumour: a controlled study' *Lancet* 355(9212): 1310–1314

Medical Research Council (1996) *The Assessment of MRC Trials 1996/1997*. London: Medical Research Council

Meeske K, Katz ER, Palmer SN, Burwinkle T & Varni JW (2004) 'Parent proxy-reported health-related quality of life and fatigue in pediatric patients diagnosed with brain tumors and acute lymphoblastic leukaemia' *Cancer* 101(9): 2116–2125

Mitby PA, Robison LL, Whitton JA, Zevon MA, Gibbs IC, Tersak JM, Meadows A *et al.* (2003) 'Utilization of special education services and educational attainment among long-term survivors of childhood cancer: a report from the Childhood Cancer Survivor Study' *Cancer* 97(4): 1115–1126

Moe PJ, Holen A, Glomstein A, Madsen B, Hellebostad M, Stokland T *et al.* (1997) 'Long-term survival and quality of life in patients treated with a national ALL protocol 15-20 years earlier: IDM/HDM and late effects?' *Pediatric Hematology Oncology* 14(6): 513–524

Mostow EN, Byrne J, Connelly RR & Mulvihill JJ (1991) 'Quality of life in long-term survivors of CNS tumors of childhood and adolescence' *Journal of Clinical Oncology* 9(4): 592–599

Mulhern RK, Phipps S & White H (2004) 'Neuropsychological outcomes' *in*: Wallace WHB & Green D (eds) *Late Effects of Childhood Cancer*. London: Arnold, pp. 18–36

Nagarajan R, Clohisy DR, Neglia JP, Yasui Y, Mitby PA, Sklar C *et al.* (2004) 'Function and quality-of-life of survivors of pelvic and lower extremity osteosarcoma and Ewing's sarcoma: the Childhood Cancer Survivor Study' *British Journal Cancer* 91(11): 1858–1865

Nayfield SG, Ganz PA, Moinpour CM, Cella DF & Hailey BJ (1992) 'Report from a National Cancer Institute (USA) workshop on quality of life assessment in cancer clinical trials', *Quality of Life Research* 1(3): 203–210

Novakovic B, Fears TR, Horowitz ME, Tucker MA & Wexler LH (1997) 'Late effects of therapy in survivors of Ewing's sarcoma family tumors' *Journal of Pediatric Hematology Oncology* 19(3): 220–225

Oeffinger KC, Mertens AC, Hudson MM, Gurney JG, Casillas J, Chen H, *et al.* (2004) 'Health care of young adult survivors of childhood cancer: a report from the Childhood Cancer Survivor Study' *Annals of Family Medicine* 2(1): 61–70

Pastore G, Mosso ML, Magnani C, Luzzatto L, Bianchi M & Terracini B (2001) 'Physical impairment and social life goals among adult long-term survivors of childhood cancer: a population-based study from the childhood cancer registry of Piedmont, Italy' *Tumori* 87(6): 372–378

Pui CH, Cheng C, Leung W, Rai SN, Rivera GK, Sandlund JT, Ribeiro RC *et al.* (2003) 'Extended follow-up of long-term survivors of childhood acute lymphoblastic leukemia' *New England Journal of Medicine* 349 (7): 640–649

Punyko JA, Mertens AC, Gurney JG, Yasui Y, Donaldson SS, Rodeberg D *et al.* (2005) 'Long-term medical effects of childhood and adolescent rhabdomyosarcoma: A report from the childhood cancer survivor study' *Pediatric Blood Cancer* 44(7): 643–653

Ruffer JU, Flechtner H, Tralls P, Josting A, Sieber M, Lathan B & Diehl V (2003) 'Fatigue in long-term survivors of Hodgkin's lymphoma: a report from the German Hodgkin Lymphoma Study Group (GHSG)' *European Journal of Cancer* 39(15): 2179–2186

Schipper H, Clinch JJ & Olweny C (1996) 'Quality of life studies: Definitions and conceptual issues' *in*: B. Spilker (ed.) *Quality of Life and Pharmacoeconomics in Clinical Trials*. Philadelphia, PA: Lippincott-Raven, pp. 11–23

Schwartz L & Drotar D (2005) 'Posttraumatic stress and related impairment in survivors of childhood cancer in early adulthood compared to healthy peers' *Journal of Pediatric Psychology*

Seitzman RL, Glover DA, Meadows AT, Mills JL, Nicholson HS *et al.* (2004) 'Self-concept in adult survivors of childhood acute lymphoblastic leukemia: a cooperative Children's Cancer Group and National Institutes of Health study' *Pediatric Blood Cancer* 42(3): 230–240

Smets EM, Visser MR, Willems-Groot AF, Garssen B, Schuster-Uitterhoeve AL & de Haes J C (1998) 'Fatigue and radiotherapy: (B) experience in patients 9 months following treatment' *British Journal of Cancer* 78(7): 907–912

Stam H, Grootenhuis MA & Last BF (2005) 'The course of life of survivors of childhood cancer' *Psycho-oncology* 14(3): 227–238

Teta MJ, Del Po MC, Kasl SV, Meigs JW, Myers MH & Mulvihill JJ (1986) 'Psychosocial consequences of childhood and adolescent cancer survival' *Journal of Chronic Diseases* 39(9): 751–759

Vann JC, Biddle AK, Daeschner CW, Chaffee S & Gold SH (1995) 'Health insurance access to young adult survivors of childhood cancer in North Carolina' *Medical Pediatric Oncology* 25(5): 389–395

Zebrack BJ & Chesler MA (2002) 'Quality of life in childhood cancer survivors' *Psychooncology* 11(2): 132–141

Zebrack BJ, Chesler M & Penn A (2005) 'Psychosocial issues in adolescent cancer: patients' and survivors' current problems' *Pediatric and Adolescent Health* 35(5): 195-201

Zeltzer LK, Chen E, Weiss R, Guo MD, Robison LL, Meadows AT, Mills J *et al.* (1997) 'Comparison of psychologic outcome in adult survivors of childhood acute lymphoblastic leukemia versus sibling controls: a cooperative Children's Cancer Group and National Institutes of Health Study' *Journal of Clinical Oncology* 15(2): 547–556

Index

Note: Page references in *italics* refer to Figures; those in **bold** refer to Tables

Cancer in Children and Young People   Edited by Faith Gibson and Louise Soanes
© 2008 John Wiley & Sons, Ltd